The Palgrave Handbook of Positive Psychology and Health

Fuschia M. Sirois
Editor

The Palgrave Handbook of Positive Psychology and Health

palgrave
macmillan

Editor
Fuschia M. Sirois
Department of Psychology
Durham University
Durham, UK

ISBN 978-3-031-89094-9   ISBN 978-3-031-89095-6 (eBook)
https://doi.org/10.1007/978-3-031-89095-6

This Palgrave Macmillan imprint is published by the registered company Springer Nature Switzerland AG.
The registered company address is: Gewerbestrasse 11, 6330 Cham, Switzerland

If disposing of this product, please recycle the paper.

Contents

Notes on Contributors

Heather R. Altier is a research postdoctoral fellow in the Department of Psychiatry and Behavioral Sciences at Johns Hopkins University School of Medicine. She obtained her PhD in Clinical Psychology from East Tennessee State University and completed her doctoral internship at University of Washington School of Medicine in 2023. Her research investigates the influence of positive psychological traits and health behaviour engagement on physiological and psychological health in individuals with chronic illness and at risk for poor health outcomes. Outcomes of interest in both her research, and her clinical work in integrated medical settings, include sleep quality, chronic pain, functional impairment, and depression.

Meaghan A. Barlow is an Assistant Professor of Developmental Psychology at Wilfrid Laurier Psychology. Her research examines the age-related consequences of emotional experiences and self-regulatory processes across the adult lifespan. Her work has been published in scholarly journals such as Emotion, Psychology and Aging, and Health Psychology.

Emily S. Beadle is a Post-Doctoral Research Fellow in kidney health inequalities at the University of Hertfordshire. Her PhD was on the development of a measure of body compassion and its application to health behaviours (in particular physical activity and eating behaviour). She has taught and supervised research in health psychology and health behaviour and has research interests in expressive writing, self- and body-compassion, health inequalities, moral injury, and eating disorders.

Marios Biskas is a Research Associate in Psychology at Bradford University. His expertise is in emotions and well-being, with his recent research focusing on uncovering the barriers to being self-compassionate and identifying ways to promote self-compassion. He also investigates the psychological dynamics of nostalgia focusing on the implications that nostalgia has on people's life.

James Borenstein-Laurie is a doctoral candidate in Clinical Psychology at Concordia University. His research examines the ways in which optimism and pessimism can separately contribute to a person's subjective well-being and physical health.

Colette J. Brown is a doctoral candidate in Psychological Science with an emphasis in health psychology at the University of California, Irvine. Her research examines modifiable factors (e.g., daily activity, social support) for cognitive and physical health among older adults.

Maria Inês Caçador has an MSc in Clinical and Health Psychology from the University of Coimbra, Portugal, where she is currently a PhD student. Her research focuses on transdiagnostic mechanisms, Internet-based interventions, mental health promotion in the transition to college, and on the Unified Protocol for Transdiagnostic Treatment of Emotional Disorders.

Jane E. Cha MHealthPsych., is a PhD candidate in the Department of Psychological Medicine at the University of Auckland. Her research focuses on understanding the mediating pathways of self-compassion to benefit both intra- and inter-personal outcomes. She is dedicated to advancing both empirical and theoretical research in this area. At the core of her academic pursuits, she is driven by understanding how we can enhance our relationship with ourselves and the world; to build stronger connections with others in developing more compassionate communities. In addition to her PhD, she is training to become a Clinical Health Psychologist. Beyond academia, she enjoys Pilates and spending time in nature.

Susan T. Charles is Professor of Psychological Science and Professor of Nursing Science and Associate Dean of Academic Programs in the School of Social Ecology at the University of California, Irvine. Her research examines social and emotional processes across the adult life span. She is interested in how affective experience varies across the life course, and how socioemotional experiences are related to differences in cognitive and physical and mental health. She is a fellow of the Gerontological Society of America and the Association for Psychological Science.

Léandre Alexis Chénard-Poirier is a Professor of Organizational Behaviour in the Department of Management at HEC Montréal. His research interests lie at the intersection of managerial behaviours (i.e., leadership and abusive behaviours), motivational processes, and well-being at work. Throughout his research, a focus is given on advanced statistical methods that offer new tools to explore novel questions or gain a different insight on more established theories. Professor Chénard-Poirier's work has been published in several scientific journals and book chapters.

Nathan S. Consedine is a health psychologist in the School of Medicine at the University of Auckland. His training is in emotion and emotion regulation, with current research foci including disgust in health, mindfulness, and (self) compassion in healthcare. In addition to teaching in health psychology and the medical programme, he supervises numerous research students conducting interventions in patient samples as well as with clinician and student researchers examining how patient, physician, clinical, and environmental factors impact medical compassion. Nathan has published more than 180 scientific works and is an Associate Editor and reviewer for numerous international journals. He enjoys fishing, playing tennis, and listening to the sort of music that his colleagues dislike.

Christopher G. Davis is a Professor of Psychology at Carleton University, where he conducts research on the cognitive and emotional adaptations people make following life-changing experiences, including those associated with loss of significant others (e.g., bereavement), injury (e.g., spinal cord injury), chronic debilitating health conditions (such as tinnitus), as well as those experiences most people look forward to (e.g., transition to parenthood). His research examines how people find meaning in loss and transitions of this sort and how these factors promote personal growth and well-being.

Nate T. Deichert received his PhD in Experimental Social-Health Psychology from Kent State University. His current research focuses on the psychological and physical health benefits associated with the experience of gratitude. He is currently a faculty member in the Psychology and Integrative Genomics Programs at Black Hills State University in Spearfish, South Dakota.

Desiree R. Delgadillo is a first-generation college graduate and Postdoctoral Researcher at UCLA's School of Medicine. As a graduate student, Desi earned numerous fellowships and awards including the National Science Foundation's Graduate Research Fellowship and the President's Postdoctoral Fellowship. As a Health Psychologist, her programme of research focuses on the interplay between emotions, stress, close relationships, psychophysiology, and the composition of the microbiome in both children and adults. Desi's research aims to reveal mind-gut-microbiome connections that improve quality of life across socioeconomic status, ethnic groups, and health statuses across the lifespan. As an interdisciplinary researcher, her goal is to help create a new, integrated understanding of how microbial and psychological systems may work together to mutually perpetuate wellness.

Jessie Dezutter is an Associate Research Professor at the KU Leuven (Belgium). She conducts research on the nexus of existential psychology, positive psychology, and gerontology. She directs the Meaning Research Late Life Lab. Her current research lines focus on how meaningfulness is related to late life mental health, how existential givens are experienced at highly advanced age, and whether forgiveness, grace, and gratitude can function as strengths when ageing.

Erin N. Fekete received her PhD in Social and Health Psychology from Kent State University and completed post-doctoral training in health psychology at the University of Miami. Her current research focuses on factors that help individuals become more resilient to the negative effects of health-related stigma. She currently serves as the Dean for Arts and Sciences at Lakeland Community College in Kirtland, Ohio.

Peter R. Harris is Emeritus Professor of Psychology at the University of Sussex, UK. His principal research interest is in how people cope with information and events that threaten the self. He has published extensively on self-affirmation, especially as applied to health and well-being, exploring empirically and theoretically its potential to promote greater open-mindedness.

Patrick L. Hill is an Associate Professor in the Department of Psychological and Brain Sciences at Washington University in St. Louis. He received his MA and PhD in Psychology from the University of Notre Dame, and his BA in Psychology and Economics at Indiana University. His research examines the role of sense of purpose, and other individual differences, in explaining adaptive lifespan developmental trajectories.

Jameson K. Hirsch is a Professor and Assistant Chair of Research, in the Department of Psychiatry and Behavioral Sciences, Quillen College of Medicine, at East Tennessee State University (ETSU) in the United States, and he serves as the Director of the Gwen Fleming Research Laboratory for Psychiatry and Behavioral Sciences and the Laboratory of Resiliency in Psychological and Physical Health at ETSU. His research interests and expertise focus on the intersection between psychopathology and physical health, and on the role of adaptive characteristics in mitigating risk for poor health outcomes, in vulnerable populations including persons with chronic illness, veterans, older adults, and LGBTQ individuals. Dr. Hirsch has published over 200 peer-reviewed articles and book chapters, and presented more than 400 times at professional conferences, on the topic of resilience in the context of psychopathology and disease.

Olivia Hughes is a Research Associate in the School of Psychology, Cardiff University, Wales, UK. Her research interests include psychodermatology and investigating the use of mindfulness-based interventions to support the psychological well-being of children and families affected by skin conditions.

Donna C. Jessop is a Senior Lecturer in Health Psychology at the University of Sussex, UK. Her research focuses on the application of social psychological theory and positive psychology to the promotion of health and well-being. She has published multiple papers exploring the implications of self-affirmation theory for these outcomes.

Julie A. Kircher is a doctoral candidate at the University of California, Irvine in the Psychological Science PhD programme and specializes in health psychology. Her current research focuses on understanding potential psychological and physiological mechanisms involved in how emotional experience relate to cognitive function, in both momentary and longitudinal contexts.

Niko Kohls has over 20 years' experience in both research and business environments with a focus in health promotion and medical psychology. He holds a diploma in psychology (1998) and a PhD (2004) from the University of Freiburg as well as habilitation thesis (Dr. habil. med.) in medical psychology from the University of Munich (2012). As a postdoc he has worked at the University Hospital Freiburg and at the University of Northampton in Great Britain, until he earned a prestigious Samueli-Rockefeller Scholar in 2007. From 2008 until 2014 Niko was responsible for co-directing and managing the Generation Research Program, a think tank of the University of Munich responsible for finding solutions for dealing with the sociodemographic change. Employing his research skills Niko has devised and pilot tested mindfulness-based stress reduction and diversity management programmes for business enterprises and non-profit organizations alike. Since 2013 he has been employed as a professor at the University of Applied Sciences and Arts in Coburg, Germany.

Michail Mantzios is Professor in Applied and Experimental Psychology at Birmingham City University. His research interests range widely across mindful eating, mindfulness, self-compassion, and Philotimo; all in an attempt to contribute towards health behaviour change. His passion for alternative methods employing meditative and non-meditative secular practices has led him on a research journey on mindful eating, linking, and redrafting the theory of understanding mindful eating, especially its methods, validity, and scope for health and well-being.

Logan T. Martin is a graduate student in Affective Science at the University of California, Irvine. He has published on the interactions between emotion, stress, and cortisol. His research focuses on emotion, physical health, and research methods.

Joy McLeod is a PhD student in the Department of Psychology at Carleton University. Her research examines the psychological factors that influence the adjustment process among individuals living with spinal cord injuries. Her other line of research focuses on the positive and negative experiences associated with informal caregiving (such as personal growth and burnout).

Helena Moreira is a clinical psychologist and has an MSc and PhD in Psychology from the University of Coimbra (UC), Portugal. She is an Associate Professor at the Faculty of Psychology and Education Sciences of UC and an integrated member of the Center for Research in Neuropsychology and Cognitive-Behavioral Intervention of the UC. Her primary research interests include the areas of perinatal mental health and the application of mindfulness and compassion to the study of parenting. She has been involved in several research projects aiming at testing the efficacy of group and Internet-based interventions for mothers in the postpartum period and children with emotional disorders, among other populations.

Quang Anh Nguyen is a graduate student in the community psychology programme at DePaul University. He earned his bachelor's degree at Luther College and was a member of the Laboratory for the Investigation of Mind, Body, and Spirit. He has held a full-time position as a research coordinator at Mayo Clinic, and his research interests are in health, marginalized populations, substance abuse, mental health stigma, culturally specific approaches, and positive psychology.

Martin Offenbächer is currently the clinical and research director of the Gastein Healing Gallery in Bad Gastein, Austria. His medical field is physical medicine and rehabilitation with special interests in musculoskeletal disorders and chronic pain as well as holistic medicine. Recently he has been appointed as a senior researcher at the institute of ecomedicine at the Paracelsus Medical University in Salzburg, Austria. He set up a working group 'health resort medicine' with the aim to develop and to evaluate nature-based therapies and health promotion including positive psychology interventions in this setting.

Ana I. Orejuela Dávila Affiliated with the US Department of Veteran Affairs, Dr. Orejuela-Dávila holds a PhD in Psychology and has extensive experience in both research and teaching. Dr. Orejuela-Dávila's research interests revolve around health/medical psychology, and cognitive psychology with a focus on posttraumatic growth, memory, and emotion regulation following adversity and trauma. Dr. Orejuela-Dávila has published numerous research articles in reputable journals and actively contributes to the advancement of knowledge in her field.

Crystal L. Park is Professor of Clinical Psychology at the University of Connecticut. With her graduate students in the Spirituality Meaning and Health Lab, she conducts research on stress, coping, the psychology of religion, and yoga. She is currently conducting an NCCIH-funded clinical trial of yoga and emotion regulation.

Gabrielle N. Pfund is a postdoctoral researcher at Northwestern University studying the connection between personality and health across the adult lifespan. She received her PhD in Psychological and Brain Sciences from Washington University in St. Louis in 2022. Her research interests meet at the intersection of sense of purpose, health, and aging, with a focus on how short-term change maps onto long-term development.

Sarah T. Pressman is a Professor of Psychological Science and the Associate Dean of Undergraduate Education at the University of California, Irvine. She has published extensively on the beneficial effects of emotional and social well-being for physical health and the mechanisms by which these experiences "get under the skin" to influence biology. She has received numerous awards for her research and has been elected as a Fellow of the Academy of Behavioral Medicine Research, the Society for Personality and Social Psychology, and the American Psychosomatic Society.

Veronica Ramirez is a National Academies Ford Fellow and PhD student in Psychological Science at the University of California, Irvine and works in the laboratories of Drs. Stephen Schueller and Sarah Pressman. Veronica received her BA in Psychology from the University of San Diego and was a National Institutes of Health UGSP Scholar and Post Baccalaureate Research Fellow. Her work focuses on the biological and physiological factors underlying negative and positive emotions, and addictive behaviours. She uses wearable technologies to study individuals in laboratory and real-world settings, with the underlying goal of understanding the mechanisms linking emotions to health.

Jesse Renaud is an Assistant Professor in the Department of Psychiatry at McGill University. She is also a clinical psychologist and the team leader of the Centre for Cognitive Behavioural Therapy Research, Training, and Intervention at the McGill University Health Centre. Her research examines individual differences that promote psychological well-being and psychotherapy treatment outcomes.

Georgina Rowse is an Honorary Research Fellow at the Clinical and Applied Psychology Unit in the Department of Psychology at the University of Sheffield. Georgina leads research in the field of emotional well-being and Inflammatory Bowel Disease (IBD), including sleep, coping, health behaviours, and interventions to impact both psychological and physical health in IBD. She is highly published, has worked closely with IBD charities and presented her research at international conferences.

Melanie Schellekens is a senior researcher at the Helen Dowling Institute for psycho-oncological services. She is also affiliated as a researcher to the Department of Medical and Clinical Psychology at Tilburg University. Her research focuses on the dynamic resilience process, personalizing psycho-oncological care, mindfulness-based interventions, and methodological innovations.

Maya Schroevers is a psychologist, certified mindfulness trainer, and Associate Professor in Health Psychology at the Department of Health Sciences at the University of Groningen/University Medical Centre Groningen. Using quantitative and qualitative approaches, her research focuses on (predictors of) adaptation to illness, emotion regulation and coping processes, mindfulness and compassion, care needs, and the efficacy of psychological interventions.

Anthony Scioli is professor of psychology at Keene State College, the liberal arts division of the University System of New Hampshire (USA). He has previously authored two books on hope and is currently co-editing *The Oxford Compendium of Hope*, expected in 2024. Dr. Scioli is a licensed clinical psychologist and founder of the Hope Institute (www.gainhope.com).

Fuschia M. Sirois is a Professor in Social and Health Psychology at Durham University, and a former Canada Research Chair in Health and Well-being. She is also the co-Editor in Chief of the British Journal of Health Psychology. Prof Sirois' research focuses on understanding the psychological factors and qualities that help or hinder people in their efforts to regulate their emotions, thoughts, and behaviours when dealing with life's challenges. Her research has a particular focus on how positive psychological factors, including self-compassion, meaning, and gratitude, can foster taking a strengths-based approach to self-regulation issues to improve overall health and well-being.

C. Sophie Skoggard is in her final year at Naropa University's Masters in Somatic Body Psychotherapy programme. She earlier served in the Peace Corps in Botswana and intends to use her passion and expertise to make the world a better place.

Richard G. Tedeschi is Professor Emeritus in the Department of Psychological Science at the University of North Carolina at Charlotte, and Executive Director of the Boulder Crest Institute for Posttraumatic Growth in Bluemont, Virginia. A licensed psychologist, Dr. Tedeschi has extensive experience in clinical practice, specializing in bereavement and trauma. He is a consultant to the American Psychological Association on trauma and resilience, and a subject matter expert for the US Army's Comprehensive Soldier Fitness Program. His work has significantly advanced the understanding of how individuals can experience positive psychological change following adversity.

Andrew R. Thompson is the Director of the South Wales Clinical Psychology training programme. He is the co-editor in chief of the British Journal of Health Psychology. His research focusses on conditions that affect appearance and he has an interest in psychodermatology. He has supported the work of charities, including the Vitiligo Society, the Katie Piper Foundation, and he is a Trustee to the charity Changing Faces.

Loren L. Toussaint is a professor of psychology at Luther College in Decorah, Iowa. He is chair of the Discover Forgiveness Advisory Council for the Templeton World Charity Foundation, president of the Forgiveness Foundation, associate director of the Sierra Leone Forgiveness Project, a consultant to Mayo Clinic, Cancer Treatment Centers of America, and Boise State University, and a visiting professor at the Katholische Universität Eichstätt-Ingolstadt. Dr. Toussaint's research examines virtues, especially forgiveness, and how they are related to health and well-being. He and colleagues recently published a compendium of research titled "Forgiveness and Health: Scientific Evidence and Theories Relating Forgiveness to Better Health" (Springer). Dr. Toussaint directs the Laboratory for the Investigation of Mind, Body, and Spirit at Luther College (https://www.luther.edu/faculty/loren-toussaint/). He encourages "everyday forgiveness" to build resilience and minimize stress in families, schools, healthcare, workplaces, and communities.

Inês A. Trindade is an Associate Senior Lecturer at the School of Law, Psychology and Social Work, Örebro, Sweden, and an integrated member of the Center for Research in Neuropsychology and Cognitive-Behavioral Intervention of the University of Coimbra (UC). She holds an MSc and PhD in Clinical Psychology from UC, and is a licensed Clinical Psychologist. Inês' main research interests are related to contextual behavioural science and behavioural medicine topics (in particular, psycho-gastroenterology and psycho-oncology). She conducts research on factors that influence clinical and patient-reported outcomes in populations with medical conditions, and on the development and evaluation of face-to-face and digital contextual behavioural interventions for these populations.

Nick A. Troop is an Associate Professor of Clinical Psychology at the University of Plymouth. He began his work on life events, coping, and social rank in eating disorders at the Institute of Psychiatry, Psychology and Neuroscience. Since then, he has taught and supervised research in health psychology at Essex University, London Metropolitan University, and the University of Hertfordshire. This has included work on expressive writing and self- and body-compassion, as well as health and health behaviours in a range of conditions including eating disorders, posttraumatic stress disorder, haemophilia, and heart disease.

Miguel A. Vallejo is a clinical psychologist, and Full Professor of Cognitive Behavior Therapy at National University of Distance Education (UNED), Madrid, Spain. He specializes in the study and psychological treatment of chronic pain and rheumatologic conditions. He is interested in health psychology and the use of Internet information technologies to promote heath in several areas, including emotion regulation and health behaviours related to addictions.

Robert J. Vallerand is currently Full Professor of Psychology at the Université du Québec à Montréal where he holds a Canada Research Chair in Motivational Processes and Optimal Functioning and is Director of the Research Laboratory on Social Behavior. Professor Vallerand is recognized as a leading international expert on motivational processes where he has developed theories dealing with intrinsic and extrinsic motivation, as well as passion for activities. He has published 12 books and monographs and over 400 scientific articles and book chapters.

Marije van der Lee is a psychologist and head of the Research Department at the Helen Dowling Institute for psycho-oncological services. She is also affiliated as professor to the Center of Research on Psychological Disorders and Somatic diseases (CoRPS), Department of Medical and Clinical Psychology at Tilburg University. Her research focuses on network approach to psychological disorders, personalizing psychological treatment, implementation of eHealth interventions and mindfulness-based interventions in psycho-oncology.

Jon R. Webb is an Associate Professor and the Addictive Disorders and Recovery Studies Program Director in the Department of Community, Family, and Addiction Sciences at Texas Tech University. He is a licensed clinical psychologist, with research interests focused on spirituality and health, including ritualistic, theistic, and existential spirituality, forgiveness, temptation, existangst, suicidal behaviour, and addiction recovery. He is currently working on a contracted edited book, entitled *Handbook of Spirituality, Health, and Well-Being: A Psychological Perspective.*

Thomas L. Webb is Professor of Psychology at the University of Sheffield in the UK. He has published extensively on the role of motivation, monitoring progress, and planning in shaping behaviour; as well as understanding how people regulate their own, and others', emotions. His recent work applies these insights to understand how people can live more sustainably.

Alex M. Wood is a Professor in Psychology at Leeds Trinity University and a Visiting Professor at the London School of Economics and Political Science (LSE). In 2013 he was awarded an Honorary Chair at the University of Manchester in recognition of lifetime contributions to health psychology. Alex's research into well-being takes a distinctly holistic approach, (a) focusing on the whole continuum from clinically impaired mental health to positive psychological functioning, and (b) integrating approaches across psychology, behavioural sciences, economics, education, health sciences, management and marketing, psychiatry, and sport—each area in which he has published. Alex is one of the most cited researchers globally in behavioural science, economic, clinical, personality, and health psychology.

Carsten Wrosch is a Professor in the Department of Psychology at Concordia University. He examines motivational and personality processes in the context of lifespan development. His theoretical and empirical work covered the importance of control, goal adjustment, and optimism for subjective well-being and physical health.

Rebecca Yeates is a Lecturer in Clinical Psychology at the University of Leeds. Rebecca teaches on the Doctorate of Clinical Psychology postgraduate research programme. Rebecca conducts research in the area of adolescence and young adult mental health and her doctoral thesis investigated the potential benefits of trait self-compassion for young people diagnosed with Inflammatory Bowel Disease. She has recently concluded a pilot and feasibility trial of a mindfulness and self-compassion intervention for young people diagnosed with the chronic condition.

List of Figures

List of Tables

1

Introduction: Why Is Taking a Positive Psychology Approach to Health Important?

Fuschia M. Sirois

Introduction

When the idea for this handbook was first conceived, a key question that arose was why do we need to bring together a collection of scholarly chapters with a focus on positive psychological approaches to health? Arguably, the importance of health psychology has come into the spotlight in recent years due in part to its value during and after the COVID-19 pandemic. Across the globe health psychologists rose to the call to help address the behavioural and social challenges of reducing transmission of the virus (Chater et al., 2020; Freedland et al., 2020; Michie et al., 2021), as well as the needs of the overburdened health-care staff and frontline workers who dealt with the care of those infected (Zaka et al., 2020). But why take a positive psychological approach to understanding health-related issues and outcomes then? Although there are a number of notable reasons, the growing emphasis on the need to restore, preserve, and enhance well-being and empower people to manage their health is a natural fit with the aims of positive psychology, as will be discussed later in this chapter. For example, in the aftermath of the pandemic, the importance of building resilience for future crises and maintaining well-being during turbulent times came into sharp focus. Although positive psychology is not limited to these themes, they are nonetheless reflective of an

F. M. Sirois (✉)
Department of Psychology, Durham University, Durham, UK
e-mail: fuschia.sirois@durham.ac.uk

F. M. Sirois (ed.), *The Palgrave Handbook of Positive Psychology and Health*,
https://doi.org/10.1007/978-3-031-89095-6_1

ongoing surge of interest in recent years in taking a strengths-based approached to dealing with challenges, including those relevant for physical health.

This handbook brings together the two important and not entirely disparate subfields of psychology, namely health psychology and positive psychology, to provide the latest developments in theory, research, and practice focused on positive psychological approaches to promoting, maintaining, and dealing with health issues and contexts. After brief reviews of the relevant tenets of health psychology and positive psychology, we will then return to address the question of why a handbook of positive psychology and health is needed. The chapter will end with an overview of the structure of the Handbook.

What is Health Psychology?

Compared to other subfields of psychology, health psychology is a relative newcomer. It is generally agreed that health psychology became a recognised subfield somewhere around the late 1970's and early 1980's, arising as a more comprehensive psychological perspective on health than its predecessor, behavioural medicine, which focused more on the behavioural aspects of health (Taylor et al., 2023). Health psychology in contrast aimed to draw upon a number of psychological factors beyond just behaviours to understand health, including social, individual, cognitive, emotional, and biological influences that contributed to health states, for better or worse. In short, Health Psychology aimed to provide a comprehensive and psychological view of the mind-body relationship.

The emerging field of health psychology was guided by the biopsychosocial model, which takes a holistic and synergistic view of health (Engel, 1977) in contrast to the prevailing biomedical model of health and illness. According to the biomedical model the mind-body relationship is essentially dualistic, with mind and body being separate entities that have little influence upon one another (Taylor et al., 2023). It also views health through a reductionistic, single factor lens, with the causes of illness reduced down to low level causes such as chemical imbalances and cellular dysfunction. Importantly, the focus of the biomedical model is almost exclusively on illness and the factors that cause it rather than those that might support and promote health.

On the other hand, the biopsychosocial model provides a framework that considers the multiplicity of factors that contribute to health, the lower- and higher-level processes involved in health states, and the inseparability of body and mind, while emphasising both health and illness (Taylor et al., 2023). In these respects, the biopsychosocial model is consistent with the revised definition of health from the World Health Organization (1948), which states that health is "a complete state of physical, mental, and social well-being and not merely the absence of disease or infirmity." Accordingly, the biopsychosocial model views health as arising from the interface of biological, social, and psychological systems, and therefore reflects the importance of maintaining balance of physical, social, and mental well-being. This s psychology.

The aims of health psychology can be grouped into four main themes (see Fig. 1.1; Taylor et al., 2023). First, health psychology focuses on the promotion and maintenance of health, including the behaviours that people engage in to stay healthy, such as healthy eating, regular physical exercise, good sleep behaviours, and stress management. Second, the prevention and treatment of illness is a key focus for health psychology. This includes screening behaviours for those at risk for disease, treatment seeking once symptoms appear, and psychological and behavioural approaches for managing illness once diagnosed. Third, health psychology is concerned with the role of psychological factors in the etiology and correlates of health, illness, and dysfunction. Understanding how social, individual, behavioural, and emotional factors are implicated in the development and experience of both good and ill health is a key focus. Lastly, health psychology is also concerned with the influence of health professionals on people's behaviour, including how the patient-provider relationship impacts individuals' health behaviours and recovery from illness. With the exception of Chap. 23, which explicitly focuses on health professionals, the chapters of this Handbook address topics relevant to the first three themes of health psychology.

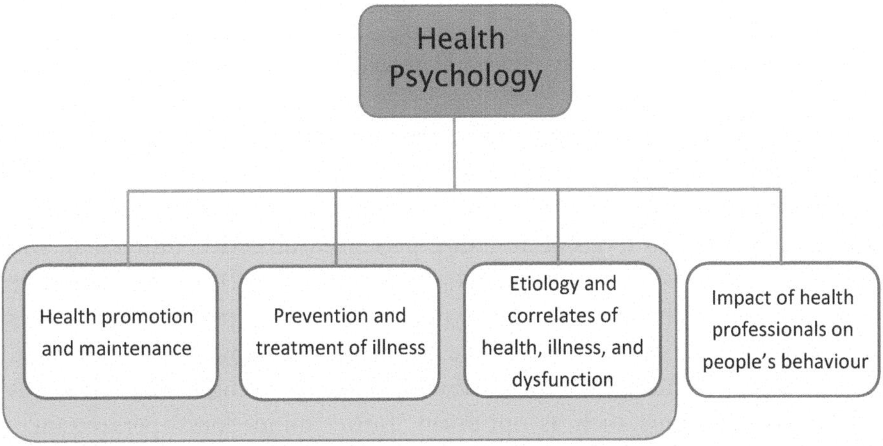

Fig. 1.1 The four key areas of health psychology, and the three that will be the focus of most of the chapters of this handbook in relation to positive psychology (adapted from Taylor et al., 2023, with permission)

What Is Positive Psychology?

Similar to health psychology, Positive Psychology is a relatively new subfield that has seen increased interest in recent years. Although the roots of Positive Psychology arguably evolved from the ideas put forth by humanist psychology theorists, such as Abraham Maslow and Carl Rogers, it is widely recognised that its start as a formal subdiscipline began in 1998. Martin Seligman, then president of the American Psychological Association (APA), recognised that the field of psychology had become pre-occupied with the study of damage, weakness, and pathology, neglecting the other side of human needs, which involved nurturing strengths, flourishing, and preventive approaches to build competencies and foster virtues (Seligman, 2019).

In January 1998, Seligman gathered with flow pioneer Mihaly Csikszentmihalyi, chief executive officer of APA, Ray Fowler, and their families to brainstorm what the possibility of a more positive psychology might look like (Seligman, 2019). Over the next week they laid the foundations of what we now know as Positive Psychology, detailing the focus of a more positive approach to psychology, and who would be involved in creating the momentum needed to launch and lead this new field. The result was a new branch of psychology that would take a strengths-based view of human nature with the goal of understanding and finding ways to optimise human functioning and well-being. This view was in contrast to the deficits-based approach that focused on human weaknesses and mental illness that had dominated the field. Martin Seligman proposed that:

> *The aim of positive psychology is to begin to catalyze a change in the focus of psychology from preoccupation only with repairing the worst things in life to also building positive qualities.* (Seligman & Csikszentmihalyi, 2000, p. 5)

In essence, positive psychology reflected a new science of happiness, well-being, and flourishing.

This new psychology of positive human functioning was proposed to function at three different levels of human experience, subjective, individual, and group (Seligman & Csikszentmihalyi, 2000; see Fig. 1.2). At the subjective level, positive psychology considers valued subjective experiences and states such as happiness, well-being, positive emotions, and flow. At the individual level, positive psychology is concerned with character strengths and virtues, as well as positive traits such as optimism, future mindedness, perseverance, courage, and forgiveness. Lastly, at the group level, positive psychology is about positive institutions and communities and the civic virtues that they

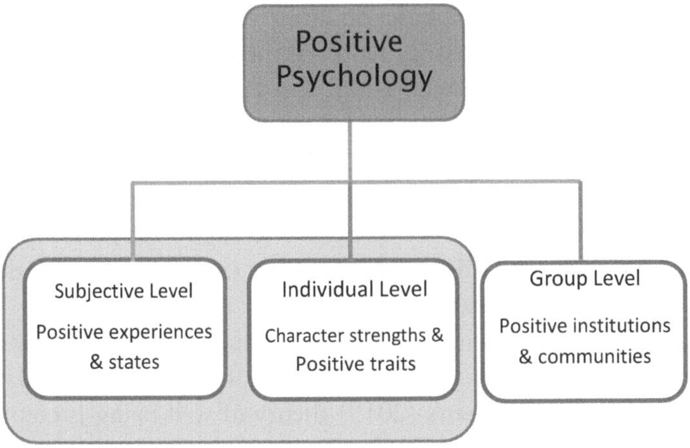

Fig. 1.2 The three main levels of positive psychology

foster, including altruism, civility, and tolerance (Seligman & Csikszentmihalyi, 2000). Although optimising human functioning at the group level is an important aim, the chapters in the Handbook focus mainly on the Positive Psychological concepts at the subjective and individual levels and how these can be applied for enhancing physical health.

It is crucial to note that positive psychology takes a scientifically informed perspective on human happiness and flourishing, doing so through the lens of one or more theoretical frameworks on the nature of well-being. Defining well-being, however, is often a hotly debated topic, as competing models emphasise different perspectives (e.g., Biswas-Diener et al., 2009; Kashdan et al., 2008; Waterman, 2008). Overall, these models are informed by one or both of the two key conceptions of what constitutes *A Good Life* according to ancient Greek philosophy (Waterman, 1993). Hedonic happiness captures the subjective experience of pleasure and is characterised by high levels of positive affective states that arise when personal needs are satisfied. In contrast, eudaimonic happiness is aligned with the teachings of Aristotle, reflects the experience of well-being that comes from living in alignment with one's true self, and emerges from engaging in activities that contribute to self-realisation (Waterman, 2008). In this respect, eudaimonic well-being is often viewed as being synonymous with flourishing.

Several conceptualisations of well-being have emerged from these perspectives and are commonly used in positive psychological research. Subjective well-being (SWB) refers to experiencing higher levels and more frequent positive emotions and lower levels and less frequent negative emotions alongside an evaluation of one's life as being satisfying (e.g., high levels of satisfaction with life). Because of the emphasis on affective states and need satisfaction, SWB is often viewed as primarily reflecting hedonic well-being (Waterman, 2008; Ryff, 2014; Ryff & Singer, 2008) concept of psychological well-being (PWB) provides an alternative perspective on positive functioning that includes six core dimensions: (1) personal growth, (2) positive relations with others, (3) purpose in life, (4) autonomy, (5) environmental mastery, and (6) self-acceptance. Although it was not created to align with philosophical conceptions of well-being, PWB nonetheless most closely aligns with the eudaimonic perspective (Waterman, 2008).

Other models of well-being span both hedonic and eudaimonic views of well-being, suggesting that they may operate in tandem (Kashdan et al., 2008). For example, Seligman's (2019) theory of well-being is comprised of five key elements that aims to provide a comprehensive framework for understanding the core components of flourishing and positive human functioning. Named after the acronym for each of its components, the PERMA model includes Positive emotions, Engagement, (positive) Relationships, Meaning, and Accomplishment, with positive emotions aligning with hedonic views of well-being, and the remaining elements reflecting more eudaimonic aspects of well-being. Self-determination theory (SDT) (Deci & Ryan, 2000) similarly includes key components that map onto both hedonic and eudaimonic well-being. SDT posits that humans have basic psychological needs, that when satisfied in a balanced manner will result in optimal levels of well-being. These include autonomy, the need to feel that one is in control of one's own behaviour, competence, the need to be effective in dealing with the environment and to have a sense of mastery within a valued life domain, and relatedness, the need to feel a sense of both attachment to other people and of belonging amongst other people (Deci & Ryan, 2000). Although these dimensions have clear relevance for eudaimonic well-being, Biswas-Deiner and colleagues (2009) have also argued that the experience of feeling good when such needs are satisfied can also reflect hedonic well-being.

Why Positive Psychology and Health?

It is notable that only two decades separates the formal arrivals of positive psychology and health psychology as important and rapidly developing subfields of psychology. Yet, the interest in positive psychological approaches to understanding and improving health pre-date the launch of the field of positive psychology. In 1985, Scheier and Carver (1985) conducted the first study investigating the implications of optimism for physical health in undergraduate students, tracking the links between optimism and physical symptoms over 4 weeks across the term. As expected, students higher in optimism reported fewer physical symptoms across the term than those low in optimism, even after taking into account initial levels of physical symptoms. Four years later the beneficial effects of optimism for health were replicated using objective health measures in patients recovering from heart surgery (Scheier et al., 1989). As early as 1986, researchers were starting to link positive emotions to enhanced immune system functioning (Dillon et al., 1986). And by 1998, there was evidence that induced positive emotional states had a restorative effect on cardiovascular activation (Fredrickson & Levenson, 1998), which was in line with Frederickson's (1998) newly proposed broaden and build model of positive emotions.

In the years following this pioneering research, the body of evidence demonstrating that positive psychological factors can have direct physiological effects that can improve and maintain physical health has continued to evolve, albeit sporadically, with the focus often being more on psychological well-being than on contexts and outcomes with relevance for physical health and well-being. Nonetheless, research that has focused on physical health has highlighted a number of important and timely benefits for taking a strengths-based approach to understanding and addressing health, as well as investigating the pathways and mechanisms involved. In particular, viewing health through the lens of positive psychology is important for three key reasons.

1. *Empowerment*: Focusing on strengths and capabilities as opposed to deficits and weaknesses can empower individuals to take ownership of their health, enhance their self-advocacy in health-related decisions, and promote self-regulation skills, which are essential for supporting health behaviours (Baumeister et al., 1994). Health behaviours, such as healthy eating and physical activity, play a central role in promoting good health, reducing obesity and therefore the risk of developing disease, and supporting self-management of chronic illness (World Health Organisation, 2024). This behavioural route is therefore a key process through which positive psychological factors can influence health-related outcomes.
2. *Proactive approach to health*: Whereas empowerment involves supporting personal agency, being proactive can be viewed as a natural outcome of feeling more agentic (Miao & Gan, 2019). Approaches that build on and highlight existing strengths can therefore promote taking a more proactive approach to healthy lifestyle habits, and encourage setting and pursuing health goals (e.g., Zhou et al., 2013). Being proactive about health can

equip individuals with the skills and motivation to prevent future health issues or reduce the risk of disease development among high-risk groups.

3. *Building resources*: As noted above, strength-based approaches to health can support improved health outcomes, which may be explained in part by the creation and bolstering of the internal and external resources known to contribute to health. From a biopsychosocial perspective these can include enhancing resilience, healthy coping skills, and emotion regulation skills, each of which can reduce both subjective and objective stress and thus have positive downstream effects on inflammatory processes, physical symptoms, and physical health status more generally (Butler, 2011; Carver & Connor-Smith, 2010; Cohen et al., 2012). Positive psychological approaches to health include promoting positive relationships with others, which as decades of research on social support have demonstrated, can play a key role in key health processes such as coping and stress reduction, health-promoting behaviours (Reblin & Uchino, 2008), and even treatment adherence (Middleton et al., 2013). These resources are also crucial for managing chronic health conditions (Maguire et al., 2021), and for supporting those who deliver health care (Sirois & Owens, 2021).

To the extent that physical health status is a key component of optimal human functioning, then understanding the implications and connections between positive psychological factors and physical health is essential. The aim of this Handbook is therefore to bring together the latest scientific theory and evidence on the potential benefits of positive psychological approaches for enhancing physical health via key pathways in the mind-body relationship. The chapters in this Handbook will consider how positive psychological qualities and factors relate to health behaviours, coping and emotion regulation, and stress mechanisms, each of which play a critical role in the three key areas of health psychology. In addition to theoretical perspectives, the chapters in the Handbook also highlight how positive psychology principles can be implemented to enhance both health outcomes and adjustment to ongoing health issues to promote physical well-being and thriving. A number of positive psychological interventions (PPIs) have been developed in recent years and are increasingly being applied to address issues with relevance for physical health (Carr et al., 2024), such as health behaviour change (Kukucska et al., 2023), adjustment to chronic health conditions (Mistretta & Davis, 2022), sleep quality (Boggiss et al., 2020), and stress reduction and management (Boggiss et al., 2020; Meyer & Stutts, 2024).

Overview of the Handbook

The Handbook is organised into four parts that reflect three key established areas within Positive Psychology, along with a relatively new topic area. As noted previously, subjective level positive experiences and states, or well-being, can be further viewed as focused on the experience of pleasant, in the moment states or happiness (hedonic well-being), or as positive experiences that arise from focusing on meaning and purpose in life (eudaimonic well-being). Parts I and II of the Handbook address how well-being constructs may play a role in health, doing so from the hedonic and eudaimonic perspectives, respectively. Part III turns to the next key area within positive psychology, character strengths, also often referred to as positive traits.

In Part IV we venture into a slightly different perspective on positive psychological factors and their relevance for health. The chapters in this part present theory and research on positive qualities and practices in relation to health outcomes and processes that have their roots situated primarily in Eastern rather than Western traditions. Mindfulness and self-compassion are two such positive qualities for which there continues to be a fast-growing evidence base in relation to health-related outcomes, and therefor receive their due attention in this part.

This introductory chapter is purposefully brief, especially with regards to the details of what to expect from the contributions in each chapter. This is because each part of the Handbook is prefaced with a more detailed overview of the chapters within, their focus, themes, and the issues that they address to help orient the reader. Although the very brief introduction to Health Psychology and Positive Psychology in this chapter only scratches the surface in terms of relevant theories, concepts, and debates, the Handbook chapters will provide more nuanced and involved discussions and applications of positive psychology for understanding health.

References

Baumeister, R. F., Heatherton, T. F., & Tice, D. M. (1994). *Losing control: How and why people fail at self-regulation*. Academic Press.

Biswas-Diener, R., Kashdan, T. B., & King, L. A. (2009). Two traditions of happiness research, not two distinct types of happiness. *The Journal of Positive Psychology, 4*(3), 208–211. https://doi.org/10.1080/17439760902844400

Boggiss, A. L., Consedine, N. S., Brenton-Peters, J. M., Hofman, P. L., & Serlachius, A. S. (2020). A systematic review of gratitude interventions: Effects on physical health and health behaviors. *Journal of Psychosomatic Research, 135*, 110165. https://doi.org/10.1016/j.jpsychores.2020.110165

Butler, E. A. (2011). Three views of emotion regulation and health. *Social and Personality Psychology Compass, 5*(8), 563–577. https://doi.org/10.1111/j.1751-9004.2011.00372.x

Carr, A., Finneran, L., Boyd, C., Shirey, C., Canning, C., Stafford, O., Lyons, J., Cullen, K., Prendergast, C., Corbett, C., Drumm, C., & Burke, T. (2024). The evidence-base for positive psychology interventions: A mega-analysis of meta-analyses. *The Journal of Positive Psychology, 19*(2), 191–205. https://doi.org/10.1080/17439760.2023.2168564

Carver, C. S., & Connor-Smith, J. (2010). Personality and coping. *Annual Review of Psychology, 61*, 679–704.

Chater, A., Whittaker, E., Lewis, L., Arden, M., Byrne-Davis, L., Chadwick, P., Drury, J., Epton, T., Hart, J., Kamal, A., McBride, E., O'Connor, D., Shorter, G. W., Swanson, V., & Armitage, C. (2020). Health psychology, behavioural science and Covid-19 disease prevention. *Health Psychology Update, 29*(29), 3–9. https://doi.org/10.53841/bpshpu.2020.29.3.3

Cohen, S., Janicki-Deverts, D., Doyle, W. J., Miller, G. E., Frank, E., Rabin, B. S., & Turner, R. B. (2012). Chronic stress, glucocorticoid receptor resistance, inflammation, and disease risk. *Proceedings of the National Academy of Sciences*. https://doi.org/10.1073/pnas.1118355109

Deci, E. L., & Ryan, R. M. (2000). The "what" and "why" of goal pursuits: Human needs and the self-determination of behavior. *Psychological Inquiry, 11*(4), 227–268. https://doi.org/10.1207/S15327965PLI1104_01

Dillon, K. M., Minchoff, B., & Baker, K. H. (1986). Positive Emotional States and Enhancement of the Immune System. *The International Journal of Psychiatry in Medicine, 15*(1), 13–18. https://doi.org/10.2190/r7fd-urn9-pq7f-a6j7

Engel, G. L. (1977). The need for a new medical model: A challenge for biomedicine. *Science, 196*(4286), 129–136. https://doi.org/10.1126/science.847460

Fredrickson, B. L. (1998). What good are positive emotions? *Review of General Psychology, 2*(3), 300–319. https://doi.org/10.1037/1089-2680.2.3.300

Fredrickson, B. L., & Levenson, R. W. (1998). Positive emotions speed recovery from the cardiovascular Sequelae of negative emotions. *Cognition and Emotion, 12*(2), 191–220. https://doi.org/10.1080/026999398379718

Freedland, K. E., Dew, M. A., Sarwer, D. B., Burg, M. M., Hart, T. A., Ewing, S. W. F., Fang, C. Y., Blozis, S. A., Puterman, E., Marquez, B., & Kaufmann, P. G. (2020). Health psychology in the time of COVID-19. *Health Psychology, 39*(12), 1021–1025. https://doi.org/10.1037/hea0001049

Kashdan, T. B., Biswas-Diener, R., & King, L. A. (2008). Reconsidering happiness: The costs of distinguishing between hedonics and eudaimonia. *The Journal of Positive Psychology, 3*(4), 219–233. https://doi.org/10.1080/17439760802303044

Kukucska, D., Whitehall, J., Shorter, G. W., Howlett, N., Wyld, K., & Chater, A. M. (2023). A systematic review of positive psychology interventions (PPIs) to improve the health behaviours, psychological wellbeing and/or physical health of police staff. *Journal of Police and Criminal Psychology, 38*(3), 728–742. https://doi.org/10.1007/s11896-023-09579-1

Maguire, R., Hanly, P., & Maguire, P. (2021). Living well with chronic illness: How social support, loneliness and psychological appraisals relate to well-being in a population-based European sample. *Journal of Health Psychology, 26*(10), 1494–1507. https://doi.org/10.1177/1359105319883923

Meyer, H. H., & Stutts, L. A. (2024). The impact of single-session gratitude interventions on stress and affect. *The Journal of Positive Psychology, 19*(2), 315–322. https://doi.org/10.1080/17439760.2023.2170823

Miao, M., & Gan, Y. (2019). How does meaning in life predict proactive coping? The self-regulatory mechanism on emotion and cognition. *Journal of Personality, 87*(3), 579–592. https://doi.org/10.1111/jopy.12416

Michie, S., West, R., Pidgeon, N., Reicher, S., Amlôt, R., & Bear, L. (2021). Staying 'Covid-safe': Proposals for embedding behaviours that protect against Covid-19 transmission in the UK. *British Journal of Health Psychology, 26*(4), 1238–1257. https://doi.org/10.1111/bjhp.12557

Middleton, K. R., Anton, S. D., & Perri, M. G. (2013). Long-Term Adherence to Health Behavior Change. *American Journal of Lifestyle Medicine (AJLM), 7*(6), 395–404. https://doi.org/10.1177/1559827613488867

Mistretta, E. G., & Davis, M. C. (2022). Meta-analysis of self-compassion interventions for pain and psychological symptoms among adults with chronic illness. *Mindfulness, 13*(2), 267–284. https://doi.org/10.1007/s12671-021-01766-7

Reblin, M., & Uchino, B. N. (2008). Social and emotional support and its implication for health. *Current Opinion in Psychiatry, 21*(2), 201–205. https://doi.org/10.1097/YCO.0b013e3282f3ad89

Ryff, C. D. (2014). Psychological well-being revisited: Advances in the science and practice of eudaimonia. *Psychother Psychosom, 83*(1), 10–28. https://doi.org/10.1159/000353263

Ryff, C. D., & Singer, B. H. (2008). Know thyself and become what you are: A eudaimonic approach to psychological well-being. *Journal of Happiness Studies: An Interdisciplinary Forum on Subjective Well-Being, 9*(1), 13–39. https://doi.org/10.1007/s10902-006-9019-0

Scheier, M. F., & Carver, C. S. (1985). Optimism, coping, and health: Assessment and implications of generalized outcome expectancies. *Health Psychology, 4*(3), 219–247. https://doi.org/10.1037/0278-6133.4.3.219

Scheier, M. F., Matthews, K. A., Owens, J. F., Magovern, G. J., Lefebvre, R. C., Abbott, R. A., & Carver, C. S. (1989). Dispositional optimism and recovery from coronary artery bypass surgery: The beneficial effects on physical and psychological well-being. *Journal of Personality and Social Psychology, 57*(6), 1024–1040. https://doi.org/10.1037/0022-3514.57.6.1024

Seligman, M. E. P. (2019). Positive psychology: A personal history. *Annual Review of Clinical Psychology, 15*, 1–23. https://doi.org/10.1146/annurev-clinpsy-050718-095653

Seligman, M. E. P., & Csikszentmihalyi, M. (2000). Positive psychology: An introduction. *American Psychologist, 55*(1), 5–14. https://doi.org/10.1037/0003-066X.55.1.5

Sirois, F. M., & Owens, J. (2021). Factors associated with psychological distress in health-care workers during an infectious disease outbreak: A rapid systematic review of the evidence [Systematic Review]. *Frontiers in Psychiatry, 11*. https://doi.org/10.3389/fpsyt.2020.589545

Taylor, S. E., Stanton, A. L., Sirois, F. M., & Andersen, J. (2023). *Health psychology* (6th Canadian edition ed.). McGraw-Hill Ryerson.

Waterman, A. S. (1993). Two conceptions of happiness: Contrasts of personal expressiveness (eudaimonia) and hedonic enjoyment. *Journal of Personality and Social Psychology, 64*(4), 678–691. https://doi.org/10.1037/0022-3514.64.4.678

Waterman, A. S. (2008). Reconsidering happiness: A eudaimonist's perspective. *The Journal of Positive Psychology, 3*(4), 234–252. https://doi.org/10.1080/17439760802303002

World Health Organisation. (2024). *Obesity and overweight Fact sheet*. WHO. Retrieved April 14, 2025 from https://www.who.int/news-room/fact-sheets/detail/obesity-and-overweight

World Health Organization. (1948). Definition of Health. Preamble to the Constitution of the World Health Organization as Adopted by the International Health Conference. *Official Records of the World Health Organization, 2*(100). http://www.who.int/about/.

Zaka, A., Shamloo, S. E., Fiorente, P., & Tafuri, A. (2020). COVID-19 pandemic as a watershed moment: A çall for systematic psychological health care for frontline medical staff. *Journal of Health Psychology, 25*(7), 883–887. https://doi.org/10.1177/1359105320925148

Zhou, G., Gan, Y., Knoll, N., & Schwarzer, R. (2013). Proactive coping moderates the dietary intention–planning–behavior path. *Appetite, 70*, 127–133. https://doi.org/10.1016/j.appet.2013.06.097

Part I

Preface: Hedonic Well-Being and Health (Positive Emotional States)

Fuschia M. Sirois

This section of the Handbook brings together different perspectives on hedonic well-being and specifically the role of positive emotions in health. There is a longstanding view that positive emotional states are a key aspect of well-being. For example, from the hedonic perspective, well-being is closely aligned with the ancient Greek Epicurean conceptions of the purpose in life and the nature of living the "Good Life". Well-being is achieved by maximizing pleasure—"hedonia"—and minimizing pain. Positive emotions therefore reflect positive hedonic states arising from pleasurable experiences, however those experiences are defined.

Like other emotions, positive emotions can range from lower (calm, serenity) to higher (excitement, joy) levels of arousal reflecting lower to higher levels of intensity of pleasurable experiences. Yet research into the health effects of positive emotions is only beginning to examine the issue of whether different positive emotions along the spectrum of arousal (e.g. low arousal positive emotions such as serenity versus high arousal positive emotions such as excitement) have meaningfully distinct influences on physical health, or whether the effects are similar enough that making such distinctions are unnecessary for understanding the role of positive emotions in health. It is possible that there are meaningful distinctions between those positive emotions that lie at the opposite ends of the arousal spectrum, but not for those in the mid-range compared to the extremes. Distinctions could also exist with respect to the health-related outcomes associated with the positive emotions, the pathways and mechanisms that explain their links, or both.

The five chapters included in this section present theory and evidence on the potential of positive emotions—broadly construed—for health, as well as emerging research on specific emotional states such as passion and gratitude in the context of health. Collectively this theory and research highlights the multiple and often intertwined psychophysiological and behavioural pathways through which positive emotions can contribute to improved health. They also highlight the role of positive emotions for offsetting the deleterious effects of negative emotions on health, and the roles of intra- and interpersonal factors in the genesis and enhancement of the impact of positive emotions on health.

Chapters 2 and 3 focus on the role of positive emotions in physical health more generally and from different perspectives. In Chap. 2, Charles and colleagues provide a theoretical overview of the key pathways linking positive emotional states to health outcomes, how positive emotion interventions can be harnessed to combat negative emotions and improve health, and the contextual factors that may contour the effects of positive emotions on health. Chapter 3 continues the theme of the value of positive affect for health. Ramirez and colleagues view the contribution of positive emotions to health from the lens of psychophysiology, and note the relevance of the interconnections between the endocrine, immune, and cardiovascular systems in the physiological responses linked to positive affect.

Although there is clear value in understanding how general positive affective states can contribute to physical health, it is equally important to recognize the value of specific positive emotions, whether momentary or as more stable tendencies. Chapters 4, 5 and 6 focus on the relevance of specific positive emotions for understanding health-related pathways and outcomes. Research is increasingly demonstrating that gratitude is one positive emotion that has a number of relevant links to health in both medical and non-medical populations. In Chap. 4, Deichert and Feket provide an overview of this emerging research and highlight the potential physiological and stress-related pathways through which gratitude may exert its beneficial effects on health. Chapter 5 builds on these insights to further examine how and why gratitude can impact health through behavioural pathways. Sirois and Wood propose that affective states work alongside temporal thinking to play a key role in explaining why gratitude may support the practice of health-promoting behaviours and extend current theory to support this new perspective.

This section concludes by introducing how passion can contribute to important outcomes relevant for a more holistic sense of health and well-being. In Chap. 6, Chénard-Poirier and Vallerand draw upon insights from different theoretical perspective of well-being and combine these with passion theory to provide novel insights into the potential of adaptive passion for promoting health and optimal functioning in society. The role of passion for health-related outcomes is an emerging and promising new area of research that will hopefully continue to grow in years to come.

2

Positive Emotions and Health

Susan T. Charles, Colette J. Brown, and Julie A. Kircher

A popular theme in science fiction is the distinction between artificial and human life, where characters must wrestle with defining what it means to be human. Invariably, emotions play a pivotal role. Yet, one of the first documents positing that emotions are inherent in all animals was not fiction, but a treatise on the theory of evolution (Darwin, 1859). Emotions are imprinted

S. T. Charles (✉)
Department of Psychological Science, 4200 Social & Behavioral Sciences Gateway, University of California, Irvine, CA, USA
e-mail: scharles@uci.edu

C. J. Brown
Department of Psychological Science, 4200 Social & Behavioral Sciences Gateway, University of California, Irvine, CA, USA

Department of Family Medicine, University of California, San Diego, San Diego, CA, United States
e-mail: coletteb@uci.edu

J. A. Kircher
Department of Psychological Science, 4200 Social & Behavioral Sciences Gateway, University of California, Irvine, CA, USA

Department of Biobehavioral Health, The Pennsylvania State University, University Park, PA, United States
e-mail: jkircher@uci.edu

F. M. Sirois (ed.), *The Palgrave Handbook of Positive Psychology and Health*,
https://doi.org/10.1007/978-3-031-89095-6_2

in our DNA and expressed in the structure of the brain, and they influence our thoughts, behaviors, and health. Health psychologists posit that emotions are integral to our survival, and they study how the emotions people experience in their daily lives influence physical health.

A growing number of studies find that emotions impact daily activities, thoughts, and physiological functioning that, in turn, shape both short- and long-term health outcomes. Many of these studies focus on the damaging effects of stress and other negative emotions on our physiology. In the past few decades, however, an increasing number of studies have documented the power of positive emotions on health. People who report experiencing more frequent positive emotions in their lives reported fewer physical symptoms, better immune functioning, and fewer chronic conditions—living longer and in better physical health than their less happy peers (Folkman, 2008; Lyubomirsky et al., 2005). The central question now in positive psychology and health is not as much whether positive emotions influence health, but the mechanisms explaining this link.

To answer this question, scientists have examined the effects of specific emotions separately from broader psychological processes (e.g., the emotions derived from social interactions as opposed to the presence of social partners), differentiated the effect of positive from negative emotions, and charted the physiological and behavioral pathways linking positive emotional experiences to physical health. In this chapter, we provide an overview of the current understanding of how positive emotions are related to physical health. We begin by defining positive emotions and how they differ in function and role from negative emotions. We next discuss the pathways through which positive emotions relate to physical health, and briefly outline interventions that harness the power of positive emotions to boost health. We then discuss sociocultural influences that shape these mechanisms, and how these processes unfold across the adult life span. We conclude by offering some future directions for this growing area of research.

Defining Emotions

Emotion theorists argue over every aspect of emotional experience, including its very definition (e.g., Mulligan & Scherer, 2012). These debates are still active, but for the purpose of this chapter we define emotion as a relatively brief experience involving physiological, cognitive, behavioral, and subjective components that occur in response to an environmental stimulus. Most studies we review, however, focus on self-reported emotional experience (referred to as affective responses). Affective responses can refer to one-time self-reported specific emotional states (e.g., happiness), or to the reports of multiple emotional experiences throughout the day (e.g., feeling cheerful, content, and happy) that are generally either positively (positive affect) or negatively (negative affect) valanced. We use the terms emotions or emotional experiences when referring to emotion theories or laboratory studies that involve both subjective and physiological components, but we use the term affect when discussing the subjective component of a person's emotional experience. We also briefly discuss more stable personality traits that include emotional dispositions—or the tendency to experience certain emotion(s) for a sustained period of time.

In addition to discrepancies in the use of terms for emotional experiences, theorists have also debated their structure. It is generally agreed upon that those emotions are characterized by at least two dimensions: arousal and valence. Although arousal is commonly accepted to represent a single dimension, with high and low activation levels on opposite ends (e.g., alert vs. calm), there has been less of a consensus regarding the underlying structure of valence. Some theorists posit that emotional valence is structured along a single dimension with positive and negative poles, while others support a bivalent view, with positive and negative emotional valences each structured along independent dimensions (Larsen et al., 2001; see Barrett and Russell (1999) for a review of the debate and nature of positive and negative valence). Early neurological research has also supported the bivalent view by demonstrating select brain pathways for approach- and withdrawal-related emotional states (see Gray, 2004; Carver & Scheier, 1990 for a more nuanced view). The debate is still ongoing (e.g., Itkes et al., 2019; Petrolini & Viola, 2020; Russell, 2017), but the bivalent view has received growing support, with studies documenting separate processes for the two valences that can be activated individually or simultaneously (e.g., feeling both happy and sad; Vaccaro et al., 2020). Thus, since its inception, discourse on positive emotions has been intertwined with that of negative emotions, a tête-à-tête that is also reflected in theories explaining the role of positive emotions for physical health.

Theories Linking Positive Emotions to Health

Positive emotions took a backseat in early theories of emotion and health. Negative emotions were pivotal in these early evolutionary theories, where emotions such as anger or fear were posited to motivate fight or flight responses that enabled us to survive hostile environments. When theorists considered the role of positive emotions, survival benefits were explained in service to negative emotions. Positive emotions functioned to undo the damaging physiological effects of fight-or-flight arousal (Fredrickson & Levenson, 1998; Fredrickson et al., 2000), but on their own were not believed to have any immediate impact on physical health. One exception to the dominant focus of negative emotions were the early motivational conflict theories that distinguished between approach versus avoidance goals (e.g., Lewin et al., 1931). The greatest challenge to the emphasis on negative emotions, however, came later when Fredrickson (2001) proposed that an entirely different theoretical framework would be required to understand the evolved function of positive emotions.

The Broaden and Build theory was the first to outline the unique function of positive emotions for survival and thriving, describing how discrete positive emotions not only serve to undo negative emotional states, but also facilitate unique behaviors and outcomes that build health resources (Fredrickson, 2001). According to this theory, positive emotions motivate thoughts and behaviors to explore, create, and discover that build social, psychological, and physical resources – creating "upward spirals" that ultimately promote healthy survival. The majority of research supporting this theory has examined relatively short-term health effects on attention, general cognition, social cognition, and health behaviors (e.g., Sekerka et al., 2012), but these upward spirals are theorized to have long-term health implications and contribute to a more positive disposition over time (Fredrickson, 2013). The theory of Broaden and Build provides insight into how positive emotions foster survival over time through personal growth and development of resources that can make us more equipped to overcome harder times ahead (Fredrickson, 2003).

Through this theoretical lens, the undoing effect can be understood as a by-product of the broadening function of positive emotions (Fredrickson, 2013). The broadened thought-action repertoires derived from positive emotions can counteract, or undo, the narrowed tendencies produced by negative emotions. The undoing effect is supported in studies where people who are exposed to acute stressors (e.g., experimentally induced anxiety before giving a speech), immediately followed by exposure to positive stimuli (as opposed to negative), recover from negative arousal more quickly. Having illustrated the function of positive emotions both in and outside the context of negativity, these theories sparked a wealth of scientific inquiry to identify the direct and indirect pathways through which positive emotions influence physical health.

Pathways Explaining the Effects of Positive Emotion on Physical Health

Researchers have documented several pathways to explain how positive emotions could lead to better health outcomes—namely, via behavioral, psychosocial, and biological systems (Ong, 2010; Pressman & Cohen, 2005). Two major theoretical models are commonly used to understand how positive emotions operate on or through these systems to impact health. The main effects model describes how positive emotions directly bolster health behaviors, physiological functioning, and psychosocial wellness. Main effects are generally understood to result from positive emotions that endure with relative stability over time, or at least that last long enough to establish sustained boosts in health. Alternatively, the stress-buffering model proposes that positive emotions benefit health indirectly by helping to mitigate the harmful effects of stressful life events. Stress-buffering is hypothesized to result from both long-term and short-term positive emotional experience, but the key difference between the two models is that the second suggests that the health benefits of positive emotions occur primarily in the context of stress.

Health Behaviors

Positive affect is prospectively related to a number of health-promoting behaviors among both young and older adults and ranging from those with no chronic illnesses to those recovering from life-threatening disease. These behaviors include healthier profiles of exercise, tobacco use, sleep, medication adherence, and eating habits (Bassett et al., 2019; Sin et al., 2015). For example, Sin and colleagues found that, among patients with stable coronary heart disease, experiencing greater levels of positive affect was associated with higher levels of physical exercise, lower rates of smoking, improved sleep quality, and increased adherence to medication. Another study by White et al. (2013) assessed young adults' daily experiences of negative and positive affect and food consumption. On days when young adults experienced greater levels of positive affect, they reported consuming more fruits and vegetables. Interestingly, the consumption of healthy foods predicted improvements in affective experiences the next day, suggesting a bilateral relationship between eating behavior and positive affect.

Although the balance weighs in the direction of positive emotions related to healthier behaviors, there are a few exceptions to this rule. For example, positive emotions are related to more social behavior, and socializing is sometimes accompanied by alcohol and tobacco use. Several studies have found that extraversion, a disposition related to greater sociability and higher levels of positive affect, is indeed related to greater alcohol consumption (e.g., Fairbairn et al., 2015). The effect of positive emotions on poor health behaviors, however, varies across demographic factors such as gender and socioeconomic status. For example, tobacco use is related to greater sociability among individuals lower in socioeconomic status (Leischow et al., 2000), but related to stress reduction among those higher in socioeconomic status (Businelle et al., 2010). In addition, people with stronger behavioral activating systems (the system that is activated when you are having a positive experience) often report more positive emotions, but they also have reported greater alcohol and drug use (Voigt et al., 2009).

Psychosocial Pathways

Emotions are elicited by the environment, yet researchers have found that people are not passive vessels exposed to random vagaries of life. Our emotional states or dispositions undoubtedly play a role in determining the types of environments we seek out, the way we interact with others, and how others respond to us. Happier people tend to engage in more exploratory and social activities, experience more controllable and desirable life events, and have more and better-quality social relationships compared to their less happy peers (Fredrickson, 2013; Pressman & Cohen, 2005; Saudino et al., 1997). Consistent with the main effects model, these psychosocial processes, when boosted by positive emotions, have a direct impact on physical health, including brain health. For example, exploration of novel activities (e.g., learning a new language or instrument) helps to build more flexible, efficient neural networks that are more resilient to damage or diseases related to dementia (known as the cognitive reserve hypothesis; Stern, 2013). Furthermore, simply engaging in more diverse common daily activities (e.g., reading, driving, shopping) is related to better cognitive functioning both cross-sectionally and over time (Lee et al., 2020). Active and engaged lifestyles are also closely tied to one's sense of social belonging, and social integration is robustly related to mortality (Holt-Lunstad et al., 2010).

These psychosocial boosts not only have a main effect on health, but also build resources to cope with stressful life events. For example, people with personality traits that are associated with more positive and less negative affect (e.g., higher levels of extraversion and openness, and lower levels of neuroticism) report less negative affect on the day a stressor occurs, and they perceive stressors as less threatening and more controllable (Leger et al., 2016). Perceptions and appraisals have a powerful influence on the situations we select and how we interpret the events around us. In a study describing this self-fulfilling prophecy, Voss et al. (2017) found that positive (or negative) future self-views were reinforced by subsequent life events of corresponding valence, such that life events appeared to confirm people's expectations for their older selves, for better or worse. These findings suggest that our levels of positivity and outlook on life partially determines the quality of our experiences, and importantly, our ability to navigate those situations in ways most optimal for our health.

Biological Pathways

Positive emotions are related to health indirectly by helping undo the physiological effects of stress. The term "stress" was coined by Selye in the 1930s to name the psychological distress that leads to physiological dysregulation and disease. When a person perceives their environment as threatening—either real or imagined—a cascade of physiological response ensues. They may notice their heart racing, the effect of a fast-acting sympathetic adrenal-medullary axis (SAM) that releases adrenaline and noradrenaline, which in turn causes multiple changes in the system (e.g., increased heart rate and blood pressure). The slower activation of the hypothalamic-pituitary-adrenal (HPA) axis ends with the release of cortisol, which also influences a variety of processes (e.g., inflammation and other neuroimmunological changes). These effects produce short-term benefits for rapid action to prepare for either a fight or flight reaction. Over time, however, chronic stress reactions produce wear and tear on the body that leads to a variety of stress-related diseases (Agorastos & Chrousos, 2022).

Positive emotions help to combat the dangers of long-term activation of the stress response. The undoing effects of positive emotions help speed recovery to homeostasis (i.e., their pre-stress levels of physiological functioning; Fredrickson, 2001), which is consistent with the stress-buffering model. Other studies examining the effects of positive affect on states of distress imply that health will be better with the shorter duration of stress. Some studies have examined these effects with objective indicators of health. Papa and Bonanno (2008) studied how "smiling in the face of adversity" leads to better health outcomes. Their findings indicated that when genuine smiles were present among participants, they had better long-term adjustment, and negative emotion was decreased through the undoing effect. In another study, researchers assessed whether positive affect buffers the effects of acute stress on wound healing (Robles et al., 2009). Participants went through a procedure that disrupted their normal skin barrier, and then half were randomly assigned to complete a social stress task involving an arithmetic task and speech while being evaluated and harassed. After completing the psychological stressor, those with higher levels of positive affect were able to recover faster.

Robles et al. (2013) demonstrated this effect again in another wound healing study using couples—the researchers found that feeling satisfied with their relationship and having positive attachment was associated with better skin recovery. Some studies suggest that psychological interventions to alleviate stress may benefit wound healing. Robinson et al. (2017) conducted a systematic review to probe whether psychological interventions are aiding in a variety of types of wound healing (e.g., experimentally created wounds, surgical patients, burn wounds, etc.). Across the studies reviewed, improved wound healing was associated with relaxation interventions; however, more research is needed to assess the efficacy of positive psychological interventions and wound healing.

In addition, researchers have examined the role of arousal in positive emotions, examining how reports of high arousal emotions (e.g., excitement, enthusiasm) and low arousal emotions (e.g., calm, contentment) are related to health. Some studies find that high arousal emotions more than low arousal emotions are related to greater longevity (Pressman & Cohen, 2012). Moreover, this salutary effect did not change when taking into consideration social integration, optimism, and other affective experiences—exemplifying the main effects model. Conversely, other studies have found benefits in either type (high or low arousal) of positive emotions on health (Armon et al., 2014), with low arousal positive affect exhibiting associations with desirable changes in physiological functioning, such as lowered heart rate and systolic blood pressure. Such findings indicate a main effect between positive affect and reduced risk of cardiovascular disease.

Combating Negative Emotions: Positive Interventions

As indicated by the overview above, people who experience high levels of positive emotions report greater number of positive events and fewer negative events; they appraise negative events more positively, and they recover from negative experiences more rapidly from negative events (Sin & Almeida,

2018). Additionally, a meta-analysis which included 51 positive interventions, found that these interventions enhance well-being and reduce depressive symptoms (Sin & Lyubomirsky, 2009). Given the benefits of positive emotions, researchers have examined interventions to increase overall levels of positive affect, positive behaviors, and positive cognitions. Interventions include such activities as yoga, focusing on gratitude, and practicing mindfulness, and types of interventions. For example, Rash et al. (2011) studied the efficacy of a gratitude intervention in improving one's well-being. The intervention was a 4-week pre- and post-intervention design where participants either completed a gratitude intervention or a memorable events intervention. In the gratitude group, people were asked to think about "items, people or events for which you are particularly grateful" and then were instructed to attempt to maintain any experience of gratitude that they felt. They asked participants to engage in this reflection two times a week for a total of eight reflection days. The memorable events group followed the same protocol with one difference: although the, group's journal reflection entries were the same, only they were instead asked to "think of a memorable event" and then provide a reflection on that event. Findings revealed the gratitude group experienced significantly higher life satisfaction and self-esteem compared to the meaningful event group, adding evidence for the role of gratitude in inducing positive emotions and well-being.

Other researchers have studied the effects of "happiness" interventions among people with diagnosed health problems. For example, Moskowitz et al. (2017) designed a positive intervention for individuals recently diagnosed with HIV. Participants learned about positive emotion-eliciting strategies such as positive reappraisal of stressful events, listing a personal strength, or savoring a positive event. Fifteen months after the intervention, the intervention group had a lower viral load (i.e., a lower amount of the HIV virus in the body, calculated by the number of HIV RNA copies per milliliter of blood) than the control group. Other researchers have engaged in positive emotion interventions among breast cancer survivors (Casellas-Grau et al., 2014; Casellas-Grau et al., 2016). In a review of these interventions, they found that, overall, the positive therapies of mindfulness and hope therapy were able to enhance patient's quality of life, well-being, hope, life satisfaction, and benefit finding (Casellas-Grau et al., 2014).

When designing happiness interventions, researchers caution that no one size fits all, and people need to select the intervention that feels most natural and effective for them (Sin & Lyubomirsky, 2009). To design a successful intervention, the types of variations that exist across sociodemographics such as age and culture also need to be considered.

Variation in Relationships Between Affect and Health

In view of the evidence presented in the chapter thus far, it can be generally understood that happiness is good medicine. A more nuanced view, however, reveals that the strength and direction of these associations can vary depending on several contextual factors. Below, we discuss how culture and aging are two factors that may influence the extent to which positive emotions influence physical health.

Cultural Differences in Emotional Experience

Cultural context can alter the link between emotions and health in numerous ways. For one, broad cultural differences in the value of independence (focus on oneself) versus interdependence (focus on social balance) can shape the types of emotions that people value. Much of this chapter has focused on the health effects of how people actually feel, but a person's actual affect is not always aligned with the types of emotional experiences that they value or prefer to feel. *Affect valuation theory* holds that ideal affect is strongly shaped by cultural context, and that it influences people's behavior and the health effects of their actual affect (Tsai, 2017). For example, in cultural contexts that value a balance of both positive and negative affect, such as in Germany and Japan, experiencing negative emotions is less harmful to health. Such values may also give insight as to why the experience of mixed emotions occurs more frequently in some cultures compared to others (An et al., 2017). A greater discrepancy between ideal and actual affect (e.g., when people do not feel the way they want to feel) is associated with poor health outcomes. Among older adults who value calm states (i.e., low arousal positive affect), for example, meeting that emotional goal was associated with fewer physical symptoms, even after adjusting for actual affect (Scheibe et al., 2013). Together, these studies highlight the importance of cultural values, and whether those values are met, in determining the health-effects of positive emotions.

Culture and social relationships. Emotions are foundational to developing and maintaining relationships. Given that relationships can provide positive emotional experiences, they are an integral part of outcomes in disease, mortality, and health behaviors (Campos, 2015). The sociocultural variation of relationships has long been recognized (Mesquita et al., 1997); however, the field lacks studies assessing sociocultural variation in the context of health and relationships (Campos, 2015). Even less studied is the role of positive emotion in relationships and health associations. Campos (2015) posits that couples who are in satisfied relationships would have similar patterns of relationships and health across cultures, such that positive relationship processes (e.g., emotional positivity of interactions) are generally related to healthier outcomes (e.g., more health behaviors). However, research has yet to test and examine this model in culturally diverse samples, and these phenomena should be studied across more than two cultural contexts for appropriate variation. In addition, researchers have also implicated cultural diversity of familial relationships as influential to health, most especially collectivist cultures (such as east Asian and Latino; Campos & Kim, 2017). Although this topic is currently an understudied research area, culture is increasingly becoming recognized as an important component in emotions and health.

Positive Emotions and Health Across the Adult Life Span

With few exceptions (e.g., Ong, 2010), emotions and emotional constructs have similar relationships with health outcomes across the adult life span. The number of social relationships predict mortality in both younger and older adults, and the affect reactivity is related to risk of chronic physical and mental health problems similarly in middle-aged and older adults (Charles et al., 2013; Piazza et al., 2007). Positive emotions do not necessarily hold more power to influence health later in life, but health goals may be more salient to people who are more physiologically vulnerable.

The prevalence of chronic illnesses increases with age. Fortunately, older adults often experience high levels of emotional well-being, a phenomenon explained by socioemotional selectivity theory (SST; Carstensen et al., 1999). SST posits that time perspective—or the time people perceive remaining in their lives—governs life goals. Younger adults, recognizing a long life ahead for which they must plan and prepare, often select goals that will help them accrue resources they will need for their future. For older adults, however, a growing awareness of the ephemerality of life and their ability to focus on the present instead of a distant future shifts their preferences to emotionally meaningful goals. Time perspective changes with age; even when asked about their focus on the present, older adults report these thoughts more frequently, and these thoughts have stronger associations with well-being than they do among younger adults (Mahlo & Windsor, 2021). This present mindfulness is related to better health outcomes (Shook et al., 2017), and older adults are more focused on the present than younger adults. This priority on emotional goals may offset their greater physical vulnerability given their increased prevalence of chronic illnesses, but this conjecture has not been tested.

Future Directions in Positive Emotions and Health Research

The past two decades have witnessed a number of studies on positive emotions, providing foundational knowledge regarding the strong links between positive emotions and health across age groups and cultures. This foundation has expanded what we know, but also illuminated gaps in this knowledge. For example, several studies provide support for health behaviors as a direct pathway linking positive emotions and physical health, but more work is needed to examine direct physiological pathways. A number of studies find support for the undoing effect on self-reported negative affect, but fewer studies have examined this effect on physiological arousal. A review of this research has called for more research on the physiological mechanisms in this hypothesis (Cavanagh & Larkin, 2018). In addition, a couple of studies have examined the physiological effects of positive affect in the absence of strong negative emotions (Pressman & Cohen, 2005). For example, laughter and humor are associated with decreased stress hormones and the dopaminergic reward system (Savage et al., 2017). It is unclear, however, whether this physiological pathway operates as a main effect, or only in the context of undoing the effects of negative emotions.

Health psychologists also discuss the role of exposure to more positive events and fewer negative events as another pathway explaining the link between positive emotions and health. Although studies have documented that these links exist, fewer studies have examined the reasons for this differential exposure. Voss et al. (2017), in their study examining the role of appraisals in this process, is a notable exception to this gap in the research. But more research is needed to study the appraisals, decisions, and behaviors that lead to this differential exposure.

Additionally, further research is needed on the role of specific positive emotions, and the constellations of reported emotions that are related to health outcomes. For example, laboratory studies have documented the salubrious effects of amusement or happiness. The effects of other emotions that are difficult to experimentally manipulate in the laboratory, such as pride or love, or high-arousal positive emotions such as excitement, remain unclear. In addition, the report of co-occurring emotional states across the day, called affective diversity or emo-diversity, has been related to better physical health in some studies, but not in others (e.g., Urban-Wojcik et al., 2020). More research is necessary to understand these conflicting findings.

Finally, more work is needed to understand the varied contexts in which the association between positive emotions and health is either stronger, attenuated, or not present. The majority of this research has been done in Western-dominant cultures. Given that a study on Japan found no association between positive emotions and health (Kitayama et al., 2010), more research is needed to understand cultural differences in these associations. In addition, cultural differences need to be examined across a variety of daily life contexts, as indicated by research showing differences in emotions expressed during social situations between European Americans and Latin Americans (Campos & Kim, 2017). Age also provides its own "culture within a culture." The importance of emotions changes with age, as posited by socioemotional selectivity theory. More research is needed to understand how age differences in the value of emotions play a role in the emotion-health link.

Conclusion

Emotions are woven in the fabric of humanity, hardwiring our brains, and making survival impossible without them. Emotions are intimately linked to physical well-being, a tenet first discussed by Darwin, and then articulated in Nobel-award winning work by Selye. Yet, the work establishing these associations has focused predominantly on negative emotions. In the past two decades, researchers have produced a number of studies examining links between positive emotions and health, beginning to offset this imbalance. We have a solid foundation for claims that positive emotions are important for physical health, but we also must continue addressing the gaps in our knowledge. Happiness makes us healthy, and understanding all the pathways explaining this link will enable us to design interventions to elevate both our physical and our mental well-being.

References

Agorastos, A., & Chrousos, G. P. (2022). The neuroendocrinology of stress: the stress-related continuum of chronic disease development. *Molecular Psychiatry, 27*(1), 502–513. https://doi.org/10.1038/s41380-021-01224-9

An, S., Ji, L.-J., Marks, M., & Zhang, Z. (2017). Two sides of emotion: Exploring positivity and negativity in six basic emotions across cultures. *Frontiers in Psychology, 8*(610), 1–14. https://doi.org/10.3389/fpsyg.2017.00610

Armon, G., Melamed, S., Berliner, S., & Shapira, I. (2014). High arousal and low arousal work-related positive affects and basal cardiovascular activity. *The Journal of Positive Psychology, 9*(2), 146–154. https://doi.org/10.1080/17439760.2013.848375

Barrett, L. F., & Russell, J. A. (1999). The structure of current affect: Controversies and emerging consensus. *Current Directions in Psychological Science, 8*(1), 10–14. https://doi.org/10.1111/1467-8721.00003

Bassett, S. M., Schuette, S. A., O'Dwyer, L. C., & Moskowitz, J. T. (2019). Positive affect and medication adherence in chronic conditions: A systematic review. *Health Psychology, 38*(11), 960–974. https://doi.org/10.1037/hea0000778

Businelle, M. S., Kendzor, D. E., Reitzel, L. R., Costello, T. J., Cofta-Woerpel, L., Li, Y., Mazas, C. A., Vidrine, J. I., Cinciripini, P. M., Greisinger, A. J., & Wetter, D. W. (2010). Mechanisms linking socioeconomic status to smoking cessation: A structural equation modeling approach. *Health Psychology, 29*(3), 262–273. https://doi.org/10.1037/a0019285

Campos, B. (2015). What is the role of culture in the association of relationships with health? *Social and Personality Psychology Compass, 9*(11), 661–677. https://doi.org/10.1111/spc3.12226

Campos, B., & Kim, H. S. (2017). Incorporating the cultural diversity of family and close relationships into the study of health. *American Psychologist, 72*(6), 543–554. https://doi.org/10.1037/amp0000122

Carstensen, L. L., Isaacowitz, D. M., & Charles, S. T. (1999). Taking time seriously: A theory of socioemotional selectivity. *American Psychologist, 54*(3), 165. https://doi.org/10.1037/0003-066X.54.3.165

Carver, C. S., & Scheier, M. F. (1990). Origins and functions of positive and negative affect. *Psychological Review, 97*(1), 19–35. https://doi.org/10.1037/0033-295X.97.1.19

Casellas-Grau, A., Font, A., & Vives, J. (2014). Positive psychology interventions in breast cancer. A systematic review. *Psycho-Oncology, 23*(1), 9–19. https://doi.org/10.1002/pon.3353

Casellas-Grau, A., Vives, J., Font, A., & Ochoa, C. (2016). Positive psychological functioning in breast cancer: An integrative review. *Breast, 27*, 136–168. https://doi.org/10.1016/j.breast.2016.04.001

Cavanagh, C. E., & Larkin, K. T. (2018). A critical review of the "undoing hypothesis": Do positive emotions undo the effects of stress? *Applied Psychophysiology and Biofeedback, 43*, 259–273. https://doi.org/10.1007/s10484-018-9412-6

Charles, S. T., Piazza, J. R., Mogle, J., Sliwinski, M. J., & Almeida, D. M. (2013). The wear and tear of daily stressors on mental health. *Psychological Science, 24*(5), 733–741. https://doi.org/10.1177/0956797612462222

Darwin, C. (1859). *On the origin of species by means of natural selection, or the preservation of Favoured races in the struggle for life*. John Murray.

Fairbairn, C. E., Sayette, M. A., Wright, A. G. C., Levine, J. M., Cohn, J. F., & Creswell, K. G. (2015). Extraversion and the rewarding effects of alcohol in a social context. *Journal of Abnormal Psychology, 124*(3), 660–673. https://doi.org/10.1037/abn0000024

Folkman, S. (2008). The case for positive emotions in the stress process. *Anxiety, Stress, and Coping, 21*(1), 3–14. https://doi.org/10.1080/10615800701740457

Fredrickson, B. L. (2001). The role of positive emotions in positive psychology: The broaden-and-build theory of positive emotions. *American Psychologist, 56*(3), 218–226. https://doi.org/10.1037/0003-066X.56.3.218

Fredrickson, B. L. (2003). The value of positive emotions: The emerging science of positive psychology is coming to understand why it's good to feel good. *American Scientist, 91*(4), 330–335. https://www.jstor.org/stable/27858244

Fredrickson, B. L. (2013). Positive emotions broaden and build. In *Advances in experimental social psychology* (Vol. 47, pp. 1–53). https://doi.org/10.1016/B978-0-12-407236-7.00001-2

Fredrickson, B. L., & Levenson, R. W. (1998). Positive emotions speed recovery from the cardiovascular sequelae of negative emotions. *Cognition & Emotion, 12*(2), 191–220. https://doi.org/10.1080/026999398379718

Fredrickson, B. L., Mancuso, R. A., Branigan, C., & Tugade, M. M. (2000). The undoing effect of positive emotions. *Motivation and Emotion, 24*(4), 237–258.

Gray, J. R. (2004). Integration of emotion and cognitive control. *Current Directions in Psychological Science, 13*(2), 46–48. https://doi.org/10.1111/j.0963-7214.2004.00272.x

Holt-Lunstad, J., Smith, T. B., & Layton, J. B. (2010). Social relationships and mortality risk: A meta-analytic review. *PLoS Medicine, 7*(7). https://doi.org/10.1371/journal.pmed.1000316

Itkes, O., Eviatara, Z., & Kron, A. (2019). Semantic and affective manifestations of ambi(valence). *Cognition and Emotion, 33*(7), 1356–1369. https://doi.org/10.1080/02699931.2018.1564249

Kitayama, S., Markus, H. R., & Kurokawa, M. (2010). Culture, emotion, and well-being: Good feelings in Japan and the United States. *Cognition and Emotion, 14*(1), 93–124. https://doi.org/10.1080/026999300379003

Larsen, J. T., McGraw, A. P., & Cacioppo, J. T. (2001). Can people feel happy and sad at the same time? *Journal of Personality and Social Psychology, 81*(4), 684–696. https://doi.org/10.1037/0022-3514.81.4.684

Lee, S., Charles, S. T., & Almeida, D. M. (2020). Change is good for the brain: Activity diversity and cognitive functioning across adulthood. *Journals of Gerontology, Series B: Psychological Science, 76*(6), 1036–1048. https://doi.org/10.1093/geronb/gbaa020

Leger, K. A., Charles, S. T., Turiano, N. A., & Almeida, D. M. (2016). Personality and stressor-related affect. *Journal of Personality and Social Psychology, 111*(6), 917–928. https://doi.org/10.1037/pspp0000083

Leischow, S. J., Ranger-Moore, J., & Lawrence, D. (2000). Addressing social and cultural disparities in tobacco use. *Addictive Behaviors, 25*(6), 821–831. https://doi.org/10.1016/S0306-4603(00)00123-4

Lewin, K. (1931). The conflict between approach and avoidance. In C. Murchison (Ed.), *Handbook of Child Psychology* (2nd ed., pp. 1–46). Clark University Press.

Lyubomirsky, S., King, L., & Diener, E. (2005). The benefits of frequent positive affect: Does happiness lead to success? *Psychological Bulletin, 131*(8), 803–855. https://doi.org/10.1037/0033-2909.131.6.803

Mahlo, L., & Windsor, T. D. (2021). Older and more mindful? Age differences in mindfulness components and well-being. *Aging & Mental Health, 25*(7), 1320–1331. https://doi.org/10.1080/13607863.2020.1734915

Mesquita, B., Frijda, N. H., & Scherer, K. (1997). Culture and emotion. In J. W. Berry, P. R. Dasen, & T. S. Saraswathi (Eds.), *Handbook of cross-cultural psychology* (Vol. 2, 2nd ed., pp. 255–297). Allyn & Bacon.

Moskowitz, J. T., Carrico, A. W., Duncan, L. G., Cohn, M. A., & M.A., Cheung, E. O, Batchelder, A., Martinez, L., Segawa, E., Acree, M., & Folkman, S. (2017). Randomized controlled trial of a positive affect intervention for people newly diagnosed with HIV. *Journal of Consulting and Clinical Psychology, 85*(5), 409–423. https://doi.org/10.1037/ccp0000188

Mulligan, K., & Scherer, K. R. (2012). Toward a working definition of emotion. *Emotion Review, 4*(4), 345–357. https://doi.org/10.1177/1754073912445818

Ong, A. D. (2010). Pathways linking positive emotion and health in later life. *Current Directions in Psychology, 19*(6), 358–362. https://doi.org/10.1177/0963721410388805

Papa, A., & Bonanno, G. A. (2008). Smiling in the face of adversity: The interpersonal and intrapersonal functions of smiling. *Emotion, 8*(1), 1–12. https://doi.org/10.1037/1528-3542.8.1.1

Petrolini, V., & Viola, M. (2020). Core affect dynamics: Arousal as a modulator of valence. *Review of Philosophy and Psychology, 11*, 783–801. https://doi.org/10.1007/s13164-020-00474-w

Piazza, J. R., Charles, S. T., & Almeida, D. M. (2007). Living with chronic health conditions: Age differences in affective well-being. *The Journals of Gerontology Series B: Psychological Sciences and Social Sciences, 62*(6), P313–P321. https://doi.org/10.1093/geronb/62.6.P313

Pressman, S. D., & Cohen, S. (2005). Does positive affect influence health? *Psychological Bulletin, 131*(6), 925–971. https://doi.org/10.1037/0033-2909.131.6.925

Pressman, S. D., & Cohen, S. (2012). Positive emotion word use and longevity in famous deceased psychologists. *Health Psychology, 31*(3), 297–305. https://doi.org/10.1037/a0025339

Rash, J. A., Matsuba, M. K., & Prkachin, K. M. (2011). Gratitude and well-being: Who benefits the most from a gratitude intervention? *Applied Psychology: Health and Well-Being, 3*(3), 350–369. https://doi.org/10.1111/j.1758-0854.2011.01058.x

Robinson, H., Norton, S., Jarrett, P., & Broadbent, E. (2017). The effects of psychological interventions on wound healing: A systematic review of randomized trials. *British Journal of Health Psychology, 22*(4), 805–835. https://doi.org/10.1111/bjhp.12257

Robles, T. F., Brooks, K. P., & Pressman, S. D. (2009). Trait positive affect buffers the effects of acute stress on skin barrier recovery. *Health Psychology, 28*(3), 373–378. https://doi.org/10.1037/a0014662

Robles, T. F., Brooks, K. P., Kane, H. S., & Schetter, C. D. (2013). Attachment, skin deep? Relationships between adult attachment and skin barrier recovery. *International Journal of Psychophysiology, 88*(3), 241–252. https://doi.org/10.1016/j.ijpsycho.2012.04.007

Russell, J. A. (2017). Mixed emotions viewed from the psychological constructionist perspective. *Emotion Review, 9*(2), 111–117. https://doi.org/10.1177/1754073916639658

Saudino, K. J., Pedersen, N. L., Lichtenstein, P., McClearn, G. E., & Plomin, R. (1997). Can personality explain genetic influences on life events? *Journal of Personality and Social Psychology, 72*(1), 196–206.

Savage, B. M., Lujan, H. I., Thipparthi, R. R., & Dicarlo, S. E. (2017). Humor, laughter, learning, and health! A brief review. *Advances in Physiology Education, 41*, 341–347. https://doi.org/10.1152/advan.00030.2017

Scheibe, S., English, T., Tsai, J. L., & Carstensen, L. L. (2013). Striving to feel good: Ideal affect, actual affect, and their correspondence across adulthood. *Psychology and Aging, 28*(1), 160–171. https://doi.org/10.1037/a0030561

Sekerka, L.E., Vacharkulksemsuk, T., & Fredrickson, B. L. (2012). Positive emotions: Broadening and building upward spirals of sustainable enterprise. In (Online Eds.), *The Oxford handbook of positive organizational scholarship.* https://doi.org/10.1093/oxfordhb/9780199734610.013.0013.

Shook, N. J., Ford, C., Strough, J., Delaney, R., & Barker, D. (2017). In the moment and feeling good: Age differences in mindfulness and positive affect. *Translational Issues in Psychological Science, 3*(4), 338–347. https://doi.org/10.1037/tps0000139

Sin, N. L., & Almeida, D. M. (2018). Daily positive experiences and health: Biobehavioral pathways and resilience to daily stress. In (Online Eds.), *The Oxford handbook of integrative health science.* https://doi.org/10.1093/oxfordhb/9780190676384.013.10.

Sin, N. L., & Lyubomirsky, S. (2009). Enhancing well-being and alleviating depressive symptoms with positive psychology interventions: A practice-friendly meta-analysis. *Journal of Clinical Psychology, 65*(5), 467–487. https://doi.org/10.1002/jclp.20593

Sin, N. L., Moskowitz, J. T., & Whooley, M. A. (2015). Positive affect and health behaviors across five years in patients with coronary heart disease: The heart and soul study. *Psychosomatic Medicine, 77*(9), 1058–1066. https://doi.org/10.1097/PSY.0000000000000238

Stern, Y. (2013). Cognitive reserve: Implications for assessment and intervention. *Folia Phoniatrica et Logopaedica, 65*(2), 49–54. https://doi.org/10.1159/000353443

Tsai, J. L. (2017). Ideal affect in daily life: Implications for affective experience, health, and social behavior. *Current Opinion in Psychology, 17*, 118–128. https://doi.org/10.1016/j.copsyc.2017.07.004

Urban-Wojcik, E. J., Mumford, J. A., Almeida, D. M., Lachman, M. E., Ryff, C. D., Davidson, R. J., & Schaefer, S. M. (2020, April 9). Emodiversity, health, and well-being in the Midlife in the United States (MIDUS) daily diary study. *Emotion*. Online First Publication. https://doi.org/10.1037/emo0000753.

Vaccaro, A. G., Kaplan, J. T., & Damasio, A. (2020). Bittersweet: The neuroscience of ambivalent affect. *Perspectives on Psychological Science, 15*(5), 1187–1199. https://doi.org/10.1177/1745691620927708

Voigt, D., Dillard, J., Braddock, K., Anderson, J. W., Sopory, P., & Stephenson, M. (2009). Carver and White's (1994) BIS/BAS scales and their relationship to risky health behaviours. *Personality and Individual Differences, 47*, 89–93. https://doi.org/10.1016/j.paid.2009.02.003

Voss, P., Kornadt, A. E., & Rothermund, K. (2017). Getting what you expect? Future self-views predict the valence of life events. *Developmental Psychology, 53*(3), 567–580. https://doi.org/10.1037/dev0000285

White, B. A., Horwath, C. C., & Conner, T. S. (2013). Many apples a day keep the blues away - daily experiences of negative positive affect and food consumption in young adults. *British Journal of Health Psychology, 18*, 782–798. https://doi.org/10.1111/bjhp.12021

3

Physiological Pathways Connecting Positive Affect and Health

Veronica Ramirez, Desiree R. Delgadillo, Logan T. Martin, and Sarah D. Pressman

Connecting Positive Affect to Physiological Function

Early theories about the physiology underlying human reason and emotions can be traced back to ancient history, with Greek philosophers like Aristotle suggesting that the mind resided in the heart (Smith, 2013). As psychology developed into a scientific field, William James, the father of psychology, emphasized that physiological processes were necessary for the experience of emotions (James, 1884). To date, modern theorists and researchers have been able to empirically demonstrate the link between physiology and positive emotions, which are a central focus to the understanding of positive affect (PA), and how it could influence health outcomes, longevity, and well-being. This relation between PA with mental and physical health has been established extensively over the past 30 years (Jenkins et al., 2018; Pressman et al., 2019; Steptoe, 2019). In this chapter, we review the three most researched physiological systems that play a role in linking PA to health: the cardiovascular, endocrine, and immune systems. While there are other pathways that could be described in-depth (see Pressman and Cohen, 2005 for examples), the goal of this chapter is to review the most likely physiological pathways by which positive emotions "get under the skin" to influence health, also focusing on those with the most evidence at this point. Before the review of the

V. Ramirez (✉) • D. R. Delgadillo • L. T. Martin • S. D. Pressman
Department of Psychological Science, University of California, Irvine, CA, USA

F. M. Sirois (ed.), *The Palgrave Handbook of Positive Psychology and Health*,
https://doi.org/10.1007/978-3-031-89095-6_3

literature, we outline definitions of our variables of interest, relevant theories that might help with the understanding of the affect-physiology connection and provide the reader with a wide view of the physical systems that will be discussed.

Affect, Emotions, and PA

Affect is an umbrella term that encompasses emotions, mood, and emotion-related traits. The main features of emotions include the subjective experience (i.e., perception), the physiological response (i.e., changes in respiration or sweating), and the behavioral responses (i.e., crying or smiling). The duration of emotions determines whether they are dispositional in nature, lasting weeks, months, and even throughout people's lifespan (i.e., trait affect), or short-lasting and temporary (i.e., state affect). Emotions can also be categorized by arousal or physiological activation (i.e., high arousal and low arousal), as well as valence (i.e., positive, or negative) (Larsen 2009; Russell 1980). Relevant to this chapter, state and trait PA or positive *valenced* emotions have been described as feelings that reflect pleasurable engagement with oneself and the environment (Clark et al., 1989). Considering arousal levels is important to this chapter because they produce distinct bodily responses with likely differences in downstream health outcomes. Commonly studied low arousal positive emotions include: calm, content, serene, at ease, proud, and satisfied). They contrast with high arousal positive emotions (e.g., elated, peppy, excited, joyful, enthusiastic, and happy), which are characterized by higher alertness, increased energy, pronounced facial expressions, and more robust physiological activation, like increased heart rate and respiration rate. As we will learn in this chapter, arousal levels in PA can distinctly influence health outcomes due to differences in how they are processed physiologically.

In this chapter, non-affect but PA-related constructs (e.g., optimism) will sometimes be discussed to illustrate contrasting or supporting examples of emotion-physiology associations. Negative affect (NA) is also important to consider because it too alters physiological states. While PA and NA are typically negatively correlated, certain measurements allow for independence of constructs (Watson et al., 1988), especially when assessed over longer periods of time (Diener & Emmons, 1984). It is important to assess both PA and NA in physiological and health research, however, because of their typical measurement overlap, and the need to understand whether health or physiological changes are due to the presence or absence of one type of valence, or some combination of both, as well as whether the effects are independent of one another (Pressman & Cohen, 2005). While research has revealed many deleterious effects of stress and NA on health (Cohen et al., 2007), there is compelling evidence that independent of NA, PA is associated with a wide range of better health outcomes (Pressman & Cohen, 2005), such as increased longevity (Diener & Chan, 2011), and lower mortality (Chida & Steptoe, 2008). Although the focus of this chapter is on positive emotions, we will still include some relevant research findings of stress and/or NA to demonstrate how they contrast or interact with PA in terms of physiology and health outcomes, or when they are used as covariates in research studies. This will allow us to provide a more global understanding of the link between PA and health and its underlying physiological mechanisms.

Theories Connecting PA and Health

Various theoretical frameworks have been developed to explain how PA may affect physical health (see Table 3.1). We review these because physiology is a pathway for many of these theories, which will help the reader understand why these biomarkers (i.e., cardiovascular, hormonal, immunological) are so important, and the role they likely play in connecting PA to physical well-being. First, the Main Effect Model (Pressman & Cohen, 2005) hypothesizes that PA influences health outcomes through its effects on physiology, but also via social relationships and health behaviors that impact physiological function. This model guides our understanding and expectations of interesting and relevant interconnections between PA and outcomes, like levels of antibodies, cardiac, or hormonal activity in day-to-day life and their possible downstream health benefits. The Stress Buffering Hypothesis of PA, on the other hand, proposes that social support "buffers" or shields individuals from the negative pathological influence of stressful events. Similarly, PA is beneficial by lessening the occurrence of stress and mitigating its negative impact on physiology and health (Pressman & Cohen, 2005; Cohen & Wills, 1985). This model helps to understand the contributions of PA in the presence of NA and daily life stressors, and why individuals with higher PA and with PA-related resources, like social support, can remain shielded from the negative consequences of stress. The Undoing Hypothesis, like the Stress-Buffering Hypothesis, posits that PA helps ameliorate the deleterious stress effects by hastening stress *recovery* towards resting levels of physical function (Fredrickson et al., 2001). While the main effect and stress-related models are distinct, both are likely true. That is, PA is expected to both influence health via day-to-day differences in physical function, but also to be especially helpful during stress.

Table 3.1 Theoretical frameworks linking PA to health and their physiological pathways

Theories	Concepts definitions	Examples
Stress Buffering Hypothesis (Cohen & Wills, 1985; Pressman & Cohen, 2005)	PA "buffers" or shields individuals from the negative pathological influence of stressful events Through social, psychological, and physical resources, PA mitigates the effect of stress on the body and thus health This model focuses on a PA x stress interaction rather than a direct effect of PA on health. PA moderates (i.e., decreases the strength) the relation between stress and health outcomes by altering stress perceptions, reactions, and recovery	Higher daily state PA was also associated with lower blood pressure during a stressful task and faster recovery to baseline afterward (Steptoe et al., 2007) – Naturally occurring PA is negatively correlated with cortisol during naturalistic responses to stress (Joseph et al., 2021) – Higher self-reported trait PA is associated with lower reactivity (i.e., cortisol responses) to stress (Bostock et al., 2011) – PA during induced stress was protective against depressive symptoms one year later, a relation mediated by markers of inflammation (Aschbacher et al., 2012) – In a stress-inducing task, smiling was associated with a lower heart rate during recovery when compared with a neutral non-smiling group (Kraft & Pressman, 2012)
Main Effect Model (Pressman & Cohen, 2005)	PA *directly* affects health outcomes. This model emphasizes a main effect or link between trait PA and ANS and HPA, social ties, and health practices. These in turn influence immune and cardiovascular systems and thus health outcomes This model emphasizes the biological and behavioral pathways that connect PA to disease	– Trait PA is positively correlated with higher physical activity (Ryff et al., 2004) – Trait PA and laboratory-induced PA is negatively correlated with levels of epinephrine and norepinephrine (Cohen et al., 2003) – Higher trait PA is associated with lower waking-day cortisol concentration (Polk et al., 2005) – Higher trait PA is linked to lower C-reactive protein, an inflammatory marker associated with less optimal health (Ridker, 2005)

(*continued*)

Table 3.1 (continued)

Theories	Concepts definitions	Examples
Undoing Hypothesis of Positive Emotions (Fredrickson & Levenson, 1998)	The Undoing Hypothesis posits that PA helps ameliorate deleterious stress effects by hastening stress *recovery* toward resting levels of physical function. It posits that some positive emotions "restore autonomic activity" It focuses on state PA rather than trait PA. The dampening effects of positive emotions on physiological activation are said to closely follow episodes of stress or state NA. This means that this model applies when NA precedes PA, highlighting a temporal component not present in other models	– Faster cardiovascular recovery from NA when subsequently induced to experience state PA (Fredrickson & Levenson, 1998) – Higher state PA measured in naturalistic settings was associated with better diastolic BP recovery and lower acute cortisol response to stress tasks (Bostock et al., 2011) – Social connectedness predicted PA, lower blood pressure at baseline, lower diastolic blood pressure reactivity, and faster blood pressure recovery from daily state NA (Ong & Allaire, 2005)
Broaden-and-Build Theory (Fredrickson, 2013)	PA broadens individuals' attentional scope, leading to novel ideas and resource accrual (e.g., developing new friendships, hobbies, skills). It focuses on state and trait PA as they unfold in people's lifetimes This model focuses on how PA facilitates long-term health behaviors through the upward spiral theory of lifestyle change, where PA during health behaviors leads to unconscious motives and engagement of health behaviors, which in turn build psychological, physiological, and social resources	– In an experimental study, a group with increased daily state PA showed increased PA resources, like social support, purpose, and reduced illness symptoms: including less pain, congestion, and weakness compared to a control group (Fredrickson et al., 2008) – Increased state PA predicted increased vagal tone, and this association was explained by a higher perception of social connections (Kok et al., 2013) – PA experienced during physical activity led to increased positive thoughts, which increased engagement in physical activity (Van Cappellen et al., 2018)

(continued)

Table 3.1 (continued)

Theories	Concepts definitions	Examples
Allostatic (Over) Load (McEwen & Stellar, 1993)	Adapting to stress is important and healthy, but the over-accumulation of defensive physiological responses to perceived threats disrupts homeostasis and can ultimately harm the body Allostatic overload mostly occurs through overly intense stress responses, overly frequent stress responses, or inadequate recovery after stress	– PA was positively associated with healthier allostatic load profiles in a large-scale study of the general population of the Netherlands (Schenk et al., 2018) – PA is negatively associated with chronically high cortisol secretion, which is one biomarker of allostatic load models (Steptoe et al., 2008) – PA is negatively associated with allostatic load, indexed by multisystem dysfunction in hypothalamic-pituitary-adrenal axis function, immune function, anabolic activity, and cardiovascular activity in a group of community older adults (Kobrosly et al., 2014)

(*continued*)

Table 3.1 (continued)

Theories	Concepts definitions	Examples
Polyvagal Theory of Emotions (Porges, 1995, 2007)	This theory highlights an evolutionary perspective on emotions and physiological function centered on the vagus nerve It posits that the autonomic nervous system and the vagal nerve underlies mechanisms of emotions, like PA expression that allow for social enrichment and creativity and the ability to optimally respond and adapt to the demands of the environment, like sources of threat or stressors Processes like attention, emotions, and communication can be traced to the vagus nerve and how it integrates with other systems. For example, social engagement is supported by the vagus nerve that innervates facial and head muscles and inhibits sympathetic and HPA axis activity, optimizing social engagement	– Longitudinal naturalistic studies showed that higher RSA at baseline predicts positive emotions in response to social experiences and increased social activity (Isgett et al., 2017) – Higher HRV is associated with better emotion regulation (Thayer & Lane, 2000) – Higher trait PA is associated with higher HRV (Geisler et al., 2010)

Note: In this table, we provide a description of theoretical frameworks on the physiological pathways linking PA and health. We explain the main concepts of these models, and on the right column, we provide examples of research studies that have supported these models; these findings are both correlational and causal evidence of how PA influences health their relevant physiological markers. Note that although we have categorized the examples of research findings that best fit specific models, these theories are not always exclusive, so they can apply to the same research studies

Abbreviations: PA: Positive Affect; ANS: Autonomic Nervous System; HPA: Hypothalamic Pituitary Adrenal

While not specific to health and physiology, another theory is also helpful in understanding these complex physiological connections: Fredrickson's Broaden-and-Build Theory (Fredrickson, 2013). The idea here is that PA broadens one's attentional scope, leading to novel ideas and resource accrual (e.g., developing new friendships, hobbies, skills). This might connect to physiology because, for example, playing sports could increase cardiovascular capacity, and friendships could provide arousal-reducing support and comfort under duress. This provides further support for the importance of studying PA and NA separately since NA's role is thought to be focused on supporting momentary defense actions (and narrowing of focus) as opposed to a broadened awareness and activity that is beneficial long term. To understand why this is the case, it is necessary to understand the mechanisms underlying physiological responses to stress. Thus, we will next provide a brief review of human physiological processes relevant to affect and health connections.

Basic Physiological Function

The autonomic nervous system (ANS) is highly involved in the physiological manifestations of emotions by controlling largely involuntary bodily actions that are necessary for survival. Two branches encompass the ANS: the sympathetic and parasympathetic nervous systems (SNS and PNS, respectively). The PNS is mainly responsible for, but not limited to controlling homeostatic functions (i.e., rest and digest) via the vagus nerve. This large nerve spans throughout the body and connects to the brain, vital organs and the immune and endocrine networks. Through this nerve, the PNS aids involuntary processes like digestion, salivation, inflammation, and immune processes, etc. During stress, PNS withdrawal also allows the SNS to activate (i.e., fight or flight) as a defense response (McCorry, 2007). When the PNS and SNS dynamics are imbalanced, the ANS is thought to be rigid, and this lack of flexibility makes the organism less adaptable to respond or recover from stressful events or illness and disease (Thayer & Lane, 2007), and thus be more vulnerable to mental and physical health problems.

The cardiovascular system supports all essential bodily functions, from breathing and digesting to physiological responses to emotions. Most popular cardiovascular assessments (e.g., blood pressure, heart rate) tap both SNS and PNS contributions (Shaffer & Ginsberg, 2017). When experiencing stress, the body prepares to run and escape through PNS withdrawal *and* SNS activation, resulting in respiration and heart rate increases, as well as blood pressure and blood vessel changes that together result in increased oxygen consumption and elevated blood flow, as well as redirected blood flow to the extremities (i.e., muscles) to prepare for the expected fight and flight. After the stress episode is over, the SNS reduces its activity level, and the PNS becomes more dominant.

The endocrine system also plays a role in basic bodily functions during stress and rest. It releases chemicals (i.e., hormones) into the bloodstream for several purposes such as regulating homeostatic processes (e.g., hunger, thirst, circadian rhythms), regulating metabolism, and critically for health, influencing inflammation and immune function as well as stress responses. Finally, the immune system is a network of disease-fighting substances and proteins (e.g., cytokines, antibodies), cells, and organs that protect the body from infection but can destroy the body's own abnormal cells (e.g., cancer cells) as a defense mechanism (Delves, 2000). There are two branches of the immune system: the innate immune system mounts an immediate response to invading pathogenic microbes that enter the body to prevent infection, and the acquired immune system, which is more targeted and rapid and acts once the body has learned to specifically fight off specific invaders in a highly effective manner. Like the cardiovascular system, immune and endocrine processes change during stress and emotional responses, primarily to maximize the likelihood of survival. While the ANS responds within seconds to influence cardiac activity, the endocrine's hypothalamic-pituitary-adrenal (HPA) axis activates and results in cortisol release minutes later to enhance and prolong acceleration of heart rate (HR) (Rotenberg & McGrath, 2016). Cortisol is also thought to increase with stress because the body senses the presence of chronic stressors, and its release is needed to store energy for extended periods. Immune function similarly traffics energy to processes that are helpful in a flight or fight event, as opposed to slower-moving immune activities which are downregulated at rest (Segerstrom & Miller, 2004).

How do these physiological systems work together to support affective states and/or impact health? These systems are all under the influence of overlapping brain and autonomic networks that are essential for self-regulation and affective processes (Thayer & Lane, 2000, 2007). Specifically, the ANS is linked to the endocrine's HPA axis, which allows them to work together during stress or at rest (Lopez et al., 2018). When the body experiences stress, disease, infection, or damage, the vagal nerve communicates with the brain and the endocrine system, resulting in immune activation and inflammation. Interestingly, the brain can also exert anti-inflammatory action back into the body through the ANS and subsequent cortisol release (Borovikova et al., 2000). Because cortisol functions as an immunosuppressive glucocorticoid, its release can attenuate or decrease immune function. When there is dysregulation in the body, such as a lack of recovery period or heightened and prolonged activation of these systems, there can be resulting tissue damage (Cooper et al., 2015), immune disruption, or harm to the cardiovascular system (Fava et al., 2019; B. McEwen, 2000). While brief changes in immune, endocrine, and heart function can be helpful in the short term, when these physiological responses to stress occur too often and too frequently, the result could entail health damage in the long term (Buford & Willoughby, 2008).

Theories of Physiological Mechanisms Underlying Affect and Health

While not specific to PA, there are several theoretical frameworks that further our understanding of affective psychophysiology, the role of stress, and how these fit into PA and health more broadly. First, the Polyvagal Theory of Emotions is an evolutionary model on affective processes and social connection, and it highlights the role of the ANS and the vagus nerve (Porges, 2009). It is thought that the ANS and the vagal nerve underlies mechanisms of PA expression that allow for social enrichment and creativity and the ability to optimally respond and adapt to the demands of the environment, like sources of threat or stressors. Social engagement is supported by the vagus nerve that innervates facial and head muscles and inhibits sympathetic and HPA activity, optimizing social engagement. Porges' social engagement system is marked by safety cues and allows for free expression and positive engagements characteristic of PA.

On the other hand, imbalance of the ANS marked by prolonged and hyperactive SNS keeps the body in a state of unsafety, leading to the overuse of physiological systems that are not meant to be in a state of stress for extended periods. A second framework focuses on the wear and tear on the body due to the "damaging effects of biological responses to stress," which is referred to as Allostatic Load (McEwen & Stellar, 1993). According to this model, an over-accumulation of defensive physiological responses to perceived threats disrupts homeostasis and can ultimately harm the body (e.g., hypertension, autoimmune disorders). Although physiological responses to stress are functional and imperative for survival, chronic stress leads to aversive effects. For instance, acute stress can promote immune function through cortisol, but constant cortisol release due to chronic stress results in immunological suppression (McEwen, 2005). We will next provide conceptual and empirical PA-physiology research evidence that supports these theoretical frameworks.

Research Methods in the Study of Affect and Physiology

We now provide a brief overview of commonly used methods in affect-related research, which will help the reader better understand scientific findings and concepts of physiological pathways underlying PA and health outcomes. First, researchers often study state affect through experimental procedures that induce emotions while simultaneously capturing physiological changes, also referred to as physiological reactivity. Studies that manipulate emotion are imperative to our understanding of causal effects of PA on physiology, for example, in studies examining whether the experience of PA can alter stress physiology (via buffering or undoing). Experimental studies are typically performed in highly controlled laboratory environments to ensure participants are not influenced by confounds that may influence the results (e.g., presence of others, social context, ambiance noise and visual distractors of natural environments, physical and contextual characteristics of the geographical location) can impact affective psychophysiological outcomes. Common mood manipulation methods include using emotion-laden pictures or film clips (Bond, 1998; Sinha et al., 1992), positive mental imagery (Sinha, 1996), and behavior or action-related methods that alter emotions, like induced smiles, as in the Facial Feedback Hypothesis (Buck, 1980; Kraft & Pressman, 2012).

Second, studies on naturally occurring state and trait affect, on the other hand, allow researchers to ask questions about PA in a variety of settings, social contexts, and over longer periods of time. While causation cannot be established, prospective longitudinal studies that account for baseline levels of affect and resting physiological function, with subsequent changes in physiology assessed, can at least hint at precedent relevant factors. Most of these non-experimental studies rely on self-report (e.g., state PA as assessed by how someone feels in the moment, or trait PA by how one feels for weeks or longer), which can then be correlated with physiological data (e.g., salivary assays, blood samples, electrocardiograms) obtained in the laboratory, at participants' homes, or even as individuals go about their day-to-day activities in the real world while using portable sampling kits or wearable devices. These methods allow for a wide array of possible research questions to be asked and answered, as we will see next.

Below, we review how trait PA and state PA (both induced and naturally occurring), examined in laboratory and real-world settings, are associated with cardiovascular, endocrine, and immune function. For each system, we overview the mechanistic features of their physiology, describing briefly how they might relate to health, and most critically how these behave in connection with PA and related constructs. We also delineate methodological factors and limitations that need to be addressed in future research. For this review, we focus primarily on recent articles published over the last 15 years, but also include older and classic studies that provide context and important supporting evidence on the PA-physiology connection. Thus, this review is not comprehensive, but it does aim to capture the breadth of research findings on these topics and utilize representative studies that reflect what the broader literature says.

Cardiovascular System

PA has been consistently associated with a wide range of cardiovascular measures and health outcomes (Kubzansky et al., 2018), making it imperative to understand this association. Emotions are known to have an impact on cardiac activity, reflected in fluctuations of HR, blood pressure (BP), and heart rate variability (HRV), but the reverse is also true: cardiovascular physiology can influence emotions through a range of interoception mechanisms (Pace-Schott et al., 2019). Below we describe a range of study methods and outcomes that have been used to explore PA-cardiovascular interconnections.

Blood Pressure

BP is a key feature of cardiovascular health; it is the force of the blood passing through blood vessels, and it is influenced by cardiac output and peripheral resistance. Balanced levels of BP are important for maintaining optimal physical health since chronically elevated BP increases the risk for cardiovascular disease (Ettehad et al., 2016; Kearney et al., 2005). Because emotions, particularly those high in arousal, induce rapid changes in HR and BP, these cardiac markers can be used to measure physiological reactivity (Ifeagwazi et al., 2018). In cross-sectional studies, we generally find that lower (i.e., healthy) levels of BP are associated with higher PA and a wide range of more optimal psychological well-being measures (Appleton et al., 2013; Kubzansky et al., 2018). One example can be drawn from a global scale survey study that showed that trait PA was negatively associated with increased hypertension (i.e., elevated blood pressure) across numerous countries; in other words, the happier the country, the less risk for hypertension was observed (Blanchflower & Oswald, 2008);

The above cross-sectional results echo findings from other large-scale naturalistic studies. For example, BP has been found to be lower during state PA as compared to anger and anxious states captured in real-world settings in a population of over a thousand borderline hypertensive individuals (James et al., 1986). Similarly, in an ambulatory study that assessed BP every 20 minutes throughout the day, BP was negatively associated with PA (i.e., happiness) even after adjusting for NA and demographics (Steptoe & Wardle, 2005). This provides evidence that it is the presence of PA, and not simply the lack of NA, that is tied to healthier BP levels. In another study by the same researchers, higher daily state PA was also associated with lower BP during a stress task and faster BP recovery to baseline afterward (Steptoe et al., 2007); this study provides support for the stress-buffering hypothesis (Pressman & Cohen, 2005). Furthermore, it aligns with Fredrickson's Undoing Hypothesis and her classic laboratory study using films to induce emotions: participants experienced faster cardiovascular recovery from negative emotions when subsequently induced to experience PA (Fredrickson & Levenson, 1998).

Heart Rate (HR)

Another popular cardiovascular biomarker is HR, or the number of times the heart contracts or beats per minute (bpm) to deliver oxygenated blood to the body. HR is an easy to assess biomarker that fluctuates with a wide range of stimuli including physical movement, metabolic and cognitive processes, and changes in emotions, explaining its wide use in health and emotion research. Like resting BP, resting HR is negatively associated with PA, that is, lower HR (within normative ranges) is associated with higher PA as well as a range of other healthy behaviors (e.g., regular exercise, not smoking) and outcomes (e.g., longer lifespan) (Amutio et al., 2015; Kobau et al., 2011). Yet experiencing strong emotions, even positive ones, can also lead to vagal withdrawal, resulting in increased HR (Thayer & Sternberg, 2006). Prolonged elevated HR results in disrupted flow mechanisms and dysregulated blood demand/supply to body organs (Malcolm et al., 2008), and it is linked to a higher risk for disease and all-cause mortality (Jensen et al., 2013). That said, transient increases in HR (such as those occurring with brief emotion changes) are healthy responses to environmental stimuli, and not typically problematic for health. Rather, it is prolonged elevations (e.g., such as those seen in chronic stress) (Taylor, 2010; Valentini & Parati, 2009) that are most tied to ill health due to the lasting strain on the arteries and internal organs.

When we do see ties between higher HR and higher state PA, it is typically because of the arousal level of the emotion. For example, in studies of naturally occurring PA and NA, both elatedness and anxiousness (high arousal emotions) were correlated with increases in HR recorded as participants went about their daily lives (Jacob et al., 1999). HR increases have also been demonstrated repeatedly in mood induction experiments on mid arousal PA (happiness; Marci et al., 2007) and high arousal emotions like enthusiasm (Shiota et al., 2011). Similarly, studies that induced amusement have also shown significant increases in HR (Giuliani et al., 2008; Mauss et al., 2005). On the other hand, lower arousal PA, like awe, produces smaller HR fluctuations that are not significantly different from the baseline state (Shiota et al., 2011). Thus, we see that arousal plays a role in how PA relates to autonomic activity. As described above, this type of PA-related HR increase is not thought to be harmful given that it is less robust of an increase than with NA, as well as shorter lived (Brosschot & Thayer, 2003; Ehlers et al., 2010), thus not causing long term harm on blood vessels and the heart (Chida & Steptoe, 2008; Peçanha et al., 2014). Moreover, PA is also thought to specifically prevent these long-lasting elevations since it serves as an "undoer" of NA or stress, although it is likely that low arousal PA, like feelings of calm, are more effective in these cases (Acevedo et al., 2020).

Heart Rate Variability (HRV)

The interactions between the PNS and SNS result in time variation between heartbeats. Measurement of the change in the amount of time between beats is referred to as heart rate variability (HRV) (Thayer et al., 2012). Low HRV reflects a less variable interval pattern between heartbeats and can be an index of autonomic imbalance and is tied with higher perceived difficulties to regulate one's emotions (Williams et al. 2015). In contrast, high HRV is indicative of autonomic balance and flexibility (Cheng et al., 2019; Holzman & Bridgett, 2017), and it is strongly linked with better emotion regulation (Thayer & Lane, 2000), psychological well-being (Drury et al., 2019), and higher trait PA (Geisler et al., 2010; Schwerdtfeger & Gerteis, 2014).

Respiratory Sinus Arrhythmia (RSA) is a measure of HRV that is mediated by the parasympathetic branch, reflecting vagal tone. At baseline, higher RSA is positively associated with trait PA (Oveis et al., 2009). High RSA reflects flexible and adaptive responses to stressors that allow individuals to experience social engagement, which we know is important for cultivating and maintaining PA (Fredrickson, 2013). Longitudinal naturalistic studies have demonstrated that higher RSA at baseline predicts positive emotions in response to social experiences and increased social activity (Isgett et al., 2017). This index of autonomic flexibility is also positively associated with prosocial behaviors and social well-being and connectedness, which is key for broadening the mindset that produces positive experiences and results in higher PA (Kok & Fredrickson, 2010). A causal relation between PA and enhanced vagal tone has been supported by positive psychology interventions (Kok et al., 2013), which showed that a positive emotion increasing loving kindness meditation intervention led to an increase in social connectedness and increased high-frequency HRV levels. This aligns with the assertions that positive emotions can lead to a cascade of health-related benefits through social engagement that are reflected in efficient vagal tone, although it is also important to note that several criticisms of this study have been raised (Heathers et al., 2015).

Summary

PA is associated with healthy cardiovascular functioning such as sustained healthy levels of BP and HR, which may be a pathway explaining increased longevity and reduced risk for disease among people with high PA. Similarly, higher levels of HRV are associated with both positive mental and positive physical health outcomes, pointing at other possible pathways to more optimal health via cardiovascular differences in people with high PA. Although positive emotions can lead to heightened cardiovascular activity, higher arousal levels are the most responsible for these changes, and they are not at a level (e.g., not high enough or long lasting enough) that would result in damage. While much of the literature is consistent, showing benefits of PA for cardiovascular function and health (see review by Boehm & Kubzansky, 2012 for further discussion), there are some inconsistencies in the literature. For example, mixed studies have discussed whether high HRV does serve as a marker of PA and well-being (Kogan et al., 2013), and of course, many naturalistic studies do not address the directionality of this connection. Thus, further work is needed to unpack some of the newer findings as well as other new and interesting possibilities such as curvilinear PA-physiological function relationships (see discussion in Pressman & Cohen, 2005).

Endocrine System

Another physiological pathway by which PA may affect health is through the endocrine system. The endocrine system includes the pituitary gland, adrenal gland, adrenal cortex, thyroid, and gonads (Hiller-Sturmhöfel, 1998). The limbic system, which regulates emotional responses, interfaces with the endocrine system, which then releases health and metabolic chemicals into the bloodstream that regulates important homeostasis processes (e.g., hunger, thirst, circadian rhythms). There are various endocrine hormones that could connect PA to health, but those that have been most studied in the context of emotions are cortisol, alpha amylase, and catecholamines (i.e., epinephrine/norepinephrine). These hormones are relevant for metabolic and immune function and can have downstream effects on health outcomes such as hypertension, cancer mortality, bone density, and obesity (Adam et al., 2017; Sephton & Kraemer, 2000). Here we review the links between PA and health-relevant hormones. Because cortisol studies are much more prevalent and techniques used to examine it are more varied and nuanced than other chemicals, this section will review cortisol studies, separated by meaningful differences in analysis procedures, with the rest of this section covering the remaining chemicals, without those nuanced methodological distinctions.

Cortisol

Cortisol is a hormone that is an indicator of activity of the endocrine's HPA axis, a central nervous system (CNS) stress response system. Cortisol regulates many physiological processes (McEwen, 2019), but its most studied health effects are deregulating the HPA axis (Weckesser et al., 2014), or inhibiting inflammation and appropriate immune responses (Adam et al., 2017). Cortisol may be collected in a range of methods (i.e., saliva, hair, blood, or urine), each with its own measurement issues due to a range of possible confounds and timing concerns. For example, blood samples may cause stress themselves (i.e., from the needle) which is problematic for studies assessing emotion or stress themselves (Weckesser et al., 2014). Urine samples indicate total cortisol for the preceding 12 or 24-hour period (Turpeinen & Hämäläinen, 2013), limiting questions that can be asked, and its collection can be very challenging given that *all* urine must be collected over the time period of interest. Thus, it is not surprising that saliva sampling is by far the most popular approach in psychological studies given its simplicity, non-invasiveness, and the ability to be collected in a range of locations. Different measurement approaches determine which analyses techniques are possible because of the issues and temporal resolutions of each method, thus researchers need to think through methods and possible confounds carefully before diving into data collection (Dickerson & Kemeny, 2004). Below we review the PA-cortisol literature divided by different assessment approaches.

Area Under the Curve

The area under the curve (AUC) represents the total amount of cortisol produced over the period assessed (Pruessner et al., 2003). PA is typically negatively associated with AUC. For example, in a well-powered longitudinal study, Steptoe and colleagues reported that PA in older adults predicted lower AUC cortisol three years later (Steptoe & Wardle, 2005). Also hinting at the directionality of this association, a quasi-experimental study revealed a 25% decrease in cortisol AUC for participants who underwent a positive psychology intervention (McCraty et al., 1998). Cross-sectional naturalistic studies typically replicate this association of higher PA and lower cortisol production (Chida & Steptoe, 2008; Lai et al., 2005; Smyth et al., 1998), although notable exceptions exist (Steptoe et al., 2007). That said, studies that do not replicate often have methodological issues such as failed manipulation checks for increases in PA in experimental studies (Salzmann et al., 2018) and the use of nontraditional PA measures (Miller et al., 2016). Interestingly, urinary cortisol (Ryff et al., 2006; Szcepanski et al., 1997) does not appear to replicate the patterns of findings drawn from salivary assessments, which highlights the importance of considering methods carefully when attempting to replicate or combine findings in biomarker research.

Awakening Response

Cortisol awakening response (CAR) assesses the peak level of cortisol that occurs shortly after wake (e.g., 0 min, 30 min, and 45 min later after waking up). CAR represents the body's metabolic response to the anticipated day ahead and is an indicator of HPA axis activity that is distinct from cortisol released later in the day (Stalder et al., 2016). Higher CAR has been associated with people who are generally less healthy, as measured by a wide variety of symptoms and diseases (Kudielka & Kirschbaum, 2003). Higher PA is typically tied to smaller awakening responses. For example, Brummett and colleagues reported that PA predicted lower CAR on the next day, with a unique factor analytic approach to calculating PA scores (Brummett et al., 2009). Similarly, both self and informant-reported PA predict lower CAR (Miller et al., 2016) with other well-powered studies replicating this finding (Polk et al., 2005; Sin et al., 2017).

Diurnal Slope

Diurnal slope analysis gauges the cortisol slope (which declines after wake-up response) over the day. Diurnal rhythms are positively skewed with the highest level shortly after wake (CAR) and a gradual decline until sleep (Turner et al., 2020). This slope is an important index of stress regulation (Adam et al., 2017) and a predictor of future health (Sephton & Kraemer, 2000). PA is sometimes associated with a healthier steeper decline in diurnal slope, but findings are mixed. For example, it was reported that PA was associated with a steeper declining slope, but this effect was only observed in one time-point out of four time-points (Lai et al., 2005). Miller and colleagues found the steeper slope-PA connection (Miller et al., 2016), but several other studies reported null or contradicting findings (Brummett et al., 2009; Ryff et al., 2006; van Eck et al., 1996). One possible reason for this discrepancy is that most studies not finding slope associations utilize far fewer time points to determine slope, most commonly utilizing a 3-times-a-day approach versus a 4–12 times per day in studies that have indeed found associations (see Steptoe et al., 2007 for an exception). This suggests that more samples over the same periods could increase the precision of effect estimates and the resulting likelihood of detecting an effect, pointing to methodological factors to be considered in future research.

Stress Reactivity

Like the cardiovascular reactivity measures discussed above, cortisol can also be used as an indicator of acute physiological responses to stress (Endrighi et al., 2011). As would be expected from the Stress Buffering and Undoing Hypotheses described earlier, PA is typically associated with more adaptive cortisol responses to acute stress. The most convincing evidence is that a recent meta-analytic review of 20 studies reported that transient naturally occurring PA is negatively associated with cortisol during naturalistic responses to stress (Joseph et al., 2021). Similarly, associations between PA and less reactivity or better recovery to stress in the laboratory have been reported

(Bostock et al., 2011; Codispoti et al., 2003), but like many cortisol studies, these studies had small samples. While distinct from PA, optimism has also been tied to faster stress recovery (Puig-Perez et al., 2015), indicating broad benefits of positivity on cortisol during stress.

Catecholamines

Epinephrine and norepinephrine are catecholamines that are indicators of the sympathetic-adrenal-medullary (SAM) system. The SAM system is the ANS's stress response system. Deregulation of the SAM system may affect inflammation responses and increase hypertension and coronary heart disease risk (O'Connor et al., 2021). Epinephrine and norepinephrine are typically assessed in blood and urine, which as mentioned earlier, have methodological drawbacks for PA studies. PA has been associated with both epinephrine and norepinephrine, but the majority of studies report conflicting or null findings. For example, Cohen and colleagues reported catecholamines were negatively associated with PA (Cohen et al., 2003), while a positive association between PA and norepinephrine was found in other studies (Brummett et al., 2009; Codispoti et al., 2003), and null findings have also been reported (Ryff et al., 2004, 2006; Szcepanski et al., 1997). These findings suggest that further research is still needed to detangle the role of these neurochemicals.

Salivary Alpha-Amylase

Salivary Alpha-Amylase (SAA) is an enzyme that is considered an index of SNS activity, with some PNS contributions (Ali & Nater, 2020). Like cortisol, SAA's AUC, awakening response, diurnal rhythm, and reactivity can be assessed to indicate regulation of the SAM stress response. There is early evidence of connections between PA and SAA. For example, a pilot study reported that positive orientation was positively associated with SAA CAR (Pasquali et al., 2020). Children with high trait PA also have better SAA recovery after stress (Jenkins et al., 2018). Finally, researchers reported a marginal positive association between state PA and SAA in a naturalistic diary of university students (Nater et al., 2007). While this is promising, null findings connecting PA to SAA have also been reported (Het & Wolf, 2007), and given the few studies in this new area, more research needs to be done and replicated to understand the full nature of the association.

Summary

There is strong evidence that PA is negatively associated with total cortisol and CAR. Those reporting higher PA secrete less cortisol overall throughout the day and during their morning peak, and thus, may be less likely to suffer from allostatic load in their HPA axis, lowering their risk for a variety of health problems. Although PA is typically negatively associated with both cortisol assessments, there is evidence that they are indicators of different health-relevant mechanisms (Stalder et al., 2016). There is weaker, but some, evidence that PA is associated with steeper diurnal slopes or adaptive cortisol responses to stress. Studies on PA and catecholamines do not seem as promising as cortisol or SAA, but this may be at least partially due to the limitations of blood and urine sampling. That said, the SAM system remains a potentially important mechanism through which PA could affect health and should be studied more extensively.

Immune System

The immune system is a complex and dynamic network of organs and cells that permeates every part of the body. It may be helpful to imagine this all-encompassing system as an ecosystem that requires balance to thrive. For instance, the short-term elevation of inflammation in response to pathogens is necessary to ward off infection (e.g., to traffic immune cells to the right parts of the body), but prolonged and unnecessarily elevated levels of inflammation have detrimental consequences over time, including an increased risk for various diseases and increased mortality (Ridker, 2005). Interestingly, research suggests that naturally occurring and induced PA are both linked to immune function and may foster adaptive immune responses. In this section, we provide a snapshot of the literature, organizing studies by outcome, design, and study context.

Various assessments can be used to measure immune function, including counting all white blood cells (WBC; cells that fight off pathogens) or specific types of WBCs such as B-cells, T-cells, monocytes, neutrophils, and natural killer (NK) cells that kill off harmful cells (i.e., cancerous, infected, or abnormal) (Folds & Schmitz, 2003), as well as assessing their function (e.g., killing capacity). Other immune cells can also be measured, including those that are specific to certain illnesses (e.g., T-cells for HIV) and antibodies (i.e., the highly specific immunoglobulin [Ig] proteins released from some WBCs to attack invaders) which protect against bacterial and viral infections. Typically, more immune cells equal greater protection, but prolonged or excessively high levels of certain immune markers in the absence of a threat can be maladaptive, resulting in damage to healthy tissue and even disease (e.g., autoimmune disorders). The key here is that like high stress reactivity, where return to baseline/rest is key, the immune system also relies on balance and homeostasis, but short-term activity/increases in immune activity can be seen as healthy.

Below as we review a number of immune markers, the assumption should be that these include both blood and saliva assessments, the primary methods of immune function monitoring. We do not review all possible immune parameters but instead focus on those most linked to PA. More in-depth but older reviews are also available, and these discuss an array of other immune parameters such as a range of white blood cell total counts, allergic responses, white blood cell proliferation in response to challenge, and more, with many studies showing immune benefits connected to higher PA (Pressman & Black, 2012).

Inflammatory Markers

Numerous experimental studies using inflammatory markers as a health outcome have revealed that PA may promote better immune function, consistent with the main effect model of PA discussed earlier (Bartlett et al., 1993; see review by Jones & Graham-Engeland, 2021). For example, participants who listened to positive mood-inducing music showed an increase in the pro-inflammatory cytokine interleukin (IL)-1 (Bartlett et al., 1993). As in the section on cardiovascular reactivity to certain mood inductions, we see a brief increase in markers of inflammation and thus a boost in immune function, which is usually interpreted as adaptive in healthy samples (Pressman & Black, 2012). While these experimental studies support the main effect model of PA, other evidence suggests that the stress buffering hypothesis of PA is also supported in studies of PA and inflammation as evidenced by a recent review of 28 studies (Jones & Graham-Engeland, 2021). For example, one laboratory experiment showed that the positive relation between stress and levels of pro-inflammatory cytokines (IL-1β and IL-6) became stronger as levels of PA decreased. Further, in a laboratory study, being able to maintain PA during induced stress was protective against depressive symptoms one year later, a relation mediated by markers of inflammation (Aschbacher et al., 2012).

Thus, it is likely that both the stress buffering and main effect models apply in terms of how PA might be connecting with inflammation.

Naturalistic studies have shown that one-time measures of trait PA, as well as other lasting well-being constructs (e.g., life satisfaction), are linked to lower C-reactive protein (CRP), an inflammatory marker tied to less optimal health (Ridker, 2005). For example, in one nationwide survey, individuals with low PA had a greater risk of presenting clinically high levels of CRP (Ironson & Hayward, 2008). This association has also been found in numerous large correlational studies (Okely et al., 2017). Importantly, this effect may be bi-directional since prolonged, heightened levels of inflammation can also lead to worsened mood and even clinical depression (Berk et al., 2013). Higher IL-6, a pro-inflammatory marker intricately connected to CRP, has similarly been tied inversely to self-reported trait PA (Brouwers et al., 2013; Stellar et al., 2015). Other proinflammatory (i.e., inflammation enhancing) markers have also been correlated inversely to PA (e.g., TNFr2, TNFα, fibrinogen) (Brouwers et al., 2013; Hamer & Chida, 2011).

Emerging research suggests that PA-inflammation links are sensitive to numerous contexts. For example, findings may vary depending on when and how PA is measured (Graham-Engeland et al., 2018). While rare, some studies have examined which types of PA were most tied to IL-6 and CRP. Interestingly, one study found that feelings of awe were the strongest predictor, as compared to other PA types, like happiness, joy, contentment, and pride (Stellar et al., 2015). Another study focused on breast cancer survivors found that low arousal PA was positively associated with lower levels of CRP (Moreno et al., 2016). Taken together, studies assessing PA and inflammation suggest that PA is linked to adaptive immune function, as demonstrated in a brief (i.e., healthy) boost in immune activation in response to a stimulus followed by a return to homeostasis (Bartlett et al., 1993).

Antibodies

PA has been assessed a great deal in the context of changes in secretory immunoglobulin A (sIgA), an antibody that fights illness and infection. SIgA is most found in mucosal surfaces (e.g., saliva, ear wax, mucus, tears) and is easily and accurately measured in saliva making it relatively easy to study across numerous designs. The association between higher PA and increases in sIgA has been repeatedly replicated and observed in various populations, throughout the lifespan, and across cultures (see review by Pressman & Black, 2012). Of note, both high and low arousal PA seem to be beneficial to increasing sIgA levels, as exposing individuals to both humorous films and relaxing music has resulted in SIgA elevations (Burns, 2001). The evidence for positive linkages between PA and sIgA is also not limited to adults. For instance, in an intervention study on healthy children and children with respiratory tract infections, those assigned to a relaxation condition displayed increases in sIgA (Hewson-Bower & Drummond, 2001), indicating sIgA benefits of low arousal PA across the lifespan. The experimental evidence is compelling, but what about the real world?

Naturalistic research on older adults has revealed positive associations between state PA on influenza vaccination day and higher levels of vaccine-specific antibodies following vaccination (Ayling et al., 2018), indicating a more robust immunization response. Similarly, higher PA-related brain activity in older adults was associated with higher levels of antibody titers in response to a flu vaccination as compared to those with more NA-related brain activity (Rosenkranz et al., 2003). This is especially important since older adults have worse immune function on average than younger populations, indicating possible additional vaccination protection for this higher risk sample. Further, this association appears to be replicated for other vaccine types. For example, higher PA was associated with higher antibodies in response to hepatitis B in younger adults (Marsland et al., 2006). This provocative evidence might suggest promise for PA-enhancing interventions delivered at vaccination sites or around the time of vaccination with the goal of maximizing immunization effectiveness.

Summary

There is strong evidence to suggest that PA is associated with optimal immune function. This includes regulation of inflammatory cytokines, increased titers, and antibodies. PA-immune associations are observed throughout the lifespan, across cultures, and in healthy and clinical populations. These immune changes likely lead to important differences in health given the many studies showing associations between PA and immune-related health indices such as reduced infectious illness upon experimental exposure (e.g., Cohen et al., 2003) and faster wound healing (Robles et al., 2009; Broadbent & Koschwanez, 2012). One possible reason for these immune benefits is that PA may lead to a mindset of resource building which in turn fosters increased access to health strengthening resources (e.g., physical, intellectual, and social) as suggested by Fredrickson's theory. PA may also directly affect major body systems (e.g., endocrine, cardiovascular) which could influence immune function (Pressman

& Cohen, 2005), supporting the main effects model, at least in the inflammation literature (Jones & Graham-Engeland, 2021). Future work should explore in even greater depth the mechanisms by which PA and immune function are connected.

Main Conclusions and Future Directions

In this chapter, we have described the physiological mechanisms associated with PA, and how they may lead to positive health outcomes. Based on scientific literature spanning at least three decades, findings drawn from naturalistic and laboratory-based studies demonstrate how cardiovascular, endocrine, and immune systems can serve as pathways between PA and health. Overall, these studies provide evidence, both correlational and experimental, that support the theoretical frameworks hypothesizing that PA can influence health through the ANS and the HPA axis that collectively influence immunity and downstream health. Evidence also supports that PA aids health via shielding individuals from the negative impact of stress and NA (e.g., via improving physiological recovery processes). In general, baseline levels of cardiovascular markers, like HR and BP, as well as endocrine markers, like cortisol and SAA tend to be lower in people with higher trait PA. This can be beneficial for health because, as discussed, overactivity of these markers and imbalanced autonomic function could lead to higher inflammation as well as other dysregulations. Further, while not discussed as much in this chapter, PA benefits on health and physiology could also be enhanced via PA-associated higher levels of healthy behaviors (e.g., sleeping better, eating well, not drinking to excess) and better quality social environments (e.g., higher social support, higher quality relationships), also known to enhance physical well-being. That said, much research is still needed to assess how these factors may moderate or mediate this phenomenon.

In the cardiovascular context, the most compelling literature showed extensive evidence on how the cardiovascular system changes upon the experience of emotions, particularly high arousal emotions. High arousal PA and NA can alter various cardiac markers through PNS withdrawal, but NA reactivity typically lasts longer, delaying recovery, putting a strain on the body, resulting in deleterious effects on the body and a negative impact on health, especially when NA is prolonged or repeated. Fortunately, PA can ameliorate these negative effects by buffering and undoing the effect of stress on these systems. In the context of physiological reactivity and recovery, it is most likely that low arousal, rather than high arousal PA, is more advantageous to aid or speed up cardiovascular stress recovery, as evidenced by a recent experimental study on this topic (Acevedo et al., 2020). Finally, cross-sectional correlations between trait PA and cardiovascular biomarkers were consistent across outcomes: higher PA was associated with healthier circulatory and cardiovascular function such as lower HR, lower BP, and higher HRV. While some studies did not always find these results, this is likely due to differences and sometimes problems in research designs, samples studied, variance in PA measures, or cardiovascular assessment methods.

For the endocrine results, there is strong evidence for a relationship between cortisol secretion and PA. Specifically, PA is generally associated with lower total cortisol production when measured as cortisol AUC. It was also the case that PA was negatively associated with CAR. There was weaker evidence for a link between PA and a steeper cortisol slope throughout the rest of the day or better stress recovery. Taken together, these findings indicate that individuals with higher PA, either trait or state, have a healthier (i.e., better regulated) HPA Axis, which could lead to better downstream health by reducing the possibility of allostatic load, immune suppression, and chronic pain or disease. At this point, a relationship between PA and catecholamines is not supported by the current literature. Early work on SAA indicates some possible connections with PA, which may be due to stress-buffering and/or recovery effects of PA, as opposed to direct effects.

In the immune literature, PA is generally associated with increased antibodies in response to vaccination, regulation of markers of inflammation, and beneficial effects on inflammation linked pathologies, such as arthritis and chronic heart failure (Ayling et al., 2018; Brouwers et al., 2013). Indeed, numerous experimental and naturalistic studies suggest that PA may enhance immune function. Inconsistencies found in the literature may be because most studies create a mean score for PA that includes various types of PA without distinguishing arousal (e.g., awe, joy, calm, happiness, contentment), which may sometimes make a difference in results, as was clearly shown in the cardiovascular section. That said, in at least some outcomes, both high and low arousal PA were beneficial for immune function. Researchers should approach PA-immune questions with these methodological nuances in mind to better understand downstream illness impacts and whether immunity is a mediator of the PA-health connection. In sum, there are many open-ended questions in this area of research, but also much promising evidence that provides a sound foundation to build upon.

As the field of positive psychology continues to illuminate how different physiological systems interact with affect and behaviors that result in better physical and mental health, methodological issues continue to be a focus of scientists to better explain these dynamics. As shown throughout this chapter, studying the causal effect of emotions and physiology remains limited to laboratory experiments that can focus on few variables at a time in specific environments. As a result, the directionality of the relations between health, numerous physiological markers, and PA is still not proven and is likely circular since it is well established that the arrows go both ways between these variables (e.g., happiness can lead to health, but the opposite is also true). That said, proving causality will not be an easy task due to the complexity of human life: countless variables are at play and fluctuate constantly, like major and minor life events and stressors, society, age, cultural/ethnic/racial background, socioeconomic status, etc. Capturing the interaction of these factors is an ever-changing playing field. So, there is a need to optimize research methods, tools, and statistical techniques, to capture the causal relationship between emotion and underlying mechanisms in real-time and real-world settings.

Finally, it is important to note that the compelling evidence of the link between PA and health has led to a surge in positive psychology intervention programs that help us determine its causality (Sin & Lyubomirsky, 2009). Generating applied intervention programs is a critical step to apply basic research findings in practical settings and communities. That said, there is still a great need for well-designed inclusive interventions that consider the influence of race, cultural background, socioeconomic status, and other psychosocial factors. More relevant to this review, it is also key to test out different positive psychology interventions and better understand how different approaches distinctly influence arms of the autonomic system, especially those relevant to specific diseases. Can certain types of well-being measures be beneficial to reduce the risk for one disease but increase it for another? Are there key time periods in disease when it is ideal to intervene based on physiological mechanisms? The compelling evidence described here suggests it is worth it for us to keep addressing these physiology-related questions. As epidemiological studies continue to alert us on the associations between affect and health, the race to find how positive psychology interventions can increase quantity and quality of life is still on, as is the race to understand whether these interventions can play a pivotal factor to help reduce health disparities, and ultimately reduce the burden of disease across all groups of our society.

References

Acevedo, A. M., Leger, K. A., Jenkins, B. N., & Pressman, S. D. (2020). Keep calm or get excited? Examining the effects of different types of positive affect on responses to acute pain. *The Journal of Positive Psychology*, 1–10. https://doi.org/10.1080/17439760.2020.1858338

Adam, E. K., Quinn, M. E., Tavernier, R., McQuillan, M. T., Dahlke, K. A., & Gilbert, K. E. (2017). Diurnal cortisol slopes and mental and physical health outcomes: A systematic review and meta-analysis. *Psychoneuroendocrinology, 83*, 25–41. https://doi.org/10.1016/j.psyneuen.2017.05.018

Ali, N., & Nater, U. M. (2020). Salivary Alpha-Amylase as a biomarker of stress in behavioral medicine. *International Journal of Behavioral Medicine, 27*(3), 337–342. https://doi.org/10.1007/s12529-019-09843-x

Amutio, A., Martínez-Taboada, C., Hermosilla, D., & Delgado, L. C. (2015). Enhancing relaxation states and positive emotions in physicians through a mindfulness training program: A one-year study. *Psychology, Health & Medicine, 20*(6), 720–731. https://doi.org/10.1080/13548506.2014.986143

Appleton, A. A., Buka, S. L., Loucks, E. B., Rimm, E. B., Martin, L. T., & Kubzansky, L. D. (2013). A prospective study of positive early-life psychosocial factors and favorable cardiovascular risk in adulthood. *Circulation, 127*(8), 905–912. https://doi.org/10.1161/CIRCULATIONAHA.112.115782

Aschbacher, K., Epel, E., Wolkowitz, O. M., Prather, A. A., Puterman, E., & Dhabhar, F. S. (2012). Maintenance of a positive outlook during acute stress protects against pro-inflammatory reactivity and future depressive symptoms. *Brain, Behavior, and Immunity, 26*(2), 346–352. https://doi.org/10.1016/j.bbi.2011.10.010

Ayling, K., Fairclough, L., Tighe, P., Todd, I., Halliday, V., Garibaldi, J., Royal, S., Hamed, A., Buchanan, H., & Vedhara, K. (2018). Positive mood on the day of influenza vaccination predicts vaccine effectiveness: A prospective observational cohort study. *Brain, Behavior, and Immunity, 67*, 314–323. https://doi.org/10.1016/j.bbi.2017.09.008

Bartlett, D., Kaufman, D., & Smeltekop, R. (1993). The effects of music listening and perceived sensory experiences on the immune system as measured by interleukin-1 and cortisol. *Journal of Music Therapy, 30*(4), 194–209. https://doi.org/10.1093/jmt/30.4.194

Berk, M., Williams, L. J., Jacka, F. N., O'Neil, A., Pasco, J. A., Moylan, S., Allen, N. B., Stuart, A. L., Hayley, A. C., Byrne, M. L., & Maes, M. (2013). So depression is an inflammatory disease, but where does the inflammation come from? *BMC Medicine, 11*(1), 200. https://doi.org/10.1186/1741-7015-11-200

Blanchflower, D. G., & Oswald, A. J. (2008). Hypertension and happiness across nations. *Journal of Health Economics, 27*(2), 218–233. https://doi.org/10.1016/j.jhealeco.2007.06.002

Boehm, J. K., & Kubzansky, L. D. (2012). The heart's content: The association between positive psychological well-being and cardiovascular health. *Psychological Bulletin, 138*(4), 655–691. https://doi.org/10.1037/a0027448

Bond, C. V. A. (1998). Personal relevance is an important dimension for visceral reactivity in emotional imagery. *Cognition and Emotion, 12*(2), 231–242. https://doi.org/10.1080/026999398379736

Borovikova, L. V., Ivanova, S., Zhang, M., Yang, H., Botchkina, G. I., Watkins, L. R., Wang, H., Abumrad, N., Eaton, J. W., & Tracey, K. J. (2000). *Vagus nerve stimulation attenuates the systemic in˜ammatory response to endotoxin., 405*, 5.

Bostock, S., Hamer, M., Wawrzyniak, A. J., Mitchell, E. S., & Steptoe, A. (2011). Positive emotional style and subjective, cardiovascular and cortisol responses to acute laboratory stress. *Psychoneuroendocrinology, 36*(8), 1175–1183. https://doi.org/10.1016/j.psyneuen.2011.02.009

Broadbent, E., & Koschwanez, H. E. (2012). The psychology of wound healing. *Current Opinion in Psychiatry, 25*(2), 135–140. https://doi.org/10.1097/YCO.0b013e32834e1424

Brosschot, J. F., & Thayer, J. F. (2003). Heart rate response is longer after negative emotions than after positive emotions. *International Journal of Psychophysiology, 50*(3), 181–187. https://doi.org/10.1016/S0167-8760(03)00146-6

Brouwers, C., Mommersteeg, P. M. C., Nyklíček, I., Pelle, A. J., Westerhuis, B. L. W. J. J. M., Szabó, B. M., & Denollet, J. (2013). Positive affect dimensions and their association with inflammatory biomarkers in patients with chronic heart failure. *Biological Psychology, 92*(2), 220–226. https://doi.org/10.1016/j.biopsycho.2012.10.002

Brummett, B. H., Boyle, S. H., Kuhn, C. M., Siegler, I. C., & Williams, R. B. (2009). Positive affect is associated with cardiovascular reactivity, norepinephrine level, and morning rise in salivary cortisol. *Psychophysiology, 46*(4), 862–869. https://doi.org/10.1111/j.1469-8986.2009.00829.x

Buck, R. (1980). Nonverbal behavior and the theory of emotion: The facial feedback hypothesis. *Journal of Personality and Social Psychology, 38*(5), 811–824. https://doi.org/10.1037/0022-3514.38.5.811

Buford, T. W., & Willoughby, D. S. (2008). Impact of DHEA(S) and cortisol on immune function in aging: A brief review. *Applied Physiology, Nutrition, and Metabolism, 33*(3), 429–433. https://doi.org/10.1139/H08-013

Burns, D. S. (2001). The effect of the bonny method of guided imagery and music on the mood and life quality of cancer patients. *Journal of Music Therapy, 38*(1), 51–65. https://doi.org/10.1093/jmt/38.1.51

Cheng, Y.-C., Huang, Y.-C., & Huang, W.-L. (2019). Heart rate variability as a potential biomarker for alcohol use disorders: A systematic review and meta-analysis. *Drug and Alcohol Dependence, 204*, 107502. https://doi.org/10.1016/j.drugalcdep.2019.05.030

Chida, Y., & Steptoe, A. (2008). Positive psychological well-being and mortality: A quantitative review of prospective observational studies. *Psychosomatic Medicine, 70*(7), 741–756. https://doi.org/10.1097/PSY.0b013e31818105ba

Clark, L. A., Watson, D., & Leeka, J. (1989). Diurnal variation in the positive affects. *Motivation and Emotion, 13*(3), 205–234. https://doi.org/10.1007/BF00995536

Codispoti, M., Gerra, G., Montebarocci, O., Zaimovic, A., Augusta Raggi, M., & Baldaro, B. (2003). Emotional perception and neuroendocrine changes. *Psychophysiology, 40*(6), 863–868. https://doi.org/10.1111/1469-8986.00104

Cohen, S., Doyle, W. J., Turner, R. B., Alper, C. M., & Skoner, D. P. (2003). Emotional style and susceptibility to the common cold. *Psychosomatic Medicine, 65*(4), 652–657. https://doi.org/10.1097/01.PSY.0000077508.57784.DA

Cohen, S., Janicki-Deverts, D., & Miller, G. E. (2007). Psychological stress and disease. *JAMA, 298*(14), 1685. https://doi.org/10.1001/jama.298.14.1685

Cohen, S., & Wills, T. A. (1985). Stress, social support, and the buffering hypothesis. *Psychological Bulletin, 98*(2), 310–357. https://doi.org/10.1037/0033-2909.98.2.310

Cooper, T. M., McKinley, P. S., Seeman, T. E., Choo, T.-H., Lee, S., & Sloan, R. P. (2015). Heart rate variability predicts levels of inflammatory markers: Evidence for the vagal anti-inflammatory pathway. *Brain, Behavior, and Immunity, 49*, 94–100. https://doi.org/10.1016/j.bbi.2014.12.017

Delves, P. J. (2000). The immune system. *Advances in Immunology, 13*.

Dickerson, S. S., & Kemeny, M. E. (2004). Acute stressors and cortisol responses: A theoretical integration and synthesis of laboratory research. *Psychological Bulletin, 130*(3), 355–391. https://doi.org/10.1037/0033-2909.130.3.355

Diener, E., & Chan, M. Y. (2011). Happy people live longer: Subjective well-being contributes to health and longevity: Health benefits of happiness. *Applied Psychology: Health and Well-Being, 3*(1), 1–43. https://doi.org/10.1111/j.1758-0854.2010.01045.x

Diener, E., & Emmons, R. A. (1984). The independence of positive and negative affect. *Journal of Personality and Social Psychology, 47*(5), 1105–1117. https://doi.org/10.1037/0022-3514.47.5.1105

Drury, R. L., Porges, S., Thayer, J., & Ginsberg, J. P. (2019). Editorial: Heart rate variability, health and well-being: A systems perspective. *Frontiers in Public Health, 7*, 323. https://doi.org/10.3389/fpubh.2019.00323

Ehlers, A., Suendermann, O., Boellinghaus, I., Vossbeck-Elsebusch, A., Gamer, M., Briddon, E., Martin, M. W., & Glucksman, E. (2010). Heart rate responses to standardized trauma-related pictures in acute posttraumatic stress disorder. *International Journal of Psychophysiology, 78*(1), 27–34. https://doi.org/10.1016/j.ijpsycho.2010.04.009

Endrighi, R., Hamer, M., & Steptoe, A. (2011). Associations of trait optimism with diurnal neuroendocrine activity, cortisol responses to mental stress, and subjective stress measures in healthy men and women. *Psychosomatic Medicine, 73*(8), 672–678. https://doi.org/10.1097/PSY.0b013e31822f9cd7

Ettehad, D., Emdin, C. A., Kiran, A., Anderson, S. G., Callender, T., Emberson, J., Chalmers, J., Rodgers, A., & Rahimi, K. (2016). Blood pressure lowering for prevention of cardiovascular disease and death: A systematic review and meta-analysis. *The Lancet, 387*(10022), 957–967. https://doi.org/10.1016/S0140-6736(15)01225-8

Fava, G. A., McEwen, B. S., Guidi, J., Gostoli, S., Offidani, E., & Sonino, N. (2019). Clinical characterization of allostatic overload. *Psychoneuroendocrinology, 108*, 94–101. https://doi.org/10.1016/j.psyneuen.2019.05.028

Folds, J. D., & Schmitz, J. L. (2003). 24. Clinical and laboratory assessment of immunity. *Journal of Allergy and Clinical Immunology, 111*(2), S702–S711. https://doi.org/10.1067/mai.2003.122

Fredrickson, B. L. (2013). Positive emotions broaden and build. In *Advances in experimental social psychology* (Vol. 47, pp. 1–53). Elsevier. https://doi.org/10.1016/B978-0-12-407236-7.00001-2

Fredrickson, B. L., Cohn, M. A., Coffey, K. A., Pek, J., & Finkel, S. M. (2008). Open hearts build lives: Positive emotions, induced through loving-kindness meditation, build consequential personal resources. *Journal of personality and social psychology, 95*(5), 1045–1062. https://doi.org/10.1037/a0013262

Fredrickson, B. L., & Levenson, R. W. (1998). Positive emotions speed recovery from the cardiovascular sequelae of negative emotions. *Cognition and Emotion, 12*(2), 191–220. https://doi.org/10.1080/026999398379718

Fredrickson, B. L., Mancuso, R. A., Branigan, C., & Tugade, M. M. (2001). The undoing effect of positive emotions. *Motivation and Emotion, 22.*

Geisler, F. C. M., Vennewald, N., Kubiak, T., & Weber, H. (2010). The impact of heart rate variability on subjective well-being is mediated by emotion regulation. *Personality and Individual Differences, 49*(7), 723–728. https://doi.org/10.1016/j.paid.2010.06.015

Giuliani, N. R., McRae, K., & Gross, J. J. (2008). The up- and down-regulation of amusement: Experiential, behavioral, and autonomic consequences. *Emotion, 8*(5), 714–719. https://doi.org/10.1037/a0013236

Graham-Engeland, J. E., Sin, N. L., Smyth, J. M., Jones, D. R., Knight, E. L., Sliwinski, M. J., Almeida, D. M., Katz, M. J., Lipton, R. B., & Engeland, C. G. (2018). Negative and positive affect as predictors of inflammation: Timing matters. *Brain, Behavior, and Immunity, 74*, 222–230. https://doi.org/10.1016/j.bbi.2018.09.011

Hamer, M., & Chida, Y. (2011). Life satisfaction and inflammatory biomarkers: The 2008 Scottish Health Survey1: Life satisfaction and C-reactive protein. *Japanese Psychological Research, 53*(2), 133–139. https://doi.org/10.1111/j.1468-5884.2011.00460.x

Heathers, J. A., Brown, N. J., Coyne, J. C., & Friedman, H. L. (2015). The elusory upward spiral: A reanalysis of Kok et al. (2013). *Psychological Science, 26*(7), 1140–1143. https://doi.org/10.1177/0956797615572908

Het, S., & Wolf, O. T. (2007). Mood changes in response to psychosocial stress in healthy young women: Effects of pretreatment with cortisol. *Behavioral Neuroscience, 121*(1), 11–20. https://doi.org/10.1037/0735-7044.121.1.11

Hewson-Bower, B., & Drummond, P. D. (2001). Psychological treatment for recurrent symptoms of colds and flu in children. *Journal of Psychosomatic Research, 51*(1), 369–377. https://doi.org/10.1016/S0022-3999(01)00212-4

Hiller-Sturmhöfel, S. (1998). The Endocrine System. *Research World, 22*(3), 12.

Holzman, J. B., & Bridgett, D. J. (2017). Heart rate variability indices as bio-markers of top-down self-regulatory mechanisms: A meta-analytic review. *Neuroscience & Biobehavioral Reviews, 74*, 233–255. https://doi.org/10.1016/j.neubiorev.2016.12.032

Ifeagwazi, C. M., Egberi, H. E., & Chukwuorji, J. C. (2018). Emotional reactivity and blood pressure elevations: Anxiety as a mediator. *Psychology, Health & Medicine, 23*(5), 585–592. https://doi.org/10.1080/13548506.2017.1400670

Ironson, G., & Hayward, H. (2008). Do positive psychosocial factors predict disease progression in HIV-1? A review of the evidence. *Psychosomatic Medicine, 70*(5), 546–554. https://doi.org/10.1097/PSY.0b013e318177216c

Isgett, S. F., Kok, B. E., Baczkowski, B. M., Algoe, S. B., Grewen, K. M., & Fredrickson, B. L. (2017). Influences of oxytocin and respiratory sinus arrhythmia on emotions and social behavior in daily life. *Emotion, 17*(8), 1156–1165. https://doi.org/10.1037/emo0000301

Jacob, R. G., Thayer, J. F., Manuck, S. B., Muldoon, M. F., Tamres, L. K., Williams, D. M., Ding, Y., & Gatsonis, C. (1999). Ambulatory blood pressure responses and the circumplex model of mood: A 4-Day Study. *Psychosomatic Medicine, 15.*

James, G. D., Yee, L. S., Harshfield, G. A., Blank, S. G., & Pickering, T. G. (1986). The influence of happiness, anger, and anxiety on the blood pressure of borderline hypertensives. *Psychosomatic Medicine, 48*(7), 502–508. https://doi.org/10.1097/00006842-198609000-00005

James, W. (1884). II.—what is an emotion ? *Mind, os-IX*(34), 188–205. https://doi.org/10.1093/mind/os-IX.34.188

Jenkins, B. N., Granger, D. A., Roemer, R. J., Martinez, A., Torres, T. K., & Fortier, M. A. (2018). Emotion regulation and positive affect in the context of salivary alpha-amylase response to pain in children with cancer. *Pediatric Blood & Cancer, 65*(6), e26973. https://doi.org/10.1002/pbc.26973

Jensen, M. T., Suadicani, P., Hein, H. O., & Gyntelberg, F. (2013). Elevated resting heart rate, physical fitness and all-cause mortality: A 16-year follow-up in the Copenhagen Male Study. *Heart, 99*(12), 882–887. https://doi.org/10.1136/heartjnl-2012-303375

Jones, D. R., & Graham-Engeland, J. E. (2021). Positive affect and peripheral inflammatory markers among adults: A narrative review. *Psychoneuroendocrinology, 123*, 104892. https://doi.org/10.1016/j.psyneuen.2020.104892

Joseph, N. T., Jiang, Y., & Zilioli, S. (2021). Momentary emotions and salivary cortisol: A systematic review and meta-analysis of ecological momentary assessment studies. *Neuroscience & Biobehavioral Reviews, 125*, 365–379. https://doi.org/10.1016/j.neubiorev.2021.02.042

Kearney, P. M., Whelton, M., Reynolds, K., Muntner, P., Whelton, P. K., & He, J. (2005). Global burden of hypertension: Analysis of worldwide data. *Lancet, 365*, 7.

Kobau, R., Seligman, M. E. P., Peterson, C., Diener, E., Zack, M. M., Chapman, D., & Thompson, W. (2011). Mental health promotion in public health: Perspectives and strategies from positive psychology. *American Journal of Public Health, 101*(8), e1–e9. https://doi.org/10.2105/AJPH.2010.300083

Kobrosly, R. W., van Wijngaarden, E., Seplaki, C. L., Cory-Slechta, D. A., & Moynihan, J. (2014). Depressive symptoms are associated with allostatic load among community-dwelling older adults. *Physiology & Behavior, 123*, 223–230.

Kogan, A., Gruber, J., Shallcross, A. J., Ford, B. Q., & Mauss, I. B. (2013). Too much of a good thing? Cardiac vagal tone's nonlinear relationship with well-being. *Emotion, 13*(4), 599–604. https://doi.org/10.1037/a0032725

Kok, B. E., Coffey, K. A., Cohn, M. A., Catalino, L. I., Vacharkulksemsuk, T., Algoe, S. B., Brantley, M., & Fredrickson, B. L. (2013). How positive emotions build physical health: Perceived positive social connections account for the upward spiral between positive emotions and vagal tone. *Psychological Science, 24*(7), 1123–1132. https://doi.org/10.1177/0956797612470827

Kok, B. E., & Fredrickson, B. L. (2010). Upward spirals of the heart: Autonomic flexibility, as indexed by vagal tone, reciprocally and prospectively predicts positive emotions and social connectedness. *Biological Psychology, 85*(3), 432–436. https://doi.org/10.1016/j.biopsycho.2010.09.005

Kraft, T. L., & Pressman, S. D. (2012). Grin and bear it: The influence of manipulated facial expression on the stress response. *Psychological Science, 23*(11), 1372–1378. https://doi.org/10.1177/0956797612445312

Kubzansky, L. D., Huffman, J. C., Boehm, J. K., Hernandez, R., Kim, E. S., Koga, H. K., Feig, E. H., Lloyd-Jones, D. M., Seligman, M. E. P., & Labarthe, D. R. (2018). Positive psychological well-being and cardiovascular disease. *Journal of the American College of Cardiology, 72*(12), 1382–1396. https://doi.org/10.1016/j.jacc.2018.07.042

Kudielka, B. M., & Kirschbaum, C. (2003). Awakening cortisol responses are influenced by health status and awakening time but not by menstrual cycle phase. *Psychoneuroendocrinology, 28*(1), 35–47. https://doi.org/10.1016/S0306-4530(02)00008-2

Lai, J. C. L., Evans, P. D., Ng, S. H., Chong, A. M. L., Siu, O. T., Chan, C. L. W., Ho, S. M. Y., Ho, R. T. H., Chan, P., & Chan, C. C. (2005). Optimism, positive affectivity, and salivary cortisol. *British Journal of Health Psychology, 10*(4), 467–484. https://doi.org/10.1348/135910705X26083

Larsen, R. (2009). The contributions of positive and negative affect to emotional well-being. *Psihologijske teme, 18*(2), 247–266.

Lopez, R. B., Denny, B. T., & Fagundes, C. P. (2018). Neural mechanisms of emotion regulation and their role in endocrine and immune functioning: A review with implications for treatment of affective disorders. *Neuroscience & Biobehavioral Reviews, 95*, 508–514. https://doi.org/10.1016/j.neubiorev.2018.10.019

Malcolm Arnold, J., Fitchett, D. H., Howlett, J. G., Lonn, E. M., & Tardif, J.-C. (2008). Resting heart rate: A modifiable prognostic indicator of cardiovascular risk and outcomes? *Canadian Journal of Cardiology, 24*, 3A–15A. https://doi.org/10.1016/S0828-282X(08)71019-5

Marci, C. D., Glick, D. M., Loh, R., & Dougherty, D. D. (2007). Autonomic and prefrontal cortex responses to autobiographical recall of emotions. *Cognitive, Affective, & Behavioral Neuroscience, 7*(3), 243–250. https://doi.org/10.3758/CABN.7.3.243

Marsland, A. L., Cohen, S., Rabin, B. S., & Manuck, S. B. (2006). Trait positive affect and antibody response to hepatitis B vaccination. *Brain, Behavior, and Immunity, 20*(3), 261–269. https://doi.org/10.1016/j.bbi.2005.08.009

Mauss, I. B., Levenson, R. W., McCarter, L., Wilhelm, F. H., & Gross, J. J. (2005). The tie that binds? Coherence among emotion experience, behavior, and physiology. *Emotion, 5*(2), 175–190. https://doi.org/10.1037/1528-3542.5.2.175

McCorry, L. K. (2007). Physiology of the autonomic nervous system. *American Journal of Pharmaceutical Education, 11*.

McCraty, R., Barrios-Choplin, B., Rozman, D., Atkinson, M., & Watkins, A. D. (1998). The impact of a new emotional self-management program on stress, emotions, heart rate variability, DHEA and cortisol. *Integrative Physiological and Behavioral Science, 33*(2), 151–170. https://doi.org/10.1007/BF02688660

McEwen, B. (2000). Allostasis and allostatic load implications for Neuropsychopharmacology. *Neuropsychopharmacology, 22*(2), 108–124. https://doi.org/10.1016/S0893-133X(99)00129-3

McEwen, B. S. (2005). Stressed or stressed out: What is the difference? *Journal of Psychiatry and Neuroscience, 30*(5), 315.

McEwen, B. S. (2019). What is the confusion with cortisol? *Chronic Stress, 3*, 247054701983364. https://doi.org/10.1177/2470547019833647

McEwen, B. S., & Stellar, E. (1993). Stress and the individual: Mechanisms leading to disease. *Archives of Internal Medicine, 153*(18), 2093–2101.

Miller, K. G., Wright, A. G. C., Peterson, L. M., Kamarck, T. W., Anderson, B. A., Kirschbaum, C., Marsland, A. L., Muldoon, M. F., & Manuck, S. B. (2016). Trait positive and negative emotionality differentially associate with diurnal cortisol activity. *Psychoneuroendocrinology, 68*, 177–185. https://doi.org/10.1016/j.psyneuen.2016.03.004

Moreno, P. I., Moskowitz, A. L., Ganz, P. A., & Bower, J. E. (2016). Positive affect and inflammatory activity in breast cancer survivors: Examining the role of affective arousal. *Psychosomatic Medicine, 78*(5), 532–541. https://doi.org/10.1097/PSY.0000000000000300

Nater, U. M., Rohleder, N., Schlotz, W., Ehlert, U., & Kirschbaum, C. (2007). Determinants of the diurnal course of salivary alpha-amylase. *Psychoneuroendocrinology, 32*(4), 392–401. https://doi.org/10.1016/j.psyneuen.2007.02.007

O'Connor, D. B., Thayer, J. F., & Vedhara, K. (2021). Stress and health: A review of psychobiological processes. *Annual Review of Psychology, 72*(1), 663–688. https://doi.org/10.1146/annurev-psych-062520-122331

Okely, J. A., Weiss, A., & Gale, C. R. (2017). Well-being and arthritis incidence: The role of inflammatory mechanisms. Findings from the English longitudinal study of ageing. *Psychosomatic Medicine, 79*(7), 742–748. https://doi.org/10.1097/PSY.0000000000000480

Ong, A. D., & Allaire, J. C. (2005). Cardiovascular intraindividual variability in later life: The influence of social connectedness and positive emotions. *Psychology and aging, 20*(3), 476. https://doi.org/10.1037/0882-7974.20.3.476

Oveis, C., Cohen, A. B., Gruber, J., Shiota, M. N., Haidt, J., & Keltner, D. (2009). Resting respiratory sinus arrhythmia is associated with tonic positive emotionality. *Emotion, 9*(2), 265–270. https://doi.org/10.1037/a0015383

Pace-Schott, E. F., Amole, M. C., Aue, T., Balconi, M., Bylsma, L. M., Critchley, H., Demaree, H. A., Friedman, B. H., Gooding, A. E. K., Gosseries, O., Jovanovic, T., Kirby, L. A. J., Kozlowska, K., Laureys, S., Lowe, L., Magee, K., Marin, M.-F., Merner, A. R., Robinson, J. L., et al. (2019). Physiological feelings. *Neuroscience & Biobehavioral Reviews, 103*, 267–304. https://doi.org/10.1016/j.neubiorev.2019.05.002

Pasquali, V., Ghiciuc, C. M., Castellani, V., Caprara, G. V., Alessandri, G., D'Amelio, R., Ziparo, V., Scarinci, F., & Patacchioli, F. R. (2020). Salivary cortisol and α-amylase production at awakening is associated with positivity (POS) levels in healthy young subjects. *Journal of Happiness Studies*. https://doi.org/10.1007/s10902-020-00314-9

Peçanha, T., Silva-Júnior, N. D., & Forjaz, C. L. de M. (2014). Heart rate recovery: Autonomic determinants, methods of assessment and association with mortality and cardiovascular diseases. *Clinical Physiology and Functional Imaging, 34*(5), 327–339. https://doi.org/10.1111/cpf.12102

Polk, D. E., Cohen, S., Doyle, W. J., Skoner, D. P., & Kirschbaum, C. (2005). State and trait affect as predictors of salivary cortisol in healthy adults. *Psychoneuroendocrinology, 30*(3), 261–272. https://doi.org/10.1016/j.psyneuen.2004.08.004

Porges, S. W. (1995). Orienting in a defensive world: Mammalian modifications of our evolutionary heritage. A polyvagal theory. *Psychophysiology, 32*(4), 301–318. https://doi.org/10.1111/j.1469-8986.1995.tb01213.x

Porges, S. W. (2007). The polyvagal perspective. *Biological Psychology, 74*(2), 116–143. https://doi.org/10.1016/j.biopsycho.2006.06.009

Porges, S. W. (2009). The polyvagal theory: New insights into adaptive reactions of the autonomic nervous system. *Cleveland Clinic Journal of Medicine, 76*(4 suppl 2), S86–S90. https://doi.org/10.3949/ccjm.76.s2.17

Pressman, S. D., & Black, L. L. (2012). *Positive emotions and immunity*. Oxford University Press. https://doi.org/10.1093/oxfordhb/9780195394399.013.0006

Pressman, S. D., & Cohen, S. (2005). Does positive affect influence health? *Psychological Bulletin, 131*(6), 925–971. https://doi.org/10.1037/0033-2909.131.6.925

Pressman, S. D., Jenkins, B. N., & Moskowitz, J. T. (2019). Positive affect and health: What do we know and where next should we go? *Annual Review of Psychology, 70*(1), 627–650. https://doi.org/10.1146/annurev-psych-010418-102955

Pruessner, J. C., Kirschbaum, C., Meinlschmid, G., & Hellhammer, D. H. (2003). Two formulas for computation of the area under the curve represent measures of total hormone concentration versus time-dependent change. *Psychoneuroendocrinology, 28*(7), 916–931. https://doi.org/10.1016/S0306-4530(02)00108-7

Puig-Perez, S., Villada, C., Pulopulos, M. M., Almela, M., Hidalgo, V., & Salvador, A. (2015). Optimism and pessimism are related to different components of the stress response in healthy older people. *International Journal of Psychophysiology, 98*(2), 213–221. https://doi.org/10.1016/j.ijpsycho.2015.09.002

Ridker, P. M. (2005). C-reactive protein, inflammation, and cardiovascular disease. *The Texas Heart Institute Journal, 32*(3), 384–386.

Robles, T. F., Brooks, K. P., & Pressman, S. D. (2009). Trait positive affect buffers the effects of acute stress on skin barrier recovery. *Health Psychology, 28*(3), 373–378. https://doi.org/10.1037/a0014662

Rosenkranz, M. A., Jackson, D. C., Dalton, K. M., Dolski, I., Ryff, C. D., Singer, B. H., Muller, D., Kalin, N. H., & Davidson, R. J. (2003). Affective style and in vivo immune response: Neurobehavioral mechanisms. *Proceedings of the National Academy of Sciences, 100*(19), 11148–11152. https://doi.org/10.1073/pnas.1534743100

Rotenberg, S., & McGrath, J. J. (2016). Inter-relation between autonomic and HPA axis activity in children and adolescents. *Biological Psychology, 117*, 16–25. https://doi.org/10.1016/j.biopsycho.2016.01.015

Russell, J. A. (1980). A circumplex model of affect. *Journal of Personality and Social Psychology, 39*(6), 1161–1178. https://doi.org/10.1037/h0077714

Ryff, C. D., Dienberg Love, G., Urry, H. L., Muller, D., Rosenkranz, M. A., Friedman, E. M., Davidson, R. J., & Singer, B. (2006). Psychological well-being and ill-being: Do they have distinct or mirrored biological correlates? *Psychotherapy and Psychosomatics, 75*(2), 85–95. https://doi.org/10.1159/000090892

Ryff, C. D., Singer, B. H., & Dienberg Love, G. (2004). Positive health: Connecting well–being with biology. *Philosophical Transactions of the Royal Society of London. Series B: Biological Sciences, 359*(1449), 1383–1394. https://doi.org/10.1098/rstb.2004.1521

Salzmann, S., Euteneuer, F., Strahler, J., Laferton, J. A. C., Nater, U. M., & Rief, W. (2018). Optimizing expectations and distraction leads to lower cortisol levels after acute stress. *Psychoneuroendocrinology, 88*, 144–152. https://doi.org/10.1016/j.psyneuen.2017.12.011

Schenk, H. M., Jeronimus, B. F., van der Krieke, L., Bos, E. H., de Jonge, P., & Rosmalen, J. G. (2018). Associations of positive affect and negative affect with allostatic load: A lifelines cohort study. *Psychosomatic Medicine, 80*(2), 160–166.

Schwerdtfeger, A. R., & Gerteis, A. K. S. (2014). The manifold effects of positive affect on heart rate variability in everyday life: Distinguishing within-person and between-person associations. *Health Psychology, 33*(9), 1065–1073. https://doi.org/10.1037/hea0000079

Segerstrom, S. C., & Miller, G. E. (2004). Psychological stress and the human immune system: A meta-analytic study of 30 years of inquiry. *Psychological Bulletin, 130*(4), 601–630. https://doi.org/10.1037/0033-2909.130.4.601

Sephton, S. E., & Kraemer, H. C. (2000). Diurnal cortisol rhythm as a predictor of breast cancer survival. *Journal of the National Cancer Institute, 92*(12), 7.

Shaffer, F., & Ginsberg, J. P. (2017). An overview of heart rate variability metrics and norms. *Frontiers in Public Health, 5*, 258. https://doi.org/10.3389/fpubh.2017.00258

Shiota, M. N., Neufeld, S. L., Yeung, W. H., Moser, S. E., & Perea, E. F. (2011). Feeling good: Autonomic nervous system responding in five positive emotions. *Emotion, 11*(6), 1368–1378. https://doi.org/10.1037/a0024278

Sin, N. L., & Lyubomirsky, S. (2009). Enhancing well-being and alleviating depressive symptoms with positive psychology interventions: A practice-friendly meta-analysis. *Journal of Clinical Psychology, 65*(5), 467–487. https://doi.org/10.1002/jclp.20593

Sin, N. L., Ong, A. D., Stawski, R. S., & Almeida, D. M. (2017). Daily positive events and diurnal cortisol rhythms: Examination of between-person differences and within-person variation. *Psychoneuroendocrinology, 83*, 91–100. https://doi.org/10.1016/j.psyneuen.2017.06.001

Sinha, R. (1996). Multivariate response patterning of fear and anger. *Cognition & Emotion, 10*(2), 173–198. https://doi.org/10.1080/026999396380321

Sinha, R., Lovallo, W. R., & Parsons, O. A. (1992). Cardiovascular differentiation of emotions. *Psychosomatic Medicine, 54*(4), 422–435. https://doi.org/10.1097/00006842-199207000-00005

Smith, C. U. M. (2013). Cardiocentric neurophysiology: The persistence of a delusion. *Journal of the History of the Neurosciences, 22*(1), 6–13. https://doi.org/10.1080/0964704X.2011.650899

Smyth, J., Ockenfels, M. C., Porter, L., Kirschbaum, C., Hellhammer, D. H., & Stone, A. A. (1998). Stressors and mood measured on a momentary basis are associated with salivary cortisol secretion. *Psychoneuroendocrinology, 23*(4), 353–370. https://doi.org/10.1016/S0306-4530(98)00008-0

Stalder, T., Kirschbaum, C., Kudielka, B. M., Adam, E. K., Pruessner, J. C., Wüst, S., Dockray, S., Smyth, N., Evans, P., Hellhammer, D. H., Miller, R., Wetherell, M. A., Lupien, S. J., & Clow, A. (2016). Assessment of the cortisol awakening response: Expert consensus guidelines. *Psychoneuroendocrinology, 63*, 414–432. https://doi.org/10.1016/j.psyneuen.2015.10.010

Stellar, J. E., John-Henderson, N., Anderson, C. L., Gordon, A. M., McNeil, G. D., & Keltner, D. (2015). Positive affect and markers of inflammation: Discrete positive emotions predict lower levels of inflammatory cytokines. *Emotion, 15*(2), 129–133. https://doi.org/10.1037/emo0000033

Steptoe, A. (2019). Happiness and health. *Annual Review of Public Health, 40*(1), 339–359. https://doi.org/10.1146/annurev-publhealth-040218-044150

Steptoe, A., Leigh Gibson, E., Hamer, M., & Wardle, J. (2007). Neuroendocrine and cardiovascular correlates of positive affect measured by ecological momentary assessment and by questionnaire. *Psychoneuroendocrinology, 32*(1), 56–64. https://doi.org/10.1016/j.psyneuen.2006.10.001

Steptoe, A., O'Donnell, K., Badrick, E., Kumari, M., & Marmot, M. (2008). Neuroendocrine and inflammatory factors associated with positive affect in healthy men and women: The Whitehall II study American. *Journal of Epidemiology, 167*(1), 96–102. https://doi.org/10.1093/aje/kwm252

Steptoe, A., & Wardle, J. (2005). Positive affect and biological function in everyday life. *Neurobiology of Aging, 26*(1), 108–112. https://doi.org/10.1016/j.neurobiolaging.2005.08.016

Szcepanski, R., Napolitano, M., Feaganes, J. R., Barefoot, J. C., Luecken, L., Swoap, R., Kuhn, C., Suarez, E., Siegler, I. C., Williams, R. B., & Blumenthal, J. A. (1997). Relation of mood ratings and neurohormonal responses during daily life in employed women. *International Journal of Behavioral Medicine, 4*(1), 1–16. https://doi.org/10.1207/s15327558ijbm0401_1

Taylor, C. B. (2010). Depression, heart rate related variables and cardiovascular disease. *International Journal of Psychophysiology, 78*(1), 80–88. https://doi.org/10.1016/j.ijpsycho.2010.04.006

Thayer, J. F., Åhs, F., Fredrikson, M., Sollers, J. J., & Wager, T. D. (2012). A meta-analysis of heart rate variability and neuroimaging studies: Implications for heart rate variability as a marker of stress and health. *Neuroscience & Biobehavioral Reviews, 36*(2), 747–756. https://doi.org/10.1016/j.neubiorev.2011.11.009

Thayer, J. F., & Lane, R. D. (2000). A model of neurovisceral integration in emotion regulation and dysregulation. *Journal of Affective Disorders, 61*(3), 201–216. https://doi.org/10.1016/S0165-0327(00)00338-4

Thayer, J. F., & Lane, R. D. (2007). The role of vagal function in the risk for cardiovascular disease and mortality. *Biological Psychology, 74*(2), 224–242. https://doi.org/10.1016/j.biopsycho.2005.11.013

Thayer, J. F., & Sternberg, E. (2006). Beyond heart rate variability: Vagal regulation of allostatic systems. *Annals of the New York Academy of Sciences, 1088*(1), 361–372. https://doi.org/10.1196/annals.1366.014

Turner, A. I., Smyth, N., Hall, S. J., Torres, S. J., Hussein, M., Jayasinghe, S. U., Ball, K., & Clow, A. J. (2020). Psychological stress reactivity and future health and disease outcomes: A systematic review of prospective evidence. *Psychoneuroendocrinology, 114*, 104599. https://doi.org/10.1016/j.psyneuen.2020.104599

Turpeinen, U., & Hämäläinen, E. (2013). Determination of cortisol in serum, saliva and urine. *Best Practice & Research Clinical Endocrinology & Metabolism, 27*(6), 795–801. https://doi.org/10.1016/j.beem.2013.10.008

Valentini, M., & Parati, G. (2009). Variables influencing heart rate. *Progress in Cardiovascular Diseases, 52*(1), 11–19. https://doi.org/10.1016/j.pcad.2009.05.004

Van Cappellen, P., Rice, E. L., Catalino, L. I., & Fredrickson, B. L. (2018). Positive affective processes underlie positive health behaviour change. *Psychology & Health, 33*(1), 77–97. https://doi.org/10.1080/08870446.2017.1320798

Van Eck, M., Berkhof, H., Nicolson, N., & Sulon, J. (1996). The effects of perceived stress, traits, mood states, and stressful daily events on salivary cortisol. *Psychosomatic Medicine, 58*(5), 447–458. https://doi.org/10.1097/00006842-199609000-00007

Watson, D., Anna, L., & Tellegen, A. (1988). Development and validation of brief measures of positive and negative affect: The PANAS scales. *Journal of Personality and Social Psychology, 54*, 1063–1070.

Weckesser, L. J., Plessow, F., Pilhatsch, M., Muehlhan, M., Kirschbaum, C., & Miller, R. (2014). Do venepuncture procedures induce cortisol responses? A review, study, and synthesis for stress research. *Psychoneuroendocrinology, 46*, 88–99. https://doi.org/10.1016/j.psyneuen.2014.04.012

Williams, D. P., Cash, C., Rankin, C., Bernardi, A., Koenig, J., & Thayer, J. F. (2015). Resting heart rate variability predicts self-reported difficulties in emotion regulation: A focus on different facets of emotion regulation. *Frontiers in Psychology, 6*. https://doi.org/10.3389/fpsyg.2015.00261

4

Gratitude and Physical Health

Nathan T. Deichert and Erin M. Fekete

Since Seligman and Csikszentmihalyi's (2000) seminal article introducing positive psychology, a burgeoning literature has developed within the field, including extensive research on the concept of gratitude. Although research examining gratitude's impact on health has mainly focused on the relationship between gratitude and psychological functioning, research has started exploring how gratitude relates to physical well-being. While less extensive, evidence suggests gratitude has positive effects on physical health and the underlying physiological mechanisms associated with health, although results are mixed (Boggiss et al., 2020; Jans-Beken et al., 2019). In this chapter, we review research examining the link between gratitude and physical health. We first discuss how gratitude is conceptualized, the different methods of assessing gratitude, and several theories explaining the functions of gratitude. Next, we summarize research investigating the link between gratitude and physical health, focusing on the cardiovascular, immune, and neuroendocrine systems. We conclude with a discussion of the psychosocial mechanisms through which gratitude may influence physical health, specifically highlighting gratitude's effects on stress, social support, and coping behaviors.

N. T. Deichert (✉)
Department of Psychology, Black Hills State University, Spearfish, SD, USA
e-mail: Nathan.Deichert@bhsu.edu

E. M. Fekete
College of Applied Behavioral Sciences, University of Indianapolis,
Indianapolis, IN, USA

F. M. Sirois (ed.), *The Palgrave Handbook of Positive Psychology and Health*,
https://doi.org/10.1007/978-3-031-89095-6_4

Conceptualizing Gratitude

Gratitude is commonly conceptualized as a positive reaction to a gift or benefit provided by an intentional agent (e.g., Fredrickson, 2004). Others view gratitude more broadly as a "generalized tendency to recognize and respond with grateful emotion" (McCullough et al., 2002, p. 112) as well as being a "part of a wider life orientation towards noticing and appreciating the positive in the world" (Wood et al., 2010, p. 891). Such conceptualizations are important as they highlight factors to consider when examining the relationship between gratitude and physical health. First, gratitude is primarily viewed as a positive affective experience. Second, gratitude has been conceptualized as both a cognitive and emotional reaction as well as a "general tendency" to experience gratitude. Thus, gratitude can be examined as a trait (i.e., disposition) and as a state (i.e., emotion). Finally, gratitude has been conceptualized as a more general sense of appreciation, thus broadening its definition beyond transactional experiences between a beneficiary and benefactor. Even though research has explored whether gratitude and appreciation are unique constructs (Fagley, 2016; Wood et al., 2008b) and has also started examining whether gratitude is an exclusively positive experience (e.g., Wood et al., 2016), we focus the remainder of this section on the distinction between trait and state experience of gratitude as this is the most common issue regarding the conceptualization of gratitude in the current research on gratitude and health.

The Trait and State Experience of Gratitude

Gratitude, like other emotions, can be studied on multiple interrelated levels of affective experience: traits, moods, and emotions (Rosenberg, 1998). According to Rosenberg, traits are relatively stable attributes hypothesized to impact emotional experiences and cognitive processes. Conversely, emotions are consciously experienced affective states consisting of brief but more intense psychophysiological changes often with an identifiable cause. The third level of affective experience, moods, are longer lasting but less intense than emotions and more transient than traits, and therefore, more likely to be consciously experienced.

Research supports the experience of gratitude at these various affective levels (McCullough et al., 2004; Watkins, 2014b). This is most clearly demonstrated in a series of daily diary studies by McCullough et al. (2004) using samples of patients with neuromuscular diseases and healthy undergraduate students. Both studies found trait gratitude predicted grateful mood over time, with individuals higher in trait gratitude reporting increased grateful mood even after controlling for personality factors and positive and negative affect. In addition to studying the impact of traits on mood, McCullough et al. (2004, Study 2) also examined the relationship between grateful emotion and mood. Results indicated that greater emotional intensity caused by gratitude eliciting events predicted higher levels of grateful moods. Interestingly, this was true only for people *low* in trait gratitude, which suggests individuals higher in trait gratitude may not be as impacted by daily events because their grateful moods are likely elevated due to higher trait gratitude. More recent research continues to support a link between trait and state affective experiences by showing that trait gratitude is positively correlated with grateful mood (Solom et al., 2017) and grateful emotional states[1] (Deichert et al., 2021).

The distinction between trait and state gratitude is important in relation to physical health as they may differentially predict outcomes. For example, an eight-week longitudinal study found no direct association between trait gratitude and health-related quality of life (HRQoL), which included aspects of physical functioning (McGuire et al., 2020). Instead, results revealed that trait gratitude predicted elevated weekly state gratitude, which was associated with better HRQoL. Similarly, greater state, but not trait, gratitude was linked to lower systolic blood pressure increases in response to a laboratory stressor (Gallagher et al., 2020). Taken together, research in this area suggests it may be beneficial for future research to examine state and trait gratitude independently, given their differential associations with health outcomes.

Measuring Gratitude

Due to the multifaceted nature of gratitude, different methods have been used for its assessment, including free response, attribution measures, and self-report measures (Emmons et al., 2019). Free response methods allow participants to report their thoughts about gratitude free from the influence of researcher expectations (e.g., Lambert et al., 2009a; Morgan et al., 2014), whereas attribution measures have participants read vignettes about hypothetical situations in which a beneficiary is provided a benefit and rate the extent to which gratitude would likely be experienced (e.g., Tsang, 2006;

[1] The correlation between trait gratitude and current grateful emotion assessed at baseline prior to the gratitude writing task was $r = 0.476$, $p < 0.001$.

Wood et al., 2008c). Although the use of free-response and vignette paradigms provide important insights into the experience of gratitude, the most commonly used method of assessing gratitude in the context of health research is self-report measures, with the most frequently used measures being the Gratitude Questionnaire (GQ-6: McCullough et al., 2002), the Gratitude Adjective Checklist (GAC: McCullough et al., 2002), the Gratitude, Resentment, and Appreciation Test (GRAT: Watkins et al., 2003), and the revised GRAT Short-Form (GRAT-SF: Thomas & Watkins, 2003). The GQ-6 is a six-item survey developed to measure an individual's disposition toward experiencing feelings of gratitude and is the most widely used self-report measure of trait gratitude. Questions were designed to assess different aspects of gratitude, including its intensity (i.e., how strongly gratitude is felt), frequency (i.e., how often gratitude is felt), span (i.e., breadth of situations that elicit gratitude), and density (i.e., size of the social network to which one feels grateful). The Gratitude Adjective Checklist (GAC), which was developed in the same study as the GQ-6, is a 3-item questionnaire composed of three adjectives, *grateful*, *thankful*, and *appreciative,* with overall scores calculated by summing the extent to which participants reported experiencing each feeling. The GAC is flexible as it can be used to assess gratitude as a trait (McCullough et al., 2002), a mood (i.e., "over the past few weeks," Froh et al., 2011), or an emotion (Deichert et al., 2021). The GRAT and the GRAT-SF, which consist of 44 and 16 items, respectively, differ from the GG-6 and the GAC in that they conceptualize gratitude as a trait consisting of three underlying factors: sense of abundance, appreciation of others, and simple appreciation.

Psychometric Properties of Self-Report Gratitude Measures

Research examining the psychometric properties of these self-report measures support the proposed factor structures and found these measures had adequate reliability for individuals over the age of 14 (Card, 2019; Emmons et al., 2019; Froh et al., 2011; McCullough et al., 2002; Watkins et al., 2003). In addition to being reliable measures of gratitude, these self-report measures show strong construct validity. Specifically, scores on these measures were found to correlate positively with life satisfaction, hope, and happiness, and negatively correlate with materialism, depressive symptoms, and narcissism (Diessner & Lewis, 2007; McCullough et al., 2002; Watkins et al., 2003). Translations of the GQ-6, the GRAT, and the GRAT-SF into German, Chinese, Dutch, Portuguese, and Spanish have also been shown to be reliable and valid measures of gratitude (Chen et al., 2009; Gouveia et al., 2019; Hudecek et al., 2020; Jans-Beken et al., 2015; Langer et al., 2016; Lin & Huang, 2016).

Gratitude Interventions

In addition to assessing gratitude through the methods previously described, researchers testing the health benefits of gratitude have also induced gratitude through intrapersonal and interpersonal interventions. *Intrapersonal* interventions refer to inducing feelings of gratitude by having individuals focus their thoughts on situations or individuals for whom they are grateful. Examples of such interventions include briefly writing about situations for which one is grateful (i.e., journaling) or generating lists of events that elicited feelings of gratitude. *Interpersonal* interventions promote gratitude through interpersonal interactions. Gratitude visits are an example of this type of intervention, where a person visits someone and expresses their gratitude by reading a detailed letter about a situation for which they are grateful. Gratitude interventions may also include a psychoeducational component during which individuals meet regularly to cover factors associated with gratitude (e.g., Bai et al., 2019; Froh et al., 2014).

There is research to suggest gratitude interventions improve psychological well-being. Several meta-analyses have shown gratitude is linked to increased psychological well-being, happiness, life satisfaction, positive affect, and decreased symptoms of depression and anxiety, although such effects tend to be small (Cregg & Cheavens, 2020; Davis et al., 2016; Dickens, 2017). Moreover, in addition to the psychological benefits, evidence suggests these interventions promote the experience of gratitude (Davis et al., 2016; Dickens, 2017). Importantly, the impact of gratitude interventions appear to depend on the activities engaged in by the control groups, specifically, the positive effects of gratitude interventions tended to be larger when compared to control conditions that were not psychologically active (i.e., waitlist controls: Cregg & Cheavens, 2020) or to negative interventions (i.e., listing daily hassles: Dickens, 2017). However, the effects of gratitude interventions were equivalent to other psychologically active conditions that promoted positive well-being, suggesting that while gratitude interventions may positively impact psychological functioning compared to not engaging in such activities, these effects do not exceed those observed in other positive psychological interventions.

Moderators. Although evidence suggests gratitude interventions can produce positive outcomes, it is possible that the effects of these interventions could be positively or negatively impacted by the presence of moderators. According to the positive-activity model (Lyubomirsky & Layous, 2013), engaging in positive activities (e.g., gratitude journals) increases positive emotions, thoughts, and behaviors, resulting in increased well-being. These associations, however, are influenced by features of both the activity and the person. Regarding personal factors, older individuals have been shown to benefit more from gratitude interventions than younger individuals (Dickens, 2017). Personality traits may also be important to consider in this context. For example, curiosity was associated with increased engagement in a gratitude intervention (Kaczmarek et al., 2014b), while dispositional gratitude has been shown to moderate the psychological effects of gratitude eliciting events and interventions (McCullough et al., 2004; Rash et al., 2011). Dispositional gratitude was also found to indirectly influence an individual's intentions to participate in a gratitude intervention through attitudes and beliefs about the activity and one's self (Kaczmarek et al., 2015). Finally, given the social nature of gratitude, it is important to consider how cultural norms may impact its experience. For example, individuals from collectivistic cultures may not respond as positively to gratitude interventions relative to individuals from more individualistic cultures (Boehm et al., 2011; Shin et al., 2020).

Although gratitude interventions are typically thought to promote positive psychological states such as feelings of gratitude and positive physical health outcomes, some factors may inhibit the utility of such interventions. For example, Watkins (2014a) speculated that factors such as suspiciousness of a benefactor's motives, feelings of indebtedness that arise after receiving benefits, envy, materialism, and narcissism might prevent individuals from experiencing gratitude. In fact, research examining the relationship between gratitude and these inhibiting factors do indeed suggest a negative correlation (Diessner & Lewis, 2007; Solom et al., 2017; Tsang, 2006; Watkins, 2014a). Another factor that may moderate the effectiveness of interventions to enhance feelings of gratitude is ambivalence over emotional expression. Research has found that the relationship between gratitude and positive psychological outcomes such as quality of life and happiness were moderated by individuals' ambivalence over emotional expression (Chen et al., 2012, 2015). Specifically, the association between gratitude and psychological outcomes was weaker for individuals reporting greater levels of emotional ambivalence.[2]

[2] Interestingly, in Chen et al. (2012, Study 2) the opposite finding emerged for negative outcomes such as depression and loneliness, in which case higher emotional ambivalence *strengthened* the association

In addition to psychological outcomes, research has shown that gratitude was associated with increased perceptions of social support over three months in a sample of women living with metastatic breast cancer, but only for women low in emotional ambivalence (Algoe & Stanton, 2012). Taken together, research indicates that while gratitude interventions are capable of producing positive outcomes, it is important to consider moderators that may enhance or diminish the impact of these efforts.

In addition to personal factors, aspects of the activity are also important to consider. For example, providing information to participants about expected challenges to completing a gratitude intervention and ways to address these challenges actually *decreased* individuals' initial engagement in an intervention (Kaczmarek et al., 2014a). In another study, individuals were more likely to engage in a gratitude intervention when assigned to a journal condition instead of a condition where they were asked to write a letter (Kaczmarek et al., 2015). Taken together, these studies show that the effectiveness of gratitude interventions depends on aspects of the person, the activity, and the fit between the two as posited by the positive-activity model and suggest that interventions would be more effective when carefully considering these different factors.

Gratitude Theories

Evolutionary Function of Gratitude. Expressions of gratitude occur across cultures and languages (McCullough et al., 2008). Gratitude has several moral functions. First, gratitude functions as a moral barometer, by alerting individuals (i.e., a beneficiary) to situations where they have benefited from altruistic or prosocial acts of others (i.e., a benefactor). Gratitude may also motivate beneficiaries to continue engaging in prosocial behaviors and reinforce the importance of engaging in prosocial behaviors (McCullough et al., 2001).

From an evolutionary perspective, these moral functions are essential because they promote prosocial behaviors beyond kin relationships. For example, gratitude motivates beneficiaries to acknowledge and appreciate acts of altruism from benefactors, and in turn, engage in altruistic acts toward their benefactors (McCullough et al., 2001; Trivers, 1971; Tsang, 2007). Thus, this 'reciprocal altruism' encourages us to develop relationships with individuals unrelated to us (Bar-Tal et al., 1977). Evolutionary theorists also posit that gratitude encourages beneficiaries to engage in upstream reciprocity

---

between gratitude and the respective outcomes.

or engage in altruistic acts towards individuals other than one's benefactor, enhancing the fitness of the population (Nowak & Roch, 2007).

Broaden and Build Theory. Current theoretical approaches to gratitude focus on the function of gratitude as an emotion. Traditional theories of emotion suggest that two primary functions of emotions are to draw attention to a unique situation and coordinate a response to that situation. These responses were assumed to narrow an individual's focus to a specific set of behavioral options for dealing with the emotion. However, the broaden-and-build theory of emotion suggests that while specific action tendencies are relevant for negative emotions, they are not related to the experience of positive emotions. Instead, our cognitive and behavioral responses are broadened when experiencing positive emotions. As these positive emotions allow us to be more creative and curious, we ultimately explore and experience new things and build long-lasting social resources (Fredrickson, 1998). Furthermore, the broaden-and-build theory proposes that positive emotions can "undo" the physiological effects of negative emotions, suggesting one way positive emotions promote physical health.

Although the original broaden-and-build theory did not explicitly highlight gratitude, more recent research has suggested gratitude encourages individuals to broaden their thinking and build social resources (Fredrickson, 2004). Indeed, over time, gratitude was related to increased perceptions of social support and more adaptive coping styles (Lin, 2015; Wood et al., 2008a). Taken together, these findings suggest that gratitude allows individuals to seek out and build psychosocial resources, and these resources may have important benefits for physical well-being.

Find-Remind-and-Bind Theory. More recently, the find-remind-and-bind theory was proposed, which complements the broaden-and-build theory by incorporating theories of relationship science, and acknowledging that gratitude is a social emotion that is both experienced and expressed (Algoe, 2012). This theory suggests gratitude draws our attention to high-quality relationships and signals these relationships are worth investing in and improving. More specifically, when gratitude is experienced due to receiving some gift from a benefactor, beneficiaries experience a shift in their cognition about the world and their benefactor. The beneficiary is motivated to not only express gratitude towards their benefactor but also to engage in behavior to build and strengthen their relationship with the benefactor. These expressions of gratitude provide the benefactor with information that the recipient is responsive and cares for them (Algoe, 2012).

For example, Algoe et al. (2008) found that newly initiated sorority sisters (i.e., beneficiaries) reported experiencing gratitude after receiving gifts from an unknown big sister (i.e., benefactor). These feelings of gratitude predicted the quality of their relationship with their benefactors one month later. Moreover, the perceived responsiveness of the gift, or the extent to which the beneficiary felt valued, understood, or cared for, was a stronger predictor of gratitude than other factors such as the cost or effort that went into purchasing the gift (Algoe et al., 2008). Gratitude has also been associated with increased perceived social support, but only in women who were not ambivalent about expressing their emotions (Algoe & Stanton, 2012). These theories suggest that an important function of gratitude is to develop and strengthen social bonds. These feelings of social connectedness may be a key mechanism in explaining how gratitude is associated with better health.

Links Between Gratitude and Physical Health

Although a large body of research acknowledges the benefits of gratitude on psychological well-being, less research has focused on the links between gratitude and physical health. One review of the literature found that although both trait gratitude and gratitude interventions appeared to positively impact cardiovascular outcomes, inflammatory biomarkers, and sleep, there was less evidence suggesting gratitude predicted health outcomes or decreased pain perceptions (Jans-Beken et al., 2019). Another recent systematic review found promising results for the effects of gratitude interventions on improved sleep quality but mixed results for other health outcomes and behaviors (Boggiss et al., 2020). For example, although gratitude interventions produced significant improvements in cardiovascular (e.g., blood pressure) and endocrine (e.g., glycemic control) health outcomes, mixed results were found for inflammatory markers as well as self-reported health and health behaviors. Over one-third of the gratitude interventions produced improvements in physical symptoms, illness-related symptoms, and workplace absence. Fewer studies found improvements in health behaviors (Boggiss et al., 2020).

Cardiovascular Health. Dispositional gratitude has been associated with better health and healthier behaviors in patients with existing cardiovascular disease (Cousin et al., 2021). In patients diagnosed with acute coronary syndrome (ACS), dispositional gratitude was associated with lower levels of TNF-α (Huffman et al., 2016). Other research found that gratitude was associated with reduced inflammatory biomarkers and lower levels of endothelial dysfunction, both of which are known to cause adverse cardiovascular events (Celano et al., 2017; Mills et al., 2015). Gratitude was also related to better adherence to health behavior recommendations (e.g., steps per day, dietary, exercise, stress reduction) at six months post-ACS diagnosis (Millstein et al., 2016).

Gratitude interventions have also been effective in producing cardiovascular health benefits. A pilot study found that patients with asymptomatic heart failure who participated in a gratitude journaling intervention in addition to their standard treatment had increased parasympathetic heart rate variability responses and reduced inflammatory biomarkers compared to participants who only received their standard treatment (Redwine et al., 2016). Other studies have found that gratitude is linked to lower blood pressure and attenuated reactivity to stress (Gallagher et al., 2020; Jackowska et al., 2016).

Immune and Endocrine Function. Although research generally shows positive emotions are associated with enhanced immune function (Marsland et al., 2007), less is known about how gratitude impacts the immune system. One study examined gratitude as a moderator of the links between low SES (e.g., income, education) on IL-6 and found that higher levels of gratitude mitigated the negative impact of low SES on IL-6 (Hartanto et al., 2019). Another study examining spiritual gratitude, or feelings of gratitude toward a higher power, was associated with longer survival times in people living with HIV, even after controlling for health behaviors and social support (Ironson et al., 2016). Other studies have found that gratitude is linked to better health behaviors, well-being, and quality of life outcomes in patients with cancer, multiple sclerosis, and HIV (Crouch et al., 2020; Ma et al., 2013; Ruini & Vescovelli, 2013; Sztachańska et al., 2019)

A paucity of research has examined links between gratitude and endocrine function. The research that does exist has focused on disease markers (i.e., HbA1c) of metabolic disorders such as diabetes. For example, higher levels of gratitude were associated with lower HbA1c and lower risk of having an HbA1c level in the diabetic range in a nationally representative sample of adults (Krause et al., 2017). However, participants who took part in a gratitude intervention showed no improvements in cortisol levels (Jackowska et al., 2016).

Physical Health and Health Behaviors. A handful of studies highlight the benefits of gratitude for physical health and health behaviors. Gratitude has been linked to better self-reported physical health, and this relationship appeared to be explained by psychological well-being, healthy activities, and support-seeking behaviors. These links were more robust in older individuals than in younger individuals (Hill et al., 2013). Moreover, participants taking part in gratitude interventions have shown improvements in sleep quality and report fewer perceived sleep difficulties (Jackowska et al., 2016; Southwell & Gould, 2017) and reduced pain perception (Swain et al., 2020).

Proposed Mechanisms

Stress. While research suggests there may be a link between gratitude and physical health, less is known about the mechanisms through which gratitude promotes health. Given the importance of stress in relation to physical well-being, we propose that gratitude exerts its effects on health by positively impacting the coping process, thereby reducing stress and its negative consequences, ultimately leading to improved health outcomes (see Fig. 4.1). Generally, research has found gratitude is associated with decreased levels of stress (Corona et al., 2020; Jans-Beken et al., 2019; Lee et al., 2018; Wood et al., 2008a). Not only is gratitude associated with less stress, but growing evidence suggests gratitude acts as a stress buffer (Krejtz et al., 2016; Lee et al., 2018), with several studies examining this in relation to physical health outcomes. For example, Krause (2006) found that the stress of living in deteriorating neighborhoods predicted poorer self-reported physical health, but only for individuals with low levels of gratitude. Similarly, and more recently, a study involving college students found stressful life events and self-reported physical symptoms were positively correlated for college students, but only for those low in appreciation for what others had done for them (Deichert et al., 2019). Taken together, studies in this area show gratitude is not only associated with less stress but also buffers the negative effects of stress on self-reported physical health. Given the link between stress and health, this is a likely pathway through which gratitude may "undo" negative health consequences. Although limited, research supports this notion. Specifically, stress has been shown to mediate the relationship between gratitude and

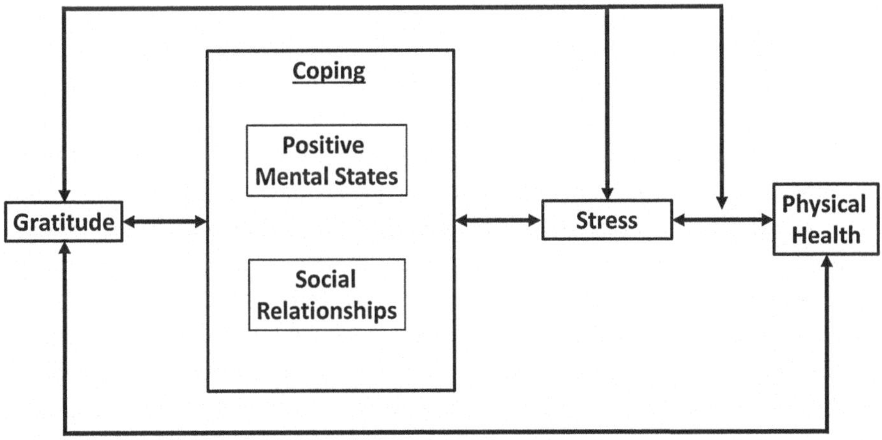

Fig. 4.1 Pathways linking gratitude and physical health

self-reported physical health and quality of life (O' Connell & Killeen-Byrt, 2018; Valikhani et al., 2019).

Coping and Positive Reframing. One reason grateful people may experience less stress and suffer fewer health issues in response to stressful events may be due to differences in how they cope with stress. Studies examining the association between gratitude and coping generally find that gratitude is associated with greater use of positive coping strategies and decreased use of maladaptive strategies. One of the first studies on this topic found that gratitude predicted greater use of active coping, planning, positive reinterpretation, social support, and decreased behavioral disengagement and denial (Wood et al., 2007). Furthermore, coping partially mediated the relationship between gratitude and perceived stress, suggesting coping is a pathway through which gratitude influences stress. More recent studies show consistent results, finding that gratitude promotes the utilization of active coping strategies such as problem-solving, positive reappraisal, acceptance, and religious coping and decreased usage of passive coping strategies such as avoidance (Lau & Cheng, 2017; Lin, 2015; Lin & Yeh, 2014; Sun et al., 2019).

One coping strategy important to consider in relation to gratitude is positive reframing or altering one's appraisals of situations so that events are viewed less negatively. Such interpretations of events are important to consider, given that appraisals are a key factor in determining whether one experiences stress (Lazarus & Folkman, 1984). Several studies by Lambert and colleagues provide support for a connection between gratitude and positive reframing. Specifically, baseline levels of trait gratitude were found to predict greater engagement in positive reframing over time in multiple studies (Lambert et al., 2012; Lambert et al., 2009b). Additional research in this area has found that gratitude is linked to a more positive interpretation of events (i.e., benefit-finding) in the context of physical health, including inflammatory bowel disease (Sirois & Wood, 2017) and COVID-19 (Tong & Oh, 2021). Importantly, research suggests that positive reframing helps account for the relationship between gratitude and stress (Wood et al., 2007). Given that gratitude leads to less negative interpretations of events, including in the context of health, and that such interpretations are associated with decreased stress, we believe positive reappraisals remain an important pathway to investigate as a possible mechanism linking gratitude and health.

Social Relationships. In addition to positively influencing cognitive appraisals, gratitude also has implications for social relationships, which is another important coping resource proposed as a link between gratitude and physical health (Alkozei et al., 2018; Lavelock et al., 2016). Research demonstrates a robust association between gratitude and social relationships, with gratitude consistently linked to greater social resources (e.g., Algoe et al., 2008). In addition, expressions of gratitude predicted increased perceptions of communal strength within a relationship (Lambert et al., 2010) and greater engagement in relationship maintenance behaviors over a year in married couples (Kubacka et al., 2011). Furthermore, research has demonstrated a link between gratitude and social support, with gratitude predicting greater perceptions and use of social support (Wood et al., 2007, 2008a). More recently, gratitude predicted increased social support over time in a sample of breast cancer patients. However, this relationship was found only for women who were not ambivalent about expressing emotion (Algoe & Stanton, 2012). In addition, gratitude has been associated with an increased likelihood of seeking help for mental and physical health problems (Hill et al., 2013).

Intervention studies also suggest that gratitude positively impacts the development of social resources. For example, a 2-week gratitude intervention was found to significantly increase social connectedness in a sample of individuals waiting to receive psychological services (Kerr et al., 2015). More recently, a 2-week gratitude intervention in a sample of women with breast cancer found that daily gratitude positively correlated with social support and spending time with others. However, this result was observed across both intervention and control conditions (Sztachańska et al., 2019). Importantly, these gains in social resources may be accounted for by increased levels of gratitude. Specifically, an intervention by O'Connell et al. (2018) found that a gratitude intervention was linked to increased friendship quality over time and that increased feelings of gratitude accounted for this relationship.

Given the stress-buffering effects of social support and the positive impact relationships have on physical health, social resources may be a pathway through which gratitude promotes physical well-being. Social relationships have been shown to mediate the association between gratitude and psychological well-being (Kong et al., 2015; Lin & Yeh, 2014; for an exception, see Wood et al., 2008a). There is preliminary evidence to suggest the same may be true regarding physical health. For example, feelings of loneliness have been found to mediate the relationship between trait gratitude and physical health symptoms (Bartlett & Arpin, 2019; O' Connell & Killeen-Byrt, 2018). Consistent with previous research, gratitude has been positively linked with social resources, which in turn have been demonstrated to predict better psychological and physical well-being.

Enhanced Social Support. Although social support has been shown to have positive associations with health, it is important to note that relationship quality has been theorized to increase the effectiveness of social support, and research reinforces this notion (Rini et al., 2006, 2011; Rini & Dunkel

Schetter, 2010). Given the impact gratitude has on various relationship characteristics, such as increased feelings of trust and intimacy (Dunn & Schweitzer, 2005; Gino & Schweitzer, 2008; Murray & Hazelwood, 2011) and viewing support providers as more genuine and sincere (Wood et al., 2008c), such changes may enhance the effectiveness of support provided by others. In fact, research shows that gratitude is associated with fewer adverse psychological reactions to receiving support. In a study of breast cancer patients, gratitude was negatively correlated with feelings of obligation and positively correlated with a willingness to accept support from others (Algoe & Stanton, 2012). More recently, social support was found to mediate the relationship between gratitude and benign and malicious envy, suggesting that gratitude is positively associated with how individuals respond to receiving help from others (Xiang et al., 2018).

Further evidence of gratitude enhancing the effectiveness of support comes from several of our studies. In one study, we found that perceived stress mediated the relationship between social support and health-compromising dietary behaviors (e.g., eating fast foods), depression, and anxiety. More importantly, we found that gratitude moderated these indirect effects. The links between social support, stress, and our outcomes were only significant for individuals with moderate to high levels of gratitude (Deichert et al., 2018). In an experimental study directly examining whether gratitude enhances support effectiveness, gratitude was induced through a brief writing task before giving a speech (Deichert et al., 2021). During the speech, approximately half of the participants received support from the research assistant, and the other half did not. Following the speech, participants rated the stressfulness of the situation. In line with our hypothesis that gratitude enhances support effectiveness, our results revealed a significant interaction. Individuals who wrote about someone they were grateful for and received support during the speech perceived the speech task as the least stressful.

Conclusions and Future Directions

Although still an emerging area of study, current research examining the link between gratitude and physical health has shown that gratitude, whether studied as a trait, a state, or through interventions, can positively impact physical health, particularly as it relates to cardiovascular and immune biomarkers. Furthermore, studies suggest gratitude promotes the development of coping resources, particularly social support, which has been shown to buffer the experience of stress and may be one avenue through which gratitude impacts physical health. While preliminary research offers some promise, future research should continue to examine what effects gratitude has on other physiological systems, particularly endocrine function. Given that stress is a pathway through which gratitude may influence physical health and impact cortisol, it may be prudent to begin by examining this association.

There is also a limited amount of research on clinically relevant variables in chronic patient populations. Due to the psychological, physical, and financial costs associated with

chronic pain, rehospitalizations, recurrence, and mortality, research should examine whether gratitude offers any protective effects given such interventions are easy and cost-effective to administer and could therefore help reach a broader range of patient populations. In addition to potential clinical benefits, there are methodological advantages to studying gratitude in such populations. First, many studies on gratitude and health utilize healthy populations, risking the possibility of ceiling effects. Studying the impact of gratitude and health in chronically ill populations may reduce the possibility of having ceiling effects in positive psychological health outcomes (e.g., positive affect), which would more easily allow researchers to discern how gratitude impacts health. A second benefit to using patient populations may be that there could be larger effect sizes in patient populations, which may also help clarify how gratitude impacts health.

Lastly, future research should continue to examine the nature of gratitude and how it relates to health. For example, research should examine whether state and trait gratitude influence health through the same pathways or distinct mechanisms. Additionally, researchers should explore whether more generalized views of gratitude relate differentially to health outcomes than narrower or transactional views of gratitude. Finally, researchers should continue to examine personal attributes as well as aspects of gratitude interventions that may impact the effectiveness of the intervention such as personality and dispositional characteristics, the types of activity, and more macrolevel processes such as culture to determine how such factors impact the link between gratitude and health.

References

Algoe, S. B. (2012). Find, remind, and bind: The functions of gratitude in everyday relationships. *Social and Personality Psychology Compass, 6*(6), 455–469. https://doi.org/10.1111/j.1751-9004.2012.00439.x

Algoe, S. B., Haidt, J., & Gable, S. L. (2008). Beyond reciprocity: Gratitude and relationships in everyday life. *Emotion, 8*(3), 425–429. https://doi.org/10.1037/1528-3542.8.3.425

Algoe, S. B., & Stanton, A. L. (2012). Gratitude when it is needed most: Social functions of gratitude in women with metastatic breast cancer. *Emotion, 12*(1), 163–168. https://doi.org/10.1037/a0024024

Alkozei, A., Smith, R., & Killgore, W. D. S. (2018). Gratitude and subjective wellbeing: A proposal of two causal frameworks. *Journal of Happiness Studies, 19*(5), 1519–1542. https://doi.org/10.1007/s10902-017-9870-1

Bai, C.-F., Cui, N.-X., Xu, X., Mi, G.-L., Sun, J.-W., Shao, D., Li, J., Jiang, Y.-Z., Yang, Q.-Q., Zhang, X., & Cao, F.-L. (2019). Effectiveness of two guided self-administered interventions for psychological distress among women with infertility: A three-armed, randomized controlled trial. *Human Reproduction, 34*(7), 1235–1248. https://doi.org/10.1093/humrep/dez066

Bar-Tal, D., Bar-Zohar, Y., Greenberg, M. S., & Hermon, M. (1977). Reciprocity behavior in the relationship between donor and recipient and between harm-doer and victim. *Sociometry, 40*(3), 293. https://doi.org/10.2307/3033537

Bartlett, M. Y., & Arpin, S. N. (2019). Gratitude and loneliness: Enhancing health and well-being in older adults. *Research on Aging, 41*(8), 772–793. https://doi.org/10.1177/0164027519845354

Boehm, J. K., Lyubomirsky, S., & Sheldon, K. M. (2011). A longitudinal experimental study comparing the effectiveness of happiness-enhancing strategies in Anglo Americans and Asian Americans. *Cognition & Emotion, 25*(7), 1263–1272. https://doi.org/10.1080/02699931.2010.541227

Boggiss, A. L., Consedine, N. S., Brenton-Peters, J. M., Hofman, P. L., & Serlachius, A. S. (2020). A systematic review of gratitude interventions: Effects on physical health and health behaviors. *Journal of Psychosomatic Research, 135*, 110165. https://doi.org/10.1016/j.jpsychores.2020.110165

Card, N. A. (2019). Meta-analyses of the reliabilities of four measures of gratitude. *The Journal of Positive Psychology, 14*(5), 576–586. https://doi.org/10.1080/17439760.2018.1497690

Celano, C. M., Beale, E. E., Beach, S. R., Belcher, A. M., Suarez, L., Motiwala, S. R., Gandhi, P. U., Gaggin, H., Januzzi, J. L., Healy, B. C., & Huffman, J. C. (2017). Associations between psychological constructs and cardiac biomarkers after acute coronary syndrome. *Psychosomatic Medicine, 79*(3), 318–326. https://doi.org/10.1097/PSY.0000000000000404

Chen, L. H., Chen, M. Y., Kee, Y. H., & Tsai, Y. M. (2009). Validation of the gratitude questionnaire (GQ) in Taiwanese undergraduate students. *Journal of Happiness Studies, 10*(6), 655–664. https://doi.org/10.1007/s10902-008-9112-7

Chen, L. H., Chen, M. Y., & Tsai, Y. M. (2012). Does gratitude always work? Ambivalence over emotional expression inhibits the beneficial effect of gratitude on well-being. *International Journal of Psychology, 47*(5), 381–392. https://doi.org/10.1080/00207594.2011.632009

Chen, L. H., Wu, C. H., & Chen, S. (2015). Gratitude and athletes' life satisfaction: A intra-individual analysis on the moderation of ambivalence over emotional expression. *Social Indicators Research, 123*(1), 227–239. https://doi.org/10.1007/s11205-014-0737-0

Corona, K., Senft, N., Campos, B., Chen, C., Shiota, M., & Chentsova-Dutton, Y. E. (2020). Ethnic variation in gratitude and well-being. *Emotion, 20*(3), 518–524. https://doi.org/10.1037/emo0000582

Cousin, L., Redwine, L., Bricker, C., Kip, K., & Buck, H. (2021). Effect of gratitude on cardiovascular health outcomes: A state-of-the-science review. *Journal of Positive Psychology, 16*(3), 348–355. https://doi.org/10.1080/17439760.2020.1716054

Cregg, D. R., & Cheavens, J. S. (2020). Gratitude Interventions: Effective self-help? A meta-analysis of the impact on symptoms of depression and anxiety. *Journal of Happiness Studies.* https://doi.org/10.1007/s10902-020-00236-6

Crouch, T. A., Verdi, E. K., & Erickson, T. M. (2020). Gratitude is positively associated with quality of life in multiple sclerosis. *Rehabilitation Psychology, 65*(3), 231–238. https://doi.org/10.1037/rep0000319

Davis, D. E., Choe, E., Meyers, J., Wade, N., Varjas, K., Gifford, A., Quinn, A., Hook, J. N., Van Tongeren, D. R., Griffin, B. J., & Worthington, E. L. (2016). Thankful for the little things: A meta-analysis of gratitude interventions. *Journal of Counseling Psychology, 63*(1), 20–31. https://doi.org/10.1037/cou0000107

Deichert, N. T., Fekete, E. M., & Craven, M. (2018). Gratitude enhances the beneficial effects of social support on health in women. *Paper Presented at the 88th Annual Meeting of the Rocky Mountain Psychological Association.*

Deichert, N. T., Fekete, E. M., & Craven, M. (2021). Gratitude enhances the beneficial effects of social support on psychological well-being. *The Journal of Positive Psychology, 16*(2), 168–177. https://doi.org/10.1080/17439760.2019.1689425

Deichert, N. T., Prairie Chicken, M., & Hodgman, L. (2019). Appreciation of others buffers the associations of stressful life events with depressive and physical symptoms. *Journal of Happiness Studies, 20*(4), 1071–1088. https://doi.org/10.1007/s10902-018-9988-9

Dickens, L. R. (2017). Using gratitude to promote positive change: A series of meta-analyses investigating the effectiveness of gratitude interventions. *Basic and Applied Social Psychology, 39*(4), 193–208. https://doi.org/10.1080/01973533.2017.1323638

Diessner, R., & Lewis, G. (2007). Further validation of the Gratitude, Resentment, and Appreciation Test (GRAT). *The Journal of Social Psychology, 147*(4), 445–447.

Dunn, J. R., & Schweitzer, M. E. (2005). Feeling and believing: The influence of emotion on trust. *Journal of Personality and Social Psychology, 88*(5), 736–748. https://doi.org/10.1037/0022-3514.88.5.736

Emmons, R. A., Froh, J., & Rose, R. (2019). *Gratitude. In Positive psychological assessment: A handbook of models and measures* (2nd ed., pp. 317–332). American Psychological Association. https://doi.org/10.1037/0000138-020

Fagley, N. S. (2016). The construct of appreciation: It is so much more than gratitude. In D. Carr (Ed.), *Perspectives on gratitude: An interdisciplinary approach* (pp. 70–84). Routledge.

Fredrickson, B. L. (1998). What good are positive emotions? *Review of General Psychology, 2*(3), 300–319.

Fredrickson, B. L. (2004). Gratitude, like other positive emotions, broadens and builds. In R. A. Emmons & M. E. McCullough (Eds.), *The psychology of gratitude* (pp. 145–166). Oxford University Press.

Froh, J. J., Bono, G., Fan, J., Emmons, R. A., Henderson, K., Harris, C., Leggio, H., & Wood, A. M. (2014). Nice thinking! An educational intervention that teaches children to think gratefully. *School Psychology Review, 43*(2), 132–152. https://doi.org/10.1080/02796015.2014.12087440

Froh, J. J., Fan, J., Emmons, R. A., Bono, G., Huebner, E. S., & Watkins, P. (2011). Measuring gratitude in youth: Assessing the psychometric properties of adult gratitude scales in children and adolescents. *Psychological Assessment, 23*(2), 311–324. https://doi.org/10.1037/a0021590

Gallagher, S., Solano, A. C., & Liporace, M. F. (2020). State, but not trait gratitude is associated with cardiovascular responses to acute psychological stress. *Physiology and Behavior, 221*, 112896. https://doi.org/10.1016/j.physbeh.2020.112896

Gino, F., & Schweitzer, M. E. (2008). Blinded by anger or feeling the love: How emotions influence advice taking. *The Journal of Applied Psychology, 93*(5), 1165–1173. https://doi.org/10.1037/0021-9010.93.5.1165

Gouveia, V. V., Ribeiro, M. G. C., de Aquino, T. A. A., Loureto, G. D. L., Nascimento, B. S., & Rezende, A. T. (2019). Gratitude Questionnaire (GQ-6): Evidence of construct validity in Brazil. *Current Psychology, June 2020*. https://doi.org/10.1007/s12144-019-00197-x

Hartanto, A., Lee, S. T. H., & Yong, J. C. (2019). Dispositional gratitude moderates the association between socioeconomic status and Interleukin-6. *Scientific Reports, 9*(1), 802. https://doi.org/10.1038/s41598-018-37109-1

Hill, P. L., Allemand, M., & Roberts, B. W. (2013). Examining the pathways between gratitude and self-rated physical health across adulthood. *Personality and Individual Differences, 54*(1), 92–96. https://doi.org/10.1016/j.paid.2012.08.011

Hudecek, M. F. C., Blabst, N., Morgan, B., & Lermer, E. (2020). Measuring gratitude in Germany: Validation study of the German version of the Gratitude Questionnaire-Six Item Form (GQ-6-G) and the Multi-Component Gratitude Measure (MCGM-G). *Frontiers in Psychology, 11*(October), 1–11. https://doi.org/10.3389/fpsyg.2020.590108

Huffman, J. C., Beale, E. E., Celano, C. M., Beach, S. R., Belcher, A. M., Moore, S. V., Suarez, L., Motiwala, S. R., Gandhi, P. U., Gaggin, H. K., & Januzzi, J. L. (2016). Effects of optimism and gratitude on physical activity, biomarkers, and readmissions after an acute coronary syndrome: The Gratitude Research in Acute Coronary Events Study. *Circulation: Cardiovascular Quality and Outcomes, 9*(1), 55–63. https://doi.org/10.1161/CIRCOUTCOMES.115.002184

Ironson, G., Kremer, H., & Lucette, A. (2016). Relationship between spiritual coping and survival in patients with HIV. *Journal of General Internal Medicine, 31*(9), 1068–1076. https://doi.org/10.1007/s11606-016-3668-4

Jackowska, M., Brown, J., Ronaldson, A., & Steptoe, A. (2016). The impact of a brief gratitude intervention on subjective well-being, biology and sleep. *Journal of Health Psychology, 21*(10), 2207–2217. https://doi.org/10.1177/1359105315572455

Jans-Beken, L., Jacobs, N., Janssens, M., Peeters, S., Reijnders, J., Lechner, L., & Lataster, J. (2019). Gratitude and health: An updated review. *Journal of Positive Psychology*. https://doi.org/10.1080/17439760.2019.1651888

Jans-Beken, L., Lataster, J., Leontjevas, R., & Jacobs, N. (2015). Measuring gratitude: A comparative validation of the Dutch Gratitude Questionnaire (GQ6) and Short Gratitude, Resentment, and Appreciation Test (SGRAT). *Psychologica Belgica, 55*(1), 19–31. https://doi.org/10.5334/pb.bd

Kaczmarek, L. D., Goodman, F. R., Drążkowski, D., Kashdan, T. B., Połatyńska, K., & Komorek, J. (2014a). Instructional support decreases desirability and initiation of a gratitude intervention. *Personality and Individual Differences, 64*, 89–93. https://doi.org/10.1016/j.paid.2014.02.022

Kaczmarek, L. D., Kashdan, T. B., Drazkowski, D., Bujacz, A., & Goodman, F. R. (2014b). Why do greater curiosity and fewer depressive symptoms predict gratitude intervention use? Utility beliefs, social norm, and self-control beliefs. *Personality and Individual Differences, 66*, 165–170. https://doi.org/10.1016/j.paid.2014.03.032

Kaczmarek, L. D., Kashdan, T. B., Drazkowski, D., Enko, J., Kosakowski, M., Szäefer, A., & Bujacz, A. (2015). Why do people prefer gratitude journaling over gratitude letters? The influence of individual differences in motivation and personality on web-based interventions. *Personality and Individual Differences, 75*, 1–6. https://doi.org/10.1016/j.paid.2014.11.004

Kerr, S. L., O'Donovan, A., & Pepping, C. A. (2015). Can gratitude and kindness interventions enhance well-being in a clinical sample? *Journal of Happiness Studies, 16*(1), 17–36. https://doi.org/10.1007/s10902-013-9492-1

Kong, F., Ding, K., & Zhao, J. (2015). The relationships among gratitude, self-esteem, social support and life satisfaction among undergraduate students. *Journal of Happiness Studies, 16*(2), 477–489. https://doi.org/10.1007/s10902-014-9519-2

Krause, N. (2006). Gratitude toward God, stress, and health in late life. *Research on Aging, 28*(2), 163–183.

Krause, N., Emmons, R. A., Ironson, G., & Hill, P. C. (2017). General feelings of gratitude, gratitude to god, and hemoglobin A1c: Exploring variations by gender. *The Journal of Positive Psychology, 12*(6), 639–650. https://doi.org/10.1080/17439760.2017.1326520

Krejtz, I., Nezlek, J. B., Michnicka, A., Holas, P., & Rusanowska, M. (2016). Counting one's blessings can reduce the impact of daily stress. *Journal of Happiness Studies, 17*(1), 25–39. https://doi.org/10.1007/s10902-014-9578-4

Kubacka, K. E., Finkenauer, C., Rusbult, C. E., & Keijsers, L. (2011). Maintaining close relationships: Gratitude as a motivator and a detector of maintenance behavior. *Personality and Social Psychology Bulletin, 37*(10), 1362–1375. https://doi.org/10.1177/0146167211412196

Lambert, N. M., Clark, M. S., Durtschi, J., Fincham, F. D., & Graham, S. M. (2010). Benefits of expressing gratitude: Expressing gratitude to a partner changes one's view of the relationship. *Psychological Science, 21*(4), 574–580. https://doi.org/10.1177/0956797610364003

Lambert, N. M., Fincham, F. D., & Stillman, T. F. (2012). Gratitude and depressive symptoms: The role of positive reframing and positive emotion. *Cognition and Emotion, 26*(4), 615–633. https://doi.org/10.1080/02699931.2011.595393

Lambert, N. M., Graham, S. M., & Fincham, F. D. (2009a). A prototype analysis of gratitude: Varieties of gratitude experiences. *Personality & Social Psychology Bulletin, 35*(9), 1193–1207. https://doi.org/10.1177/0146167209338071

Lambert, N. M., Graham, S. M., Fincham, F. D., & Stillman, T. F. (2009b). A changed perspective: How gratitude can affect sense of coherence through positive reframing. *The Journal of Positive Psychology, 4*(6), 461–470. https://doi.org/10.1080/17439760903157182

Langer, Á. I., Ulloa, V. G., Aguilar-Parra, J. M., Araya-Véliz, C., & Brito, G. (2016). Validation of a Spanish translation of the Gratitude Questionnaire (GQ-6) with a Chilean sample of adults and high schoolers. *Health and Quality of Life Outcomes, 14*(1), 1–10. https://doi.org/10.1186/s12955-016-0450-6

Lau, B. H. P., & Cheng, C. (2017). Gratitude and coping among familial caregivers of persons with dementia. *Aging and Mental Health, 21*(4), 445–453. https://doi.org/10.1080/13607863.2015.1114588

Lavelock, C. R., Griffin, B. J., Worthington, E. L., Benotsch, E. G., Lin, Y., Greer, C. L., Garthe, R. C., Coleman, J. A., Hughes, C. M., Davis, D. E., & Hook, J. N. (2016). A qualitative review and integrative model of gratitude and physical health. *Journal of Psychology and Theology, 44*(1), 55–86. https://doi.org/10.1177/009164711604400105

Lazarus, R. S., & Folkman, S. (1984). *Stress, appraisal, and coping*. Springer.

Lee, J. Y., Kim, S. Y., Bae, K. Y., Kim, J. M., Shin, I. S., Yoon, J. S., & Kim, S. W. (2018). The association of gratitude with perceived stress and burnout among male firefighters in Korea. *Personality and Individual Differences, 123*(March 2017), 205–208. https://doi.org/10.1016/j.paid.2017.11.010

Lin, C. C. (2015). Impact of gratitude on resource development and emotional well-being. *Social Behavior and Personality, 43*(3), 493–504. https://doi.org/10.2224/sbp.2015.43.3.493

Lin, C. C., & Yeh, Y. C. (2014). How gratitude influences well-being: A structural equation modeling approach. *Social Indicators Research, 118*(1), 205–217. https://doi.org/10.1007/s11205-013-0424-6

Lin, S.-H., & Huang, Y.-C. (2016). Psychometric properties and factorial structure of the Chinese version of the gratitude resentment and appreciation test. *British Journal of Guidance and Counselling, 44*(3), 347–361. https://doi.org/10.1080/03069885.2015.1119234

Lyubomirsky, S., & Layous, K. (2013). How do simple positive activities increase well-being? *Current Directions in Psychological Science, 22*(1), 57–62. https://doi.org/10.1177/0963721412469809

Ma, M., Kibler, J. L., & Sly, K. (2013). Gratitude is associated with greater levels of protective factors and lower levels of risks in African American adolescents. *Journal of Adolescence, 36*(5), 983–991. https://doi.org/10.1016/j.adolescence.2013.07.012

Marsland, A. L., Pressman, S., & Cohen, S. (2007). Positive affect and immune function. In R. Ader (Ed.), *Psychoneuroimmunology, 4E* (pp. 761–779). Elsevier.

McCullough, M. E., Emmons, R., & Tsang, J.-A. (2002). The grateful disposition: A conceptual and empirical topography. *Journal of Personality and Social Psychology, 82*(1), 112–127. https://doi.org/10.1037/0022-3514.82.1.112

McCullough, M. E., Kilpatrick, S. D., Emmons, R. A., & Larson, D. B. (2001). Is gratitude a moral affect? *Psychological Bulletin, 127*(2), 249–266. https://doi.org/10.1037/0033-2909.127.2.249

McCullough, M. E., Kimeldorf, M. B., & Cohen, A. D. (2008). An adaptation for altruism? The social causes, social effects, and social evaluation of gratitude. *Current Directions in Psychological Science, 17*(4), 281–285. https://doi.org/10.1111/j.1467-8721.2008.00590.x

McCullough, M. E., Tsang, J.-A., & Emmons, R. A. (2004). Gratitude in intermediate affective terrain: Links of grateful moods to individual differences and daily emotional experiences. *Journal of Personality and Social Psychology, 86*(2), 295–309. https://doi.org/10.1037/0022-3514.86.2.295

McGuire, A. P., Szabo, Y. Z., Murphy, K. M., & Erickson, T. M. (2020). Direct and indirect effects of trait and state gratitude on health-related quality of life in a prospective design. *Psychological Reports, 123*(6), 2248–2262. https://doi.org/10.1177/0033294119868784

Mills, P. J., Redwine, L., Wilson, K., Pung, M. A., Chinh, K., Greenberg, B. H., Lunde, O., Maisel, A., Raisinghani, A., Wood, A., & Chopra, D. (2015). The role of gratitude in spiritual well-being in asymptomatic heart failure patients. *Spirituality in Clinical Practice, 2*(1), 5–17. https://doi.org/10.1037/scp0000050

Millstein, R. A., Celano, C. M., Beale, E. E., Beach, S. R., Suarez, L., Belcher, A. M., Januzzi, J. L., & Huffman, J. C. (2016). The effects of optimism and gratitude on adherence, functioning and mental health following an acute coronary syndrome. *General Hospital Psychiatry, 43*, 17–22. https://doi.org/10.1016/j.genhosppsych.2016.08.006

Morgan, B., Gulliford, L., & Kristjánsson, K. (2014). Gratitude in the UK: A new prototype analysis and a cross-cultural comparison. *Journal of Positive Psychology, 9*(4), 281–294. https://doi.org/10.1080/17439760.2014.898321

Murray, A. J., & Hazelwood, Z. J. (2011). Being grateful: Does it bring us closer? Gratitude, attachment and intimacy in romantic relationships. *Journal of Relationships Research, 2*(01), 17–25. https://doi.org/10.1375/jrr.2.1.17

Nowak, M. A., & Roch, S. (2007). Upstream reciprocity and the evolution of gratitude. *Proceedings of the Royal Society B: Biological Sciences, 274*(1610), 605–609. https://doi.org/10.1098/rspb.2006.0125

O' Connell, B. H., & Killeen-Byrt, M. (2018). Psychosocial health mediates the gratitude-physical health link. *Psychology, Health & Medicine*. https://doi.org/10.1080/13548506.2018.1469782

O' Connell, B. H., O' Shea, D., & Gallagher, S. (2018). Examining psychosocial pathways underlying gratitude interventions: Randomized controlled trial. *Journal of Happiness Studies, 19*(8), 2421–2444. https://doi.org/10.1007/s10902-017-9931-5

Rash, J. A., Matsuba, M. K., & Prkachin, K. M. (2011). Gratitude and well-being: Who benefits the most from a gratitude intervention? *Applied Psychology: Health and Well-Being, 3*(3), 350–369. https://doi.org/10.1111/j.1758-0854.2011.01058.x

Redwine, L. S., Henry, B. L., Pung, M. A., Wilson, K., Chinh, K., Knight, B., Jain, S., Rutledge, T., Greenberg, B., Maisel, A., & Mills, P. J. (2016). Pilot randomized study of a gratitude journaling intervention on heart rate variability and inflammatory biomarkers in patients with Stage B heart failure. *Psychosomatic Medicine, 78*(6), 667–676. https://doi.org/10.1097/PSY.0000000000000316

Rini, C., & Dunkel Schetter, C. (2010). The effectiveness of social support attempts in intimate relationships. In K. T. Sullivan & J. Davila (Eds.), *Support processes in intimate relationships* (pp. 26–67). Oxford University Press.

Rini, C., Dunkel Schetter, C., Hobel, C. J., Glynn, L. M., & Sandman, C. A. (2006). Effective social support: Antecedents and consequences of partner support during pregnancy. *Personal Relationships, 13*, 207–229. 1350-4126=06

Rini, C., Redd, W. H., Austin, J., Mosher, C. E., Meschian, Y. M., Isola, L., Scigliano, E., Moskowitz, C. H., Papadopoulos, E., Labay, L. E., Rowley, S., Burkhalter, J. E., Schetter, C. D., & Duhamel, K. N. (2011). Effectiveness of partner social support predicts enduring psychological distress after hematopoietic stem cell transplantation. *Journal of Consulting and Clinical Psychology, 79*(1), 64–74. https://doi.org/10.1037/a0022199

Rosenberg, E. L. (1998). Levels of analysis and the organization of affect. *Review of General Psychology, 2*(3), 247–270.

Ruini, C., & Vescovelli, F. (2013). The role of gratitude in breast cancer: Its relationships with post-traumatic growth, psychological well-being and distress. *Journal of Happiness Studies, 14*(1), 263–274. https://doi.org/10.1007/s10902-012-9330-x

Seligman, M. E. P., & Csikszentmihalyi, M. (2000). Positive psychology: An introduction. *American Psychologist, 55*(1), 5–14. https://doi.org/10.1037/0003-066X.55.1.5

Shin, L. J., Armenta, C. N., Kamble, S. V., Chang, S. L., Wu, H. Y., & Lyubomirsky, S. (2020). Gratitude in collectivist and individualist cultures. *Journal of Positive Psychology, 00*(00), 598–604. https://doi.org/10.1080/17439760.2020.1789699

Sirois, F. M., & Wood, A. M. (2017). Gratitude uniquely predicts lower depression in chronic illness populations: A longitudinal study of inflammatory bowel disease and arthritis. *Health Psychology, 36*(2), 122–132. https://doi.org/10.1037/hea0000436

Solom, R., Watkins, P. C., McCurrach, D., & Scheibe, D. (2017). Thieves of thankfulness: Traits that inhibit gratitude. *Journal of Positive Psychology, 12*(2), 120–129. https://doi.org/10.1080/17439760.2016.1163408

Southwell, S., & Gould, E. (2017). A randomised wait list-controlled pre–post–follow-up trial of a gratitude diary with a distressed sample. *Journal of Positive Psychology, 12*(6), 579–593. https://doi.org/10.1080/17439760.2016.1221127

Sun, P., Sun, Y., Jiang, H., Jia, R., & Li, Z. (2019). Gratitude and problem behaviors in adolescents: The mediating roles of positive and negative coping styles. *Frontiers in Psychology, 10*(JULY), 1–8. https://doi.org/10.3389/fpsyg.2019.01547

Swain, N., Lennox Thompson, B., Gallagher, S., Paddison, J., & Mercer, S. (2020). Gratitude Enhanced Mindfulness (GEM): A pilot study of an internet-delivered programme for self-management of pain and disability in people with arthritis. *Journal of Positive Psychology, 15*(3), 420–426. https://doi.org/10.1080/17439760.2019.1627397

Sztachańska, J., Krejtz, I., & Nezlek, J. B. (2019). Using a gratitude intervention to improve the lives of women with breast cancer: A daily diary study. *Frontiers in Psychology, 10*. https://doi.org/10.3389/fpsyg.2019.01365

Thomas, M., & Watkins, P. (2003). Measuring the grateful trait: Development of revised GRAT. *Paper Presented at the Annual Convention of the Western Psychological Association.*

Tong, E. M. W., & Oh, V. Y. S. (2021). Gratitude and adaptive coping among Chinese Singaporeans during the beginning of the COVID-19 pandemic. *Frontiers in Psychiatry, 11*(January), 1–8. https://doi.org/10.3389/fpsyt.2020.628937

Trivers, R. L. (1971). The evolution of reciprocal altruism. *The Quarterly Review of Biology, 46*(1), 35–57. https://doi.org/10.1086/406755

Tsang, J. A. (2006). The effects of helper intention on gratitude and indebtedness. *Motivation and Emotion, 30*(3), 198–204. https://doi.org/10.1007/s11031-006-9031-z

Tsang, J. A. (2007). Gratitude for small and large favors: A behavioral test. *Journal of Positive Psychology, 2*(3), 157–167. https://doi.org/10.1080/17439760701229019

Valikhani, A., Ahmadnia, F., Karimi, A., & Mills, P. J. (2019). The relationship between dispositional gratitude and quality of life: The mediating role of perceived stress and mental health. *Personality and Individual Differences, 141*, 40–46. https://doi.org/10.1016/j.paid.2018.12.014

Watkins, P. C. (2014a). What inhibits gratitude? In *Gratitude and the good life: Toward a psychology of appreciation* (pp. 213–224). Springer.

Watkins, P. C. (2014b). What is gratitude and how can it be measured? In *Gratitude and the Good Life: Toward a Psychology of Appreciation*. https://doi.org/10.1007/978-94-007-7253-3

Watkins, P. C., Woodward, K. K., Stone, T., & Kolts, R. L. (2003). Gratitude and happiness: Development of a measure of gratitude, and relationships with subjective well-being. *Social Behavior and Personality, 31*(5), 431–452.

Wood, A. M., Emmons, R. A., Algoe, S. B., Froh, J. J., Lambert, N. M., & Watkins, P. (2016). A dark side of gratitude? Distinguishing between beneficial gratitude and its harmful impostors for the positive clinical psychology of gratitude and well-being. In A. M. Wood & J. Johnson (Eds.), *The Wiley handbook of positive clinical psychology* (pp. 137–151). Wiley. https://doi.org/10.1002/9781118468197.ch10

Wood, A. M., Froh, J. J., & Geraghty, A. W. A. (2010). Gratitude and well-being: A review and theoretical integration. *Clinical Psychology Review, 30*(7), 890–905. https://doi.org/10.1016/j.cpr.2010.03.005

Wood, A. M., Joseph, S., & Linley, P. A. (2007). Coping style as a psychological resource of grateful people. *Journal of Social and Clinical Psychology, 26*(9), 1076–1093. https://doi.org/10.1521/jscp.2007.26.9.1076

Wood, A. M., Maltby, J., Gillett, R., Linley, P. A., & Joseph, S. (2008a). The role of gratitude in the development of social support, stress, and depression: Two longitudinal studies. *Journal of Research in Personality, 42*(4), 854–871. https://doi.org/10.1016/j.jrp.2007.11.003

Wood, A. M., Maltby, J., Stewart, N., & Joseph, S. (2008b). Conceptualizing gratitude and appreciation as a unitary personality trait. *Personality and Individual Differences, 44*, 619–630. http://www.sciencedirect.com/science/article/pii/S0191886907003431

Wood, A. M., Maltby, J., Stewart, N., Linley, P. A., & Joseph, S. (2008c). A social-cognitive model of trait and state levels of gratitude. *Emotion, 8*(2), 281–290. https://doi.org/10.1037/1528-3542.8.2.281

Xiang, Y., Chao, X., & Ye, Y. (2018). Effect of gratitude on benign and malicious envy: The mediating role of social support. *Frontiers in Psychiatry, 9*, 1–7. https://doi.org/10.3389/fpsyt.2018.00139

5

Gratitude and Health Behaviour Change: A Self-regulation Resource Perspective

Fuschia M. Sirois and Alex M. Wood

Individual differences in gratitude have been well-studied with respect to mental health, where it has been shown to be a strong and unique predictor of a wide variety of mental health conditions (Wood et al., 2010). Whether defined as a momentary state of appreciation or an enduring orientation towards noticing and appreciating the positive in life (Wood et al., 2008b), gratitude has also emerged as an important positive quality for understanding other consequential health outcomes in recent years, including health behaviours. Attempts to understand how and why gratitude may be linked to health-related outcomes have drawn upon classic personality and health theory (Smith, 2006), as well as models linking positive psychological constructs to health (Schache et al., 2019). Common to both these perspectives is that health behaviours are a key pathway through which gratitude may operate to improve physical health outcomes. However, theoretical perspectives on *why* gratitude may promote engaging in health-promoting behaviours are scarce, despite established theory and evidence on the central role of self-regulation for initiating and maintaining health behaviours.

F. M. Sirois (✉)
Department of Psychology, Durham University, Durham, UK
e-mail: fuschia.sirois@durham.ac.uk

A. M. Wood
School of Psychology and Therapeutic Studies, Leeds Trinity University, Leeds, UK

F. M. Sirois (ed.), *The Palgrave Handbook of Positive Psychology and Health*,
https://doi.org/10.1007/978-3-031-89095-6_5

In this chapter we address this important gap by proposing for the first time that gratitude promotes the practice of health-promoting behaviours because it is linked to resources that can enhance self-regulation. In particular, we suggest that affective states and future time perspective, an orientation towards considering the future when making decisions, are two key self-regulation resources that link gratitude to health behaviours. This prediction is consistent with the Temporal Affective Self-regulation Resource (TASRR) model of health behaviours (Sirois, 2014, 2015a, 2015b; Sirois & Hirsch, 2015).

After first reviewing current evidence linking gratitude to health and health behaviours specifically, we then present a self-regulation resource view of gratitude that situates it as a quality that can strengthen resources that support self-regulation and mitigate factors that can interfere with self-regulation. We then present a critical discussion of the implications of a self-regulation view of gratitude for understanding and changing health behaviours, and end with a proposed extension to the self-regulation resource model, and a research agenda for progressing future research on gratitude and health behaviours.

The Relevance of Gratitude for Health

Although gratitude is often viewed as a positive social emotion that is experienced in response to receiving aid from others (Wood et al., 2011), it can also be viewed as a life orientation (Wood et al., 2008b). This latter conceptualisation posits that gratitude can be a tendency "towards noticing and appreciating the positive in the world" which can manifest as a trait-like quality that might be expected to have strong links to health and well-being (Wood et al., 2010). As a trait, gratitude involves the experience of gratitude frequently, intensely, and across a variety of situations (McCullough et al., 2002). Importantly, this life orientation towards being grateful is something that can be cultivated and maintained over time through engaging in reflective daily gratitude practices (e.g., Cheng et al., 2015). Thus, as a target point for intervention, gratitude holds promise as a potential means of improving health outcomes.

From this life orientation perspective of gratitude, it is not surprising that a growing evidence base has demonstrated that gratitude is associated with a range of better health-related outcomes. With respect to mental health, gratitude is associated with lower depression in both non-clinical and medical populations (Sirois & Wood, 2017; Wood et al., 2010; Wood et al., 2008a), as well as lower anxiety (Cregg & Cheavens, 2021; Ruini & Vescovelli, 2013).

Further, gratitude has a unique relationship between both life satisfaction and positive well-being, with this relationship being independent of the 30 personality facets of the Five Factor model which comprise some of the most studied traits in psychology (Wood, Joseph, & Maltby, 2009b; Wood et al., 2008b). The physical health outcomes linked to gratitude include better sleep (Wood et al., 2009a), health-related quality of life (Toussaint et al., 2017), improved blood pressure, glycaemic control, and asthma control (Boggiss et al., 2020), as well as better cardiovascular health outcomes (Cousin et al., 2021) (see also Chap. 4).

Gratitude and Health Behaviours

Health behaviours are crucial for promoting and maintaining health. As modifiable risk factors for the development of obesity and disease, health behaviours are common targets in health promotion and disease prevention efforts. Although health behaviours are often viewed as a unitary construct that includes both health-promoting (e.g., healthy eating, exercise, and getting adequate sleep) and health risk behaviours (e.g., smoking, alcohol, and substance misuse), theory and research have demonstrated that these two categories of health behaviours form distinct and replicable dimensions (Lippke et al., 2012; Vickers et al., 1990).

Although there is limited research on the role of gratitude for promoting positive health behaviours, the current evidence is promising. Much of this initial research has focused on the associations of trait gratitude with an array of behaviours relevant for promoting health. For example, in one study, gratitude, as assessed by the GQ6 (McCullough et al., 2002), was associated engaging in health-promoting activities, such as healthy eating and exercise in a large sample of adults (Hill et al., 2013). Similar results were found in two longitudinal studies of patients who had experienced acute coronary syndrome (ACS; Legler et al., 2019; Millstein et al., 2016). Dispositional gratitude at 2 weeks post ACS was associated with better medical adherence to health behaviour recommendations at the 6-month follow-up. These results remained significant after accounting for the effects of potentially confounding medical and social variables in one study (Millstein et al., 2016), but not the other (Legler et al., 2019).

Recent research has built on these initial findings by testing whether state gratitude induced via gratitude interventions might also promote better engagement with positive health behaviours. Gratitude interventions are relatively straightforward to implement and commonly involve list writing (i.e., three things you are grateful for), keeping a gratitude diary, or writing a gratitude letter (Wood et al., 2010). Further, they have been shown to be as effective in reducing worry (Geraghty et al., 2010b) and body dissatisfaction (Geraghty et al., 2010a) than a technique based around identifying and changing negative cognitions, whilst having a lower dropout rate from the intervention that may suggest grater patient acceptability.

Although gratitude interventions have been tested across a variety of contexts and domains (Dickens, 2017), their effectiveness for increasing health behaviours is only recently attracting interest from researchers. At the time of this writing, there were only five published studies that investigated the effects of a gratitude intervention for health-relevant behaviours. One of the earliest investigations was conducted by Emmons and McCullough (2003) that included a series of studies that examined the effects of gratitude lists on a variety of health behaviours over a two-week period. The two studies that examined the effects of gratitude on health-promoting behaviours (number of minutes spent exercising or engaging in daily exercise) did not find any significant effects. Given the short study period, it is possible there wasn't enough time for expected changes in health behaviour.

Recent research provides mixed support for this explanation. Across two studies, a gratitude writing intervention was effective for improving eating habits in both undergraduate students, and high school students (Fritz et al., 2019). Notably, the study with university students was conducted over a one-week period. However, the sample was highly motivated to change their eating habits, and the findings from the between group comparisons to the control group were non-significant. State gratitude post intervention collapsed across both groups did, however, predict healthier eating behaviour at the one-week follow-up. The results from the sample of high school students were more robust, as the findings demonstrated that the gratitude letter was effective in increasing healthy eating behaviour compared to the control group at the four-week follow-up. Taken together, these results suggest that the effects of gratitude interventions on health behaviours require a sufficient time frame for any expected behaviour changes to occur.

Investigations with medical populations also provide some preliminary support for the notion that gratitude interventions can be effective for changing health behaviours in the context of challenging health conditions. One proof-of-concept trial tested the effects of a telephone-delivered positive psychology intervention on health behaviours in people with mild to moderate heart failure (Celano et al., 2018). Although the intervention was multifaceted and included several positive psychology interventions, the expressing gratitude component predicted large improvements in both health behaviours and medication adherence from the pre to post period. However, there were mixed results in one pilot randomised controlled trial of an 8-week gratitude intervention aimed at improving self-care behaviours and glycaemic control among adolescents with Type 1 diabetes (Schache et al., 2020). There were no differences between the intervention and control groups with respect to diabetes self-care (i.e., monitoring, insulin use, diet, and exercise), nor any significant changes in $HbA1_{c,}$ a measure of glycaemic control. The lack of significant effects might be explained by several factors. For example, baseline gratitude levels were relatively high, 25 percent of the participants did not complete the study, and less than half of the participants fully engaged with the daily gratitude journal, with almost 30 percent completing it once a week or less over the 8 weeks of the intervention. A further analysis suggested that those who adhered to the intervention had small but significant improvements in glycaemic control compared to those who did not adhere (Schache et al., 2020). Because glycaemic control relies largely up diet behaviours, these findings suggest that further investigations are needed with this population.

There is also some evidence that gratitude interventions can help reduce unhealthy behaviours. In one study of female undergraduate students, a 14-day gratitude list intervention was found to be more effective in reducing dysfunctional eating behaviour (e.g., binging, purging, dieting) compared to the cognitive restructuring intervention, or the control group (Wolfe & Patterson, 2017). Although the mechanisms of change were not directly examined, the analyses also revealed that negative mood decreased and positive mood significantly increased as a result of the gratitude intervention. In contrast, there were no significant changes in mood for either the cognitive restructuring or the control conditions.

The evidence for gratitude in reducing health risk behaviours is much more limited, yet still promising. Cross-sectional studies have found that trait gratitude was associated with abstinence from drug and alcohol use in adolescents (Ma et al., 2013), with less drug use among drug misusers at a rehabilitation centre (Leung & Tong, 2017), and with less substance use coping (Wood et al., 2007). However, studies examining the effects of gratitude interventions on health risk behaviours are scarce. In one the few studies conducted, a positive psychology intervention that included the "three good things" exercise was tested for its efficacy as an adjunct to a standard smoking cessation programme (Kahler et al., 2014). Although a control group was not included, almost a third of the participants were able to sustain their smoking abstinence six months later.

Gratitude and the Self-regulation of Health Behaviours

Taken together, current research provides some support for the potential value of cultivating gratitude to facilitate making and maintaining positive health behaviour changes. Yet despite this evidence, the processes underlying the role of gratitude for health behaviours remains largely unexplored. We propose that applying a self-regulation lens to address this issue provides a potentially valuable perspective from which to better understand how and why gratitude may operate to improve health behaviours, especially as self-regulation is considered a key process for understanding why people may or may not engage in health behaviours.

Self-regulation is well recognised as an important capacity for understanding when and why people successfully engage in health behaviours. Self-regulation is defined as the regulation of thoughts, emotions, and behaviours directed towards reaching goals (Carver & Scheier, 1982), and it involves a series of interlinked processes. Once a goal is set, for example, to become more physically active, effort is required to monitor progress towards this goal, such a keeping track of minutes of exercise, trips to the gym, and so on, and to shield one from tempting alternatives that may lead to lapses. If there are lapses whilst working towards the goal (i.e., a scheduled run is missed), self-regulation of the cognitive, emotional, and behavioural responses to this lapse are required to maintain focus and effort, as well as reduce the chance of goal disengagement.

Health behaviours can be viewed as the prototypical self-regulation task for a number of reasons (Baumeister et al., 1994). First, they require monitoring and regulating emotions to maintain a focus on long-term health goals rather than permitting emotions to derail goal focus toward the gratification of immediate needs (Tice & Bratslavsky, 2000). Second, successfully making health behaviour changes requires thinking about the future consequences of one's current actions. Engaging in health behaviour changes requires first setting a goal for one's health to be achieved in the future, and then keeping engaging in actions that support this goal despite immediate temptations to do otherwise. Both of these self-regulation tasks require being able to readily orient one's thoughts to the future (Baird et al., 2021), a capacity which is often referred to has having a future-orientation (Zimbardo & Boyd, 1999).

To the extent that being grateful contributes to a capacity to think about the future, a self-regulation account of why gratitude may promote health behaviours is reasonable. As will be outlined in the next section, converging evidence from correlational, longitudinal, and neuroscience studies provides support for a connection between gratitude and future-oriented thinking.

Gratitude and Future-Oriented Thinking

With respect to temporal thinking, gratitude is often viewed as a past or present-oriented quality. People experience gratitude when they receive assistance from others that is valuable, perceived to be costly to the giver, and is given in spirit of genuine helpfulness (Wood et al., 2008c). Being the receiver of such benefits in the present, or recalling and reflecting on what others have done in the past, can elicit feelings of gratitude. From this perspective, it may not be apparent how or why gratitude would involve future-oriented thinking.

However, if we consider that gratitude can be viewed a prosocial emotion that arises from acts of altruism, the links to future-oriented thinking become clearer. Researchers have proposed that gratitude reinforces and maintains prosocial behaviour by motivating responding in like to either the benefactor or others (McCullough et al., 2008). For example, when an individual is the recipient of help or other beneficial acts from others, the experience of gratitude can orient them towards thinking about how they can reciprocate the act of kindness in the future. This reciprocal altruism is more likely to occur when the recipient perceives that (1) a reciprocal act would be of need to the benefactor, or (2) there would be an opportunity to repay the act of kindness in the future (Nowak & Roch, 2007). In the event that the benefactor may not need a reciprocal act (e.g., offering a ride to someone who has a car and doesn't need a ride), or the benefactor will not be available to receive a reciprocal act of kindness (e.g., there benefactor won't be encountered again), then gratitude is posited to motivate prosocial behaviour towards strangers or others who were not involved in the initial gratitude-triggering act of kindness. Evolutionary scientists have argued that this upstream altruism or "pay it forward" altruism is a by-product of the gratitude and other positive emotions that are involved in and facilitate direct altruism (Nowak & Roch, 2007).

This motivational account of the prosocial functions of gratitude provides a reasonable explanation for why future-oriented thinking may be involved in the experience of gratitude. Whether gratitude is experienced in the context of reciprocal or pay it forward altruism, thinking about whether and how one may repay the benefactor or others engages future-oriented thinking. Additionally, thoughts about *how* a repaid act of kindness may benefit others requires making predictions about outcomes, which is arguably a form of future-oriented thinking.

Although the link between gratitude and future-oriented thinking is somewhat understudied, the findings from current research are consistent with the above propositions. In correlational studies, gratitude has been linked to higher levels of future-oriented thinking (Allemand & Hill, 2016; Casu et al., 2020; Przepiorka & Sobol-Kwapinska, 2021; Szcześniak & Timoszyk-Tomczak, 2018). In one of the few longitudinal studies that have been conducted on gratitude and temporal thinking, average daily state gratitude was found to be significantly associated with higher average daily future-time perspective over a two-week period (Allemand & Hill, 2019). Although the results could not establish a causal direction between gratitude and future time perspective, it is possible that they are linked in dynamic and mutually reinforcing ways.

Not surprisingly, the findings from this correlational and longitudinal research converge with those from neuropsychological studies. Research examining the brain regions implicated in the experience of gratitude and for those high in trait gratitude has identified several key neural regions and potential mechanisms involved. In one prospective study, people who had entered psychotherapy for depression and/or anxiety were randomised to complete a gratitude writing intervention involving expressing gratitude to others once a week for the first three weeks of their counselling, or to one of two control conditions: engaging in an expressive writing task, or attending psychotherapy as usual (Kini et al., 2016). Then three months later those who were in the gratitude intervention group completed several iterations of a gratitude evoking "pay it forward" task while in an fMRI scanner, in which they were told a benefactor gave them money. They then had the choice to donate this money to a worthy cause, with the amount donated reflecting gratitude-related behaviour.

Consistent with the hypotheses (Kini et al., 2016), the results of the brain imaging analyses showed that the gratitude intervention was associated with lasting and measurable changes in brain activity. Specifically, there was greater neural activity in response to the gratitude task in the perigenual anterior cingulate cortex three months post-intervention among those who received the gratitude intervention, compared to the treatment-as-usual control group. From a functional perspective, this particular brain region is involved in predicting the outcomes and effects of one's actions (Alexander & Brown, 2011; Jahn et al., 2014). In short, it is a region involved in prospective or future-oriented thinking. This change was also consistent with participants' own self-reported increased feelings of gratitude as a result of the intervention, compared to the control group, and their behavioural expression of gratitude in the "pay it forward" task. Lastly, trait gratitude was associated with activation in the medial prefrontal cortex, a region that overlaps with the perigenual anterior cingulate cortex, and has been found to be associated with the experience of gratitude in other research (Fox et al., 2015). Collectively, the findings from current neuropsychological studies support the notion that the experience of gratitude, as well as an enduring tendency to be grateful, involve processes that engage future-oriented thinking.

Overall, current evidence links gratitude to self-reported future time orientation, and to greater activation and responsiveness in neural regions involved in predicting behavioural outcomes. It is therefore plausible to expect that when people feel grateful it may be easier for them think about not only the outcomes of acts of kindness to or from others, but also of the outcomes of their own behaviours more generally. This could extend to considering the outcomes of engaging in certain health behaviours, as future-oriented thinking is central to the self-regulatory process involved in successfully engaging in health-promoting behaviours (Baird et al., 2021).

Gratitude, Affective Resources, and Health Behaviours

In addition to temporal thinking, affective states can have important implications for the success of efforts to self-regulate health behaviour. In this respect, the affective profile of high levels of positive affect, and low levels of negative affect that characterises gratitude could explain why gratitude promotes the practice of positive health behaviours.

Gratitude involves noticing and appreciating the positives in life (Wood et al., 2010). It could be argued then that this orientation to positive stimuli can facilitate the experience of positive affective states. For example, gratitude interventions have been shown to increase positive affective states in a clinical population (Krentzman et al., 2015). However, it is important to note that this is not simply a truism or circular reasoning. Indeed, research has demonstrated that gratitude exerts its effects on consequential outcomes over and above those attributed to general positive affect (Froh et al., 2009a, 2009b), indicating that gratitude is not equivalent to positive affect.

Whether gratitude is experienced as a momentary state or a life orientation, numerous studies have demonstrated that gratitude is associated with a reduction in the negative affective states that can disrupt self-regulation. Dispositional gratitude is associated with lower levels of depression, anxiety, and stress, in cross-sectional and longitudinal research, and in both general and medical populations (Cregg & Cheavens, 2021; Sirois & Wood, 2017). For example, in one study of people with either inflammatory bowel disease or arthritis, trait gratitude predicted lower levels of depression at baseline and six months later, even after controlling for baseline depression, demographic variables, illness cognitions, changes in illness-relevant variables, and other positive psychological constructs (Sirois & Wood, 2017). Gratitude interventions provide further robust evidence that gratitude can be effective for reducing negative states (Krentzman et al., 2015; Portocarrero et al., 2020).

As noted previously, one of the key challenges in making health behaviour changes is maintaining focus and effort for the target health behaviour despite tempting alternatives, and the inevitable lapses and struggles experienced on the path towards adopting a healthier lifestyle. Negative thoughts directed towards the self are a common response to struggles, obstacles, and goal lapses, that can fuel negative mood and derail goal persistence (Wagner & Heatherton, 2015). In such instances, the negative affective states such as frustration, stress, or anxiety, that people experience, can shift their focus from achieving their long-term goal of changing their health behaviour, to the short-term goal of decreasing their negative mood. The result of this momentary reprioritisation of goals is often procrastination or even abandonment of the long-term goal as a way to reach their short-term goal of managing the negative emotions (Sirois & Pychyl, 2013). In such instances, the availability of self-regulation resources to down-regulate negative mood and maintain focus on the longer-term outcome of successfully changing health behaviours are crucial to offset these derailing effects. In short, gratitude may help facilitate the practice of health behaviours both by providing positive affective resources, and by countering goal-derailing negative affective states.

Gratitude, Temporal-Affective Resources, and Health Behaviours

The theory and research presented thus far suggest that gratitude is linked to affective states and future-oriented thinking, which in turn provide resources for supporting (or hindering) efforts aimed at the self-regulation of health behaviours. One model that has particular relevance for our discussion of the role of gratitude for providing self-regulation resources to support the practice of health behaviours is the Temporal Self-Regulation Resource model (TASRR; Sirois, 2015b, 2016). This conceptual framework highlights how temporal thinking and affective states associated with personality traits and individual differences can support or hinder the self-regulation of health behaviours. Specifically, the TASSR proposes that the extent to which certain individual differences promote or hinder engagement with health behaviours can be understood in terms of their associations with positive and negative affect, and future-oriented thinking. Individual differences and qualities that are characterised by the self-regulation resources of higher levels of positive affect and future oriented thinking, and also tend to have lower levels of negative affect, will promote greater practice of health-promoting behaviours. According to the TASSR model, trait gratitude would be considered an individual difference that can support the self-regulation of health behaviours through its connection to supportive temporal-affective resources, as illustrated in Fig. 5.1.

A key assumption of the TASSR that is relevant for understanding gratitude and health behaviours is that there is a synergy and dynamic, mutually reinforcing roles between positive and negative affect, and temporal thinking. In addition to theory highlighting the role of positive affect as an internal resource for down-regulating negative mood and supporting self-regulation (Fredrickson, 2001), positive affective states have been shown to enhance future-oriented thinking, and vice versa, by promoting abstract thinking (Critcher & Ferguson, 2011; Fredrickson, 2001; Rösch et al., 2021; Sirois

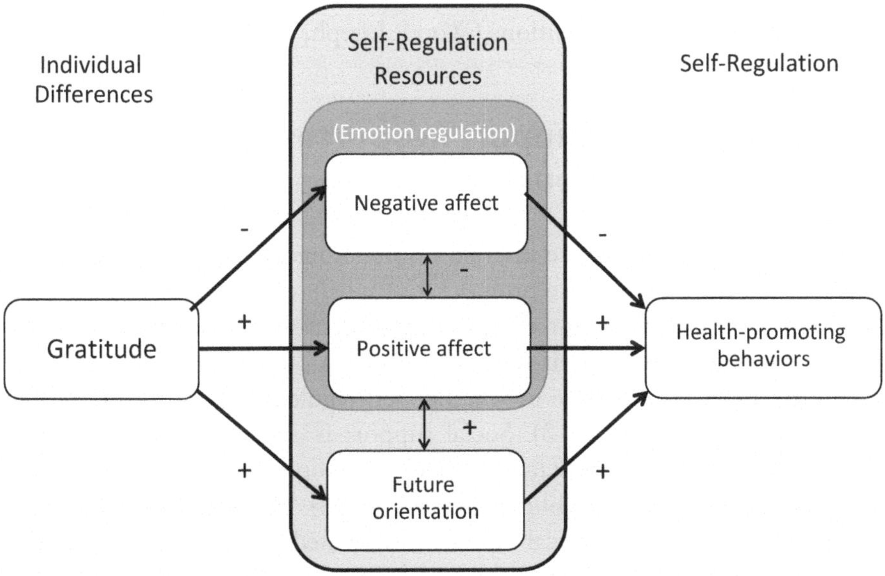

Fig. 5.1 Gratitude and health behaviours from the lens of the Temporal Affective Self-Regulation Resource Model (TASRR)

et al., 2015). Future-oriented thinking is also a key resource for promoting self-regulatory processes and outcomes in general (Baird et al., 2021) and specifically with respect to health behaviours (Dassen et al., 2016; Joireman et al., 2012). In contrast, negative affect foreshortens the action-contingency horizon, creating a temporal short-sightedness or myopia that directs attention to immediate threats and concerns at the expense of longer range goals (Sirois, 2014), such as changing health behaviours (Sirois et al., 2015). In short, it is not simply that gratitude is linked to positive affect or to future-oriented thinking alone that explains why gratitude can facilitate health behaviours, but that gratitude is associated with *both* self-regulation resources as well as low levels of negative affect.

Current research provides some support for the idea that gratitude may facilitate healthy behaviours through temporal and affective self-regulation resources as proposed by the TASRR model. In the study conducted by Fritz et al. (2019) examining the effects of a gratitude intervention on health behaviours in adolescents, those who expressed more gratitude engaged in healthier eating behaviours over time compared to a control group. Notably, this improvement in healthy eating was partially explained by reductions in average daily negative affect across the four weeks of the intervention. Similarly, a study examining the influence of trait gratitude on sleep behaviour found that those who were more grateful reported better sleep quality and duration, with these links being explained by having more positive pre-sleep cognitions, and fewer negative pre-sleep cognitions (Wood, Joseph, Lloyd, et al., 2009).

Gratitude, Social Support Resources, and Health Behaviours

In addition to supporting the internal resources necessary to regulate health behaviours, gratitude may also promote health behaviours through its links to external self-regulation resources. Increasingly researchers are acknowledging that self-regulation doesn't happen in a vacuum, and that certain external resources can play a key role in whether self-regulation is successful or not (e.g., Zaki & Williams, 2013). Social support is one such resource that is widely recognised as important for helping people initiate and maintain health behaviour change (Reblin & Uchino, 2008). Having strong social networks, often referred to as social capital, is associated with engaging in healthier behaviours in population-based research (Nieminen et al., 2013). There is also evidence that support from others can both help to prevent lapses and help people manage their responses to lapses while making health behaviour changes (Schumacher et al., 2017). Provision of social support can enhance perceptions of efficacy for adhering to lifestyle changes (Milsom et al., 2007), improve health behaviours in those who are vulnerable to poor health (Harvey & Alexander, 2012; Schulz et al., 2008), and promote long-term adherence to health behaviour change (Middleton et al., 2013). Collectively, this research highlights social support as an additional and plausible self-regulation resource pathway that can support the practice and maintenance of health behaviours.

Considering the prosocial nature of gratitude, it is possible that the fostering of, and access to, social resources may also explain why gratitude promotes healthy behaviours. Indeed, several studies have noted that dispositional gratitude is associated with higher levels of perceived social support (Chen et al., 2021; Kong et al., 2015; McGuire et al., 2021; Ni et al., 2015; You et al., 2022). Wood et al. (2008a) conducted two longitudinal studies testing the directionality of the linkages between dispositional gratitude and social support in college samples during a period of transition. Across the two studies, six models testing both directional and reciprocal causation found that the strongest support was for the model in which gratitude contributed to the development of social support over time. There is no evidence to support models in which social support increased gratitude although this may have happened were longer time frames studied. However, social support is a complicated construct which includes (a) the actual support that people receive ("received support"), (b) perceptions of the availability of support if and when needed ("perceived support"), and (c) perception of whether the actual support provided occurs when needed verses unneeded ("receive support when needed"). These three components have different empirical correlates, with only the latter two being consistently related to well-being (Melrose et al., 2015). Whilst there is strong evidence that gratitude relates to perceived support, there is less evidence as to whether gratitude relates to received support (and whether or not any such received support corresponds to an actual need). Perceptions of social support themselves relate to health behaviours, possibly through reducing stress. Additionally, it may be that gratitude also relates to received support when needed. Gratitude expressed in the context of reciprocal altruism may help develop more supportive environments, as benefactors are more likely to give further aid if their acts of kindness are appreciated. This could increase the provision of social support when needed. This proposition is also consistent with a meta-analysis of 91 studies which found that gratitude was associated with prosocial behaviour, and with studies examining gratitude in response to other's kindness showing larger effects than those examining generalised gratitude (Ma et al., 2017).

Figure 5.2 provides an extension of the TASRR model that incorporates a possible role of social support in understanding the mechanisms linking gratitude to health behaviours. In addition to the internal temporal-affective pathways, social support is a feasible and promising external self-regulation resource pathway that may provide additional explanatory power for understanding the role of gratitude in health behaviours. Although grounded in theory and research, the proposed pathway from gratitude to social support to health behaviours remains to be tested. What is also unknown is the extent to which this external self-regulation resource may operate in conjunction with internal self-regulation resources to explain the influence of gratitude on the practice, and maintenance, of health-promoting behaviours. For example, it is possible that there is a synergy between the positive affective states and social support fostered by gratitude, such that they work in reciprocal and mutually reinforcing ways to further support health behaviours beyond what each might accomplish alone. Indeed, research indicates that social support is

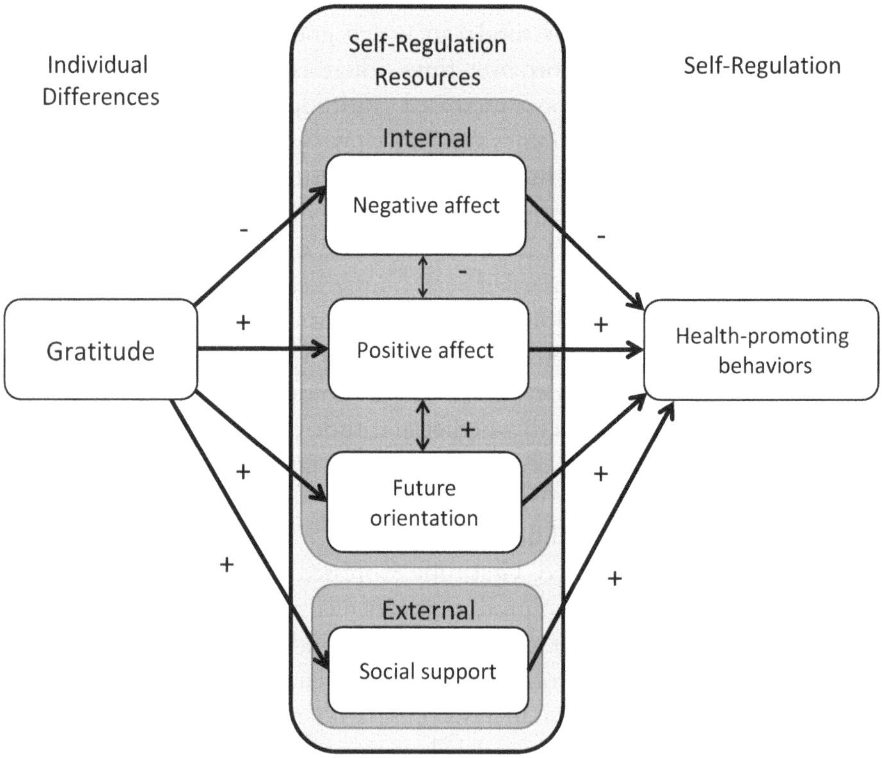

Fig. 5.2 Revised Temporal Affective Self-Regulation Resource Model (TASRR) showing expanded pathways linking gratitude to health behaviours

linked to increases in positive affect over time (Murrell et al., 1992), and has a synergistic relationship with positive affect in explaining other health outcomes (Park et al., 2018). Although there is limited evidence showing that social support is positively associated with future time perspective (e.g., Park et al., 2018), it is plausible that both positive affect and future-oriented thinking may have additional synergistic relationships with social support. These and other possible linkages between the proposed self-regulation resources in this extended TASRR model warrant further research to deepen our understanding of how and why gratitude may support the practice of healthy behaviours.

Gratitude and Health Behaviours: Next Steps and a Provisional Research Agenda

From the evidence presented thus far, it is clear that the research landscape on the role of gratitude in health behaviours is still developing. Promising initial evidence suggests that gratitude may have value for promoting health behaviours. However, there are some clear gaps that need to be addressed to both increase confidence in the preliminary findings, and to further elaborate the theoretical underpinnings that might explain why gratitude may be a valuable tool for supporting health behaviours. In this chapter we have viewed the link between gratitude from the lens of the TASRR. From this perspective we propose that there are several avenues of inquiry which may be fruitful for enhancing our understanding of the possible benefits of gratitude for health behaviours.

The majority of the research on gratitude and health behaviours to date has focused on health-promoting behaviours. With the exception of a handful of studies (Kahler et al., 2014), there has been much less attention given to whether gratitude may also be linked to positive health behaviour changes in the form of reducing health risk behaviours. Negative health behaviours, such as excessive alcohol consumption, substance use, smoking, are often driven by avoidance of negative emotional states such as distress. Gratitude may therefore support efforts to reduce these behaviours through its connections with emotion regulation and specifically the reduction of negative states. Research on the links between both trait and induced gratitude and health risk behaviours over time would expand our current understanding of the range of health-relevant behaviours linked to gratitude and provide insights into the possible affective pathways.

As noted previously, there is little research directly testing the pathways suggested by the TASRR model with respect to gratitude, and none examining our proposed extended TASRR model. Given the evidence demonstrating clear links between gratitude and emotion regulation, the role of gratitude for fostering social support, and the emerging evidence indicating that gratitude is linked to future-oriented thinking, further research examining these self-regulation pathways and their combined and relative contributions to health behaviours is warranted. For example, it's possible that the mitigating effects of gratitude on negative affect may be more salient for reducing health-risk behaviours than for increasing health-promoting behaviours. Similarly, the temporal and positive affective resources fostered by gratitude may have a greater role for supporting health-promoting behaviours than for reducing health risk behaviours. Investigations that test these propositions, as well as the potential for synergistic relationships among the pathways, are needed to gain a greater understanding of how gratitude may contribute to the self-regulation of health behaviours.

As is the case with any developing research area, the methods used to invest gratitude and health behaviours have tended to rely on less rigorous, exploratory approaches, leaving much room for improvement. Moving forward, research on gratitude and health behaviours would benefit from research designs that test this relationship and relationships with proposed pathways, over time, such as daily diary and event sampling methods, or longitudinal methods over longer periods of time. The latter is especially important to understand both whether the potential effects of gratitude on health behaviours persist over time, and to better assess the potential of gratitude to help maintain positive health behaviour changes once achieved. In the case of gratitude interventions, evidence suggests that their effects may persist for up to 6 months (Seligman et al., 2005). Understanding the duration of any effects from gratitude interventions is crucial when designing and implementing programmes that cultivate gratitude to target health behaviour change. Research on gratitude interventions further needs to carefully consider control conditions; gratitude interventions work well verses passive control or waiting lists, it is less clear how they compare to techniques already used in clinical practice (although there is some suggestion that they may compete on reducing drop-out: (Geraghty et al., 2010a, 2010b)). Establishing how gratitude interventions compared to others would both show if and when they are best deployed as well as whether increasing gratitude is the specific mechanism through which they operate.

Conclusions

Considering the role of gratitude for health behaviours provides an alternative, strengths-based approach to health behaviour change that can help address the issue of the difficulties people have translating intentions into actions. This "intention behaviour gap" is a perennial issue in health psychology that remains a challenge for public health efforts aimed at promoting health especially among vulnerable and at-risk populations. Indeed, social cognitive approaches to health behaviour change tend to focus on cognitions that strengthen health behaviour intentions, but often only show weak associations to actual health behaviour change (Sheeran & Webb, 2016). Gratitude offers a strengths-based approach to translating health behaviour intentions into actions as a promising alternative way of addressing this issue that may add value to current social cognitive approaches.

As we have outlined, gratitude may be beneficial for successfully navigating the self-regulation challenges involved in initiating and sustaining health behaviour change, including the inevitable setbacks and lapses that occur during behaviour change (e.g., Thøgersen-Ntoumani et al., 2021). It's during these moments when, for example, workouts are missed, that it can take extra effort to manage self-directed negative thoughts and feelings about the lapse, stay focused on the longer-term goal of becoming more fit, and persist rather than procrastinate or abandon health goals (Sirois & Pychyl, 2013). Because it reflects an orientation and appreciation towards the positives, gratitude may make it easier to balance negative reactions to lapses with a focus on the positive progress made, as well as the future benefits that will be achieved if efforts are continued rather than abandoned. As we have proposed, gratitude provides access to the inner and outer resources that can support self-regulation and are therefore crucial not only for the initiation of new health behaviours, but also the maintenance of health behaviour change. Given the accessibility and ease of administration of gratitude interventions, gratitude may be particularly valuable for supporting the change and maintenance of health behaviours, especially in low resource settings.

References

Alexander, W. H., & Brown, J. W. (2011). Medial prefrontal cortex as an action-outcome predictor. *Nature Neuroscience, 14*(10), 1338–1344. https://doi.org/10.1038/nn.2921

Allemand, M., & Hill, P. L. (2016). Gratitude from early adulthood to old age. *Journal of Personality, 84*(1), 21–35. https://doi.org/10.1111/jopy.12134

Allemand, M., & Hill, P. L. (2019). Future time perspective and gratitude in daily life: A Micro-longitudinal Study. *European Journal of Personality, 33*(3), 385–399. https://doi.org/10.1002/per.2201

Baird, H. M., Webb, T. L., Sirois, F. M., & Gibson-Miller, J. (2021). Understanding the effects of time perspective: A meta-analysis testing a self-regulatory framework. *Psychological Bulletin, 147*(3), 233–267. https://doi.org/10.1037/bul0000313

Baumeister, R. F., Heatherton, T. F., & Tice, D. M. (1994). *Losing control: How and why people fail at self-regulation*. Academic Press.

Boggiss, A. L., Consedine, N. S., Brenton-Peters, J. M., Hofman, P. L., & Serlachius, A. S. (2020). A systematic review of gratitude interventions: Effects on physical health and health behaviors. *Journal of Psychosomatic Research, 135*, 110165. https://doi.org/10.1016/j.jpsychores.2020.110165

Carver, C. S., & Scheier, M. F. (1982). Control theory: A useful conceptual framework for personality–social, clinical, and health psychology. *Psychological Bulletin, 92*(1), 111–135.

Casu, G., Gentili, E., & Gremigni, P. (2020). Future time perspective and perceived social support: The mediating role of gratitude. *International Journal of Environmental Research and Public Health, 17*(18). https://doi.org/10.3390/ijerph17186707

Celano, C. M., Freedman, M. E., Beale, E. E., Gomez-Bernal, F., & Huffman, J. C. (2018). A positive psychology intervention to promote health behaviors in heart failure: A proof-of-concept trial. *Journal of Nervous and Mental Disease, 206*(10), 800–808. https://doi.org/10.1097/nmd.0000000000000883

Chen, H., Yang, X., Xia, W., Li, Y., Deng, Y., & Fan, C. (2021). The relationship between gratitude and job satisfaction: The mediating roles of social support and job crafting. *Current Psychology*. https://doi.org/10.1007/s12144-021-01658-y

Cheng, S.-T., Tsui, P. K., & Lam, J. H. M. (2015). Improving mental health in health care practitioners: Randomized controlled trial of a gratitude intervention. *Journal of Consulting and Clinical Psychology, 83*, 177–186.

Cousin, L., Redwine, L., Bricker, C., Kip, K., & Buck, H. (2021). Effect of gratitude on cardiovascular health outcomes: A state-of-the-science review. *The Journal of Positive Psychology, 16*(3), 348–355. https://doi.org/10.1080/17439760.2020.1716054

Cregg, D. R., & Cheavens, J. S. (2021). Gratitude interventions: Effective self-help? A meta-analysis of the impact on symptoms of depression and anxiety. *Journal of Happiness Studies, 22*(1), 413–445. https://doi.org/10.1007/s10902-020-00236-6

Critcher, C. R., & Ferguson, M. J. (2011). Affect in the abstract: Abstract mindsets promote sensitivity to affect. *Journal of Experimental Social Psychology, 47*(6), 1185–1191. https://doi.org/10.1016/j.jesp.2011.04.014

Dassen, F. C. M., Jansen, A., Nederkoorn, C., & Houben, K. (2016). Focus on the future: Episodic future thinking reduces discount rate and snacking. *Appetite, 96*, 327–332. https://doi.org/10.1016/j.appet.2015.09.032

Dickens, L. R. (2017). Using gratitude to promote positive change: A series of meta-analyses investigating the effectiveness of gratitude interventions. *Basic and Applied Social Psychology, 39*(4), 193–208. https://doi.org/10.1080/01973533.2017.1323638

Emmons, R. A., & McCullough, M. E. (2003). Counting blessings versus burdens: An experimental investigation of gratitude and subjective well-being in daily life. *Journal of Personality and Social Psychology, 84*(2), 377–389. https://doi.org/10.1037/0022-3514.84.2.377

Fox, G. R., Kaplan, J., Damasio, H., & Damasio, A. (2015). Neural correlates of gratitude [Original Research]. *Frontiers in Psychology, 6*. https://doi.org/10.3389/fpsyg.2015.01491

Fredrickson, B. L. (2001). The role of positive emotions in positive psychology. The broaden-and-build theory of positive emotions. *American Psychologist, 56*(3), 218–226. https://doi.org/10.1037/0003-066x.56.3.218

Fritz, M. M., Armenta, C. N., Walsh, L. C., & Lyubomirsky, S. (2019). Gratitude facilitates healthy eating behavior in adolescents and young adults. *Journal of Experimental Social Psychology, 81*, 4–14. https://doi.org/10.1016/j.jesp.2018.08.011

Froh, J. J., Kashdan, T. B., Ozimkowski, K. M., & Miller, N. (2009a). Who benefits the most from a gratitude intervention in children and adolescents? Examining positive affect as a moderator. *The Journal of Positive Psychology, 4*(5), 408–422. https://doi.org/10.1080/17439760902992464

Froh, J. J., Yurkewicz, C., & Kashdan, T. B. (2009b). Gratitude and subjective well-being in early adolescence: Examining gender differences. *Journal of Adolescence, 32*(3), 633–650. https://doi.org/10.1016/j.adolescence.2008.06.006

Geraghty, A. W. A., Wood, A. M., & Hyland, M. E. (2010a). Attrition from self-directed interventions: Investigating the relationship between psychological predictors, intervention content and dropout from a body dissatisfaction intervention. *Social Science & Medicine, 71*(1), 30–37. http://www.sciencedirect.com/science/article/pii/S0277953610002327

Geraghty, A. W. A., Wood, A. M., & Hyland, M. E. (2010b). Dissociating the facets of hope: Agency and pathways predict dropout from unguided self-help therapy in opposite directions. *Journal of Research in Personality, 44*(1), 155–158. https://doi.org/10.1016/j.jrp.2009.12.003

Harvey, I. S., & Alexander, K. (2012). Perceived social support and preventive health behavioral outcomes among older women. *Journal of Cross-Cultural Gerontology, 27*(3), 275–290. https://doi.org/10.1007/s10823-012-9172-3

Hill, P. L., Allemand, M., & Roberts, B. W. (2013). Examining the pathways between gratitude and self-rated physical health across adulthood. *Personality and Individual Differences, 54*(1), 92–96. https://doi.org/10.1016/j.paid.2012.08.011

Jahn, A., Nee, D. E., Alexander, W. H., & Brown, J. W. (2014). Distinct regions of anterior cingulate cortex signal prediction and outcome evaluation. *NeuroImage, 95*, 80–89. https://doi.org/10.1016/j.neuroimage.2014.03.050

Joireman, J., Shaffer, M. J., Balliet, D., & Strathman, A. (2012). Promotion orientation explains why future-oriented people exercise and eat healthy: Evidence from the two-factor consideration of future consequences-14 scale. *Personality and Social Psychology Bulletin, 38*(10), 1272–1287. https://doi.org/10.1177/0146167212449362

Kahler, C. W., Spillane, N. S., Day, A., Clerkin, E. M., Parks, A., Leventhal, A. M., & Brown, R. A. (2014). Positive psychotherapy for smoking cessation: Treatment development, feasibility, and preliminary results. *The Journal of Positive Psychology, 9*(1), 19–29. https://doi.org/10.1080/17439760.2013.826716

Kini, P., Wong, J., McInnis, S., Gabana, N., & Brown, J. W. (2016). The effects of gratitude expression on neural activity. *NeuroImage, 128*, 1–10. https://doi.org/10.1016/j.neuroimage.2015.12.040

Kong, F., Ding, K., & Zhao, J. (2015). The relationships among gratitude, self-esteem, social support and life satisfaction among undergraduate students. *Journal of Happiness Studies, 16*(2), 477–489. https://doi.org/10.1007/s10902-014-9519-2

Krentzman, A. R., Mannella, K. A., Hassett, A. L., Barnett, N. P., Cranford, J. A., Brower, K. J., Higgins, M. M., & Meyer, P. S. (2015). Feasibility, acceptability, and impact of a web-based gratitude exercise among individuals in outpatient treatment for alcohol use disorder. *The Journal of Positive Psychology, 10*(6), 477–488. https://doi.org/10.1080/17439760.2015.1015158

Legler, S. R., Beale, E. E., Celano, C. M., Beach, S. R., Healy, B. C., & Huffman, J. C. (2019). State gratitude for one's life and health after an acute coronary syndrome: Prospective associations with physical activity, medical adherence and re-hospitalizations. *Journal of Positive Psychology, 14*(3), 283–291. https://doi.org/10.1080/17439760.2017.1414295

Leung, C.-C., & Tong, E. M. W. (2017). Gratitude and drug misuse: Role of coping as mediator. *Substance Use & Misuse, 52*(14), 1832–1839. https://doi.org/10.1080/10826084.2017.1312449

Lippke, S., Nigg, C. R., & Maddock, J. E. (2012). Health-promoting and health-risk behaviors: Theory-driven analyses of multiple health behavior change in three international samples. *International Journal of Behavioral Medicine, 19*(1), 1–13. https://doi.org/10.1007/s12529-010-9135-4

Ma, L. K., Tunney, R. J., & Ferguson, E. (2017). Does gratitude enhance prosociality?: A meta-analytic review. *Psycholological Bulletin, 143*(6), 601–635. https://doi.org/10.1037/bul0000103

Ma, M., Kibler, J. L., & Sly, K. (2013). Gratitude is associated with greater levels of protective factors and lower levels of risks in African American adolescents. *Journal of Adolescence, 36*(5), 983–991. https://doi.org/10.1016/j.adolescence.2013.07.012

McCullough, M. E., Emmons, R. A., & Tsang, J.-A. (2002). The grateful disposition: A conceptual and empirical topography. *Journal of Personality and Social Psychology, 82*(1), 112–127.

McCullough, M. E., Kimeldorf, M. B., & Cohen, A. D. (2008). An Adaptation for altruism: The social causes, social effects, and social evolution of gratitude. *Current Directions in Psychological Science, 17*(4), 281–285. https://doi.org/10.1111/j.1467-8721.2008.00590.x

McGuire, A. P., Fogle, B. M., Tsai, J., Southwick, S. M., & Pietrzak, R. H. (2021). Dispositional gratitude and mental health in the U.S. veteran population: Results from the National Health and Resilience Veterans Study. *Journal of Psychiatric Research, 135*, 279–288. https://doi.org/10.1016/j.jpsychires.2021.01.020

Melrose, K. L., Brown, G. D. A., & Wood, A. M. (2015). When is received social support related to perceived support and well-being? When it is needed. *Personality and Individual Differences, 77*, 97–105. https://doi.org/10.1016/j.paid.2014.12.047

Middleton, K. R., Anton, S. D., & Perri, M. G. (2013). Long-term adherence to health behavior change. *American Journal of Lifestyle Medicine, 7*(6), 395–404. https://doi.org/10.1177/1559827613488867

Millstein, R. A., Celano, C. M., Beale, E. E., Beach, S. R., Suarez, L., Belcher, A. M., Januzzi, J. L., & Huffman, J. C. (2016). The effects of optimism and gratitude on adherence, functioning and mental health following an acute coronary syndrome. *General Hospital Psychiatry, 43*, 17–22. https://doi.org/10.1016/j.genhosppsych.2016.08.006

Milsom, V. A., Perri, M. G., & Rejeski, W. J. (2007). Guided group support and the long-term management of obesity. In J. D. Latner & G. T. Wilson (Eds.), *Self-help approaches for obesity and eating disorders: Research and practice* (pp. 205–222). Guilford Press.

Murrell, S. A., Norris, F. H., & Chipley, Q. T. (1992). Functional versus structural social support, desirable events, and positive affect in older adults. *Psychology and Aging, 7*(4), 562–570. https://doi.org/10.1037/0882-7974.7.4.562

Ni, S., Yang, R., Zhang, Y., & Dong, R. (2015). Effect of gratitude on loneliness of Chinese college students: Social support as a mediator. *Social Behaviour and Personality: An International Journal, 43*(4), 559–566.

Nieminen, T., Prättälä, R., Martelin, T., Härkänen, T., Hyyppä, M. T., Alanen, E., & Koskinen, S. (2013). Social capital, health behaviours and health: A population-based associational study. *BMC Public Health, 13*(1), 613. https://doi.org/10.1186/1471-2458-13-613

Nowak, M. A., & Roch, S. (2007). Upstream reciprocity and the evolution of gratitude. *Proceedings of Biological Sciences, 274*(1610), 605–609. https://doi.org/10.1098/rspb.2006.0125

Park, I.-J., Kim, M., Kwon, S., & Lee, H.-G. (2018). The relationships of self-esteem, future time perspective, positive affect, social support, and career decision: A longitudinal multilevel study [original research]. *Frontiers in Psychology, 9*. https://doi.org/10.3389/fpsyg.2018.00514

Portocarrero, F. F., Gonzalez, K., & Ekema-Agbaw, M. (2020). A meta-analytic review of the relationship between dispositional gratitude and well-being. *Personality and Individual Differences, 164*, 110101. https://doi.org/10.1016/j.paid.2020.110101

Przepiorka, A., & Sobol-Kwapinska, M. (2021). People with positive time perspective are more grateful and happier: Gratitude mediates the relationship between time perspective and life satisfaction. *Journal of Happiness Studies, 22*(1), 113–126. https://doi.org/10.1007/s10902-020-00221-z

Reblin, M., & Uchino, B. N. (2008). Social and emotional support and its implication for health. *Current Opinion in Psychiatry, 21*(2), 201–205. https://doi.org/10.1097/YCO.0b013e3282f3ad89

Rösch, S. A., Stramaccia, D. F., & Benoit, R. G. (2021). Promoting farsighted decisions via episodic future thinking: A meta-analysis. *Journal of Experimental Psychology: General*, No Pagination Specified-No Pagination Specified. https://doi.org/10.1037/xge0001148

Ruini, C., & Vescovelli, F. (2013). The role of gratitude in breast cancer: Its relationships with post-traumatic growth, psychological well-being and distress. *Journal of Happiness Studies, 14*(1), 263–274. https://doi.org/10.1007/s10902-012-9330-x

Schache, K., Consedine, N., Hofman, P., & Serlachius, A. (2019). Gratitude—More than just a platitude? The science behind gratitude and health. *British Journal of Health Psychology, 24*(1), 1–9. https://doi.org/10.1111/bjhp.12348

Schache, K. R., Hofman, P. L., & Serlachius, A. S. (2020). A pilot randomized controlled trial of a gratitude intervention for adolescents with Type 1 diabetes. *Diabetic Medicine, 37*(8), 1352–1356. https://doi.org/10.1111/dme.14078

Schulz, U., Pischke, C. R., Weidner, G., Daubenmier, J., Elliot-Eller, M., Scherwitz, L., Bullinger, M., & Ornish, D. (2008). Social support group attendance is related to blood pressure, health behaviours, and quality of life in the Multicenter Lifestyle Demonstration Project. *Psychology, Health & Medicine, 13*(4), 423–437. https://doi.org/10.1080/13548500701660442

Schumacher, L. M., Arigo, D., & Thomas, C. (2017). Understanding physical activity lapses among women: Responses to lapses and the potential buffering effect of social support. *Journal of Behavioral Medicine, 40*(5), 740–749. https://doi.org/10.1007/s10865-017-9846-y

Seligman, M. E., Steen, T. A., Park, N., & Peterson, C. (2005). Positive psychology progress: Empirical validation of interventions. *American Psychologist, 60*(5), 410–421. https://doi.org/10.1037/0003-066x.60.5.410

Sheeran, P., & Webb, T. L. (2016). The Intention–Behavior Gap. *Social and Personality Psychology Compass, 10*(9), 503–518. https://doi.org/10.1111/spc3.12265

Sirois, F. M. (2014). Out of sight, out of time? A meta–analytic investigation of procrastination and time perspective. *European Journal of Personality, 28*(5), 511–520. https://doi.org/10.1002/per.1947

Sirois, F. M. (2015a). Perfectionism and health behaviors: A self-regulation resource perspective. In F. M. Sirois & D. S. Molnar (Eds.), *Perfectionism, health and well-being* (pp. 45–68). Springer.

Sirois, F. M. (2015b). A self-regulation resource model of self-compassion and health behavior intentions in emerging adults. *Preventive Medicine Reports, 2*, 218–222. https://doi.org/10.1016/j.pmedr.2015.03.006

Sirois, F. M. (2016). Perfectionism and health behaviors: A self-regulation resource perspective. In F. M. Sirois & D. S. Molnar (Eds.), *Perfectionism, health, and well-being* (pp. 45–67). Springer International Publishing. https://doi.org/10.1007/978-3-319-18582-8_3

Sirois, F. M., & Hirsch, J. K. (2015). Big Five traits, affect balance and health behaviors: A self-regulation resource perspective. *Personality and Individual Differences, 87*, 59–64. https://doi.org/10.1016/j.paid.2015.07.031

Sirois, F. M., Kitner, R., & Hirsch, J. K. (2015). Self-compassion, affect, and health-promoting behaviors. *Health Psychol, 34*(6), 661–669. https://doi.org/10.1037/hea0000158

Sirois, F. M., & Pychyl, T. (2013). Procrastination and the priority of short-term mood regulation: Consequences for future self. *Social and Personality Psychology Compass, 7*(2), 115–127. https://doi.org/10.1111/spc3.12011

Sirois, F. M., & Wood, A. M. (2017). Gratitude uniquely predicts lower depression in chronic illness populations: A longitudinal study of inflammatory bowel disease and arthritis. *Health Psychology, 36*(2), 122–132. https://doi.org/10.1037/hea0000436

Smith, T. W. (2006). Personality as risk and resilience in physical health. *Current Directions in Psychological Science, 15*(5), 227–231.

Szcześniak, M., & Timoszyk-Tomczak, C. (2018). A time for being thankful: Balanced time perspective and gratitude. *Studia Psychologica, 60*, 150–166.

Tice, D. M., & Bratslavsky, E. (2000). Giving in to feel good: The place of emotion regulation in the context of general self-control. *Psychological Inquiry, 11*(3), 149–159. https://doi.org/10.1207/S15327965PLI1103_03

Thøgersen-Ntoumani, C., Dodos, L. A., Stenling, A., & Ntoumanis, N. (2021). Does self-compassion help to deal with dietary lapses among overweight and obese adults who pursue weight-loss goals? *British Journal of Health Psychology, 26*(3), 767–788. https://doi.org/10.1111/bjhp.12499

Toussaint, L., Sirois, F., Hirsch, J., Weber, A., Vajda, C., Schelling, J., Kohls, N., & Offenbacher, M. (2017). Gratitude mediates quality of life differences between fibromyalgia patients and healthy controls. *Quality of Life Research, 26*(9), 2449–2457. https://doi.org/10.1007/s11136-017-1604-7

Vickers, R. R., Conway, T. L., & Hervig, L. K. (1990). Demonstration of replicable dimensions of health behaviors. *Preventive Medicine, 19*, 377–401.

Wagner, D. D., & Heatherton, T. F. (2015). Self-regulation and its failure: The seven deadly threats to self-regulation. In M. Mikulincer, P. R. Shaver, E. Borgida, & J. A. Bargh (Eds.), *APA handbook of personality and social psychology, Volume 1:*

Attitudes and social cognition. APA handbooks in psychology (pp. 805–842). American Psychological Association.

Wolfe, W. L., & Patterson, K. (2017). Comparison of a gratitude-based and cognitive restructuring intervention for body dissatisfaction and dysfunctional eating behavior in college women. *Eating Disorders, 25*(4), 330–344. https://doi.org/10.1080/10640266.2017.1279908

Wood, A. M., Brown, G. D. A., & Maltby, J. (2011). Thanks, but I'm used to better: A relative rank model of gratitude. *Emotion, 11*, 175–180.

Wood, A. M., Froh, J. J., & Geraghty, A. W. A. (2010). Gratitude and well-being: A review and theoretical integration. *Clinical Psychology Review, 30*(7), 890–905. http://www.sciencedirect.com/science/article/pii/S0272735810000450

Wood, A. M., Joseph, S., & Linley, P. A. (2007). Coping style as a psychological resource of grateful people. *Journal of Social and Clinical Psychology, 26*(9), 1076–1093. https://doi.org/10.1521/jscp.2007.26.9.1076

Wood, A. M., Joseph, S., Lloyd, J., & Atkins, S. (2009a). Gratitude influences sleep through the mechanism of pre-sleep cognitions. *Journal of Psychosomatic Research, 66*(1), 43–48. http://linkinghub.elsevier.com/retrieve/pii/S0022399908004224?showall=true

Wood, A. M., Joseph, S., & Maltby, J. (2009b). Gratitude predicts psychological well-being above the Big Five facets. *Personality and Individual Differences, 46*(4), 443–447. https://doi.org/10.1016/j.paid.2008.11.012

Wood, A. M., Maltby, J., Gillett, R., Linley, P. A., & Joseph, S. (2008a). The role of gratitude in the development of social support, stress, and depression: Two longitudinal studies. *Journal of Research in Personality, 42*(4), 854–871. https://doi.org/10.1016/j.jrp.2007.11.003

Wood, A. M., Maltby, J., Stewart, N., & Joseph, S. (2008b). Conceptualizing gratitude and appreciation as a unitary personality trait. *Personality and Individual Differences, 44*(3), 621–632. https://doi.org/10.1016/j.paid.2007.09.028

Wood, A. M., Maltby, J., Stewart, N., Linley, P. A., & Joseph, S. (2008c). A social-cognitive model of trait and state levels of gratitude. *Emotion, 8*, 281–290.

You, S., Lee, J., & Lee, Y. (2022). Relationships between gratitude, social support, and prosocial and problem behaviors. *Current Psychology, 41*(5), 2646–2653. https://doi.org/10.1007/s12144-020-00775-4

Zaki, J., & Williams, W. C. (2013). Interpersonal emotion regulation. *Emotion, 13*(5), 803–810. https://doi.org/10.1037/a0033839

Zimbardo, P. G., & Boyd, N. (1999). Putting time in perspective: A valid, reliable, individual-differences metric. *Journal of Personality and Social Psychology, 17*, 1271–1288.

6

The Role of Passion in Optimal Functioning in Society: Theory and Research

Léandre Alexis Chénard-Poirier and Robert J. Vallerand

We can all identify a thriving person who is in a state of heightened well-being. However, when it comes to developing a scholarly definition of well-being, the task is much more arduous. What is well-being? What is living the good life? What is thriving? What characterizes optimal human functioning? These questions have been the subject of theorizing, research, and debate for centuries. Greek philosophers like Aristotle, enlightenment thinkers like Bacon, Hobbes, Humes, or Locke, and even more contemporary figures of the field of psychology such as Rogers or Maslow, all offered their own different conceptions of well-being (for reviews on the history of well-being definition, see Compton & Hoffman, 2019; Sheldon, 2004).

Having a clear understanding of the nature of well-being is at the very core of positive psychology. Indeed, Seligman and Csikszentmihalyi (2000), two founding members of this perspective, argued that "a psychology of positive human functioning will arise that achieves a scientific understanding and effective interventions to build thriving in individuals, families and communities" (p. 13). In order to promote thriving and well-being, we suggest that it is essential to better understand its nature. There are two goals to

L. A. Chénard-Poirier (✉)
Department of Management, HEC Montréal, Montréal, QC, Canada
e-mail: leandre-alexis.chenard-poirier@hec.ca

R. J. Vallerand
Research Laboratory on Social Behavior, Psychology Department, Université du Québec à Montréal, Montréal, QC, Canada

F. M. Sirois (ed.), *The Palgrave Handbook of Positive Psychology and Health*,
https://doi.org/10.1007/978-3-031-89095-6_6

this chapter. First, following a brief overview of the various perspectives on well-being, we present a multidimensional conceptualization of well-being called "Optimal Functioning in Society" (OFIS) proposed by Vallerand (2013, 2015). This perspective posits that optimal functioning entails psychological, physical, and relational well-being, along with high performance in one's main field of endeavor (e.g., work, education, sports) and contributing to society. What sets apart the OFIS model is its aim to understand human functioning in a holistic fashion, thus arguing that we must consider physical health, along with elements of psychological and social functioning that are more commonly considered in well-being conceptualizations. Second, using the Dualistic Model of Passion (DMP; Vallerand, 2010, 2015), we suggest and provide evidence that we must consider the nature of people's engagement in significant activities to understand if such engagement fosters well-being or not. Indeed, using the OFIS perspective, this chapter shows that while some forms of passion (i.e., high-intensity engagement in an activity) may facilitate well-being, others may undermine it. Of key interest for physical well-being, we show that various types of passion may either promote people's health (e.g., general physical health and energy) or lead people to engage in extreme or dangerous behaviors that may jeopardize their health (e.g., injuries, physical symptoms, exhaustion). Thus, we feel that a more fine-grained analysis of both the nature of well-being and its determinants is necessary to move the field of positive psychology forward.

Conceptualizing Well-Being

A Brief Historical Overview of Well-Being Conceptualizations

Going back millennia, several philosophers such as Socrates (469–399 BCE) and Plato (427–347 BCE) offered their perspectives on human well-being (Compton & Hoffman, 2019). However, none had more impact on contemporary conceptualizations than Aristotle (384–322 BCE). Aristotle proposed two forms of well-being. The first one, usually referred to as hedonia or living *the* good life, suggested that happiness was achieved by obtaining a maximum amount of pleasure from wealth, physical fitness, beauty, fame, and so on. The second form of happiness was eudemonia or living *a* good life, which was achieved through a lifetime of virtuous activity. Although hedonic goals may produce positive emotions, for Aristotle, they did not represent true well-being which consisted in eudemonia (Compton & Hoffman, 2019).

This idea that well-being is considered mainly as the presence of positive emotions (i.e., hedonia) or as a way of living that brings purpose and meaning to life (i.e., eudemonia) has been pervasive throughout history (see Ryan & Deci, 2001). Philosophers, theologians, and academics have repeatedly used one perspective or the other to define well-being. For example, organized religions, mostly the major monotheistic ones, have dictated in their liturgy strict ways of living virtuously to be followed by their believers to reach true happiness in the afterlife. In contrast, enlightenment philosophers such as Bacon, Hobbes, Locke, Hume, or Smith endorsed hedonic philosophies, suggesting that the pursuit of self-interest or personal gain is considered as what is the good life and the fundamental human motivation (Sheldon, 2004).

The Conceptualizations of Hedonic and Eudemonic Well-being in Psychology

In the past decades, well-being has also been studied in the field of psychology through the lens of the hedonic and eudemonic perspectives. On the one hand, the hedonic perspective has been narrowly focused on positive emotions such as happiness and pleasure. For example, Kahneman (1999) argued that human well-being could be defined or at least measured by the simple presence of positive emotions. Similarly, Diener et al. (1999) proposed the concept of subjective well-being, which defines well-being as the presence of positive emotions, the absence of negative ones, and a perception of satisfaction with life.

On the other hand, the eudemonic position has been mostly popularized in the twentieth century by humanist psychologists like Rogers (1961) and Maslow (1971), who respectively theorized well-being as a process of realizing one's full potential and as a process of self-actualization and transcendence. In line with these theorists, others also fully endorsed the eudemonic ideas that developing a sense of meaning, direction, and purpose in life through the actualization of people's potential defines well-being (Deci & Ryan, 2008; Ryan & Deci, 2001).

Contemporary Conceptualizations of Flourishing

More recent perspectives have moved beyond the hedonic and eudemonic views to embrace a multidimensional understanding of human functioning. Such a comprehensive take on well-being is often referred to as flourishing. According to Butler and Kern (2016), flourishing refers to "a dynamic optimal state of psychosocial functioning that arises from functioning well across multiple psychosocial domains" (p. 2). These models can be divided into two broad categories.

In the first category, flourishing has been considered as a positive state of functioning that can be diagnosed in the presence of a series of positive symptoms. For example, Keyes (2002, 2005) considered that flourishing individuals display symptoms of emotional wellness (i.e., life satisfaction, happiness, and interest in life), social wellness (i.e., social integration, social actualization, social acceptance, and social coherence), and psychological wellness (i.e., self-acceptance, environmental mastery, positive relations, personal growth, autonomy, and purpose in life). Likewise, Huppert and So (2013) conceptualized flourishing as the feeling of positive emotions (i.e., life satisfaction and positive emotions) with the presence of positive characteristics (i.e., emotional stability, vitality, optimism, resilience, and self-esteem) and positive functioning indicators (i.e., engagement, competence, meaning, and positive relationships).

In the second category, individuals are flourishing if they present high levels of functioning in multiple domains. For example, Seligman (2011) viewed flourishing as the presence of five elements: positive emotions, engagement, meaning and purpose in life, positive relationships, and accomplishment. Similarly, Diener et al. (2010) considered individuals to be flourishing if they display eight functioning indicators (i.e., purposeful and meaningful life, positive relations, engagement and interest in daily activities, contributing to the happiness of others, being respected by others, perceptions of being a good person, optimism toward the future, and competence in important activities). Ryff (1989) also viewed what she called positive functioning or psychological well-being as a complex phenomenon encompassing self-acceptance, positive relations, autonomy, environmental mastery, purpose in life, and personal growth. Finally, Marsh et al. (2020) conceptualized well-being as encompassing 15 different components, which are: competence, clear thinking, emotional stability, engagement, meaning, optimism, positive emotions, positive relations, resilience, self-esteem, vitality, acceptance, autonomy, empathy, and prosocial behaviors.

From this brief and non-exhaustive review of well-being conceptualizations, we observe that well-being operationalizations, specifically flourishing models, seem to have expanded their scope. Indeed, they have moved from models that focus specifically on hedonic or eudemonic well-being to broader conceptualizations where multiple aspects or domains of psychosocial functioning are considered. However, these models present some challenges. First, as Hone et al. (2014) and Forgeard et al. (2011) argue, although there is some overlap, flourishing models disagree on which dimensions of psychosocial functioning should be considered. Indeed, Martela and Sheldon (2019) identified more than 45 different conceptualizations of well-being, which encompassed a total of 63 different dimensions. Second, the World Health Organization (1948) recommended that human well-being should include psychological, social, and physical functioning. If current multidimensional models consider aspects of psychological and social well-being, they generally omit physical health (for an exception see Blasi et al., 2013). Finally, some conceptualizations include dimensions, such as personality traits or motivational states, that could be considered as *determinants* of well-being. Making the distinction between well-being and its antecedents is crucial for positive psychology. To this end, we propose that a definition of well-being should include the main domains of human functioning and leave out its antecedents. Determinants, however, should be central to the elaboration of a theory on well-being that can be useful for promoting well-being through interventions for instance. We address these issues in the next two sections.

Optimal Functioning in Society

The OFIS model of well-being (Vallerand, 2013, 2015) *proposes that optimally functioning individuals experience high levels of psychological, physical, and social well-being, along with high levels of performance in their main field of endeavor, and a perception of contributing to the community or society at large.* In line with many leading voices in this field (e.g., Diener et al., 2010; Seligman, 2011), this definition states that to be "optimally functioning", individuals must be fully engaging with their environment at high levels across multiple important life domains. For instance, workers who are performing at work at a high level would only display OFIS if such high performance takes place along high levels of psychological, physical, and relational well-being and a contribution to their community or society at large.

The OFIS construct also focuses on the multidimensional nature of well-being. Specifically, it includes the main elements of well-being seen previously. For instance, most flourishing models reviewed previously considered psychological and social well-being, as well as performance. All models presented above integrate some form of psychological well-being indicators corresponding to hedonia, such as positive emotions or happiness (Diener et al., 1999, 2010; Huppert & So, 2013; Keyes, 2005; Marsh et al., 2020; Seligman, 2011), and eudemonia, most of the time captured by a sense of meaning, direction, or purpose in life (Diener et al., 2010; Huppert & So, 2013; Keyes,

2005; Marsh et al., 2020; Ryff, 1989; Seligman, 2011). Thus, Vallerand (2016) suggests that both hedonia and eudemonia should be considered in a complete analysis of psychological well-being, specifically happiness, and meaning and purpose in life (Chénard-Poirier et al., 2023).

In addition, most flourishing models and the OFIS construct consider relationships with others as an intricate part of optimal functioning. Indeed, flourishing conceptualizations generally assess the presence of positive relationships in a person's life (Diener et al., 2010; Huppert & So, 2013; Keyes, 2005; Marsh et al., 2020; Ryff, 1989; Seligman, 2011). More precisely, they do not consider the mere presence of relationship but rather if the person is fully benefiting from them (e.g., relationships qualified as satisfying, rewarding, trusting, loving, etc.). Of interest, research has shown that different relationships (e.g., romantic relationships or friendships) differently impact well-being (Birditt & Antonucci, 2007; Girme et al., 2016). Thus, the OFIS construct defines social well-being as the presence of high-quality relationships in multiple life spheres, namely romantic and non-romantic relationships (Chénard-Poirier et al., 2023; Vallerand, 2013, 2015).

Furthermore, the OFIS construct goes beyond relationships to affirm that people with a high level of functioning also contribute to their community or society, as they should be well integrated into their broader social group. This perspective is shared by Compton and Hoffman (2019), who suggest that well-being or functioning is not a purely individualistic phenomenon that resides within the person. Rather, a thriving self should be defined as deeply intertwined with others and the society at large. This view is also shared by Diener et al. (2010), Keyes (2005), and Marsh et al. (2020), whose conceptualizations of flourishing also include social contribution or prosocial behaviors. Furthermore, considering how people function in their collectivity has long been proposed by humanist theorist Maslow (1971), who argued that people in a higher state of well-being transcend themselves to benefit human beings in general. This perspective is supported by studies showing that helping others is a more consequential factor of health than being helped (Brown et al., 2003), and that giving is more rewarding for psychological well-being than receiving (Poulin & Holman, 2013).

Most models also include some form of accomplishment or performance as part of well-being because fully functioning people see themselves as productive and accomplished. For example, Ryff (1989) and Keyes (2005) proposed the construct of environmental mastery to convey that people should be able to adequately handle their responsibilities. Similarly, Huppert and So (2013) and Seligman (2011) consider the achievement of general goals that people have set for themselves. Likewise, Diener et al. (2010) posit that competence should be observed in activities that are important for the individual. Similarly, the OFIS model proposes that individuals should perform at high levels in their main field of endeavor in life. It seems natural that to function optimally, individuals must perform in their main occupation, which is probably the life sphere where one dedicates most of their time and energy.

Finally, in line with the World Health Organization's (1948) position on well-being, the OFIS model is one of the rare well-being conceptualizations that includes physical health. Historically, health has been posited as a foundation for human functioning. For example, Aristotle agreed that health was a condition to achieve eudemonic well-being (Ryff & Singer, 2008). Later on, Maslow (1971) positioned physiological needs as the first element of his hierarchy. Recently, many have proposed that health could be a missing core element of flourishing (Friedman & Kern, 2014; Norrish, 2015; Seligman, 2018), as it is generally highly correlated with its other dimensions (e.g., Butler & Kern, 2016). Further, research has generally supported the existence of a reciprocal interplay between physical health and other areas of functioning, such as psychological well-being (Friedman & Kern, 2014; Ryff & Singer, 2008), performance (Sonnentag, 2015), or social well-being (Holt-Lunstad, 2018; Umberson et al., 2010). Thus, we want to highlight the importance of positive psychology to consider physical health in well-being conceptualizations and posit it as central to obtaining a more complete description of the full spectrum of one's functioning.

The OFIS construct thus includes five core elements that would appear to be well substantiated by past research: psychological, physical, and social well-being, high performance, and contributing to society. In addition, the OFIS model also deliberately *excludes* determinants of well-being in its construct. The present position is that a model cannot use the same variables to refer to the determinants and the measure of optimal functioning. Determinants are those that produce changes in optimal functioning and should be treated separately from their measurement. This position is thus different from that used in other models. Indeed, many conceptualizations have included motivational states such as autonomy (Keyes, 2002, 2005; Marsh et al., 2020; Ryff, 1989) and engagement (Diener et al., 2010; Huppert & So, 2013; Marsh et al., 2020; Seligman, 2011) as part of their well-being conceptualizations. However, autonomy for example is generally seen as a determinant of optimal functioning and not as an element of well-being (Chen et al., 2015; Ryan & Deci, 2017). Similarly, some models see dispositional characteristics such as personality traits (e.g., emotional stability, optimism, resilience; Huppert & So 2013; Marsh et al., 2020) as core elements of well-being. Again, personality variables have been found to contribute to the prediction of physical (e.g., Friedman & Kern, 2014) and psychological (e.g., Diener et al., 1999, 2003) well-being and performance (e.g., Judge & Zapata, 2015) and thus should not be included as core elements of well-being.

Measuring OFIS

Taking all these elements into account, Chénard-Poirier et al. (2023) recently conceptualized and validated a new scale measuring the OFIS construct. The OFIS scale contains the following six subscales: psychological well-being (e.g., *I am generally happy*; *I understand my life's meaning*), physical health (e.g., *In general, how would you say your health is? Mediocre to excellent*), social well-being through high-quality romantic relations (e.g., *In general, my current romantic relationship [or my past ones, in general, if I am not currently involved] is enriching*), social well-being through high-quality non-romantic relations (e.g., *In general, my non-romantic relationships with the people I interact with on a regular basis are enriching*), performance in one's main endeavor in life (e.g., *I generally go beyond the call of duty to reach a very high level of performance*), and contribution to the community or society (e.g., *I have a positive impact on my community or society*).

In three studies, Chénard-Poirier et al. (2023) had students and workers complete the OFIS scale and various other scales. Results from both exploratory and confirmatory factor analysis supported the six-factor structure of the scale (*Studies 1, & 2*). These factors were also moderately correlated with each other, which is expected as they all reflect some form of well-being. Using multigroup analysis, these observations (i.e., factor structure and correlations among factors) have also been shown to be invariant across samples of participants with different main endeavors in life (i.e., workers and students), age group, gender, and relationship status (i.e., in a relationship or not). In addition, the convergent and divergent validity of the scale was supported through positive and negative correlations between each OFIS dimension and a wide variety of well-being measures (i.e., positive emotions, flourishing, vitality, satisfaction with life, and sleep satisfaction) and ill-being indicators (i.e., negative emotions, pain in daily life, and need to take medicine to function; *Study 1*). Together, these results support the validity of the OFIS scale as well as the multidimensional nature of optimal functioning it reflects.

In sum, the OFIS perspective posits that domains of human functioning include psychological and physical health, high-quality social relationships with romantic partners and with others in one's social network, performance in one's main field, and finally contribution to the community or society.

People would be optimally functioning if they present high levels of functioning in all these domains. It is important to mention that the OFIS model does not claim that these dimensions exhaustively describe human well-being (Vallerand, 2013, 2015). It rather suggests that the consideration of the five OFIS dimensions allows for a parsimonious, yet comprehensive, assessment of people's functioning.

Optimal Functioning in Society: The Perspective of the Dualistic Model of Passion

The first section of this chapter focused on defining the concept of well-being through the lens of the OFIS model (Vallerand, 2013, 2015). This model posits that a conceptualization of well-being in positive psychology should consider physical health, along with more common dimensions of psychological and social functioning. We now turn our attention to another issue in the field of positive psychology, which is the promotion of well-being. We specifically focus on the role of intentional activities in the promotion of optimal functioning. In this section, we discuss how the DMP (Vallerand, 2015; Vallerand et al., 2003) explains why intentional activities might not invariably lead to increased well-being. We do so by exploring the relationship between the concept of passion and the OFIS model.

Intentional Activities and Well-being

Intentional activities are actions or activities that people choose to engage in. Such activities typically foster well-being (Lyubomirsky et al., 2005). The Sustainable Happiness Model (Lyubomirsky et al., 2005; also see Layous & Lyubomirsky, 2014) argues that this broad category of behaviors represents the "best potential route" (p. 119) to sustained well-being because people have control over their involvement in these activities, contrary to other antecedents of well-being such as personality traits or life circumstances. In addition, these activities are also well aligned with the eudemonic perspective on well-being development. Indeed, Waterman et al. (2010) posit that well-being is attained through active involvement in meaningful activities that are expressive of people's identity, and which foster growth and a sense of purpose in life.

If intentional activities contribute to increased well-being, recent critics of the Sustainable Happiness Model have argued they may have a much smaller impact than expected (Brown & Rohrer, 2020). Lyubomirsky et al. (2005)

initially suggested that such activities would explain up to 40% of the variance of people's well-being. However, Sheldon and Lyubomirsky (2021) revised this evaluation downward, citing a meta-analysis by Klug & Maier (2015), who found the explained variance between the achievement of important personal goals and well-being (i.e., indication of an activity effect on well-being) was approximately 15%. In light of these observations, we may ask why intentional activities may not be as effective as previously thought. A possible explanation for this question comes from the DMP (Vallerand, 2015; Vallerand et al., 2003), which posits that to understand if an intentional activity will foster well-being or not, we must consider the quality of one's engagement in it. Specifically, Vallerand and colleagues and many others (see Curran et al., 2015; Vallerand, 2015; Vallerand et al., 2003; Vallerand & Houlfort, 2019) have shown in hundreds of original studies that a passion, which represents a specific type of motivational force to engage in intentional activities that can take two forms, may either enhance or hinder people's optimal functioning. Thus, not all passions are equivalent in the promotion of well-being.

The Dualistic Model of Passion

According to the DMP (Vallerand, 2015; Vallerand et al., 2003), passion is a strong inclination toward a self-defining activity that people love, find important and meaningful in their life, and in which they will invest a considerable amount of time and energy. The concept of passion perfectly taps into this idea that fully engaging in an intentional activity that one loves should lead to sustainable well-being (Vallerand, 2012). However, the DMP also posits that depending on how a passion is internalized into the identity, it may either take a harmonious form and foster optimal functioning or an obsessive form that may lead to lower levels of functioning and at times can even be detrimental to one's well-being (e.g., Philippe et al., 2010).

More specifically, harmonious passion (HP) occurs when a person freely engages in a passionate activity, which will be autonomously internalized into their identity. This takes place when the activity is internalized into the identity merely out of love for it (Vallerand, 2015). Passion is then characterized by a strong but controllable and flexible motivational force to be fully engaged in the activity, allowing the person to be mindful (St-Louis et al., 2018), and to experience a state of flow, positive emotions, satisfaction, and energy (Vallerand, 2015). In contrast, obsessive passion (OP) occurs when the activity becomes part of the identity out of love for it but also for some external contingencies, such as social acceptance or a boost of self-esteem stemming from success (e.g., Lafrenière et al., 2011; Mageau et al., 2011). Such internalization to the identity creates a compulsive urge to engage in the beloved activity in a less than mindful manner, which increases the risk of conflict with other life spheres and is accompanied by ruminative thoughts, negative emotions, and behaviors that could jeopardize one's physical health (Vallerand, 2015). It is crucial to highlight that both harmoniously and obsessively passionate individuals love their passionate activity and find it important in their lives. However, the quality of one's engagement in intentional activities (harmonious or obsessive) should determine if optimal functioning will be experienced. The research described below support this hypothesis.

Harmonious and Obsessive Passion as Determinants of Optimal Functioning in Society

Multiple studies have investigated the relationship between harmonious and obsessive passion and the OFIS dimensions. Below, we first explore how both types of passion are individually related to psychological, physical, and social well-being, as well as performance and perception of contribution to the community or society. Then, we present research that investigated the relationship between passion and all the OFIS dimensions within the realm of the same study using the OFIS scale (Chénard-Poirier et al., 2023).

Psychological Well-being. Psychological well-being has probably been one of the most researched outcomes of passion. Studies have respectively shown positive and negative associations between HP and OP and indicators of hedonic and eudemonic psychological well-being, such as life satisfaction, subjective well-being, happiness, meaning in life, and thriving (e.g., Carpentier et al., 2012; Forest et al., 2011; Lalande et al. 2017; Philippe et al., 2010; St-Cyr et al., 2021; St-Louis et al., 2021). In addition, positive associations between OP and indicators of ill-being such as negative effects, burnout, and depression have also been observed, while HP is typically negatively related to such indicators (e.g., Bélanger et al., 2015, 2020; Fernet et al., 2014; Lalande et al. 2017; St-Louis et al., 2021; Vallerand et al., 2010).

Of importance, the DMP posits that the quality of one's engagement determines if passion will have a positive effect on well-being. When passionate about a given activity, people will engage in it on average eight hours per week (e.g., Vallerand et al., 2003) and much more if one is passionate about work. Thus, what people experience during such engagement can have powerful mediating effects between passion and well-being. A number of mediators have been uncovered that explain the effects of HP and OP on psychological well-being. For example, several studies have shown that the relationships between HP and psychological well-being were mediated by the satisfaction of the three basic psychological needs of autonomy, competence, and relatedness (e.g., Curran et al., 2013; Kent et al., 2018; Forest et al., 2011). Conversely, findings regarding OP are rather inconsistent, as the mediating role of the basic psychological need—*dissatisfaction*—in the relationship between OP and well-being has been only sporadically obtained in some studies (Kent et al., 2018) but not others (Curran et al., 2013). Further, Carpentier et al. (2012) showed that HP was positively related to the experience of flow in the passionate activity and in other life activities (e.g., studies), which in turn led to higher psychological well-being. In contrast, OP was found to be positively associated with rumination about passion when doing other life activities (i.e., one's studies). This rumination was found to hinder subsequent psychological well-being. Finally, St-Louis et al. (2021) found that harmoniously and obsessively passionate individuals were also prone to adopt different emotion-regulation strategies to face adversity in their life, which in turn explained their respective positive and negative relationships with psychological well-being. Specifically, in three studies, St-Louis et al. (2021) found that harmoniously passionate individuals tended to adopt mature emotion-regulation strategies (i.e., cognitive reappraisal), while obsessively passionate people tended to adopt ineffective ones (i.e., emotional suppression).

Physical Well-being. Of particular interest, research on passion suggests that the impact of intentional activities goes beyond the realm of psychosocial functioning and affects physical health. Research supports the major hypothesis that HP for a given activity fosters overall physical health, while OP may lead to the experience of physical ill-being. For instance, Schellenberg et al. (2019, *Study 1*) showed in a study conducted among university students that HP and OP for any given activity were, respectively, positively and negatively related to a self-rated perception of general health. Similarly, multiple studies conducted among video game players showed that higher OP may lead to more physical symptoms related to video gaming (e.g., dry eyes, loss appetites, dizziness, sleep disorders, etc.), while HP was not related to such symptoms (Lafrenière et al., 2009; Schellenberg et al., 2019, *Study 2*). Research even showed that HP could be a positive resource for people who suffer from health problems. For example, Schellenberg et al. (2021) showed that HP for a meaningful activity was associated with less physical pain (e.g., stomach pain, headaches, or nausea) among breast cancer survivors within the first 20 weeks of primary treatment, while OP was unrelated to it. Thus, research shows that HP and OP have the potential to enhance or hinder people's physical well-being. Multiple pathways have been proposed to explain these relationships.

First, passion for an activity could either provide people with energy or deprive them from it. According to Vallerand (2015), people with an HP are able to be fully immersed and mindful when they engage in their passion, which allows the activity to be a source of energy in their lives. Indeed, research has repeatedly shown a positive relationship between HP and the experience of vitality while engaging in passionate activity, which comprises an energetic component (Ryan & Frederick, 1997). This association has been observed for passion for many activities such as sports (Vallerand et al., 2006, *Study 2*) or work (Forest et al., 2011; Lalande et al., 2017). Similarly, Stoeber et al. (2011) studied passion for studies among university students and showed a positive association between HP and the experience of vigor while studying. Przybylski et al. (2009) even showed that HP for video games was associated with heightened levels of energy (e.g., feeling active, energetic, vigorous, etc.) following activity engagement.

The same conclusion is not applicable to OP. If Stoeber et al. (2011) showed that OP for studies is positively associated with vigor, all the other studies cited above reported no significant relations between passion and vitality (Forest et al., 2011; Lalande et al., 2017; Vallerand et al., 2006, *Study 2*). Further, if people with an OP could feel more energy in the short term when engaging in their passion, it does not seem to be the case in the long term. Indeed, the compulsive nature of obsessively passionate people's engagement accompanied by conflicts with their other life spheres (e.g., leisure), ruminative thoughts, and negative emotions, may have in the long term a toll on health (Vallerand, 2015). Research has shown OP to be positively related to burnout, which comprises a component of exhaustion, in multiple fields such as sports (Gustafsson et al., 2011), work (Bélanger et al., 2015, *Study 2*; Fernet et al., 2014; Vallerand et al., 2010), or studies (Schellenberg et al., 2019, *Study 4*). A study by Bélanger et al. (2020) even showed that OP for any activity was related to a higher presence of depressive mood symptoms, which in turn lead to worse sleep quality, which has been identified as a major contributor to physical health (Buysse, 2014). HP on the contrary has been negatively associated with burnout (Bélanger et al., 2015, *Study 2*; Fernet et al., 2014; Gustafsson et al., 2011; Schellenberg et al., 2019, *Study 4*) and depressive moods (Bélanger et al., 2020).

Second, both types of passion may facilitate engagement in activities that foster physical well-being. For example, people often develop a passion that facilitates sustained engagement in physical activity such as exercise or a sport (Halvari et al., 2009; Parastatidou et al., 2012; Rip et al., 2006; Stephan et al.,

2009). However, while the flexible engagement of people with an HP allows them to have a more balanced and healthier lifestyle, people with an OP tend to neglect their physical health and engage in dangerous behaviors again due to the compulsive nature of their engagement. For example, people with an OP for sport may engage in their activity to a point where they will suffer injuries and other physical symptoms. Rip et al. (2006) studied passion for dance and showed that more obsessively passionate dancers were more likely to suffer from chronic injuries. They were also less likely to seek treatment out of pride and more likely to ignore the pain. On the contrary, dancers with an HP were not only less likely to suffer injuries but when injured they tended to take necessary actions to heal. They were also more likely to take action to prevent future injuries. Akehurst and Oliver (2014) also found that dancers with an OP, but not with an HP, were less likely to visit a doctor or follow treatment when injured. In a similar fashion, Stephan et al. (2009) have shown that competitive runners with an OP were more susceptible to suffer from a sport-related injury, while runners with an HP were less susceptible. Finally, Vallerand et al. (2003, *Study 3*) have shown that residents from Montreal who were passionate about cycling were more likely to continue cycling during the winter compared to harmoniously passionate cyclists. Bear in mind that cycling during the winter in a northern city such as Montreal is a very dangerous activity.

This tendency toward risky behaviors is not limited to sports and exercise. St-Louis et al. (2016) studied passion for a cause among people involved in humanitarian work. Multiple studies showed that the more humanitarian workers had an OP for their cause, the more they tended to self-neglect their health, which in turn was associated with injuries related to their involvement in the cause (*Study 2*) and physical symptoms (*Study 3*). Such associations were not observed for HP. On the contrary, harmoniously passionate people tend to pay greater attention to their physical health. For instance, Caudroit et al. (2011) showed the more teachers were harmoniously passionate about their work, the more they engaged in physical activity in their leisure time. Such association was not observed for OP.

Social Well-being. Regarding social well-being, the flexible and balanced engagement of harmoniously passionate individuals in their passionate activity has been associated with the ability to develop and maintain high-quality romantic (Carbonneau & Vallerand, 2013; Ratelle et al., 2013; Seguin-Lévesque et al., 2003; Vallerand et al., 2008b) and non-romantic relationships (Philippe et al., 2010; Utz et al., 2012). On the contrary, the rigid and compulsive nature of OP has been shown to have negative consequences on the ability of obsessively passionate individuals to develop and maintain quality relationships (Philippe et al., 2010; Seguin-Lévesque et al., 2003; Utz et al., 2012; Vallerand et al., 2008b). For example, Utz et al. (2012) showed that HP and OP were, respectively, positively and negatively related to the quality of friendships developed outside their passionate activity. Similarly, Séguin-Lévesque et al. (2003) showed that HP led to higher couple adjustment (i.e., agreement regarding various aspects of a couple's relationship) and fewer conflicts, while opposite results were observed for OP. Vallerand et al. (2008b) also showed that OP for being a soccer fan was associated with more conflicts between soccer and the couple, which in turn led to lower levels of the partner's relational satisfaction. HP did not lead to any conflict.

In addition to the flexible and rigid activity engagement that are characteristic of HP and OP, respectively, Philippe et al. (2010) have also shown that the emotions experienced while engaging in one's passionate activity may also explain why passion is related to social well-being. Specifically, positive emotions broaden the thought-action repertoires and the self of people (Fredrickson, 2001; Waugh & Fredrickson, 2006), which lead to more positive behaviors toward others (e.g., showing interest in others, encouraging, smiling, etc.). On the contrary, negative emotions narrow the thought-action repertoires and the self, which lead individuals to shut themselves from others (Waugh & Fredrickson, 2006). Philippe et al. (2010) have shown through four studies that HP was positively associated with positive emotions and negatively associated with negative emotions, whereas OP was only related to negative emotions. In turn, positive and negative emotions were, respectively, positively and negatively related to the development and maintenance of high-quality relationships perceived by the person and by an external observer in a variety of life domains such as work, education, and sports.

Performance. Research has supported the role of passion in the promotion or inhibition of performance in passionate activities. Indeed, individuals who are harmoniously passionate for an activity tend to display high performance in it (e.g., work, studies, professional sports practice; e.g., Astakhova & Porter, 2015; Ho et al., 2011; Schellenberg & Bailis, 2016; Vallerand et al., 2007, 2008a). In addition, HP for an activity (i.e., sport) has been shown to have a positive spillover effect on performance in another life activity such as work (Clohessy et al., 2020). Likewise, according to Vallerand (2015), the rigid engagement displayed by obsessively passionate people may give them the energy and motivation to perform at a high level in their passionate activity. However, this intense rigid engagement is not always sustainable over time and may even lead to burnout (Bélanger et al., 2015, *Study 2*; Fernet et al., 2014; Gustafsson et al., 2011; Schellenberg et al., 2019, *Study 4;* Vallerand et al., 2010). Thus, the association between OP and performance has been shown to be erratic in the literature. Indeed, some studies showed positive (e.g., Vallerand et al., 2007, 2008a), negative (e.g., Schellenberg & Bailis, 2016; for metanalytic observations see Curran et al., 2015), and no associations between OP and performance (e.g., Astakhova & Porter, 2015; Ho et al., 2011). Further, no positive spillover effect of OP for other activities on performance in the main endeavor in life has been observed (Clohessy et al., 2020). Vallerand (2015, chapter 10) presents a detailed analysis of how different mediators triggered by HP and OP may explain the different performance effects of passion both in the short and long term.

Contribution to the Community or Society. A number of studies looked at how passion for a cause may lead to adaptive outcomes for society. For instance, Rip et al. (2012, *Study 1*) showed that HP for politics led to adaptive behaviors such as trying to educate people and sharing information. Conversely, OP for politics fostered more radical behaviors such as engaging in subversive acts and rioting. Gousse-Lessard et al. (2013) found similar results with individuals passionate about the preservation of the environment. In another study dealing with passion for religion, Rip et al. (2012, *Study 2*) showed that OP led to extreme, violent, behaviors toward other groups who don't share their faith, whereas HP fostered sharing and forgiving. Finally, a series of studies by St-Louis et al. (2016) showed that HP for a humanitarian cause (such as Doctors Without Borders) led one to being successful in bringing solace to suffering countries while at the same time experiencing high levels of psychological and physical health. Conversely, OP did not predict success in the help provided toward the cause but led to post-traumatic stress disorder, and negative physical health problems (St-Louis et al., 2016, *Study 3*).

As Kruglanski et al. (2021) put it, contrary to HP, OP typically leads to extreme behavior, which may often turn against self and others, including society. Thus, passion may contribute positively or negatively to society, depending on its nature. Much more research is necessary on the role of passion in this important OFIS dimension.

Passion as a Determinant of the Multidimensional OFIS Construct. The research presented above is important as it shows the different roles of HP and OP for specific dimensions of the OFIS construct. However, such research did not assess all dimensions of the OFIS construct within the confines of the same study. Thus, it is not clear whether the findings remain the same while measuring *all* OFIS elements at the same time. Recent studies have done so. In one study, Bouizegarene et al. (2018, *Study 2*) assessed the relationship between passion for one's university studies and all five OFIS elements (using a preliminary version of the OFIS scale). The results showed that HP was positively related to students' psychological, physical, and social well-being, as well as their academic performance, and the perception that they contribute to their community or society. Interestingly, OP was only negatively related to social well-being measured as the presence of quality of interpersonal relationships in general. No other results were significant with OP. These results are important as they provide support for the role of the DMP. Specifically, HP led overall to higher levels of OFIS than OP.

Chénard-Poirier et al. (2023; *Study 3*) examined longitudinal directional associations between forms of passion and the OFIS dimensions with a sample of workers. They found that having an HP for one's work showed to be a positive determinant of psychological, physical, and social well-being. However, it was not related to performance at work. Further, longitudinal associations suggested a positive directional relationship from the perception of contributing to society to HP. Thus, this specific study suggested that HP might be a vector of health according to the World Health Organization (1948; physical, psychological, and social well-being), but not performance. Further, it was suggested that workers could be more prone to developing an HP when they perceive their job has an impact on their community.

This study also showed OP was a vector of poor physical health and higher performance. In addition, OP was positively related to high-quality romantic relationships and not related to the remaining OFIS dimensions. On one hand, and in line with the DMP, the compulsive engagement of obsessively passionate workers might enhance their performance to the detriment of their health. On the other hand, the association between OP and the quality of romantic relationships was quite surprising. Chénard-Poirier et al. (2023) noted that studies considering these variables generally were interested in a passion for activities other than work (e.g., sports, Vallerand et al., 2008b). They suggest that a passion for work might be much more time-consuming compared to other passionate activities. Thus, obsessively passionate individuals might prioritize their romantic relationships.

In sum, research on the role of intentional activities in the promotion of well-being supports the DMP on two counts. First, there is empirical support for a multidimensional view of well-being as described by the OFIS model and as captured by the OFIS scale (Chénard-Poirier et al., 2023). Second, in line with the DMP, research also shows that it is crucial to take into consideration the quality of people's engagement in intentional activities to accurately predict whether such engagement will have a positive or negative impact on functioning. As the research reviewed here shows, intentional activities should have a positive impact on well-being to the extent that they are fueled by HP. Engaging in such activities out of OP should lead to less adaptive, and sometimes maladaptive, effects on optimal functioning.

Concluding Remarks

This chapter sought to resolve two central issues pertaining to the relevance of positive psychology to the understanding of well-being. The first issue addressed in this chapter pertained to the conceptualization of well-being. Specifically, models of well-being in positive psychology disagree on its nature. In addition, most conceptualizations in our field omit to consider physical health. In light of these matters, this chapter makes the point that Vallerand's (2013, 2015) OFIS model represents a valid representation of human optimal functioning. Specifically, the OFIS operationalizes optimal functioning as the presence of high levels of psychological, physical, and social well-being, as well as performance in one's main endeavor in life, and contribution to the community or society. Further, the OFIS construct can be validly assessed with a new scale. Future research on OFIS using this scale would present an exciting new avenue for positive psychology. We mention one caveat. Although this model has received empirical support (Chénard-Poirier et al., 2023), much research is still needed to address a number of issues including the interplay among its five elements. Such research would help determine if lower functioning in one or more dimensions would over time have a negative impact on the others.

The second issue addressed in this chapter pertained to the role of intentional activities in the promotion of well-being. This chapter argued and reported research that showed that it is crucial to consider people's quality of engagement in intentional activities to better understand their consequences on optimal functioning. In line with the DMP, it was hypothesized and found that only intentional activities in which one freely engages out of HP promote people's OFIS. OP for such activities does not lead to the same adaptive outcomes and may even lead to ill-being, including poor physical health.

Future research should further explore the nomological network of the OFIS in at least two ways. First, we should identify how antecedents other than passion, such as personality traits, motivational states, or life circumstances relate to each dimension of the OFIS model. Second, research should further identify the mediating mechanisms explaining the associations between intentional activities and the OFIS construct. Many mediating mechanisms have been proposed to understand the relationship between passion and mostly psychological and social well-being (e.g., psychological need satisfaction, positive and negative emotions, coping mechanisms, emotion regulation strategies, flow, etc.). Future studies could investigate how these mediating variables are associated with all the OFIS dimensions, and how they are promoted or hindered by HP and OP or other determinants of well-being. Such research would be even more important for physical well-being as this dimension is understudied, even though the limited evidence indicates promising and possibly impactful contributions to the field of positive psychology.

Understanding the nature and the vicissitudes of well-being is a complex undertaking. In this chapter, we have proposed to adopt the view of the DMP (Vallerand, 2012, 2015) wherein the nature of well-being is best captured in a multidimensional perspective and passion for meaningful activities reflects a powerful determinant. We hope that such a position will generate interest in future research on these issues and help move the field of positive psychology forward.

References

Akehurst, S., & Oliver, E. J. (2014). Obsessive passion: a dependency associated with injury-related risky behaviour in dancers. *Journal of Sports Sciences, 32*(3), 259–267. https://doi.org/10.1080/02640414.2013.823223

Astakhova, M. N., & Porter, G. (2015). Understanding the work passion–performance relationship: The mediating role of organizational identification and moderating role of fit at work. *Human Relations, 68*(8), 1315–1346. https://doi.org/10.1177/0018726714555204

Bélanger, J. J., Pierro, A., Kruglanski, A. W., Vallerand, R. J., De Carlo, N., & Falco, A. (2015). On feeling good at work: The role of regulatory mode and passion in psychological adjustment. *Journal of Applied Social Psychology, 45*(6), 319–329. https://doi.org/10.1111/jasp.12298

Bélanger, J. J., Raafat, K. A., Nisa, C. F., & Schumpe, B. M. (2020). Passion for an activity: a new predictor of sleep quality. *Sleep, 43*(12), zsaa107. https://doi.org/10.1093/sleep/zsaa107

Birditt, K. S., & Antonucci, T. C. (2007). Relationship quality profiles and well-being among married adults. *Journal of Family Psychology, 21*(4), 595–604. https://doi.org/10.1037/0893-3200.21.4.595

Blasi, E., Nucera, M., Cicatiello, C., & Franco, S. (2013). Sociodemographic components of eudaimonic well-being: A survey in an Italian province. *Social Indicators Research, 2013*(113), 451–470. https://doi.org/10.1007/s11205-012-0104-y

Bouizegarene, N., Bourdeau, S., Leduc, C., Gousse-Lessard, A. S., Houlfort, N., & Vallerand, R. J. (2018). We are our passions: The role of identity processes in harmonious and obsessive passion and links to optimal functioning in society. *Self and Identity, 17*(1), 56–74. https://doi.org/10.1177/0265407519864446

Brown, N. J., & Rohrer, J. M. (2020). Easy as (happiness) pie? A critical evaluation of a popular model of the determinants of well-being. *Journal of Happiness Studies, 21*(4), 1285–1301. https://doi.org/10.1007/s10902-019-00128-4

Brown, S. L., Nesse, R. M., Vinokur, A. D., & Smith, D. M. (2003). Providing social support may be more beneficial than receiving it: Results from a prospective study of mortality. *Psychological Science, 14*(4), 320–327. https://doi.org/10.1111/1467-9280.14461

Butler, J., & Kern, M. L. (2016). The PERMA-Profiler: A brief multidimensional measure of flourishing. *International Journal of Wellbeing, 6*(3), 1–48. https://doi.org/10.5502/ijw.v6i3.526

Buysse, D. J. (2014). Sleep health: can we define it? Does it matter? *Sleep, 37*(1), 9–17. https://doi.org/10.5665/sleep.3298

Carbonneau, N., & Vallerand, R. J. (2013). On the role of harmonious and obsessive romantic passion in conflict behavior. *Motivation and Emotion, 37*(4), 743–757. https://doi.org/10.1007/s11031-013-9354-5

Carpentier, J., Mageau, G. A., & Vallerand, R. J. (2012). Ruminations and flow: Why do people with a more harmonious passion experience higher well-being? *Journal of Happiness Studies, 13*(3), 501–518. https://doi.org/10.1007/s10902-011-9276-4

Caudroit, J., Boiché, J., Stephan, Y., Le Scanff, C., & Trouilloud, D. (2011). Predictors of work/family interference and leisure-time physical activity among teachers: The role of passion towards work. *European Journal of Work and Organizational Psychology, 20*(3), 326–344. https://doi.org/10.1080/13594320903507124

Chen, B., Vansteenkiste, M., Beyers, W., Boone, L., Deci, E. L., Van der Kaap-Deeder, J., Duriez, B., Lens, W., Matos, L., Mouratidi, A., Ryan, R., Sheldon, K. M., Soenens, B., Van Petegem, S., & Verstuyf, J. (2015). Basic psychological need satisfaction, need frustration, and need strength across four cultures. *Motivation and Emotion, 39*(2), 216–236. https://doi.org/10.1007/s11031-014-9450-1

Chénard-Poirier, L. A., Vallerand, R. J., Verner-Filion, J., Houlfort, N., Forest, J., & Rinfret, N. (2023). Optimal functioning in society: A conceptualization, a measure, and a look at determinants. *Journal of Happiness Studies, 24*(2023), 857–892. https://doi.org/10.1007/s10902-023-00617-7

Clohessy, T., Whelan, E., & Paradis, K. F. (2020). Does passion for physical activity spillover into performance at work? Examining the direct and indirect effects of passion and life satisfaction on organisational performance and innovativeness. *International Journal of Sport and Exercise Psychology, 1–21*. https://doi.org/10.1080/1612197X.2020.1766537

Compton, W. C., & Hoffman, E. (2013). *Positive psychology: The science of happiness and flourishing* (2nd ed.). Wadsworth Cengage Learning.

Compton, W. C., & Hoffman, E. (2019). *Positive psychology: The science of happiness and flourishing* (3rd ed.). Sage Publications.

Curran, T., Appleton, P. R., Hill, A. P., & Hall, H. K. (2013). The mediating role of psychological need satisfaction in relationships between types of passion for sport and athlete burnout. *Journal of Sports Sciences, 31*(6), 597–606. https://doi.org/10.1080/02640414.2012.742956

Curran, T., Hill, A. P., Appleton, P. R., Vallerand, R. J., & Standage, M. (2015). The psychology of passion: A meta-analytical review of a decade of research on intrapersonal outcomes. *Motivation and Emotion, 39*(5), 631–655. https://doi.org/10.1007/s11031-015-9503-0

Deci, E. L., & Ryan, R. M. (2008). Hedonia, eudaimonia, and well-being: An introduction. *Journal of Happiness Studies, 9*(1), 1–11. https://doi.org/10.1007/s10902-006-9018-1

Diener, E., Oishi, S., & Lucas, R. E. (2003). Personality, culture, and subjective well-being: emotional and cognitive evaluations of life. *Annual Review of Psychology, 54*(1), 403–425. https://doi.org/10.1146/annurev.psych.54.101601.145056

Diener, E., Suh, E. M., Lucas, R. E., & Smith, H. L. (1999). Subjective well-being: Three decades of progress. *Psychological Bulletin, 125*(2), 276–302. https://doi.org/10.1037/0033-2909.125.2.276

Diener, E., Wirtz, D., Tov, W., Kim-Prieto, C., Choi, D., Oishi, S., & Biswas-Diener, R. (2010). New well-being measures: Short scales to assess flourishing and positive and negative feelings. *Social Indicators Research, 97*(2), 143–156. https://doi.org/10.1007/s11205-009-9493-y

Fernet, C., Lavigne, G. L., Vallerand, R. J., & Austin, S. (2014). Fired up with passion: Investigating how job autonomy and passion predict burnout at career start in teachers. *Work & Stress, 28*(3), 270–288. https://doi.org/10.1080/02678373.2014.935524

Forest, J., Mageau, G. A., Sarrazin, C., & Morin, E. M. (2011). "Work is my passion": The different affective, behavioural, and cognitive consequences of harmonious and obsessive passion toward work. *Canadian Journal of Administrative Sciences/Revue Canadienne des Sciences de l'Administration, 28*(1), 27–40. https://doi.org/10.1002/cjas.170

Forgeard, M. J. C., Jayawickreme, E., Kern, M. L., & Seligman, M. E. P. (2011). Doing the right thing: measuring well-being for public policy. *International Journal of Wellbeing, 1*(1). https://doi.org/10.5502/ijw.v1i1.15

Fredrickson, B. L. (2001). The role of positive emotions in positive psychology: The broaden-and-build theory of positive emotions. *American Psychologist, 56*(3), 218–226. https://doi.org/10.1037/0003-066X.56.3.218

Friedman, H. S., & Kern, M. L. (2014). Personality, well-being, and health. *Annual Review of Psychology, 65*(1), 719–742. https://doi.org/10.1146/annurev-psych-010213-115123

Girme, Y. U., Overall, N. C., Faingataa, S., & Sibley, C. G. (2016). Happily single: the link between relationship status and well-being depends on avoidance and approach social goals. *Social Psychological and Personality Science, 7*(2), 122–130. https://doi.org/10.1177/1948550615599828

Gousse-Lessard, A. S., Vallerand, R. J., Carbonneau, N., & Lafrenière, M. A. K. (2013). The role of passion in mainstream and radical behaviors: A look at environmental activism. *Journal of Environmental Psychology, 35*(2013), 18–29. https://doi.org/10.1016/j.jenvp.2013.03.003

Gustafsson, H., Hassmén, P., & Hassmén, N. (2011). Are athletes burning out with passion? *European Journal of Sport Science, 11*(6), 387–395. https://doi.org/10.1080/17461391.2010.536573

Halvari, H., Ulstad, S. O., Bagøien, T. E., & Skjesol, K. (2009). Autonomy support and its links to physical activity and competitive performance: Mediations through motivation, competence, action orientation and harmonious passion, and the moderator role of autonomy support by perceived competence. *Scandinavian Journal of Educational Research, 53*(6), 533–555. https://doi.org/10.1080/00313830903302059

Ho, V. T., Wong, S. S., & Lee, C. H. (2011). A tale of passion: Linking job passion and cognitive engagement to employee work performance. *Journal of Management Studies, 48*(1), 26–47. https://doi.org/10.1111/j.1467-6486.2009.00878.x

Holt-Lunstad, J. (2018). Why social relationships are important for physical health: A systems approach to understanding and modifying risk and protection. *Annual Review of Psychology, 69*(2018), 437–458. https://doi.org/10.1146/annurev-psych-122216-011902

Hone, L. C., Jarden, A., Schofield, G., & Duncan, S. (2014). Measuring flourishing: The impact of operational definitions on the prevalence of high levels of wellbeing. *International Journal of Wellbeing, 4*(1), 62–90. https://doi.org/10.5502/ijw.v4i1.4

Huppert, F. A., & So, T. T. C. (2013). Flourishing across Europe: Application of a new conceptual framework for defining well-being. *Social Indicators Research, 110*(3), 837–861. https://doi.org/10.1007/s11205-011-9966-7

Judge, T. A., & Zapata, C. P. (2015). The person–situation debate revisited: Effect of situation strength and trait activation on the validity of the big five personality traits in predicting job performance. *Academy of Management Journal, 58*(4), 1149–1179. https://doi.org/10.5465/amj.2010.0837

Kahneman, D. (1999). Objective happiness. In D. Kahneman, E. Diener, & N. Schwarz (Eds.), *Well-being: The foundations of hedonic psychology* (pp. 3–25). Russell Sage Foundation.

Kent, S., Kingston, K., & Paradis, K. F. (2018). The relationship between passion, basic psychological needs satisfaction and athlete burnout: Examining direct and indirect effects. *Journal of Clinical Sport Psychology, 12*(1), 75–96. https://doi.org/10.1123/jcsp.2017-0030

Keyes, C. L. M. (2002). The mental health continuum: From languishing to flourishing in life. *Journal of Health and Social Behavior, 43*(2), 207. https://doi.org/10.2307/3090197

Keyes, C. L. M. (2005). Mental illness and/or mental health? Investigating axioms of the complete state model of health. *Journal of Consulting and Clinical Psychology, 73*(3), 539–548. https://doi.org/10.1037/0022-006X.73.3.539

Klug, H. J., & Maier, G. W. (2015). Linking goal progress and subjective well-being: A meta-analysis. *Journal of Happiness Studies, 16*(1), 37–65. https://doi.org/10.1007/s10902-013-9493-0

Kruglanski, A. W., Szumowska, E., Kopetz, C. H., Vallerand, R. J., & Pierro, A. (2021). On the psychology of extremism: How motivational imbalance breeds intemperance. *Psychological Review, 128*(2), 264–289. https://doi.org/10.1037/rev0000260

Lafrenière, M.-A. K., Bélanger, J. J., Sedikides, C., & Vallerand, R. J. (2011). Self-esteem and passion for activities. *Personality and Individual Differences, 51*(4), 541–544. https://doi.org/10.1016/j.paid.2011.04.017

Lafrenière, M.-A. K., Vallerand, R. J., Donahue, R., & Lavigne, G. L. (2009). On the costs and benefits of gaming: The role of passion. *Cyberpsychology and Behavior, 12*(3), 285–290. https://doi.org/10.1089/cpb.2008.0234

Lalande, D., Vallerand, R. J., Lafrenière, M. A. K., Verner-Filion, J., Laurent, F. A., Forest, J., & Paquet, Y. (2017). Obsessive passion: A compensatory response to unsatisfied needs. *Journal of personality, 85*(2), 163–178. https://doi.org/10.1111/jopy.12229

Layous, K. T. I. N., & Lyubomirsky, S. (2014). The how, why, what, when, and who of happiness. In J. Gruber & J. T. Moskowitz (Eds.), *Positive emotion: Integrating the light sides and dark sides* (pp. 473–495). Oxford University Press.

Lyubomirsky, S., Sheldon, K. M., & Schkade, D. (2005). Pursuing happiness: The architecture of sustainable change. *Review of general psychology, 9*(2), 111–131. https://doi.org/10.1037/1089-2680.9.2.111

Mageau, G. A., Carpentier, J., & Vallerand, R. J. (2011). The role of self-esteem contingencies in the distinction between obsessive and harmonious passion. *European Journal of Social Psychology, 41*(6), 720–729. https://doi.org/10.1002/ejsp.798

Marsh, H. W., Huppert, F. A., Donald, J. N., Horwood, M. S., & Sahdra, B. K. (2020). The well-being profile (WB-Pro): Creating a theoretically based multidimensional measure of well-being to advance theory, research, policy, and practice. *Psychological Assessment, 32*(3), 294–313. https://doi.org/10.1037/pas0000787

Martela, F., & Sheldon, K. M. (2019). Clarifying the concept of well-being: Psychological need satisfaction as the common core connecting eudaimonic and subjective well-being. *Review of General Psychology, 23*(4), 458–474. https://doi.org/10.1177/1089268019880886

Maslow, A. H. (1971). *The farther reaches of human nature.* Viking Press.

Norrish, J. (2015). *Positive education: The Geelong Grammar School journey.* Oxford University Press. https://doi.org/10.1093/acprof:oso/9780198702580.001.0001

Parastatidou, I. S., Doganis, G., Theodorakis, Y., & Vlachopoulos, S. P. (2012). Exercising with passion: Initial validation of the Passion Scale in exercise. *Measurement in Physical Education and Exercise Science, 16*(2), 119–134. https://doi.org/10.1080/1091367X.2012.657561

Philippe, F. L., Vallerand, R. J., Houlfort, N., Lavigne, G. L., & Donahue, E. G. (2010). Passion for an activity and quality of interpersonal relationships: The mediating role of emotions. *Journal of Personality and Social Psychology, 98*(6), 917–932. https://doi.org/10.1037/a0018017

Poulin, M. J., & Holman, E. A. (2013). Helping hands, healthy body? Oxytocin receptor gene and prosocial behavior interact to buffer the association between stress and physical health. *Hormones and Behavior, 63*(3), 510–517. https://doi.org/10.1016/j.yhbeh.2013.01.004

Przybylski, A. K., Weinstein, N., Ryan, R. M., & Rigby, C. S. (2009). Having to versus wanting to play: Background and consequences of harmonious versus obsessive engagement in video games. *CyberPsychology & Behavior, 12*(5), 485–492. https://doi.org/10.1089/cpb.2009.0083

Ratelle, C. F., Carbonneau, N., Vallerand, R. J., & Mageau, G. (2013). Passion in the romantic sphere: A look at relational outcomes. *Motivation and Emotion, 37*(1), 106–120. https://doi.org/10.1007/s11031-012-9286-5

Rip, B., Fortin, S., & Vallerand, R. J. (2006). The relationship between passion and injury in dance students. *Journal of Dance Medicine & Science, 10*(1–2), 14–20.

Rip, B., Vallerand, R. J., & Lafrenière, M. A. K. (2012). Passion for a cause, passion for a creed: On ideological passion, identity threat, and extremism. *Journal of Personality, 80*(3), 573–602. https://doi.org/10.1111/j.1467-6494.2011.00743.x

Rogers, C. R. (1961). *On becoming a person: A therapist's view of psychotherapy.* Houghton Mifflin Harcourt.

Ryan, R. M., & Deci, E. L. (2001). On happiness and human potentials: A review of research on hedonic and eudaimonic well-being. *Annual Review of Psychology, 52*(1), 141–166. https://doi.org/10.1146/annurev.psych.52.1.141

Ryan, R. M., & Deci, E. L. (2017). *Self-determination theory: Basic psychological needs in motivation, development, and wellness.* Guilford Press.

Ryan, R. M., & Frederick, C. (1997). On energy, personality, and health: Subjective vitality as a dynamic reflection of well-being. *Journal of Personality, 65*(3), 529–565. https://doi.org/10.1111/j.1467-6494.1997.tb00326.x

Ryff, C. D. (1989). Happiness is everything, or is it? Explorations on the meaning of psychological well-being. *Journal of Personality and Social Psychology, 57*(6), 1069–1081.

Ryff, C. D., & Singer, B. H. (2008). Know thyself and become what you are: A eudaimonic approach to psychological well-being. *Journal of Happiness Studies, 9*(1), 13–39. https://doi.org/10.1007/s10902-006-9019-0

Schellenberg, B. J., & Bailis, D. S. (2016). The two roads of passionate goal pursuit: Links with appraisal, coping, and academic achievement. *Anxiety, Stress, & Coping, 29*(3), 287–304. https://doi.org/10.1080/10615806.2015.1036047

Schellenberg, B. J., Sabiston, C. M., Vallerand, R. J., & Gaudreau, P. (2021). Passion among breast cancer survivors: A 12-month prospective study. *Journal of Health Psychology, 26*(7), 1109–1114. https://doi.org/10.1177/1359105319860890

Schellenberg, B. J., Verner-Filion, J., Gaudreau, P., Bailis, D. S., Lafrenière, M. A. K., & Vallerand, R. J. (2019). Testing the dualistic model of passion using a novel quadripartite approach: A look at physical and psychological well-being. *Journal of Personality, 87*(2), 163–180. https://doi.org/10.1111/jopy.12378

Séguin-Lévesque, C., Laliberté, M. L. N., Pelletier, L. G., Blanchard, C., & Vallerand, R. J. (2003). Harmonious and obsessive passion for the internet: Their associations with the couple's relationship. *Journal of Applied Social Psychology, 33*(1), 197–221. https://doi.org/10.1111/j.1559-1816.2003.tb02079.x

Seligman, M. (2018). PERMA and the building blocks of well-being. *Journal of Positive Psychology, 13*(4), 333–335. https://doi.org/10.1080/17439760.2018.1437466

Seligman, M., & Csikszentmihalyi, M. (2000). Positive psychology: An introduction. *American Psychologist, 55*(1), 5–14.

Seligman, M. E. P. (2011). *Flourish: a visionary new understanding of happiness and well-being*. Free Press.

Sheldon, K. M. (2004). *Optimal human being: An integrated multi-level perspective*. Lawrence Erlbaum Associates.

Sheldon, K. M., & Lyubomirsky, S. (2021). Revisiting the sustainable happiness model and pie chart: can happiness be successfully pursued? *Journal of Positive Psychology, 16*(2), 145–154. https://doi.org/10.1080/17439760.2019.1689421

Sonnentag, S. (2015). Dynamics of Well-Being. *Annual Review of Organizational Psychology and Organizational Behavior, 2*(1), 261–293. https://doi.org/10.1146/annurev-orgpsych-032414-111347

St-Cyr, J., Vallerand, R. J., & Chénard-Poirier, L. A. (2021). The Role of Passion and Achievement Goals in Optimal Functioning in Sports. *International Journal of Environmental Research and Public Health, 18*(17), 1–9. https://doi.org/10.3390/ijerph18179023

Stephan, Y., Deroche, T., Brewer, B. W., Caudroit, J., & Le Scanff, C. (2009). Predictors of perceived susceptibility to sport-related injury among competitive runners: The role of previous experience, neuroticism, and passion for running. *Applied Psychology: An International Review, 58*(4), 672–689. https://doi.org/10.1111/j.1464-0597.2008.00373.x

St-Louis, A. C., Carbonneau, N., & Vallerand, R. J. (2016). Passion for a cause: how it affects health and subjective well-being: passion for a cause. *Journal of Personality, 84*(3), 263–276. https://doi.org/10.1111/jopy.12157

St-Louis, A. C., Rapaport, M., Chénard-Poirier, L., Vallerand, R. J., & Dandeneau, S. (2021). On emotion regulation strategies and well-being: The role of passion. *Journal of Happiness Studies, 2020*, 1–28. https://doi.org/10.1007/s10902-020-00296-8

St-Louis, A. C., Verner-Filion, J., Bergeron, C. M., & Vallerand, R. J. (2018). Passion and mindfulness: Accessing adaptive self-processes. *The Journal of Positive Psychology, 13*(2), 155–164. https://doi.org/10.1080/17439760.2016.1245771

Stoeber, J., Childs, J. H., Hayward, J. A., & Feast, A. R. (2011). Passion and motivation for studying: Predicting academic engagement and burnout in university students. *Educational Psychology, 31*(4), 513–528. https://doi.org/10.1080/01443410.2011.570251

Umberson, D., Crosnoe, R., & Reczek, C. (2010). Social Relationships and Health Behavior Across the Life Course. *Annual Review of Sociology, 36*(1), 139–157. https://doi.org/10.1146/annurev-soc-070308-120011

Utz, S., Jonas, K. J., & Tonkens, E. (2012). Effects of passion for massively multiplayer online role-playing games on interpersonal relationships. *Journal of Media Psychology, 24*(2), 77–86. https://doi.org/10.1027/1864-1105/a000066

Vallerand, R. J. (2010). On passion for life activities: The dualistic model of passion. In *Advances in experimental social psychology* (Vol. 42, pp. 97–193). Academic Press. https://doi.org/10.1016/S0065-2601(10)42003-1

Vallerand, R. J. (2012). The role of passion in sustainable psychological well-being. *Psychology of well-Being: Theory, research and practice, 2*(1), 1–21. https://doi.org/10.1186/2211-1522-2-1

Vallerand, R. J. (2013). Passion and optimal functioning in society: A eudaimonic perspective. In A. S. Waterman (Ed.), *The best within us: Positive psychology perspectives on eudaimonia* (pp. 183–206). American Psychological Association. https://doi.org/10.1037/14092-010

Vallerand, R. J. (2015). *The psychology of passion: A dualistic model.* Oxford University Press.

Vallerand, R. J. (2016). On the synergy between hedonia and eudaimonia: The role of passion. In J. Vittersø (Ed.), *Handbook of eudaimonic well-being* (pp. 191–204). Springer. https://doi.org/10.1007/978-3-319-42445-3_13

Vallerand, R. J., Blanchard, C., Mageau, G. A., Koestner, R., Ratelle, C., Léonard, M., Gagné, M., & Marsolais, J. (2003). Les passions de l'âme: On obsessive and harmonious passion. *Journal of Personality and Social Psychology, 85*(4), 756–767. https://doi.org/10.1037/0022-3514.85.4.756

Vallerand, R. J., & Houlfort, N. (2019). *Passion for work: Theory, research, and applications.* Oxford University Press.

Vallerand, R. J., Mageau, G. A., Elliot, A. J., Dumais, A., Demers, M. A., & Rousseau, F. (2008a). Passion and performance attainment in sport. *Psychology of Sport and Exercise, 9*(3), 373–392. https://doi.org/10.1016/j.psychsport.2007.05.003

Vallerand, R. J., Ntoumanis, N., Philippe, F. L., Lavigne, G. L., Carbonneau, N., Bonneville, A., Lagacé-Labonté, C., & Maliha, G. (2008b). On passion and sports fans: A look at football. *Journal of Sports Sciences, 26*(12), 1279–1293. https://doi.org/10.1080/02640410802123185

Vallerand, R. J., Paquet, Y., Philippe, F. L., & Charest, J. (2010). On the role of passion for work in burnout: A process model. *Journal of personality, 78*(1), 289–312. https://doi.org/10.1111/j.1467-6494.2009.00616.x

Vallerand, R. J., Rousseau, F. L., Grouzet, F. M., Dumais, A., Grenier, S., & Blanchard, C. M. (2006). Passion in sport: A look at determinants and affective experiences.

Journal of Sport and Exercise Psychology, 28(4), 454–478. https://doi.org/10.1123/jsep.28.4.454
Vallerand, R. J., Salvy, S. J., Mageau, G. A., Elliot, A. J., Denis, P. L., Grouzet, F. M., & Blanchard, C. (2007). On the role of passion in performance. *Journal of Personality, 75*(3), 505–534. https://doi.org/10.1111/j.1467-6494.2007.00447.x
Waterman, A. S., Schwartz, S. J., Zamboanga, B. L., Ravert, R. D., Williams, M. K., Bede Agocha, V., Yeong Kim, S., & Brent Donnellan, M. (2010). The questionnaire for eudaimonic well-being: Psychometric properties, demographic comparisons, and evidence of validity. *Journal of Positive Psychology, 5*(1), 41–61. https://doi.org/10.1080/17439760903435208
Waugh, C. E., & Fredrickson, B. L. (2006). Nice to know you: Positive emotions, self-other overlap, and complex understanding in the formation of new relationships. *Journal of Positive Psychology, 1*(2), 93–106. https://doi.org/10.1080/17439760500510569
World Health Organization. (1948). Constitution of the World Health Organization.

Part II

Preface: Eudaimonic Well-Being and Health (Meaning, Purpose, and Values)

Fuschia M. Sirois

In contrast to the hedonic perspective presented in Part I, the eudaimonic view presented in this section approaches well-being from a dynamic perspective, rejecting the notion that positive feelings alone reflect well-being and focusing instead on how active, growth-related aspects of life contribute to a trajectory of well-being. Rather than the pursuit of pleasure, the eudaimonic view proposes that well-being arises when one pursues goals that are aligned with the authentic self, or *daimon*. This view is consistent with Aristotle's notion that eudaimonia was not a subjective but in fact an objective state that derived from contemplating the best within oneself and personal excellence. To the extent that striving towards one's full potential reflects better health practices, lower physiological stress arousal, and access to health supporting psychosocial resources, eudaimonic states and traits can have relevance for understanding health outcomes.

This section of the Handbook presents theory and evidence linking eudaimonic concepts of well-such as meaning, values, and purpose in life, to health. Such approaches can be particularly beneficial for helping individuals struggling with the challenges of chronic health conditions who often have to renegotiate their goals and identity in light of functional limitations. But they can be equally important for anyone who is experiencing an existential crisis and who may therefore be more vulnerable to poor health habits, higher stress, and feelings of isolation from their support networks.

Together, the chapters in this section provide the latest critical views of how eudemonic aspects of well-being are linked to flourishing in health contexts, to promoting health behaviours, and to reducing physiological stress. In Chap. 7, Hill and Pfund begin by providing an overview of how purpose in life has been defined, noting the inevitable controversies that emerge when we consider overlap between sense of purpose and similar personality and identity-related constructs. They then review the research to date that situates purpose as an important eudaimonic construct for understanding health outcomes, health-promotion, and even mortality. Chapter 8 examines the value of a related construct, the search for meaning, and its implications for health for people who have been diagnosed with a life-threatening or life-altering condition. Davis and McLeod argue that as sense-making creatures, humans will naturally engage in meaning-making processes to cope with unexpected health issues and injuries, so as to restore a sense of purpose in life, find meaningful explanations for their health challenges, and align these disruptive experiences with their life narrative. In this respect, the search for meaning can play an important role in the adjustment process and contribute to health-related outcomes.

Reconnecting to one's values through self-affirmation is an area of research that has shown both promise and limits for understanding when and how people can make the health behaviour changes needed to reduce the risk of disease and maintain their health and reduce harmful responses to stressors. In Chap. 9, Harris and Jessop review current theory and evidence on the role of self-affirmation for improving health and the real-world factors that may enhance or limit the efficacy of self-affirmation interventions when applied to health issues.

Chapter 10, the final chapter in this section, focuses on the positive psychological changes that can occur in the wake of highly stressful events, including the diagnosis of a life-threatening or chronic illness, or a life-changing injury. Orejuela Dávila and Tedeschi argue that although such stressful events can be very challenging and disruptive to one's goals and sense of purpose, for others this disruption can set the stage for positive realizations regarding one's personal strength, a greater appreciation for life, new possibilities, new ways of relating to others, and spiritual change. They present current theory and evidence on the associations between post-traumatic growth and health outcomes across various medical challenges that highlight the potential of post-traumatic growth for mitigating the stress linked to these experiences.

7

Purposeful Living as an Essential Ingredient to a Healthy Life

Patrick L. Hill and Gabrielle N. Pfund

Tell me what you eat and I will tell you what you are.
Anthelme Brillat-Savarin (1826)

The connection between health and individual dispositions has been recognized for centuries. Often, as suggested by Brillat-Savarin, the focus has been on how an individual's well-being and disposition are impacted by whether they eat well and live a healthy life. However, the study of personality and health has provided decades of research in support of the alternative interpretation, namely, knowing who you are goes a long way toward understanding what you will eat, and your likelihood of engaging in healthy lifestyle behaviors more broadly. Most of this work has focused on a handful of personality trait dimensions, known as the Big Five (John & Srivastava, 1999), in part because they are assumed to be fairly universal descriptions

P. L. Hill (✉)
Department of Psychological and Brain Sciences,
Washington University in St. Louis, St. Louis, MO, USA
e-mail: Patrick.hill@wustl.edu

G. N. Pfund
Department of Psychological and Brain Sciences,
Washington University in St. Louis, St. Louis, MO, USA

Department of Human Development and Family Sciences,
Auburn University, Auburn, USA

F. M. Sirois (ed.), *The Palgrave Handbook of Positive Psychology and Health*,
https://doi.org/10.1007/978-3-031-89095-6_7

of who you are. For example, traits such as conscientiousness and neuroticism have been connected to exercise, drug abuse, and even longevity (Bogg & Roberts, 2013; Hampson, 2012; Turiano et al., 2012). This work has provided rich insights into the role of personality on health, but there is increasing recognition that additional personality characteristics may predict health behaviors and health outcomes.

The current chapter examines the evidence toward this claim with regard to sense of purpose, a perception that one has a life direction that directs lower-order goals and daily activities (McKnight & Kashdan, 2009; Ryff, 1989a, b; Scheier et al., 2006). Though sometimes viewed as solely a component of well-being or identity (Hill & Burrow, 2012; Ryff, 2014), more recent theory has highlighted the affective, behavioral, and cognitive patterns of sense of purpose more similarly represented in commonly studied personality traits (Pfund, 2020). Furthermore, this construct illustrates substantial rank-order and mean-level stability over years (Hill & Weston, 2019; Hill et al., 2015). The trait-like nature of sense of purpose suggests that we can evaluate the connection between this construct and health similarly to patterns that we find with personality traits like conscientiousness or neuroticism. Importantly, while sense of purpose is associated with these traits (Anglim et al., 2020; Meléndez et al., 2019; Sun et al., 2018), it predicts health outcomes beyond these and other personality traits (Hill et al., 2016b, 2019a).

Years after Brillat-Savarin's original text, his quote was employed to introduce highly purposeful individuals in the culinary field, as the opening to the Japanese cooking show "Iron Chef," a competition wherein top chefs from around the world competed. Borrowing from this program, we outline below why sense of purpose may be the secret ingredient to living a healthy life. First, we describe the evidence that sense of purpose longitudinally predicts a variety of health outcomes. Second, we discuss multiple routes and mechanisms by which sense of purpose may lead to better health. Third, we consider recent developments and next steps for researchers along this line of work. Of central importance is understanding whether the individual's purpose in life actually matters. For instance, does it matter whether individuals have a life direction that is focused on healthy living, or lifestyle choices? Regarding whether lifestyle behaviors can shape a purpose, we present the example of vegetarian identity as a self-defining choice and direction for daily activities. This final section thus considers the extent to which, if you tell us what your purpose is, we may be able to tell you what you eat. Before doing so, though, we must first define what is meant by sense of purpose, purpose in life, and purpose commitment, and how these constructs differ from conceptually related variables such as meaning in life, identity, and conscientiousness.

Definitional Matters

Purpose is a unique construct in several regards. For one, it is a psychosocial variable with both a rich theoretical and empirical history that has illustrated the predictive validity of the construct while leaving researchers with several unanswered questions (Burrow & Hill, 2020). Initial inquiry into leading a purposeful life, and the value inherent within purposeful living, dates back centuries, as part of the early philosophical discussion around eudaemonia and the life well lived (see Ryff, 2014; Ryff & Kim, 2020 for reviews). Another foundational touchstone came with the writing of Viktor Frankl (1984), who demonstrated the remarkable ability of individuals to persevere with purpose through difficult times. And yet, empirical inquiry into the construct was largely dormant until more recent decades (with a few exceptions, such as Crumbaugh & Maholick, 1964), catalyzed by the advent of Carol Ryff's efforts (Ryff, 1989a, 2014) to promote research into psychological well-being. The psychological well-being model was built by the original philosophers to underscore six central components of adaptive adult development. Of these six tenets, disproportionate attention has been paid to the component of having a sense of purpose in life, in part due to the consistent evidence for its predictive value for adult outcomes (see Pfund & Hill, 2018; Pfund & Lewis, 2020 for reviews).

To understand why the construct has garnered such reverence, one must consider another unique quirk of purpose—namely that researchers of purpose must navigate the different ways in which it can be operationalized and measured. To start, it serves as a central goal, a life direction that provides one with the guidance needed to organize daily activities toward a personally defining aim (McKnight & Kashdan, 2009). This conceptualization situates purpose as a hierarchically superordinate goal, something one presumably can articulate to an extent, and can often be understood as a *purpose in life*. However, there is potential harm in selecting a purpose that is tangible and achievable, as it could lead one to feeling at a loss should they ever succeed at their purpose. Instead, it is better to choose something that one can follow and progress toward throughout the lifespan (Damon et al., 2003).

Another consideration though is whether people feel like they are directed in life and purposeful. This conceptualization is reflected in the measurement strategy taken by Ryff's psychological well-being model (Ryff, 1989b; Ryff & Keyes, 1995), and emphasizes the extent to which an individual feels purposeful, rather than the more dichotomous expression of having a purpose or not. This approach also has been adopted by health psychologists, focused on identifying which individuals are more engaged in their lives (Scheier et al., 2006).

The focus then is on *sense of purpose* rather than what the individual's specific purpose may be. Although it neglects that potentially valuable source of idiographic data, the benefits of this methodology are fairly clear. First, it allows researchers to make between-participant score comparisons regardless of whether they hold similar or differing life aims. Second, most measures are easy to administer and are relatively short inventories. Because of these benefits, research on health psychology in particular has benefited by virtue of having the opportunity to assess purpose across hundreds of individuals and over time.

Additional efforts have conceived of purpose in related ways, sometimes as a melding of the two, capturing whether people report greater or lesser commitment to a specific purpose (Bundick et al., 2006). However, all these efforts are centered on the belief that a purpose provides some foundation and direction for living, which aligns with what is most frequently mentioned by participants when asked to define the construct (Hill et al., 2010b). This conceptualization, in turn, provides a central deviation and distinction from several related constructs. For instance, a sense of meaning in life can arise from several sources, including perhaps goal pursuit, but also the belief that life is coherent and that one matters to the world (Costin & Vignoles, 2020; Martela & Steger, 2016). Moreover, purpose and meaning appear to hold unique correlates in patient samples, such as cancer survivors (George & Park, 2013).

Another related construct is conscientiousness, a disposition that has received significant attention from the health psychology community (Bogg & Roberts, 2004, 2013; Roberts et al., 2005), but one that focuses less on having a direction and more on general tendencies to be self-controlled, organized, and industrious (Roberts et al., 2017). Past work indeed shows moderate-to-strong associations between sense of purpose and conscientiousness (Anglim et al., 2020), and yet several studies demonstrate that sense of purpose predicts important outcomes above and beyond this related trait (Hill et al., 2016c, 2019a; Pfund et al., 2020). One possible explanation is that sense of purpose emphasizes having self-defining goals more than conscientiousness. Indeed, some have characterized purpose as providing a compass for individuals (McKnight & Kashdan, 2009), and this directionality need not be present for meaning in life or conscientiousness.

In several ways, perhaps the construct most connected to purpose is neither of these candidates, and rather one's sense of identity. Indeed, a final way in which purpose is a unique construct is that it holds a multifaceted role within identity development. In his classic model, Erikson (1959) notes that the ability for goal-directed action, which he labeled as the capacity for *purpose*, is an important developmental benchmark for young children. Moreover, Erikson writes about how finding a purpose may be essential to figuring out who one is. Indeed, research has underscored the close empirical connection between identity commitment and purpose commitment both cross-sectionally (Burrow & Hill, 2011) and longitudinally (Hill & Burrow, 2012). Sumner and colleagues (Sumner et al., 2015) describe this intertwining development in that knowing "who am I?" helps to answer the question "where am I going?" and vice versa (p. 46). This point provides a final important characteristic for the construct of purpose; namely, purpose holds a place within multiple developmental theoretical foundations, including Ryff's model (1989a). Moreover, a burgeoning literature has considered how sense of purpose changes across the lifespan (see Pfund & Lewis, 2020 for a review). Couching purpose within this developmental literature is valuable for health psychologists, insofar that it provides evidence that sense of purpose is both relatively stable and yet malleable even late in the lifespan (Hill & Weston, 2019; Hill et al., 2015). These points underscore a central reason why purpose is a valuable construct for health psychologists—it is not simply a predictor of health risk or resilience but one that is potentially malleable.

A Purposeful Life is a Healthy One

A large literature has developed over the past decade to show that purposeful individuals experience better physical health outcomes. This work can be organized into four general categories: self-reported health concerns and limitations, stress reactivity, cardiovascular events, and mortality risk. As noted earlier, the research reviewed in each section will focus on sense of purpose as the predictor of interest rather than participants' specific stated purposes in life, largely given the methodological ease afforded to survey administration with sense of purpose measures. Utilizing brief sense of purpose assessments has opened the door to rich health psychology investigations that can address questions related to the prediction of the low occurrence outcomes common in this field (who is more likely to experience a heart attack in the next ten years?), as well as create opportunities for comparing patient and non-patient samples (does sense of purpose promote health similarly across groups?).

Purpose and Self-Rated Health

A number of studies have shown that participants who report a greater sense of purpose tend also to score higher on measures of self-rated (or self-reported) health, which represents an individual's perception of how poor to excellent their health is, and/or their reported concerns across different domains of health, like physical limitations or pain (Hill et al., 2019a; Scheier et al., 2006). These findings also hold when controlling for the Big Five personality traits (Hill et al., 2019a). Similarly, sense of purpose has been negatively associated with measures of physical limitations (Scheier et al., 2006). Self-rated health is a consistent predictor of mortality risk across samples (Benyamini, 2011; Idler & Benyamini, 1997), in part because it provides unique insights into the individual's personal viewpoint on their health (Jylhä, 2009). As such, these positive associations between sense of purpose and self-rated health provide an important first step in demonstrating the value of a purposeful life for health outcomes.

The associations between self-rated health and sense of purpose are relatively consistent across different populations. Toward this end, Scheier et al. (2006) investigated the measurement properties and correlates of their newly developed purpose measure across eight different samples. These samples included community-based non-patient participants as well as osteoarthritis patients and women experiencing different stages of breast cancer. For all samples, the brief six-item measure demonstrated evidence of strong measurement properties. Moreover, across non-patient and patient samples, greater sense of purpose was associated with better self-rated health and physical functioning, but lower levels of reported role disruptions due to physical health. Recent work also has compared individuals with and without a specific health ailment, namely diabetes, to see whether the associations between sense of purpose and self-rated health differ based on whether individuals have diabetes (Weston, Hill, & Mroczek, 2024). This research, conducted with thousands of participants across multiple secondary samples, again suggested a positive association between sense of purpose and self-rated health, but found little evidence for moderation of this effect by diabetes status. As such, even if purposeful individuals may be less prone to experiencing negative health issues, there is evidence to suggest that having a higher sense of purpose may prove beneficial for individuals' health regardless of whether one has a current health condition.

Purpose and Stress Reactivity

One potential explanation for why purposeful individuals report better health is that they may be less reactive to daily events. Significant evidence exists to show that how people react to their daily events impacts health outcomes in the future. For instance, daily emotional reactivity predicts inflammation (Sin et al., 2015), heart rate variability (Sin et al., 2016), as well as even premature mortality (Chiang et al., 2018; Mroczek et al., 2015). People who overreact, by experiencing greater negative affect or physical symptoms, in response to daily stressors tend to fair worse over time. In fact, overreacting in general could be problematic for individuals' health given past work that has suggested that overreacting to positive events can prove deleterious (Sin & Almeida, 2018). For example, one can imagine that individuals who react too positively may either experience detriments associated with overly frequent arousal, or perhaps it may be a sign of lack of positive stimuli in daily life for one to react so strongly to a single daily positive event.

Building from this research, work has suggested that purposeful individuals may be less reactive to both types of events in daily life. Adults who report a greater sense of purpose initially had attenuated increases in reports of physical symptoms and negative affect in their daily life relative to their peers (Hill et al., 2018). Furthermore, those more purposeful adults were relatively stable in their positive affect across days regardless of the number of positive events they experienced, countering the general pattern to increase in positive affect in response to daily positive events (Hill et al., 2022). Both effects were discussed as evidence that having a sense of purpose helps individuals to avoid being too reactive when things go astray or when unexpected events occur—both for negative and positive events. Similar evidence comes from work showing experimental manipulations that ask participants to write about purpose in life. In these experiments, those who wrote about purpose in life illustrated decreased levels of stress or anxiety reported in response to real-world events shown to potentially stress participants (Burrow & Hill, 2013; Burrow et al., 2014).

These effects also seem to hold when considering biological and behavioral indicators of the stress response system. For instance, one study (Fogelman & Canli, 2015) found that participants higher on sense of purpose who completed the Trier Social Stress Test (Kirschbaum et al., 1993) showed quicker return to pre-stressor cortisol levels. Other work also has found salivary cortisol levels (a biomarker related to stress) were negatively associated with sense of purpose (Ryff et al., 2004). Furthermore, sense of purpose has been shown to predict recovery to negative stimuli assessed using eyeblink startle response (Schaefer et al., 2013). Put together, these findings suggest that one benefit to purposeful living is a tendency to avoid overreacting to issues confronted in daily life. Again, it is likely that having a direction guiding one into the days ahead may help mitigate the impact of an event encountered. At the least, it may help individuals put these stressful events into a different perspective, indirect evidence for which comes from multiple studies finding negative associations between reports of perceived stress in the past and sense of purpose (e.g., Hill et al., 2016b; Scheier et al., 2006). The ability to deal with stress and daily events more adaptively plays a big role in explaining why being purposeful may help promote cardiovascular health.

Purpose and Heart Health

If light is in your heart, you will find your way home
—Rumi

The notion that one's heart provides one a direction has served as the starting point for movie directors, novelists, and poets, like Rumi. However, research also suggests this association may go both ways. Multiple studies have now shown that sense of purpose longitudinally predicts risk for cardiovascular issues (Cohen et al., 2016), a topic that has been reviewed elsewhere, and we alert the reader to that excellent work (Kim et al., 2019). In short, it appears that having a greater sense of purpose promotes having a healthier heart, across multiple cardiovascular indicators. We instead will add to this point on the more metaphorical sense, as alluded to by Rumi, namely whether sense of purpose may help people avoid a broken heart through the maintenance of positive romantic relationships. The intimate connection between sense of purpose and positive relationships with others has been noted throughout its empirical investigation (Ryff, 1989a, b; Ryff & Keyes, 1995). Most of this discussion has focused on the potential for connections with parents early in the lifespan (e.g., Bronk, 2012; Damon, 2008). Indeed, research supports the claim that positive parent–child relationships early in life predict later sense of purpose (Hill et al., 2019b), and that college students with more positive attachments to parents tend to be more purposeful (Hill et al., 2016a).

However, recent research also demonstrates that purposeful people may avoid heartbreak due to the romantic relationships they hold. In two large adult samples, Pfund et al. (2020) found that sense of purpose predicted a wide array of relationship quality variables, including greater relationship satisfaction, commitment, and investment. These associations were largely similar in magnitude from young to older adulthood, and even held above and beyond the role of the Big Five personality traits. While admittedly tongue-in-cheek to include this work in this section, romantic relationships and cardiovascular health are intertwined beyond the poetic domain. For instance, perceived ambivalence in partnerships has been linked to greater risks for cardiovascular health concerns (Uchino et al., 2013). Moreover, laboratory research suggests that partner contact and warmth can help reduce cardiovascular reactivity during a stressful task (Grewen et al., 2003). As such, purposeful partners may have more positive romantic relationships, which could aid in the promotion of cardiovascular health.

Purpose and Mortality Risk

While these three outcomes hold clear importance, often the gold standard for health psychology research is understanding the factors that reduce or increase the risk for early mortality. On this front, the past decade has produced multiple studies consistently demonstrating that adults with a greater sense of purpose tend to experience reduced mortality risk. Perhaps the first major investigation on this front was provided by Boyle and colleagues (Boyle et al., 2009), employing data from two studies originally designed to understand risks for normative and non-normative cognitive decline. Participants in these studies completed a sense of purpose measure at baseline and then were followed for up to five years post the initial assessment. Findings demonstrated that purposeful older adults lived longer than their counterparts, and these associations were the same across race and gender. Moreover, these findings were largely consistent when accounting for other known risk factors, such as depressive symptoms, chronic medical conditions, or neuroticism.

This study sparked greater empirical curiosity into the topic, with studies around the world testing for similar effects. Studies from Australia (Windsor et al., 2015), Japan (Sone et al., 2008), and additional US samples (Hill & Turiano, 2014) all have evidenced similar results. Although more work is needed to compare contexts, meta-analytic work also finds that the effect on mortality risk appears consistent when considering the potential for country-of-origin effects (Cohen et al., 2016). Moreover, one study found that sense of purpose held similar effects on mortality risk for younger versus older adults (Hill & Turiano, 2014). This finding is particularly informative as it provides insight into the potential multifaceted nature of mechanisms connecting sense of purpose to health outcomes. Specifically, it suggests the need to consider reasons why sense of purpose may protect against both premature mortality risk for younger adults as well as why it may prolong the lives of older adults.

A Purposeful Life is a Health-Promoting One

Toward this end, the next section of our review will be broken into three parts. First, we consider the evidence that sense of purpose promotes wellness-maintenance behaviors, which may promote healthier outcomes throughout the lifespan. This work constitutes the majority of the research on purpose and health behaviors. Second, we consider sense of purpose as a correlate of factors that may lead to premature or early mortality risk, including drug use, impulsivity, and suicidal ideation. Third, we consider work on other health-promoting factors linked to sense of purpose, including social support and socioeconomic status.

Purpose and Wellness Maintenance

To provide a grounding for common wellness-maintenance behaviors, it is worth considering those included in the well-known and commonly employed Health Behavior Checklist (Vickers et al., 1990). This measure sought to capture several behaviors presumed to be broadly beneficial for living a healthy lifestyle. Included in this scale were items capturing dietary behaviors and weight loss, dental health care, regular exercise, and getting regular checkups at the doctor's office. In a diverse sample of US adults, sense of purpose has been associated with self-reported adaptive diet choices, flossing behavior, and physical activity, all of which mediated the cross-sectional association between sense of purpose and self-rated health (Hill et al., 2019a). Beyond self-reported health behaviors, positive associations have been found between sense of purpose and more objective markers of physical activity, such as walking speed and grip strength (Kim et al., 2017). Moreover, longitudinal work now shows that older adults with a greater sense of purpose have a reduced prospective risk of becoming physically inactive and developing unhealthy BMI levels (Kim et al., 2020b). Additionally, purposeful people appear to do better at the doctor's office, and so far, sense of purpose has been shown to predict better healthcare usage over time (Kim et al., 2014).

Another behavior integral to maintaining positive health is getting better sleep. Sleep quality also was positively associated with sense of purpose, and a significant mediator, in the same investigation mentioned above (Hill et al., 2019a). Longitudinal research has demonstrated that sense of purpose predicts a reduced likelihood of sleep disturbances (Kim et al., 2015). Moreover, sense of purpose is predictive of reduced risk for later symptoms of sleep apnea and restless leg syndrome (Turner et al., 2017). In sum, sense of purpose appears associated with a wide array of wellness-maintenance behaviors, which provides a central mechanism through which purposeful individuals experience the long-term positive outcomes reviewed above.

Purpose and Risk Behaviors for Premature Mortality

Physical activity, diet, sleep, and medical care behaviors play an important role in predicting longevity at any age. However, it is worth reviewing other behaviors that may play a significant role in reducing life expectancy, such as self-harm and risk-taking activity. Purposeful individuals overall tend to report being less impulsive, as shown by research finding that purpose in life is negatively associated with hedonistic values (Crandall & Rasmussen, 1975). Furthermore, one study found that participants who scored higher on a purpose/meaning composite performed better (less risky) on a behavioral risk-taking task (Burrow & Spreng, 2016).

Importantly, purposeful individuals tend to be less likely to engage in risk-taking behaviors outside of the lab as well. For instance, during emerging adulthood, sense of purpose is linked to a reduced likelihood to report delinquent activity (Hill et al., 2016b). Sense of purpose also is associated with a reduced likelihood to misuse prescribed drugs (Kim et al., 2020a). However, future research is needed regarding purpose and drug use given some mixed results. For example, findings are inconsistent for the role of sense of purpose and smoking status (Kim et al., 2020b; Weston, Hill, & Mroczek, 2020). In addition, work is needed to understand how associations may go in both directions. For instance, there is some work suggesting that psychedelic experiences can promote a greater sense of purpose (Yaden et al., 2017).

A larger and more unequivocal literature has considered sense of purpose and suicidal ideation. Demonstrating its importance for mental health overall, several studies have found that those with a higher sense of purpose experience fewer depressive symptoms (Hill et al., 2016; Scheier et al., 2006; Windsor et al., 2015). With respect to suicidal ideation, one study (Harlow et al., 1986) found that males who scored lower on the Purpose in Life Test

(Crumbaugh & Maholick, 1964) were more likely to report thoughts of suicide. For females in that study, lower purpose scores were more related to greater substance use as a coping behavior, again pointing to the need to consider when and why sense of purpose may be linked to drug and substance use behavior.

Purpose and Other Health-Promoting Variables

There are two final pathways linking sense of purpose to positive health that are worth consideration. First, given the implications for social support on health outcomes (e.g., Reblin & Uchino, 2008; Uchino et al., 1996; Uchino, 2006), we return again to the intimate connection between sense of purpose and positive relationships with others. Recent research has shown that perceived support (and lower perceived strain) is positively associated with sense of purpose across relationship domains, including family, friends, and spouses (Weston et al., 2021). Moreover, changes in support were positively associated with changes in sense of purpose over time, whereas greater strain was linked to worse purpose longitudinally.

Another variable worth mentioning is personal wealth. Wealth plays an unfortunately large role in the quality of and opportunity for health care in several countries. As such, it is valuable to consider that sense of purpose predicts the accrual of net worth over time, even when controlling for the Big Five personality traits (Hill et al., 2018). Paired with the work showing that purposeful people in the United States are better users of the healthcare system (Kim et al., 2014), it is possible that they also are receiving higher-quality care as a result of their better socioeconomic status. That said, another possible explanation for these net worth findings is that purposeful individuals may be better able to accrue wealth because they are experiencing fewer health care costs, for all the reasons above. As such, future research is needed to understand the potential cyclical nature of these associations, insofar that purposeful people take better care of themselves, allowing for prospects to build wealth, which in turn provides greater opportunities to protect their health in the future. It is worth noting though that these explanations may be more prominent in countries where personal out-of-pocket health costs are greater. Even in these cases though, the potential still exists for personal wealth to play a role, insofar that purposeful individuals may experience fewer health-related absences or reduced productivity at work.

In sum, having a greater sense of purpose thus has been linked to a variety of positive health promoters. The crux of this work has focused on health behaviors, in line with theoretical frameworks that similarly point to behavioral pathways as the most likely route linking personality dispositions with health outcomes (Adler & Matthews, 1994; Smith, 2006). However, it also is worth noting that purposeful people are less impulsive, have better support bases, and are more likely to build financial assets. All of these associations though may be described with respect to the common thread noted at the start—in each case, they might reflect the tendency for purposeful individuals to focus on their futures and act in ways that promote a continued pursuit of their life direction. Purposeful people are likely to recognize the value of having resources to scaffold their goal pursuit, whether those resources are social, financial, or most importantly, healthful. Indeed, regardless of the life path one chooses, it would seem that better health provides a valuable ingredient for cooking a purposeful life.

Future Directions for Purpose and Health Research

While healthy living may help people pursue any purpose, a central goal for health psychology research will be to move beyond investigations focused solely on sense of purpose. This is a central concern for the purpose research field as a whole (Hill & Burrow, 2020; Pfund, 2020). However, health psychology research in particular may benefit from greater consideration of participants' specific purpose in life (i.e., the content of their life direction), given that it provides opportunities for connecting to other topics within health psychology. Researchers in particular should consider (a) the extent to which individuals espouse purposes focused on health promotion and (b) how dietary and health choices may shape an individual's purpose in life.

Health as a Purpose Orientation

Research on purpose in life has typically employed one of two approaches. First, researchers have asked individuals to define what it means to have a purpose in life, taking a qualitative lay conception methodology (Hill et al., 2010b; Ratner et al., 2019). While people do often report the promotion of happiness and well-being as part of a purposeful life, this work has yet to find much evidence that individuals think about health as definitive for the construct of purpose. Second, research has employed life goal measures for attempting to capture individuals' orientations toward certain purposes or directions for life (e.g., Hill et al., 2010a). However, this work similarly suffers from a lack of attention to health in particular, as none of the items used in that measure mention health, and related life goal scales similarly tend to avoid the construct (e.g., Roberts et al., 2004). One possibility is that these studies have tended to focus on how adolescents and emerging adults develop a sense of purpose in life, and it may be less common for individuals to prioritize health as a life direction at these developmental stages.

Lifespan theories have noted that older adulthood is a period in which individuals likely consider health maintenance as a more prominent goal (e.g., Baltes, 1987). In support, older adults tend to mention more health-related goals than younger counterparts (Heckhausen, 1997). When participants are asked about what they hope for in their possible future selves, studies also show that health becomes a more prioritized domain for middle and older adults relative to younger adults (Frazier et al., 2000; Hooker & Kaus, 1994). As such, there is a significant literature to call upon regarding health goals, and their shifts in prioritization and focus across the lifespan. However, these developmental shifts question the extent to which health serves as a lifelong purpose for individuals, rather than a lower-order goal that becomes of greater importance during ages when health losses are more common. Put differently, what is currently unclear is how many individuals across the lifespan view health promotion or physical fitness as their particular guiding purpose in life, rather than merely as a necessary means for promoting continued progress toward another aim (such as being healthy in order to continue supporting one's family). Future research should consider this point, which will likely require a mixed-methods strategy to capture participants' self-endorsed life aims.

Health Choices as a Purpose Orientation

Another possibility is that the choices one makes with respect to health may provide insight into an individual's purpose; in other words, some health-related behaviors could provide indicators of what one's guiding life direction may be. Returning to the opening quote, one example on this front comes with respect to how diet, and the promulgation of the ethical values placed on what one eats, serve as providing a life direction. Most extant research on this front has focused on vegetarianism, though the sentiments on this front likely carry into other dietary identities. Research has demonstrated that the three biggest motives provided by vegetarians for this dietary choice are for one's health, helping the environment, and promoting animal rights (Hopwood et al., 2020). In this sense, one can envision how dietary choices may provide a route to engage with purposeful aims, such as being vegetarian as part of a broader life aim focused on the environment. As such, additional work may wish to explore these motives for dietary and other health behavior choices, and how they align with different purpose orientations. Such research would align with recent calls to better integrate personality science into advocacy efforts for plant-based diets (Hopwood & Bleidorn, 2019).

A final consideration is whether these choices actually end up *being* a purpose in life. The most likely route by which this occurs is when one views a dietary or lifestyle choice as a central aspect of who one is. Again, purpose and identity are intimately intertwined (Erikson, 1959; Sumner et al,. 2015). Therefore, as an example of how choices become purpose, it may be valuable to consider the recent research on the vegetarian identity (Rosenfeld, 2020; Rosenfeld & Burrow, 2017a, 2017b). People with a stronger vegetarian identity may build from this identification as a foundation for their life goals. Toward this end, it is valuable to consider the Unified Model of Vegetarian Identity (Rosenfeld & Burrow, 2017a). This model points to how a vegetarian identity is strengthened when individuals are consistent in their thoughts, actions, and feelings related to vegetarianism, which is impacted by their environments and the opportunities for enacting this behavior. Given that a large component of sense of purpose is meaningful activity engagement (Scheier et al., 2006), it would be of interest to consider whether these actions in daily life lead vegetarians to feel greater purposefulness, which likely reflects the extent to which these individuals view vegetarianism as reflecting the common good. If so, connections can be made to purpose development theories that suggest this felt purposefulness and reflection are central to helping people find their direction in life (Moran, 2020).

General Conclusion

Purpose is a valuable commodity for several reasons, but perhaps none are as important as its potential for promoting health. People who report a greater sense of purpose are more likely to enact a wide variety of healthy lifestyle behaviors, and ultimately experience a reduced risk for major health problems. Though promising, additional work is needed to compare the different mechanistic accounts linking purpose to health noted in this review. Moreover, work is needed that moves beyond sense of purpose toward considering the other aspects of purpose, such as knowing the individual's specific life direction. In this respect, we recommend that researchers need to understand the extent to which health promotion, or choices related to health behaviors, may provide guidance for an individual's life. As one example, it is possible knowing what one eats may in fact tell a lot about who one is, and the life direction that one might have.

References

Adler, N., & Matthews, K. (1994). Health psychology: Why do some people get sick and some stay well? *Annual Review of Psychology, 45*(1), 229–259.

Anglim, J., Horwood, S., Smillie, L. D., Marrero, R. J., & Wood, J. K. (2020). Predicting psychological and subjective well-being from personality: A meta-analysis. *Psychological Bulletin, 146*(4), 279–323.

Baltes, P. B. (1987). Theoretical propositions of life-span developmental psychology: On the dynamics between growth and decline. *Developmental Psychology, 23*(5), 611–626.

Benyamini, Y. (2011). Why does self-rated health predict mortality? An update on current knowledge and a research agenda for psychologists. *Psychology & Health, 11*, 1407–1413.

Bogg, T., & Roberts, B. W. (2004). Conscientiousness and health-related behaviors: A meta-analysis of the leading behavioral contributors to mortality. *Psychological Bulletin, 130*(6), 887–919.

Bogg, T., & Roberts, B. W. (2013). The case for conscientiousness: Evidence and implications for a personality trait marker of health and longevity. *Annals of Behavioral Medicine, 45*(3), 278–288.

Boyle, P. A., Barnes, L. L., Buchman, A. S., & Bennett, D. A. (2009). Purpose in life is associated with mortality among community-dwelling older persons. *Psychosomatic Medicine, 71*(5), 574–579.

Bronk, K. C. (2012). A grounded theory of the development of noble youth purpose. *Journal of Adolescent Research, 27*(1), 78–109.

Bundick, M., Andrews, M., Jones, A., Mariano, J. M., Bronk, K. C., & Damon, W. (2006). *Revised youth purpose survey*. Unpublished instrument, Stanford Center on Adolescence. Stanford, CA.

Burrow, A. L., & Hill, P. L. (2011). Purpose as a form of identity capital for positive youth adjustment. *Developmental Psychology, 47*(4), 1196–1206.

Burrow, A. L., & Hill, P. L. (2013). Derailed by diversity? Purpose buffers the relationship between ethnic composition on trains and passenger negative mood. *Personality and Social Psychology Bulletin, 39*(12), 1610–1619.

Burrow, A. L., & Hill, P. L. (2020). Discussion: The burdens and promises of purpose inquiry. In A. L. Burrow & P. L. Hill (Eds.), *The ecology of purposeful living across the lifespan: Developmental, educational, and social perspectives* (pp. 249–255). Springer.

Burrow, A. L., & Spreng, R. N. (2016). Waiting with purpose: A reliable but small association between purpose in life and impulsivity. *Personality and Individual Differences, 90*, 187–189.

Burrow, A. L., Stanley, M., Sumner, R., & Hill, P. L. (2014). Purpose in life as a resource for increasing comfort with ethnic diversity. *Personality and Social Psychology Bulletin, 40*(11), 1507–1516.

Chiang, J. J., Turiano, N. A., Mroczek, D. K., & Miller, G. E. (2018). Affective reactivity to daily stress and 20-year mortality risk in adults with chronic illness: Findings from the National Study of Daily experiences. *Health Psychology, 37*(2), 170–178.

Cohen, R., Bavishi, C., & Rozanski, A. (2016). Purpose in life and its relationship to all-cause mortality and cardiovascular events: A meta-analysis. *Psychosomatic Medicine, 78*(2), 122–133.

Costin, V., & Vignoles, V. L. (2020). Meaning is about mattering: Evaluating coherence, purpose, and existential mattering as precursors of meaning in life judgments. *Journal of Personality and Social Psychology, 118*(4), 864–884.

Crandall, J. E., & Rasmussen, R. D. (1975). Purpose in life as related to specific values. *Journal of Clinical Psychology, 31*, 483–485.

Crumbaugh, J. C., & Maholick, L. T. (1964). An experimental study in existentialism: The psychometric approach to Frankl's concept of noogenic neurosis. *Journal of Clinical Psychology, 20*(2), 200–207.

Damon, W. (2008). *The path to purpose: Helping our children find their calling in life.* Simon and Schuster.

Damon, W., Menon, J., & Cotton Bronk, K. (2003). The development of purpose during adolescence. *Applied Developmental Science, 7*(3), 119–128.

Erikson, E. H. (1959). *Identity and the life cycle: Selected papers.* International Universities Press.

Fogelman, N., & Canli, T. (2015). 'Purpose in Life' as a psychosocial resource in healthy aging: An examination of cortisol baseline levels and response to the Trier Social Stress Test. *NPJ Aging and Mechanisms of Disease, 1*(1), 1–3.

Frankl, V. (1984). *Man's search for meaning.* Washington Square Press/Pocket Books.

Frazier, L. D., Hooker, K., Johnson, P. M., & Kaus, C. R. (2000). Continuity and change in possible selves in later life: A 5-year longitudinal study. *Basic and Applied Social Psychology, 22*(3), 237–243.

George, L. S., & Park, C. L. (2013). Are meaning and purpose distinct? An examination of correlates and predictors. *The Journal of Positive Psychology, 8*(5), 365–375.

Grewen, K. M., Anderson, B. J., Girdler, S. S., & Light, K. C. (2003). Warm partner contact is related to lower cardiovascular reactivity. *Behavioral Medicine, 29*(3), 123–130.

Hampson, S. E. (2012). Personality processes: Mechanisms by which personality traits "get outside the skin". *Annual Review of Psychology, 63*(1), 315–339.

Harlow, L. L., Newcomb, M. D., & Bentler, P. M. (1986). Depression, self-derogation, substance use, and suicide ideation: Lack of purpose in life as a mediational factor. *Journal of Clinical Psychology, 42*(1), 5–21.

Heckhausen, J. (1997). Developmental regulation across adulthood: Primary and secondary control of age-related challenges. *Developmental Psychology, 33*(1), 176–187.
Hill, P. L., & Burrow, A. L. (2012). Viewing purpose through an Eriksonian lens. *Identity, 12*(1), 74–91.
Hill, P. L., & Burrow, A. L. (2020). Introduction: The purpose of studying purpose and the need for an ecological perspective. In A. L. Burrow & P. L. Hill (Eds.), *The ecology of purposeful living across the lifespan: Developmental, educational, and social perspectives* (pp. 1–9). Springer.
Hill, P. L., Burrow, A. L., Brandenberger, J. W., Lapsley, D. K., & Quaranto, J. C. (2010a). Collegiate purpose orientations and well-being in early and middle adulthood. *Journal of Applied Developmental Psychology, 31*(2), 173–179.
Hill, P. L., Burrow, A. L., O'Dell, A. C., & Thornton, M. A. (2010b). Classifying adolescents' conceptions of purpose in life. *The Journal of Positive Psychology, 5*(6), 466–473.
Hill, P. L., Burrow, A. L., & Sumner, R. (2016a). Sense of purpose and parent-child relationships in emerging adulthood. *Emerging Adulthood, 4*, 436–439.
Hill, P. L., Edmonds, G. W., & Hampson, S. E. (2019a). A purposeful lifestyle is a healthful lifestyle: Linking sense of purpose to self-rated health through multiple health behaviors. *Journal of Health Psychology, 24*(10), 1392–1400.
Hill, P. L., Edmonds, G. W., Peterson, M., Luyckx, K., & Andrews, J. A. (2016b). Purpose in life in emerging adulthood: Development and validation of a new brief measure. *The Journal of Positive Psychology, 11*(3), 237–245.
Hill, P. L., Schultz, L. H., Jackson, J. J., & Andrews, J. A. (2019b). Parent-child conflict during elementary school as a longitudinal predictor of sense of purpose in emerging adulthood. *Journal of Youth and Adolescence, 48*(1), 145–153.
Hill, P. L., Sin, N. L., Almeida, D. M., & Burrow, A. L. (2022). Sense of purpose predicts daily positive events and attenuates their influence on positive affect. *Emotion, 22*(3), 597–602.
Hill, P. L., Sin, N. L., Turiano, N. A., Burrow, A. L., & Almeida, D. M. (2018). Sense of purpose moderates the associations between daily stressors and daily well-being. *Annals of Behavioral Medicine, 52*(8), 724–729.
Hill, P. L., & Turiano, N. A. (2014). Purpose in life as a predictor of mortality across adulthood. *Psychological Science, 25*(7), 1482–1486.
Hill, P. L., Turiano, N. A., Mroczek, D. K., & Burrow, A. L. (2016c). The value of a purposeful life: Sense of purpose predicts greater income and net worth. *Journal of Research in Personality, 65*, 38–42.
Hill, P. L., Turiano, N. A., Spiro, A., III, & Mroczek, D. K. (2015). Understanding inter-individual variability in purpose: Longitudinal findings from the VA Normative Aging Study. *Psychology and Aging, 30*(3), 529–533.
Hill, P. L., & Weston, S. J. (2019). Evaluating eight-year trajectories for sense of purpose in the health and retirement study. *Aging & Mental Health, 23*(2), 233–237.

Hooker, K., & Kaus, C. R. (1994). Health-related possible selves in young and middle adulthood. *Psychology and Aging, 9*(1), 126.

Hopwood, C. J., & Bleidorn, W. (2019). Psychological profiles of people who justify eating meat as natural, necessary, normal, or nice. *Food Quality and Preference, 75*, 10–14.

Hopwood, C. J., Bleidorn, W., Schwaba, T., & Chen, S. (2020). Health, environmental, and animal rights motives for vegetarian eating. *PloS one, 15*(4), e0230609.

Idler, E. L., & Benyamini, Y. (1997). Self-rated health and mortality: A review of twenty-seven community studies. *Journal of Health and Social Behavior, 38*, 21–37.

John, O. P., & Srivastava, S. (1999). The Big Five trait taxonomy: History, measurement, and theoretical perspectives. In *Handbook of personality: Theory and research* (2nd ed., pp. 102–138). Guilford.

Jylhä, M. (2009). What is self-rated health and why does it predict mortality? Towards a unified conceptual model. *Social Science and Medicine, 69*, 307–316.

Kim, E. S., Delaney, S. W., & Kubzansky, L. D. (2019). Sense of purpose in life and cardiovascular disease: Underlying mechanisms and future directions. *Current Cardiology Reports, 21*(11), 135.

Kim, E. S., Hershner, S. D., & Strecher, V. J. (2015). Purpose in life and incidence of sleep disturbances. *Journal of Behavioral Medicine, 38*(3), 590–597.

Kim, E. S., Kawachi, I., Chen, Y., & Kubzansky, L. D. (2017). Association between purpose in life and objective measures of physical function in older adults. *JAMA psychiatry, 74*(10), 1039–1045.

Kim, E. S., Ryff, C., Hassett, A., Brummett, C., Yeh, C., & Strecher, V. (2020a). Sense of purpose in life and likelihood of future illicit drug use or prescription medication misuse. *Psychosomatic Medicine, 82*(7), 715–721.

Kim, E. S., Shiba, K., Boehm, J. K., & Kubzansky, L. D. (2020b). Sense of purpose in life and five health behaviors in older adults. *Preventive Medicine, 139*, 106172.

Kim, E. S., Strecher, V. J., & Ryff, C. D. (2014). Purpose in life and use of preventive health care services. *Proceedings of the National Academy of Sciences, 111*(46), 16331–16336.

Kirschbaum, C., Pirke, K. M., & Hellhammer, D. H. (1993). The 'Trier Social Stress Test'–a tool for investigating psychobiological stress responses in a laboratory setting. *Neuropsychobiology, 28*(1–2), 76–81.

Martela, F., & Steger, M. F. (2016). The three meanings of meaning in life: Distinguishing coherence, purpose, and significance. *The Journal of Positive Psychology, 11*(5), 531–545.

McKnight, P. E., & Kashdan, T. B. (2009). Purpose in life as a system that creates and sustains health and well-being: An integrative, testable theory. *Review of General Psychology, 13*(3), 242–251.

Meléndez, J. C., Satorres, E., Cujiño, M. A., & Reyes, M. F. (2019). Big Five and psychological and subjective well-being in Colombian older adults. *Archives of Gerontology and Geriatrics, 82*, 88–93.

Moran, S. (2020). How practicing our purpose aims contributes to a cultural common good, and vice versa. In A. L. Burrow & P. L. Hill (Eds.), *The ecology of purposeful living across the lifespan: Developmental, educational, and social perspectives* (pp. 199–232). Springer.

Mroczek, D. K., Stawski, R. S., Turiano, N. A., Chan, W., Almeida, D. M., Neupert, S. D., & Spiro, A., III. (2015). Emotional reactivity and mortality: Longitudinal findings from the VA Normative Aging Study. *Journals of Gerontology Series B: Psychological Sciences and Social Sciences, 70*(3), 398–406.

Pfund, G. N. (2020). We meet again: The reintroduction and reintegration of purpose into personality psychology. In A. L. Burrow & P. L. Hill (Eds.), *The ecology of purposeful living across the lifespan* (pp. 11–28). Springer.

Pfund, G. N., Brazeau, H., Allemand, M., & Hill, P. L. (2020). Associations between sense of purpose and romantic relationship quality in adulthood. *Journal of Social and Personal Relationships, 37*(5), 1563–1580.

Pfund, G. N., & Hill, P. L. (2018). The multifaceted benefits of purpose in life. *The International Forum for Logotherapy, 41*, 27–37.

Pfund, G. N., & Lewis, N. A. (2020). Aging with Purpose: Developmental Changes and Benefits of Purpose in Life Throughout the Lifespan. In P. L. Hill & M. Allemand (Eds.), *Personality and healthy aging in adulthood* (pp. 27–42). Springer.

Ratner, K., Burrow, A. L., Burd, K. A., & Hill, P. L. (2019). On the conflation of purpose and meaning in life: A qualitative study of high school and college student conceptions. *Applied Developmental Science, 4*, 1–21.

Reblin, M., & Uchino, B. N. (2008). Social and emotional support and its implication for health. *Current Opinion in Psychiatry, 21*(2), 201.

Roberts, B. W., Hill, P. L., & Davis, J. P. (2017). How to change conscientiousness: The sociogenomic trait intervention model. *Personality Disorders: Theory, Research, and Treatment, 8*(3), 199–205.

Roberts, B. W., O'Donnell, M., & Robins, R. W. (2004). Goal and personality trait development in emerging adulthood. *Journal of Personality and Social Psychology, 87*(4), 541–550.

Roberts, B. W., Walton, K. E., & Bogg, T. (2005). Conscientiousness and health across the life course. *Review of General Psychology, 9*(2), 156–168.

Rosenfeld, D. L. (2020). Gender differences in vegetarian identity: How men and women construe meatless dieting. *Food Quality and Preference, 81*, 103859.

Rosenfeld, D. L., & Burrow, A. L. (2017a). The unified model of vegetarian identity: A conceptual framework for understanding plant-based food choices. *Appetite, 112*, 78–95.

Rosenfeld, D. L., & Burrow, A. L. (2017b). Vegetarian on purpose: Understanding the motivations of plant-based dieters. *Appetite, 116*, 456–463.

Ryff, C. D. (1989a). Happiness is everything, or is it? Explorations on the meaning of psychological well-being. *Journal of Personality and Social Psychology, 57*(6), 1069–1081.

Ryff, C. D. (1989b). Beyond Ponce de Leon and life satisfaction: New directions in quest of successful ageing. *International Journal of Behavioral Development, 12*(1), 35–55.

Ryff, C. D. (2014). Psychological well-being revisited: Advances in the science and practice of eudaimonia. *Psychotherapy and Psychosomatics, 83*(1), 10–28.

Ryff, C. D., & Keyes, C. L. M. (1995). The structure of psychological well-being revisited. *Journal of Personality and Social Psychology, 69*(4), 719–727.

Ryff, C. D., & Kim, E. S. (2020). Extending research linking purpose in life to health: The challenges of inequality, the potential of the arts, and the imperative of virtue. In A. L. Burrow & P. L. Hill (Eds.), *The ecology of purposeful living across the lifespan* (pp. 29–58). Springer.

Ryff, C. D., Singer, B. H., & Dienberg Love, G. (2004). Positive health: Connecting well–being with biology. *Philosophical Transactions of the Royal Society of London. Series B: Biological Sciences, 359*(1449), 1383–1394.

Schaefer, S. M., Boylan, J. M., Van Reekum, C. M., Lapate, R. C., Norris, C. J., Ryff, C. D., & Davidson, R. J. (2013). Purpose in life predicts better emotional recovery from negative stimuli. *PloS one, 8*(11), e80329.

Scheier, M. F., Wrosch, C., Baum, A., Cohen, S., Martire, L. M., Matthews, K. A., Schulz, R., & Zdaniuk, B. (2006). The life engagement test: Assessing purpose in life. *Journal of Behavioral Medicine, 29*(3), 291–298.

Sin, N. L., & Almeida, D. M. (2018). Daily positive experiences and health: Biobehavioral pathways and resilience to daily stress. In C. D. Ryff & R. F. Krueger (Eds.), *The Oxford handbook of integrative health science* (pp. 155–172). Oxford University Press.

Sin, N. L., Graham-Engeland, J. E., Ong, A. D., & Almeida, D. M. (2015). Affective reactivity to daily stressors is associated with elevated inflammation. *Health Psychology, 34*(12), 1154–1165.

Sin, N. L., Sloan, R. P., McKinley, P. S., & Almeida, D. M. (2016). Linking daily stress processes and laboratory-based heart rate variability in a national sample of midlife and older adults. *Psychosomatic Medicine, 78*(5), 573.

Smith, T. W. (2006). Personality as risk and resilience in physical health. *Current Directions in Psychological Science, 15*(5), 227–231.

Sone, T., Nakaya, N., Ohmori, K., Shimazu, T., Higashiguchi, M., Kakizaki, M., Kikuchi, N., Kuriyama, S., & Tsuji, I. (2008). Sense of life worth living (ikigai) and mortality in Japan: Ohsaki Study. *Psychosomatic Medicine, 70*(6), 709–715.

Sumner, R., Burrow, A. L., & Hill, P. L. (2015). Identity and purpose as predictors of subjective well-being in emerging adulthood. *Emerging Adulthood, 3*(1), 46–54.

Sun, J., Kaufman, S. B., & Smillie, L. D. (2018). Unique associations between Big Five personality aspects and multiple dimensions of well-being. *Journal of Personality, 86*(2), 158–172.

Turiano, N. A., Whiteman, S. D., Hampson, S. E., Roberts, B. W., & Mroczek, D. K. (2012). Personality and substance use in midlife: Conscientiousness as a moderator and the effects of trait change. *Journal of Research in Personality, 46*(3), 295–305.

Turner, A. D., Smith, C. E., & Ong, J. C. (2017). Is purpose in life associated with less sleep disturbance in older adults? *Sleep Science and Practice, 1*(1), 14.

Uchino, B. N. (2006). Social support and health: A review of physiological processes potentially underlying links to disease outcomes. *Journal of Behavioral Medicine, 29*(4), 377–387.

Uchino, B. N., Bosch, J. A., Smith, T. W., Carlisle, M., Birmingham, W., Bowen, K. S., Light, K. C., Heaney, J., & O'Hartaigh, B. (2013). Relationships and cardiovascular risk: Perceived spousal ambivalence in specific relationship contexts and its links to inflammation. *Health Psychology, 32*(10), 1067–1075.

Uchino, B. N., Cacioppo, J. T., & Kiecolt-Glaser, J. K. (1996). The relationship between social support and physiological processes: A review with emphasis on underlying mechanisms and implications for health. *Psychological Bulletin, 119*(3), 488–531.

Vickers, R. R., Jr., Conway, T. L., & Hervig, L. K. (1990). Demonstration of replicable dimensions of health behaviors. *Preventive Medicine, 19*(4), 377–401.

Weston, S. J., Hill, P., & Mroczek, D. (2020). Purpose in life is associated with health outcomes among diabetic adults. https://doi.org/10.31234/osf.io/4snbt

Weston, S. J., Lewis, N. A., & Hill, P. L. (2021). Building sense of purpose in older adulthood: Examining the role of supportive relationships. *The Journal of Positive Psychology, 16*(3), 398–406. https://doi.org/10.1080/17439760.2020.1725607

Weston, S. J., Hill, P. L., & Mroczek, D. K. (2024). Associations for sense of purpose with smoking and health outcomes among adults with diabetes. *International Journal of Behavioral Medicine, 31*(4), 538–548.

Windsor, T. D., Curtis, R. G., & Luszcz, M. A. (2015). Sense of purpose as a psychological resource for aging well. *Developmental Psychology, 51*(7), 975–986.

Yaden, D. B., Le Nguyen, K. D., Kern, M. L., Belser, A. B., Eichstaedt, J. C., Iwry, J., Smith, M. E., Wintering, N. A., Hood, R. W., & Newberg, A. B. (2017). Of roots and fruits: A comparison of psychedelic and nonpsychedelic mystical experiences. *Journal of Humanistic Psychology, 57*(4), 338–353.

8

When Your Life Is Turned Upside-Down: Searching for and Finding Meaning in Illness and Injury

Christopher G. Davis and Joy McLeod

Introduction

Humans are sense-making creatures. We implicitly or explicitly seek explanations for almost everything unusual or unexpected that happens to us and to those around us. Why is my child upset? Why has my friend not responded to my text message? Why was my paper rejected? Making sense of these experiences helps us understand ourselves (e.g., what we can and cannot do), others, and the world in which we live. Such understandings, accumulated over time and experience, form our fundamental schemas or self- and worldviews (Epstein, 1973; Horowitz, 1976; Janoff-Bulman, 1992; Park & Folkman, 1997); these are the lenses or filters through which we understand and interpret the world around us. When events in our lives are consistent with our self- and worldviews, they make sense. To the extent that unexpected or unusual events in our lives threaten these ways of seeing ourselves and the world, we seem motivated to reconcile the discrepancy—or, if the event is not particularly personally significant, dismiss it as an anomaly. However, when the event is highly significant, making sense of it—or finding meaning in it—takes on great importance. Such is the situation for most people facing

To appear in *Handbook on Positive Psychology and Health*

C. G. Davis (✉) • J. McLeod
Department of Psychology, Carleton University, Ottawa, ON, Canada
e-mail: chris.davis@carleton.ca

F. M. Sirois (ed.), *The Palgrave Handbook of Positive Psychology and Health*,
https://doi.org/10.1007/978-3-031-89095-6_8

life-threatening or life-changing illness or injury. In this chapter, we attempt to make sense of the search for meaning in the context of illness or injury. What is the search for meaning? How can we understand it? How do people make sense of their illness or injury? And how can we facilitate the process of meaning-making?

What Is the Search for Meaning?

The concept of meaning is both broad and fuzzy (Heintzelman & King, 2013). When asked what gives their life meaning, people provide answers that suggest that meaning comes from having a purpose or direction to their life, understanding how the world in which they live works (e.g., a sense of order and predictability), and feeling that they are significant to or valued by others (e.g., their life matters; King et al., 2006; Martela & Steger, 2016). People trying to cope with a chronic illness or disabling injury may be searching for such meanings in life—especially to the extent that the illness or injury has compromised or unsettled any of these life meanings. For instance, a spinal cord injury can threaten one's purpose in life (including one's ability to pursue important goals), one's sense that their life was ordered and predictable (e.g., "my world has been turned upside down"), and one's perceived value to others (e.g., change in one's role in various relationships, new dependency on others). People in this situation may be motivated to restore all three of these aspects of meaning.

In addition to restoring a sense that one's life is meaningful and purposeful, people trying to cope with serious illness or injury may also be searching for some meaning in their condition, asking themselves, "Why did this happen to me?" Although a causal or etiological explanation may help answer this question, people often seek a deeper explanation. That is, people often are unsatisfied with explanations that center on physical or physiological factors (e.g., diet, genetics, one's own or others' actions or omissions; i.e., "how" questions); they often seek an answer that provides a purpose for the illness or injury (i.e., the question of "why" or "why me?"). For instance, Christopher Reeve, the actor best known for playing Superman, describes his search for meaning following his life-altering injury:

> When I suddenly became a quadriplegic my deepest, almost overwhelming reaction was simply "It's not fair." Intellectually, I knew that life isn't fair and that bad things can happen to any of us at any time. Emotionally, I couldn't control myself. I demanded an answer to the apparently unanswerable question: Why me? (Reeve, 2002, p. 175)

Seeking an answer to the "Why" (or "Why me") question implies that one believes that there is a reason; one's illness or injury serves a purpose. The question "Why me?" has often been referred to as a question of selective incidence (e.g., Janoff-Bulman & Frieze, 1983; Park & Folkman, 1997); that is, why have I been singled out? Some turn to religious or spiritual beliefs for an explanation (e.g., citing God's will) whereas others see this as fated, or as a test or challenge to be overcome (e.g., Bulman & Wortman, 1977; Pakenham, 2007; Thompson, 1991). Many others, like Reeve, find no satisfactory reason or explanation and continue to search for many years (e.g., Tait & Silver, 1989).

Finally, the search for meaning in an illness or injury may also be understood in terms of the effect that the illness or injury has on one's "life narrative" or "life scheme" (Fife, 1994; McAdams, 2001; Thompson & Janigian, 1988). People often have a life story that connects the dots of the major events in their life (giving their life a sense of order), and the onset of a serious illness or injury may interrupt or jeopardize the arc of one's narrative and leave one feeling that the story no longer "makes sense", that the direction of one's life has changed, that goals to which one was striving are now unattainable, and the achievements of one's life till now have become meaningless or inconsequential. Finding meaning in this context involves revising the narrative or life scheme in a way that incorporates the condition one now finds oneself in. What is the story of my life now that I have this condition?

Given the breadth and fuzziness of the concept of meaning, it is perhaps not surprising that people's sense of meaning is often unstable, frequently changing and evolving over time (Davis et al., 2000; Fife, 1994). One may develop a renewed sense of purpose in one's life, but still be struggling with randomness, or the implications of the possibility that one's life will be cut short. In our longitudinal research with people with spinal cord injury (Davis & Novoa, 2013) and people coping with the loss of a loved one (Davis et al., 2000), we observed that finding meaning does not terminate the search; people continue to search for meaning even after reporting that they have made sense of their injury or loss.

Questions of meaning imply that one has lost something, even if what has been lost is hard for the individual to articulate. In some cases, the loss is fairly obvious—such as the loss of use of one's limbs may mean the loss of a desired future, or the inability to further pursue meaningful activities. But other losses may be more challenging to comprehend, including the loss of hope, the shattering of assumptions, or awakening to the possibility of a foreshortened life. For instance, asking the question, Why me? could imply that one is not deserving of the condition in which one finds oneself (bad things are not supposed to happen to good people; e.g., Lerner, 1980), or it could imply that one believes that life is supposed to unfold in a predictable order—and this diagnosis or experience violates or shatters that belief. A participant in one study who lost a family member to cancer captured this violation well:

> What I can tell you is that the part of the death that I had a hard time making sense of was—here was a woman who spiritually had a God that she believed in very strongly … Why she suffered as she did, and why she had to experience death in a very slow, painful way was the thing I couldn't accept. It deepened my questioning of spiritual belief, whether there really is any spirit that's out there looking over you, taking care of you. He certainly didn't do it for her. But, as one of my friends said, "You never question God." So we'll have to rely upon that. (quoted in Davis et al., 1998, p. 565)

Finding meaning in these cases may involve some creative reappraisal, turning the perceived loss into a challenge, or even a potential gain. A spinal cord injury may end one's football career, but one may find the same adrenalin rush and sense of accomplishment playing wheelchair rugby. One participant in our study of people with spinal cord injury who was a high school teacher before his injury found a renewed sense of purpose by becoming a special needs teacher (Davis & Porter, 2018).

In summary, the search for meaning following a life-threatening or life-changing event can be understood as a motivation to integrate the experience and its many implications into one's set of assumptions and beliefs about how the world works (assumptions about order, predictability, control, and fairness), how one's life has unfolded and where one thought one was going (goals, life narratives, meaning and purpose in life), and one's sense of self (who am I now that I have this condition?). Integration typically involves revising these assumptions and beliefs (accommodation) or changing how one understands the event (assimilation). As the implications of the illness or injury may not be evident soon after onset, the search for meaning, and the meanings found, may change over time.

Some Historical Perspective

Interest in meaning-making goes back at least to Viktor Frankl (1955/1986), who argued that people have an inherent need or "will" to assign meaning to their life. According to Frankl (1955/1986), the existential search for meaning in life is a dynamic, ongoing task of humankind. People who perceive meaning in their lives have goals toward which they are striving, possess a sense of purpose, and are likely to perceive adversity as a challenge to be overcome. For Frankl, meaninglessness stems from despair over the perceived loss of goals, ambitions, and purpose in life. To restore meaning, or to help them develop new meaning, Frankl encouraged individuals to assume responsibility for their own life meaning, professing that "man should not ask what he may expect from life, but should rather understand that life expects something from him" (1955/1986, p. xxi). From this perspective, life is a task to be mastered, and life's adversities are challenges that one must try to overcome. Thus, Frankl suggested that the process of restoring meaning hinges on adopting an appropriate attitude toward suffering. For instance, reflecting on the horror of his concentration camp imprisonment during World War II, Frankl (1959/1984) suggested that his fellow prisoners who were able to attach a deep, psychological meaning to their life that transcended their current suffering were better able to survive the inhuman degradation of that experience. Others, unable to find purpose or meaning in their suffering, seemed to him more likely to give up hope, succumb to disease, and die. In Frankl's words, "The way in which he accepts, ... what courage he manifests in suffering, what dignity he displays in doom and disaster, is the measure of his human fulfillment" (1955/1986, p. 44).

Several clinician-researchers working with hospitalized patients in the 1950s and 1960s also noted a strong desire in many of their patients and families to find some meaning in their experience with serious, life-threatening illnesses (e.g., Bard & Dyk, 1956; Chodoff et al., 1964). For instance, Chodoff et al. (1964) observed among parents of children dying of leukemia "a persistent and even urgent need ... to encompass the tragic events unfolding before them within some broad framework of meaning which could make these events comprehensible to them" (p. 746). Some of their respondents focused on causal issues, such as understanding the etiology of leukemia or considering whether there was anything that they had or had not done that might have been responsible for their child falling ill. Others' explanations were more philosophical, citing, for example, divine retribution, God's will, and the belief that their child's medical treatment, even though bound to fail, would nevertheless contribute to science.

In the 1970s, several research studies took a more systematic approach to meaning-making among people dealing with loss and life-threatening or life-changing illnesses and injuries (e.g., Andreasen & Norris, 1972; Bulman & Wortman, 1977; Parkes, 1971, 1975). Cognitive models of the process of adapting to undesirable life-changing events were introduced by Shontz (1975) and Horowitz (1976) that emphasized the gradual process of accepting and integrating the reality of one's situation. According to Horowitz

(1976, 1986), processing the trauma involves integrating the meanings and implications of the information with existing knowledge structures, what he refers to as "inner schemata of the self and the world" (1986, p. 93). He argued that such thoughts are intrusive, automatic, and ruminative, and motivated by a "completion tendency"—an implicit need to fully integrate the experience. As these thoughts tend to be highly distressing, he proposed the existence of a control mechanism that shuts down processing when the emotions become overwhelming. Thus, people will oscillate between periods of intense processing and periods where such thoughts are avoided until the information is fully integrated and one has developed inner schemata that accommodate the threatening information. This may include changes in how one sees oneself and one's roles, changes in priorities and values, and changes in how one sees the world. This processing—or "working through"—of information related to the trauma has much in common with the concept of searching for and finding meaning in one's experience.

Horowitz (1976, 1986) recognized that the working-through process does not proceed along a single track. He noted that a single traumatic event may elicit several trains of thought, and that each thought may be associated with a range of memories, goals, and aspects of the self, thus implying that the process of incorporating the event into one's schemata may be difficult and incremental. It also implies that while the process may be comparable across individuals, how one comes to make sense of the experience will be highly idiosyncratic—each individual will need to find their own way of integrating the experience. It is not surprising, then, that people continue to search for meaning after reporting finding meaning, and that reports of meanings found do not always remain consistent over time.

The integration process that Horowitz described was expanded upon by Janoff-Bulman and her colleagues in the early 1980s. Drawing on her research with women who had been raped (Janoff-Bulman, 1979) and people with spinal cord injuries (Bulman & Wortman, 1977), Janoff-Bulman noted that people who have experienced trauma often have a compelling need to understand their experience within existing knowledge structures or schemas. This may lead individuals to accept some personal responsibility or blame for their situation when it is not appropriate or rational; one can maintain a belief that one's world is ordered and predictable if one comes to accept that one could have done something to avoid the undesired outcome. Janoff-Bulman integrated the various functions that these attributions serve in her Assumptive World Theory (Janoff-Bulman & Frieze, 1983; see also Janoff-Bulman, 1992). The model proposed that people who experience traumatic and loss events are often faced with evidence that their most basic assumptions about the world may be wrong. From this perspective, the attributions one makes following the event serve generally to restore worldviews and assumptions concerning one's self-worth and the benevolence and meaningfulness of the world. Deciding after the fact that a serious injury was highly probable given one's behavior (e.g., courting danger by participating in dangerous sports or occupations; Bulman & Wortman, 1977) may help preserve the assumption that such outcomes are predictable and hence meaningful by suggesting that the event was not random and unavoidable. More specifically, Janoff-Bulman (1992) argued that traumatic events pose a significant threat to how people view themselves (e.g., self-esteem, skills, and abilities), how they view the world (e.g., belief in a just, non-random world), and how they view their place in the world (e.g., perceptions of control). In her model, adjustment to trauma involves assimilating or accommodating the information implied by the event with these pre-existing assumptions about the self and the world.

At the same time, Shelley Taylor (1983) proposed the Cognitive Adaptation Theory, which held that making sense of one's experience was one of three common strategies that people typically use to maintain a sense of mastery during times of crisis. Based largely on a study of women coping with treatment for breast cancer, Taylor (1983; Taylor et al., 1984) argued that people adapt to life-threatening events by selectively interpreting their situation so as to maintain self-esteem and a sense of mastery. According to this Cognitive Adaptation theory, people are motivated to explain or assign meaning to their adversity in ways that preserve a sense that their condition is under control and not as dire as one might expect. For instance, people with cancer may assume some responsibility for the onset of their disease, attempting to restore their belief in personal mastery which may help them believe that they can ward off a recurrence (Taylor, 1983). By attributing cancer to a poor diet, a survivor may regain a sense of mastery by adopting a healthy, balanced diet. Both the Assumptive World Theory and Cognitive Adaptation Theory suggest that people are highly motivated to understand why they developed the condition that they now face, but to do so in a way that is self-enhancing or self-protective.

Whereas Cognitive Adaptation Theory emphasizes people's motivation to explain one's condition, World Assumptions Theory focuses more on the need to resolve perceived discrepancies between one's fundamental assumptions about how the world works (its benevolence, order, and personal control) and the reality of one's situation. Resolving this discrepancy requires either changing how one views the present situation or the reasons for the condition (a reappraisal) or adjusting one's assumptions to incorporate the present situation (an accommodation). Park and Folkman (1997), building off of World

Assumptions Theory, similarly describe the meaning-making process as an attempt to resolve discrepancies between global meanings (general beliefs and assumptions about one's world, and the life goals towards which one is striving) and specific meanings (explanations for outcomes). Park and Folkman (1997, Park, 2010) argue that in finding meaning, people are eliminating the discrepancy between situational meanings (i.e., how one interprets the event, such as the diagnosis of a life-changing illness) and global meanings (general beliefs about justice, control, and predictability, as well as personal goals and self-views that collectively serve as a framework or set of schemas for interpreting one's experiences; Park & George, 2013). Consistent with other discrepancy theories, they argue that people find meaning either by reappraising the meaning of the event to be consistent with one's goals and beliefs (an assimilation process) or by changing global beliefs to accommodate the new information.

One of the empirical challenges of Park and Folkman's model concerns the assessment of global meanings. How does one show that the discrepancy between global and situational meaning is being reduced if one cannot assess it? Although considerable work has gone into trying to define and measure these assumptions and global meanings (e.g., Cann et al., 2011; Janoff-Bulman, 1989; Koltko-Rivera, 2004; Park et al., 2016), it may not be realistic to expect that a given trauma (e.g., diagnosis of a life-threatening illness) is going to implicate a common set of assumptions in people, nor is it realistic to expect that people will revise their assumptions in the same way. It may be more effective to understand from the individual's point of view what the threat means to them, and how it has impacted the pursuit of their goals and their relationships (Davis & Porter, 2018; Fife, 1994). Moreover, we are concerned that discrepancy-reduction models do not fully recognize the breadth of meanings that chronic illnesses and disabling injuries threaten. Serious illnesses and injuries have broad implications, some of which may not be realized for some time. With each newly realized implication or perceived loss, one must reconsider what the illness or injury means to them.

Processing Trauma

Whereas some researchers have focused on assessing the fundamental beliefs and assumptions that are threatened by trauma, Lepore and colleagues have focused on cognitive efforts to process the threats that accompany trauma (Lepore, 2001; Lepore & Helgeson, 1998; Roberts et al., 2006). In their view, processing the information of trauma involves confronting, contemplating, and re-evaluating the threatening information with the goal of assimilating or accommodating the information into one's mental models—similar to the process described by Horowitz, Janoff-Bulman, and Park. From this perspective, spontaneous intrusive thoughts and images regarding the trauma are signals of incomplete processing. Using the frequency with which one searched for meaning as an index of cognitive processing, Roberts et al. (2006) found in a sample of men with prostate cancer that such processing was strongly associated with intrusive thoughts (as measured by Horowitz et al.'s Intrusive thoughts subscale of the IES), and that both predicted worse health-related quality of life. Similarly, Kernan and Lepore (2009) reported that more frequent searching for meaning among women coping with breast cancer was associated with higher levels of negative affect at two time-points within the first 18 months since diagnosis. Interestingly, they found that reports of finding meaning did not have any discernible effects on negative affect.

Other researchers have, however, found that finding meaning has implications for adjustment in people coping with illness. In a large sample of individuals with multiple sclerosis (MS) and their caregivers, Pakenham (2007, 2008) assessed the extent to which these individuals reported several aspects of meaning with respect to their MS, including redefining a life purpose, changing values and priorities, and taking a spiritual perspective, and found that many were associated with improved well-being over a 12-month period. In a study of people who had a stroke and their caregivers, Thompson (1991) found that whereas more frequent "Why me?" thoughts were associated with worse adjustment, reports of finding meaning were associated with better adjustment. Davis and Morgan (2008) also found in a sample of individuals with tinnitus that more frequent "Why me?" thoughts were associated with more symptoms of depression and lower levels of psychological well-being, but that having an answer to the question was not associated with these indicators of adjustment.

Although these studies suggest that more frequent searching for meaning, like the intrusive thoughts described by Horowitz (1986), may be a sign of adjustment difficulties in people with illness or injury, it would be premature to conclude that they are more than a mere symptom of distress. Almost all the studies reviewed above use a cross-sectional design, and where studies are longitudinal, they do not shed light on whether the search for meaning contributes to or is a consequence of distress. Davis and Novoa (2013) attempted to distinguish between-person effects from within-person effects of searching for and finding meaning in their longitudinal study of people coping with a recent spinal cord injury. Assessing the extent to which people were searching for meaning at each of three points in time following their injury (2½ months,

5 months, and 13 months), and the extent to which they reported finding meaning at each of those time points, Davis and Novoa (2013) showed that when people searched for meaning more frequently than their average, their symptoms of depression also increased. And when they reported finding more meaning than their average, their symptoms decreased. Although such effects do not necessarily mean that searching for and finding meaning are causing changes in depression, they move us past the individual difference interpretation that some people who are adapting well are able to make sense of their adversity. The data also indicate that meaning-making is not an achievement—once obtained, the issue of meaning is not necessarily put to rest (see also Davis et al., 2000).

The process of integrating the threats that come with the information that one has a life-threatening or life-changing condition or injury with one's fundamental assumptions and goals creates opportunities for personal growth. We have seen evidence of this in two studies: one a cross-sectional study of people coping with tinnitus (Davis & Morgan, 2008) and the other our study of people with spinal cord injury, noted earlier. In our study of people with tinnitus, we found that the experience of negative life changes attributable to one's tinnitus predicted searching for meaning (asking "Why me?"), and that those who were able to come up with an answer to the "Why me?" question were more likely to report positive changes in life goals and philosophy of life. Likewise, in our study of people with spinal cord injury, we found that not only were those who reported finding meaning more likely to perceive growth but also that increases in reported meaning over time were associated with increases in perceived growth (Davis & Novoa, 2013). Prominent models of posttraumatic growth (Tedeschi & Calhoun, 2004) suggest that meaning-making—or cognitive processing of the trauma—is a critical step in the process of growing from adversity, and although the two concepts are empirically related, it is not always clear whether reports of growth are distinct from the meanings that people ascribe to their experience (Park, 2010). Developing a new appreciation for life, discovering new possibilities, and changes in self-understanding—frequent examples of posttraumatic growth—are also examples of meanings made (Davis & Novoa, 2013; Pakenham, 2007; Taylor, 1995). Given this conceptual overlap, we regard the integration process as providing an opportunity for individuals to work towards or realize (potential) positive change in values, self-concept, purpose, and relationships—changes that are recognized as posttraumatic growth.

Although most of the meanings that people report are positive and are generally regarded by those who report them as comforting, some are not. As one individual in a study of meaning-making among people coping with loss said,

> The sense of his death is that there is no sense. Those things just happen ... The sense of his death for me is "get ready to die." Don't be surprised when it happens. Don't think that somehow you're going to be exempt from it ... There's no underlying sense of order in the sense that things progress in an expectable pattern. Well, the pattern is that you're born and you die. (quoted in Davis et al., 1998, p. 569)

It is unclear whether such meanings should be regarded as promoting integration (or "completion" as Horowitz calls it). On the one hand, the revised worldview implied by quotes such as this suggests less meaning and purpose in life, while on the other hand, the revised worldview more readily incorporates random undesirable events and may better reflect the state of the world in which this person lives. The illusions of control, fairness, and benevolence of others (or God) may be stripped away leaving one feeling small, vulnerable, and angry, but perhaps with a more realistic view of life.

In each of our studies of individuals coping with life-threatening or life-changing events, we have observed a significant minority of individuals who report that they have not (even years afterward) ever searched for meaning following their loss or onset of their health condition (Davis & Morgan, 2008; Davis et al., 2007; Davis et al., 2000). These individuals tend to report less distress and depressive symptoms than those who do search for meaning, and in our tinnitus study (Davis & Morgan, 2008) were more likely to say that they accept their tinnitus (e.g., regard it as part of who they are, not something that has taken hold of their life; are less inclined to continue to seek a cure). When asked if they had ever asked "Why me?" they tended to respond by saying "Why NOT me?" This suggests that those who did not search for meaning possessed a worldview that was readily able to incorporate or assimilate the event they experienced and its implications. And while this worldview may not be as positive and optimistic as that of those for whom these events are more jarring, those who do not report searching for meaning nonetheless appear to be among the most resilient in the face of trauma. Further research is needed to better understand these individuals.

In contrast to those who do not search for meaning following life-changing or life-threatening events, we (Davis et al., 2000, 2007) and others (e.g., Silver et al., 1983; Tait & Silver, 1989) typically see many others who report searching for meaning even years afterward. The ongoing, prolonged search to make sense of one's situation is indicative of adjustment difficulties (e.g., Davis &

Novoa, 2013; Davis et al., 2000; Kernan & Lepore, 2009; Roberts et al., 2006), particularly when the search perseverates on a single issue (e.g., "Why me?"). Such perseverating may suggest an inability or unwillingness to give up a life goal, assumption, or belief that remains at odds with the apparent meaning of the event. In the next section, we consider interventions that help individuals resolve these meaning discrepancies.

Helping People Find Meaning

Meaning-making in the face of illness or injury is typically thought of as a deeply personal task. As Frankl (1955/1986) argued, it is ultimately the individual's responsibility to give their life meaning and purpose, even as the challenges of life thwart one's efforts. At present, we know very little about how people resolve issues of meaning. There is some preliminary evidence that meanings for loss tend to be shared within (some) families, and to the extent that there is agreement within families on the meanings, they tend to be adjusting more successfully (Davis et al., 2012; Nadeau, 1998). There is also evidence indicating that to the extent that individuals feel unable to discuss their thoughts and feelings about the situation they are facing, they tend to report more intrusive thoughts related to their situation and appear to be experiencing more depression (Lepore, 2001; Lepore et al., 1996; Roberts et al., 2006). There is also some evidence that at least some people dealing with life-threatening illnesses want help finding meaning in life and seek opportunities to talk with others about the meaning of life and death (Moadel et al., 1999). Although we suspect that resolving meaning discrepancies—or finding meaning—is largely an introspective task, discussions with others, especially those others who have had a similar experience (such as support groups), may spur important insights (Neimeyer, 2000).

In the absence of supportive others, guided expressive writing may also promote meaning-making among people coping with chronic or life-threatening illnesses, a technique pioneered by Pennebaker (for a review, see Pennebaker & Chung, 2007). The typical expressive writing paradigm involves writing about previously undisclosed emotional matters, such as one's diagnosis or illness experience, for three to five days, for up to half an hour at a time (Smyth et al., 2012). Pennebaker et al. (1997) suggest that these writing exercises help individuals form a narrative of their experience, which may facilitate meaning-making (see also Smyth et al., 2001). Research shows that expressive writing can lead to improvements in psychological health (Frattaroli, 2006; Graham et al., 2008; Lepore, 1997; Stockton et al.,

2014), physical health (Frattaroli, 2006; Frisina et al., 2004; Pennebaker et al., 1997), and physiological functioning (Petrie et al., 2004; Smyth et al., 1999) in a variety of clinical populations, such as people living with asthma and rheumatoid arthritis (Smyth et al., 1999), cancer (Rosenberg et al., 2002; Stanton & Danoff-Burg, 2002), chronic pain (Graham et al., 2008), human immunodeficiency virus (Petrie et al., 2004), fibromyalgia (Gillis et al., 2006), and cystic fibrosis (Taylor et al., 2003).

Expressive writing may change the quality—if not the quantity—of intrusive thoughts. Some researchers have found that expressive writing leads to a reduction in intrusive thoughts (Low et al., 2010; Schoutrop et al., 2002). For example, Low et al. (2010) found that women with metastatic breast cancer who lacked emotional support reported fewer intrusive thoughts following an expressive writing intervention. In contrast, Lepore (1997) found no change in the frequency of intrusive thoughts, but rather intrusive thoughts were no longer associated with depression among individuals who had completed an expressive writing task. This suggests a reduction in the emotional impact of intrusive thoughts. Stockton et al. (2014) also found that expressive writing did not change the frequency of intrusive thoughts in a sample of individuals who had experienced a traumatic event, but it did have an effect on perceptions of posttraumatic growth; those assigned to the expressive writing condition reported greater growth at a two-month follow-up than individuals who had completed a non-emotional, control writing task. In summary, people may find meaning by sharing their thoughts and feelings with empathic others or, in the absence of such support, by putting their thoughts and feelings onto paper. By expressing these thoughts and feelings, they may begin to form a narrative that makes sense to them.

Formal interventions (therapies) to promote meaning-making for people coping with life-threatening and life-changing conditions have been used for more than 50 years. Viktor Frankl's existentialist approach, developed during his captivity in a concentration camp during World War II, emphasizes the need for people to create their own meanings that give purpose and direction to their lives despite the existential challenges they are facing (Frankl, 1955/1986, 1959/1984). Meaning-making has also figured prominently in the therapeutic approaches of Rollo May (1953) and Irvin Yalom (1980) and, more recently, by Paul Wong (2009, 2015). Structured meaning-based interventions that have been developed for individuals coping with illness are intended to help the individual reframe their suffering within the context of their life narrative or schemes (e.g., Greenstein & Breitbart, 2000). In the case of terminal cancer, for example, therapists facilitate the processing of one's diagnosis and help the client integrate the threat of dying into their daily life.

There is some evidence that meaning-based therapies are effective. To our knowledge, Zuehlke and Watkins (1975) published the first empirical research on the effectiveness of meaning-based therapeutic interventions (based on Frankl's logotherapy). Their study compared six terminally ill men who received six 45-minute logotherapy sessions over the course of two weeks with a waitlist control group and found that those receiving therapy reported greater meaning in life post-treatment relative to controls, but also reported greater death anxiety. Since the early 2000s, several other meaning-based interventions have been evaluated, both for people dealing with terminal illness (Greenstein & Breitbart, 2000; Henry et al., 2010; Lee et al., 2006; Lepore, 2001; Rosenfeld et al., 2018; Wagner et al., 2016) and their spouses (Wagner et al., 2016), as the patient's spouse is often facing existential issues as their assumptions and goals are also threatened by the patient's condition.

More recently, Lee et al. (2006) and Henry et al. (2010) examined the efficacy of a short, four-session meaning-making intervention (MMi) among individuals living with early-stage breast or colorectal cancer and late-stage ovarian cancer, comparing the two groups against a no treatment control. Although under-powered, the Henry et al. study found significant improvements in meaning in life one month and three months post-intervention (Cohen's $d = 0.42$ and 0.41) and marginally significant improvements in quality of life ($d = 0.58$) and existential well-being three months post-intervention ($d = 0.56$). The intervention, however, had no impact on participants' levels of psychological distress or self-efficacy. On the other hand, the larger study by Lee et al. (2006) found that meaning-making intervention yielded modest improvements in self-esteem, optimism, and self-efficacy measured 24 hours post-intervention (ranging from $d = 0.22$–0.26). Rosenfeld et al. (2018) have also evaluated an eight-session meaning-centered group therapy for individuals with late-stage cancer. Relative to a supportive group psychotherapy control group, which focused more on coping with one's cancer, the meaning-centered group therapy used didactic discussion and experiential exercises to facilitate the meaning-making process. Rosenfeld et al. (2018) found that those in the meaning-centered group therapy had improvements in psychological well-being relative to the control group, specifically increased quality of life and decreased depression, which were maintained over the two-month post-session follow-up. Importantly, improvements were mediated by participants' enhanced sense of meaning. These results provide some support for the effectiveness of meaning-based interventions.

Conclusion

In this chapter, we have reviewed evidence that indicates that most people who have experienced a life-threatening or life-changing illness or injury search for meaning. The search for meaning takes varied forms: for some, it is an effort to find or renew purpose or significance for their life, for others it is an effort to find purpose or significance in the illness or injury itself—finding an answer to the question of Why, or Why me? Still others wrestle with an apparent threat that the illness or injury poses for assumptions that previously made their world ordered, predictable, and understandable. How does one go on when the goals and beliefs that made one's life meaningful and purposeful are no longer tenable? Finding meaning involves resolving these issues.

Our review suggests that resolving the various threats to meaning is a high priority for most, but not all people, at least soon after their diagnosis. According to Horowitz (1976, 1986), the intense, intrusive thoughts that people coping with trauma—including the trauma of learning that one has a life-threatening or life-changing condition—are a signal that the event or situation that one is dealing with does not make sense; it does not fit within one's existing knowledge structures. Making sense of one's experience reduces the frequency and intensity of these intrusive thoughts.

Although most people will, in time, be able to find answers to the existential questions brought on by these life-threatening or life-changing conditions, developing new understandings of themselves, life, and the world in which they live, in some cases individuals will need assistance. This is particularly likely in situations where individuals are isolated or feel social constraints on talking about their concerns, suggesting that meaning-making is facilitated when one shares one's thoughts and feelings with empathic support providers. In the absence of such persons, there is some evidence that guided expressive writing exercises may be helpful in these situations. Research also indicates that meaning-based individual and group therapies can be effective.

The research evidence for the role that meaning-making plays in the adjustment process is, with few exceptions, limited to self-reports. There may not be behavioral indicators of searching for or finding meaning, but we are not so limited when it comes to the outcomes of the process. Does a prolonged search for meaning predict deteriorating health, and does finding meaning predict health improvement? Research from the expressive writing paradigm indicates that expressive writing results in improved health (Pennebaker et al., 1988; Petrie et al., 2004), but to our knowledge, only two studies show that finding meaning, specifically, has implications for physical health (Affleck et al., 1987; Bower et al., 1998). Bower et al. reported that bereaved HIV-seropositive men who found meaning in their loss showed less rapid decline in health and lower rates of mortality at follow-up relative to those who had not found meaning. Affleck et al. (1987) also found in a sample of men who had experienced a heart attack that those who perceived benefits from their heart attack seven weeks post-infarction were less likely to have had another heart attack and reported less morbidity when reinterviewed eight years later than men who did not perceive benefits from their illness. It will be important for future research to consider whether finding meaning in one's illness or injury has implications for illness or injury management.

References

Affleck, G., Tennen, H., Croog, S., & Levine, S. (1987). Causal attribution, perceived benefits, and morbidity after a heart attack: An 8-year study. *Journal of Consulting and Clinical Psychology, 55*, 29–35. https://doi.org/10.1037/0022-006X.55.1.29

Andreasen, N. J. C., & Norris, A. S. (1972). Long-term adjustment and adaptation mechanisms in severely burned adults. *Journal of Nervous and Mental Disease, 154*, 352–362.

Bard, M., & Dyk, R. B. (1956). The psychodynamic significance of beliefs regarding the cause of serious illness. *Psychoanalytic Review, 43*, 146–162.

Bower, J. E., Kemeny, M. E., Taylor, S. E., & Fahey, J. L. (1998). Cognitive processing, discovery of meaning, CD4 decline, and AIDS-related mortality among bereaved HIV-seropositive men. *Journal of Consulting and Clinical Psychology, 66*, 979–986.

Bulman, R. J., & Wortman, C. B. (1977). Attributions of blame and coping in the "real world": Severe accident victims react to their lot. *Journal of Personality and Social Psychology, 35*, 351–363.

Cann, A., Calhoun, L., Tedeschi, R., Triplett, K., Vishnevsky, T., & Lindstrom, C. (2011). Assessing posttraumatic cognitive processes: The event-related rumination inventory. *Anxiety, Stress, & Coping, 24*(2), 137–156. https://doi.org/10.1080/10615806.2010.529901

Chodoff, P., Friedman, S. B., & Hamburg, D. A. (1964). Stress, defenses and coping behavior: Observations in parents of children with malignant disease. *American Journal of Psychiatry, 120*, 743–749.

Davis, C. G., Harasymchuk, C., & Wohl, M. J. A. (2012). Finding meaning in a traumatic loss: A families approach. *Journal of Traumatic Stress, 25*, 142–149.

Davis, C. G., & Morgan, M. S. (2008). Finding meaning, perceiving growth, and acceptance of tinnitus. *Rehabilitation Psychology, 53*, 128–138.

Davis, C. G., Nolen-Hoeksema, S., & Larson, J. (1998). Making sense of loss and benefiting from the experience: Two construals of meaning. *Journal of Personality and Social Psychology, 75*, 561–574.
Davis, C. G., & Novoa, D. C. (2013). Meaning-making following spinal cord injury: Individual differences and within person change. *Rehabilitation Psychology, 58*, 166–177.
Davis, C. G., & Porter, J. E. (2018). Pathways to growth following trauma and loss. In C. R. Snyder, S. J. Lopez, L. M. Edwards, & S. C. Marques (Eds.), *Oxford handbook of positive psychology* (3rd ed.). Oxford University Press.
Davis, C. G., Wohl, M. J. A., & Verberg, N. (2007). Profiles of posttraumatic growth following an unjust loss. *Death Studies, 31*, 693–712.
Davis, C. G., Wortman, C. B., Lehman, D. R., & Silver, R. C. (2000). Searching for meaning in loss: Are clinical assumptions correct? *Death Studies, 24*, 497–540.
Epstein, S. (1973). The self-concept revisited: Or a theory of a theory. *American Psychologist, 28*, 404–416.
Fife, B. (1994). The conceptualization of meaning in illness. *Social Science & Medicine, 38*(2), 309–316.
Frankl, V. E. (1955/1986). *The doctor and the soul: From psychotherapy to logotherapy* (3rd ed.). Vintage Books.
Frankl, V. E. (1959/1984). *Man's search for meaning: An introduction to logotherapy* (3rd ed.). Simon & Schuster.
Frattaroli, J. (2006). Experimental disclosure and its moderators: A meta-analysis. *Psychological Bulletin, 132*(6), 823–865.
Frisina, P., Borod, J., & Lepore, S. (2004). A meta-analysis of the effects of written emotional disclosure on the health outcomes of clinical populations. *The Journal of Nervous and Mental Disease, 192*(9), 629–634.
Gillis, M., Lumley, M., Mosley-Williams, A., Leisen, J., & Roehrs, T. (2006). The health effects of at-home written emotional disclosure in fibromyalgia: A randomized trial. *Annals of Behavioral Medicine, 32*(2), 135–146.
Graham, J., Lobel, M., Glass, P., & Lokshina, I. (2008). Effects of written anger expression in chronic pain patients: Making meaning from pain. *Journal of Behavioral Medicine, 31*(3), 201–212.
Greenstein, M., & Breitbart, W. (2000). Cancer and the experience of meaning: A group psychotherapy program for people with cancer. *American Journal of Psychotherapy, 54*(4), 486–500.
Heintzelman, S., & King, L. (2013). On knowing more than we can tell: Intuitive processes and the experience of meaning. *The Journal of Positive Psychology, 8*(6), 471–482.
Henry, M., Cohen, S., Lee, V., Sauthier, P., Provencher, D., Drouin, P., Gauthier, P., Gotlieb, W., Lau, S., Drummond, N., Gilbert, L., Stanimir, G., Sturgeon, J., Chasen, M., Mitchell, J., Huang, L., Ferland, M., & Mayo, N. (2010). The meaning-making intervention (MMi) appears to increase meaning in life in advanced ovarian cancer: A randomized controlled pilot study. *Psycho-Oncology, 19*(12), 1340–1347.

Horowitz, M. J. (1976). *Stress response syndromes*. Aronson.
Horowitz, M. J. (1986). *Stress response syndromes* (2nd ed.). Aronson.
Janoff-Bulman, R. (1979). Characterological versus behavioral self-blame: Inquiries into depression and rape. *Journal of Personality and Social Psychology, 37*, 1798–1809.
Janoff-Bulman, R. (1989). Assumptive worlds and the stress of traumatic events: Applications of the schema construct. *Social Cognition, 7*, 113–136.
Janoff-Bulman, R. (1992). *Shattered assumptions: Towards a new psychology of trauma*. Free Press.
Janoff-Bulman, R., & Frieze, I. H. (1983). A theoretical perspective for understanding reactions to victimization. *Journal of Social Issues, 39*(2), 1–17.
Kernan, W. D., & Lepore, S. J. (2009). Searching for and making meaning after breast cancer: Prevalence, patterns, and negative affect. *Social Science & Medicine, 68*(6), 1176–1182. https://doi.org/10.1016/j.socscimed.2008.12.038
King, L. A., Hicks, J. A., Krull, J. L., & Del Gaiso, A. K. (2006). Positive affect and the experience of meaning in life. *Journal of Personality and Social Psychology, 90*(1), 179–196.
Koltko-Rivera, M. (2004). The psychology of worldviews. *Review of General Psychology, 8*, 3–58.
Lee, V., Robin Cohen, S., Edgar, L., Laizner, A., & Gagnon, A. (2006). Meaning-making intervention during breast or colorectal cancer treatment improves self-esteem, optimism, and self-efficacy. *Social Science & Medicine, 62*(12), 3133–3145.
Lepore, S. (1997). Expressive writing moderates the relation between intrusive thoughts and depressive symptoms. *Journal of Personality and Social Psychology, 73*(5), 1030–1037.
Lepore, S. J. (2001). A social–cognitive processing model of emotional adjustment to cancer. In A. Baum & B. L. Andersen (Eds.), *Psychosocial interventions for cancer: Psychosocial interventions for cancer* (pp. 99–116). American Psychological Association. https://doi.org/10.1037/10402-006
Lepore, S. J., & Helgeson, V. S. (1998). Social constraints, intrusive thoughts, and mental health after prostate cancer. *Journal of Social and Clinical Psychology, 17*, 89–106. https://doi.org/10.1521/jscp.1998.17.1.89
Lepore, S. J., Silver, R. C., Wortman, C. B., & Wayment, H. A. (1996). Social constraints, intrusive thoughts, and depressive symptoms among bereaved mothers. *Journal of Personality and Social Psychology, 70*, 271–282. https://doi.org/10.1037/0022-3514.70.2.271
Lerner, M. (1980). The Belief in a Just World : A Fundamental Delusion (1st ed. 1980.). Springer US. https://doi.org/10.1007/978-1-4899-0448-5
Low, C. A., Stanton, A. L., Bower, J. E., & Gyllenhammer, L. (2010). A randomized controlled trial of emotionally expressive writing for women with metastatic breast cancer. *Health Psychology, 29*, 460–466. https://doi.org/10.1037/a0020153
Martela, F., & Steger, M. F. (2016). The three meanings of meaning in life: Distinguishing coherence, purpose, and significance. *The Journal of Positive Psychology, 11*, 531–545.

May, R. (1953). *Man's search for himself.* W. W. Norton.
McAdams, D. (2001). The psychology of life stories. *Review of General Psychology, 5*, 100–122. https://doi.org/10.1037/1089-2680.5.2.100
Moadel, A., Morgan, C., Fatone, A., Grennan, J., Carter, J., Laruffa, G., Skummy, A., & Dutcher, J. (1999). Seeking meaning and hope: Self-reported spiritual and existential needs among an ethnically-diverse cancer patient population. *Psycho-Oncology, 8*, 378–385.
Nadeau, J. W. (1998). *Families making sense of death*. Sage.
Neimeyer, R. A. (2000). Searching for the meaning of meaning: Grief therapy and the process of reconstruction. *Death Studies, 24*, 541–558. https://doi.org/10.1080/07481180050121480
Pakenham, K. (2008). The nature of sense making in caregiving for persons with multiple sclerosis. *Disability and Rehabilitation, 30*, 1263–1273.
Pakenham, K. I. (2007). Making sense of multiple sclerosis. *Rehabilitation Psychology, 52*, 380–389.
Park, C. L. (2010). Making sense of the meaning literature: An integrative review of meaning making and its effects on adjustment to stressful life events. *Psychological Bulletin, 136*, 257–301.
Park, C. L., & Folkman, S. (1997). Meaning in the context of stress and coping. *Review of General Psychology, 1*, 115–144.
Park, C. L., & George, L. (2013). Assessing meaning and meaning making in the context of stressful life events: Measurement tools and approaches. *The Journal of Positive Psychology, 8*, 483–504.
Park, C. L., Riley, K. E., George, L. S., Gutierrez, I. A., Hale, A. E., Cho, D., & Braun, T. D. (2016). Assessing disruptions in meaning: Development of the global meaning violation scale. *Cognitive Therapy and Research, 40*, 831–846. https://doi.org/10.1007/s10608-016-9794-9
Parkes, C. M. (1971). Psycho-social transitions: A field for study. *Social Science and Medicine, 5*, 101–115.
Parkes, C. M. (1975). What becomes of redundant world models? A contribution to the study of adaptation to change. *British Journal of Medical Psychology, 48*, 131–137.
Pennebaker, J. W., & Chung, C. K. (2007). Expressive writing, emotional upheavals, and health. In H. S. Friedman & R. C. Silver (Eds.), *Foundations of health psychology* (pp. 263–284). Oxford University Press.
Pennebaker, J. W., Kiecolt-Glaser, J. K., & Glaser, R. (1988). Disclosure of traumas and immune function: Health implications for psychotherapy. *Journal of Consulting and Clinical Psychology, 56*, 239–245. https://doi.org/10.1037/0022-006X.56.2.239
Pennebaker, J. W., Mayne, T. J., & Francis, M. E. (1997). Linguistic predictors of adaptive bereavement. *Journal of Personality and Social Psychology, 72*, 863–871.
Petrie, K. J., Fontanilla, I., Thomas, M. G., Booth, R. J., & Pennebaker, J. W. (2004). Effect of written emotional expression on immune function in patients with

human immunodeficiency virus infection. A randomized trial. *Psychosomatic Medicine, 66*, 272–275.

Reeve, C. (2002). *Nothing is impossible: Reflections on a new life*. Random House.

Roberts, K. J., Lepore, S. J., & Helgeson, V. (2006). Social-cognitive correlates of adjustment to prostate cancer. *Psycho-Oncology, 15*, 183–192. https://doi.org/10.1002/pon.934

Rosenberg, H. J., Rosenberg, S. D., Ernstoff, M. S., Wolford, G. L., Amdur, R. J., Elshamy, M. R., Bauer-Wu, S. M., Ahles, T. A., & Pennebaker, J. W. (2002). Expressive disclosure and health outcomes in a prostate cancer population. *International Journal of Psychiatry in Medicine, 32*, 37–53.

Rosenfeld, B., Cham, H., Pessin, H., & Breitbart, W. (2018). Why is meaning-centered group psychotherapy (MCGP) effective? Enhanced sense of meaning as the mechanism of change for advanced cancer patients. *Psycho-Oncology, 27*, 654–660.

Schoutrop, M. J., Lange, A., Hanewald, G., Davidovich, U., & Salomon, H. (2002). Structured writing and processing major stressful events: A controlled trial. *Psychotherapy and Psychosomatics, 71*, 151–157.

Shontz, F. C. (1975). *The psychological aspects of physical illness and disability*. Macmillan.

Silver, R. L., Boon, C., & Stones, M. H. (1983). Searching for meaning in misfortune: Making sense of incest. *Journal of Social Issues, 39*(2), 81–102.

Smyth, J., True, N., & Souto, J. (2001). Effects of writing about traumatic experiences: The necessity for narrative structuring. *Journal of Social and Clinical Psychology, 20*, 161–172.

Smyth, J. M., Pennebaker, J. W., & Arigo, D. (2012). What are the health effects of disclosure? In A. Baum, T. A. Revenson, & J. Singer (Eds.), *Handbook of health psychology* (2nd ed., pp. 175–191). Psychology Press.

Smyth, J. M., Stone, A. A., Hurewitz, A., & Kaell, A. (1999). Effects of writing about stressful experiences on symptom reduction in patients with asthma or rheumatoid arthritis: A randomized trial. *Journal of the American Medical Association, 281*, 1304–1309.

Stanton, A. L., & Danoff-Burg, S. (2002). Emotional expression, expressive writing, and cancer. In S. J. Lepore & J. M. Smyth (Eds.), *The writing cure: How expressive writing promotes health and emotional well-being* (pp. 31–51). American Psychological Association.

Stockton, H., Joseph, S., & Hunt, N. (2014). Expressive writing and posttraumatic growth: An internet-based study. *Traumatology, 20*, 75–83.

Tait, R., & Silver, R. C. (1989). Coming to terms with major negative life events. In J. S. Uleman & J. A. Bargh (Eds.), *Unintended thought* (pp. 351–382). The Guilford Press.

Taylor, E. J. (1995). Whys and wherefores: Adult patient perspectives of the meaning of cancer. *Seminars in Oncology Nursing, 11*, 32–40.

Taylor, L. A., Wallander, J. L., Anderson, D., Beasley, P., & Brown, R. T. (2003). Improving health care utilization, improving chronic disease utilization, health status, and adjustment in adolescents and young adults with cystic fibrosis: A preliminary report. *Journal of Clinical Psychology in Medical Settings, 10*, 9–16.

Taylor, S. E. (1983). Adjusting to threatening events: A theory of cognitive adaptation. *American Psychologist, 38*, 1161–1173.

Taylor, S. E., Lichtman, R. R., & Wood, J. V. (1984). Attributions, beliefs about control, and adjustment to breast cancer. *Journal of Personality and Social Psychology, 46*, 489–502.

Tedeschi, R. G., & Calhoun, L. G. (2004). Posttraumatic growth: Conceptual foundations and empirical evidence. *Psychological Inquiry, 15*, 1–18.

Thompson, S. C. (1991). The search for meaning following a stroke. *Basic and Applied Social Psychology, 12*, 81–96.

Thompson, S. C., & Janigian, A. S. (1988). Life schemes: A framework for understanding the search for meaning. *Journal of Social and Clinical Psychology, 7*, 260–280.

Wagner, C., Johns, S., Brown, L., Hanna, N., & Bigatti, S. (2016). Acceptability and feasibility of a meaning-based intervention for patients with advanced cancer and their spouses: A pilot study. *American Journal of Hospice & Palliative Medicine, 33*, 546–554.

Wong, P. (2009). Meaning therapy: An integrative and positive existential psychotherapy. *Journal of Contemporary Psychotherapy, 40*, 85–93.

Wong, P. (2015). Meaning therapy: Assessments and interventions. *Existential Analysis, 26*, 154–169.

Yalom, I. D. (1980). *Existential psychotherapy*. Basic Books.

Zuehlke, T., & Watkins, J. (1975). The use of psychotherapy with dying patients: An exploratory study. *Journal of Clinical Psychology, 31*, 729–732.

9

Self-Affirmation and Health

Peter R. Harris and Donna C. Jessop

In his seminal 1988 paper presenting Self-Affirmation Theory (Steele, 1988), Claude Steele used a health example—the psychological threat posed by being a cigarette smoker—throughout to illustrate his arguments. Nevertheless, it was some time before papers investigating how self-affirmation may buffer threat appeared in the research literature on the psychology of health (e.g., Sherman et al., 2000). In the subsequent two decades, however, research has flourished. In this chapter, we document the principal developments and issues as they stand after some 20 years of research.

Self-Affirmation Theory is a theory with a broad reach. The (largely beneficial) effects of self-affirmation have been documented across a range of areas, including education, health, intergroup conflict, and interpersonal relations (Cohen & Sherman, 2014). The focus of the theory's development and application has become its role in promoting adaptive change and accounting for some of the (largely defensive) processes that impede such change (Cohen & Sherman, 2014).

Self-Affirmation Theory posits that people are typically highly motivated to protect their "self-integrity". In a much-quoted passage, Steele (1988) defined self-integrity as the "phenomenal experience of the self … as adaptively and morally adequate, that is, as competent, good, coherent, unitary, stable, capable of free choice, capable of controlling important outcomes, and so on"

P. R. Harris (✉) • D. C. Jessop
School of Psychology, University of Sussex, Falmer, UK
e-mail: p.r.harris@sussex.ac.uk

F. M. Sirois (ed.), *The Palgrave Handbook of Positive Psychology and Health*,
https://doi.org/10.1007/978-3-031-89095-6_9

(p. 262). Threats to this global sense of being morally and adaptively adequate involve both major life events (e.g., divorce, redundancy, illness) and commonplace experiences (e.g., reading counter-attitudinal information, receiving minor insults or rejections). Such challenges to self-integrity have been labelled "psychological threats" (Cohen & Sherman, 2014, p. 335).

People are naturally vigilant to psychological threats and are often defensive when they respond. There is not enough space here to consider the range of defensive responses people may adopt—for a discussion, see van't Riet and Ruiter (2013). A critical feature of self-affirmation, however, is that it can protect self-integrity without promoting defensiveness.

Self-affirmation is "an act that manifests one's adequacy and thus affirms one's sense of global self-integrity" (Cohen & Sherman, 2014, p. 337). Such acts provide reassurance about one's moral or adaptive adequacy and thereby have the potential to offset the psychological threat. In everyday life, self-affirmation can be realised in diverse ways. For example, an individual may self-affirm by reminding herself that she is a good parent, or a skilled mathematician, or by thinking about a recent act of kindness that reflects her personally important values. In experimental work using Self-Affirmation Theory, self-affirmation is most often operationalised by asking people to reflect upon a personally important value.

There are several key things to note about self-affirmation. First, to be effective, a self-affirmation must be at least equivalent in its contribution to the individual's self-integrity as the threat is detrimental to it. So, for example, thinking about a recent act of kindness will offset a threat to self-integrity stemming from a reminder about one's unhealthy lifestyle if it brings to mind a value that is at least as important to the self as is the focal threat. Second, effective self-affirmations can be unrelated to the focal threat. For example, a smoker threatened by an image depicting the health dangers of smoking can offset that threat by reminding herself that she is a good friend or an honest person. She does not need to reduce the psychological threat by planning to stop or rationalising her smoking. This flexibility marks self-affirmation out from other ways in which people respond to psychological threats (Cohen & Sherman, 2014). Third, self-affirmation contains or contextualises the threat, but does not eliminate it. That is, a psychological threat seems less potent when people are reassured that they are adequately competent or moral. Therefore, the self-affirmed person should feel more secure and potentially able to confront the threat because the self-evaluative elements of the threat have been reduced or eliminated. Thus, self-affirmation may not only preserve self-integrity but also promote adaptive change. Not surprisingly, this aspect of the theory appeals to researchers and practitioners interested in finding ways to understand and promote such change.

Self-Affirmation and Health

There are three main strands of research involving self-affirmation and health (Harris et al., 2020). The first applies Self-Affirmation Theory to understanding and ameliorating defensive resistance to information about health risks and health status; the second examines whether and how self-affirmation may buffer stress; the third explores the potential for self-affirmation to protect and even promote well-being. In this chapter, we consider all three (see also Harris et al., 2020).

Self-Affirmation and Defensive Resistance to Health Information

Messages encouraging healthier behaviour come in many forms and through various media. However, such messages can induce defensive resistance: people may avoid, derogate, or downplay the information and its personal relevance (van't Riet & Ruiter, 2013). This can be especially true of those whose behaviour puts them at risk of the negative outcomes targeted in the information (e.g., Harris & Napper, 2005; Schüz et al., 2013).

From the perspective of Self-Affirmation Theory, one reason why health behaviour messages induce defensiveness is that they typically pose a self-integrity threat. As Steele himself puts it, what is disturbing about engaging in an act that has the potential to damage one's health is in part "its implication that one is foolish or unable to control important behavior" (Steele, 1988, p. 262). Accordingly, when people are confronted with such messages, they may avoid, criticise, or deny the personal relevance of the message as a means of protecting their sense of being competent and capable (Sherman & Cohen, 2006). However, by bolstering self-integrity, self-affirmation may provide an alternative way to offset the threat, leading to the hypothesis that, by self-affirming, people will become more open-minded and less defensive in response to psychologically threatening health information.

Does Self-Affirmation Promote Openness to Health-Risk Information?

That self-affirmation may reduce defensive resistance is of interest both theoretically and practically, so it is not surprising that this hypothesis has received much empirical attention. Most studies have been experimental and have induced self-affirmation using a values-affirmation task (for example, the participant might be asked to write about their most important value) before presenting participants with relevant health-risk information. The latter is usually textual and often designed to emulate a health promotion leaflet or brochure. Self-affirmed and control participants' responses to the information are typically assessed immediately afterwards, using measures of message acceptance and readiness to change behaviour as indicators of reduced defensive resistance. Some studies also assess subsequent behaviour (usually self-reported) at follow-up. Samples include community samples and patient groups (e.g., Armitage et al., 2008; Wileman et al., 2014), but to date, the modal participant is a female undergraduate.

Currently, most of the published evidence supports the hypothesis that self-affirmation does indeed render people more open-minded about personally relevant health information, as reflected in cognitive, affective, and behavioural responses, both immediately and at follow-up. Much of this evidence was evaluated in two independent meta-analyses published contemporaneously (Epton et al., 2015; Sweeney & Moyer, 2015). In their meta-analysis, for example, Epton et al. (2015) reported the following effect sizes: message acceptance ($d_+ = 0.17$; 34 studies), intentions ($d_+ = 0.14$; 64 studies), and behaviour ($d_+ = 0.32$; 46 studies). They note that these effects are comparable in magnitude to those obtained in meta-analyses of other health behaviour change interventions.

Schüz et al. (2017) extended the synthesis of the evidence relating to the behavioural effects of self-affirmation, adding a further 14 published studies to those in the above meta-analyses. They argue that, on balance, the evidence suggests stronger effects of self-affirmation on health-promoting behaviours (such as physical activity, 20 studies) and self-management behaviours (such as taking diagnostic tests, 3 studies) than on health-damaging behaviours (such as alcohol consumption, 11 studies). However, they did not test this claim statistically.

When considering behaviour, it is clear from the findings of several studies that positive effects of self-affirmation manipulations on immediate outcomes do not inevitably translate into differences in behaviour at follow-up (e.g.,

Harris & Napper, 2005; Harris et al., 2007). There is also evidence of the effects of self-affirmation manipulations on behaviour at follow-up without measurable effects on immediate outcomes (e.g., Cooke et al., 2014). Indeed, much remains to be established about the factors influencing the longer-term, and especially the behavioural, impacts of self-affirmation interventions (see Ferrer & Cohen, 2019; Harris, 2011, for discussions).

Since the publication of the meta-analyses, research has proceeded much as before, with demonstrations of the basic effects of self-affirmation plus, as we describe in the following sections, some attempts to pin down mediators and moderators. However, as the literature matures, null findings are also being published, most notably in the area of binge drinking among students (e.g., Knight & Norman, 2016). Backlash effects have also, on occasion, been reported (e.g., Good & Abraham, 2011). Nevertheless, the balance of the published literature currently supports the hypothesis that self-affirmation can reduce defensive resistance to health-risk information.

How Does Self-Affirmation Promote Openness to Health Risk Information and Behaviour Change? Possible Mediators

Various mediators of the effects of self-affirmation on outcomes have been proposed. These include variables such as more abstract construal (e.g., Schmeichel & Vohs, 2009), a broader perspective on the self (Critcher & Dunning, 2015), and other-related affect (Crocker et al., 2008). However, direct tests of these variables as mediators of the impact of self-affirmation on openness to health-risk information have rarely been conducted (see Crocker et al., 2008, for an exception).

Other proposed mediators include anticipated regret (e.g., van Koningsbruggen et al., 2014), intentions (e.g., Armitage et al., 2008; van Koningsbruggen et al., 2014), and variables that are very close to being in themselves indices of openness to the message, such as measures of message acceptance (e.g., Armitage et al., 2008), message derogation (e.g., van Koningsbruggen & Das, 2009), and response efficacy (e.g., Epton & Harris, 2008). Each has been shown to mediate the impact of self-affirmation on behavioural (or behavioural intention) outcomes, albeit evidence is typically limited to one or two studies per mediator.

A potentially interesting development involves measures of brain function. For example, Falk et al. (2015) showed that the boost to physical activity at follow-up produced by self-affirmation was mediated by activity in the ventromedial prefrontal cortex (see also Dutcher et al., 2020).

Logel and Cohen (2012) found that higher working memory capacity at follow-up mediated the effect of self-affirmation on weight loss among their participants, although their study did not provide any explicit health-related information.

In all likelihood, self-affirmation is mediated by multiple factors (Cohen & Sherman, 2014). Furthermore, the mechanisms by which self-affirmation reduces defensiveness to self-integrity threats may be common to a range of threats, whereas the mechanisms by which message acceptance is translated into sustained health-behaviour change may be different and encompass both reflective and automatic processes (Harris, 2011).

Under What Conditions Does Self-Affirmation Promote Openness to Health Risk Information? Possible Moderators

A large number of potential moderators of the effects of self-affirmation on outcomes has also been proposed. However, evidence for most moderators again rarely extends beyond one or two studies (for reviews see Cohen & Sherman, 2014; Harris et al., 2020; Schüz et al., 2017).

Notably, the two published meta-analyses in this area found limited evidence for moderation by the variables they tested. Sweeney and Moyer (2015) found insufficient evidence for moderation by whether the behaviour was health promoting or health damaging, the measurement of the behaviour was proximal or distal, the type of self-affirmation manipulation (values v kindness), or the specificity of the health message. Epton et al. (2015) found that self-affirmation was more effective in changing behaviour (but not message acceptance or intentions) when the hazard was temporally proximal rather than more distant, if the self-affirmation task was a values essay, and the sample contained fewer white participants. Outcomes were not, however, significantly moderated by the other variables they tested, such as gender, sample (student only v mixed), differences between samples in the percentage at baseline not meeting the guidelines recommended in the message (an index of risk), or indices of study quality.

In several studies, self-affirmation has been shown to have more of an impact on those whose behaviour places them at higher risk of the targeted negative health outcome (e.g., Harris & Napper, 2005; Harris et al., 2007; Zhao et al., 2014). This pattern of findings is consistent with predictions derived from Self-Affirmation Theory, as those at higher risk should be more threatened by the information and, therefore, more defensively resistant to it. Accordingly, such individuals should be most influenced by self-affirmation's apparent capacity to ameliorate such defensive responses. The finding that higher risk groups appear to benefit most is also potentially of practical importance as these groups are generally the most important to persuade but hardest to reach (Schüz, et al., 2013). However, not all studies find moderation by risk (see Epton et al., 2015) and at least one study found beneficial effects restricted to moderate levels of risk (e.g., Klein & Harris, 2009). There is also evidence that self-affirmation manipulations may produce distinctive effects, including detrimental effects, on responses among those experiencing little or no threat (e.g., Good et al., 2015; Zhao et al., 2014).

The quality of the health information may well also moderate the impact of self-affirmation on outcomes. Self-affirmation is hypothesised to promote greater readiness to engage with the information open-mindedly, so whether people are persuaded should depend on factors that influence the credibility of the material, such as the strength of the arguments. Indeed, there is evidence that self-affirmation can sensitise people to message strength (Correll et al., 2004; Klein et al., 2011) and may improve the calibration between perceived and actual risk, at least among participants high in the tendency to deny being at risk (Griffin & Harris, 2011).

There is a need for more tests of potential moderators, including those moderators that have already been proposed. It would be especially beneficial for these to be accompanied by a clear description of the link between the theory and the proposed moderation. Indeed, in a notable recent contribution, Ferrer and Cohen (2019) have developed an integrative model that proposes self-affirmation facilitates health behaviour change when three conditions are met: (1) the individual experiences psychological threat, (2) the individual has available appropriate resources to foster change, and (3) the self-affirmation intervention is timely, occurring when the person facing threat is aware of having access to resources that will support behaviour change, such as the support of family and friends, skills training, or healthy food that is affordable. This "trigger and channel" model has the potential to provide important insights into "when, where and for whom self-affirmation will be most effective" (Ferrer & Cohen, 2019, p. 1).

Self-Affirmation and Stress

Many stressors present threats to self-integrity (Sherman & Cohen, 2006). For example, losing one's job or failing a test may threaten one's view of the self as valued or capable. In such cases, self-affirmation may help reassure stressed people that they nevertheless possess self-integrity. Self-affirmation may also remind them of the "bigger picture" and even boost their perceptions of their available coping resources (Cohen & Sherman, 2014).

There is evidence that self-affirmation can mitigate responses to both lab-induced and naturalistic stressors. In the laboratory, Creswell et al. (2005) found that self-affirmed participants had significantly lower cortisol responses to an acute stressor than did their non-affirmed counterparts. Tang and Schmeichel (2015) found that insulting evaluative feedback had less impact on arterial blood pressure and heart rate in participants who self-affirmed after receiving the feedback than it did in control participants. There is also evidence that self-affirmation may affect other stress-related responses in the laboratory. Thus, Creswell et al. (2013) showed self-affirmation buffered problem solving among those high in chronic stress, and Dutcher et al. (2020) found that self-affirmation reduced self-reported stress and enhanced performance on stressful maths problems.

Outside the laboratory, Sherman, Bunyan et al. (2009) found that self-affirmed participants had reduced epinephrine responses to exam stress than did their non-affirmed counterparts. The buffering effects of self-affirmation were particularly apparent for those students most concerned about being evaluated negatively at college. Morgan and Harris (2015) explored the impact of a novel self-affirmation manipulation among employees at an educational institution undergoing organisational downsizing. Those who formed implemental, if-then, plans to self-affirm in response to work-related threats experienced lower levels of anxiety, both immediately post-intervention and at a three-week follow-up, compared to those who did not (see also Morgan & Atkin, 2016).

Naturally occurring self-affirmation (in the absence of an experimental manipulation) may also help counter the effects of stress. Controlling for the self-affirmational content of essays written by early-stage breast cancer survivors eliminated the benefits of expressive writing in reducing physical symptoms (Creswell et al., 2007), suggesting that self-affirmation might have been instrumental in those benefits. Self-affirmation was also associated with lower levels of distress immediately after each writing session (see also Niles et al., 2016).

However, in some situations, the defensive responses that are supposedly attenuated by self-affirmation may be advantageous. Jessop et al. (2018) demonstrated that self-affirmed (vs. non-affirmed) women reported increased anxiety and less positive mood after reading a stressful birth scenario and imagining themselves in the place of the woman giving birth. They argue that, when faced with a stressor occurring in a central life domain characterised by low levels of control (e.g., bereavement, terminal illness), defensive responses—such as denial and avoidance—may provide a valuable means of attenuating adverse psychological and physiological reactions. These findings suggest that self-affirmation should not be regarded as a panacea for stress.

There are plausible candidates for mediators of the effects of self-affirmation on stress among those proposed for self-affirmation effects on outcomes more generally. These include positive-affect (e.g., Koole et al., 1999), self-control (Schmeichel & Vohs, 2009), executive function (P. S. Harris, et al., 2017), and construal level (Schmeichel & Vohs, 2009). However, none has yet been tested. Likewise, it seems plausible that the benefits of self-affirmation might be particularly apparent for those who are most in need, either in terms of being most vulnerable to the stressor or most at risk of engaging in suboptimal coping (e.g., Sherman, Bunyan et al., 2009). However, it also seems likely that benefits of self-affirmation will be restricted to situations in which (a) reminding individuals of the bigger picture is likely to be advantageous and helps to contextualise the threat (rather than simply highlighting the severity of the situation) and (b) the defensive processes ameliorated by self-affirmation are not valuable and beneficial (Jessop et al., 2018). Research is also needed to explore the longer-term impact of self-affirmation in stressful situations.

Self-Affirmation and Well-Being

Well-being is an umbrella term used to depict a sense of physical and mental health that has captured the popular imagination. Researchers frequently distinguish between hedonic well-being, which broadly corresponds to the experience of pleasure and happiness, and eudaimonic well-being, which relates to finding meaning and purpose in life, for example through fulfilment of core psychological needs such as autonomy, competence, and relatedness (e.g., Nelson et al., 2014).

Some recent research attention has been paid to whether self-affirmation confers direct benefits for well-being (Howell, 2016). Nelson et al. (2014) found that self-affirmation can have positive implications for both eudaimonic and hedonic well-being in student samples. Armitage (2016) reported that older women who completed a brief self-affirmation manipulation subsequently experienced less of a decline in subjective well-being relative to their control counterparts. Relatedly, Lannin et al. (2018) found that self-affirmation was more effective at reducing psychological distress than a well-established intervention (expressive writing).

Uncovering the mediators and moderators of any direct effects of self-affirmation on well-being represents an important goal for future research.

With regard to potential mediators, there is evidence that self-affirmation can promote positive affect (e.g., Creswell et al., 2013; Koole et al., 1999), a component of hedonic well-being. Furthermore, self-affirmation has been shown to activate regions of the brain associated with rewards and self-related processing (e.g., Dutcher et al., 2020; Falk et al., 2015), further indicating links to positive affective experiences that may map on to hedonic outcomes.

Self-affirmation manipulations have also been shown to boost variables that may affect eudaimonic well-being. For example, self-affirmation has been associated with improved executive function (P. S. Harris et al., 2017), which could facilitate the fulfilment of the core psychological need of competence. Self-affirmation has also been shown to reduce the likelihood of self-control failure (Schmeichel & Vohs, 2009) and boost beliefs relating to self-control and self-efficacy (e.g., Churchill et al., 2018; Jessop et al., 2009), each of which might augment autonomy-related need fulfilment. Crocker et al. (2008) have demonstrated that self-affirmation boosts feelings of connectedness to others, which may well contribute to need fulfilment in the domain of relatedness.

In summary, there is evidence that self-affirmation may protect or even boost well-being, although this research is in its infancy and many issues remain unaddressed (Howell, 2016; Schüz & Schüz, 2017).

Self-Affirmation as a Practical Intervention

Naturally, given the evidence that self-affirmation can reduce resistance to health risk information, mitigate negative physiological and psychological responses to stressors, and potentially bolster well-being, researchers and practitioners have been keen to examine its potential role in real-world interventions (see Schüz, et al., 2017; van Koningsbruggen et al., 2016) and for public policy (see Klein et al., 2015). Overall, initial findings have been promising, but there are obvious risks to employing self-affirmation as an intervention when we know relatively little about its mechanism(s) of action, the potential boundary conditions to its efficacy, and its potential for backfire effects (though see Ferrer & Cohen, 2019).

One practical benefit of self-affirmation is that it can be used alongside existing health-promotion materials. However, for self-affirmation to be applied in certain everyday contexts, it would be useful to develop reliable ways of self-affirming that are easy to implement; currently, there are few such self-affirmation manipulations available. The brief 10-item kindness questionnaire has been used successfully in at least one group of patients (e.g.

Wileman et al., 2014); another questionnaire-based manipulation developed by Napper et al. (2009) has also had some positive effects (see also Zhu & Yzer, 2019).

Attempts have been made to affirm participants using mobile devices (Springer et al., 2018; Taber et al., 2019). However, there is some evidence of backfire effects when using such media (Taber et al., 2019), illustrating the difficulties inherent in translating self-affirmation manipulations to real-world contexts. Other methods are novel and await further testing (e.g., Arpan et al., 2016; Klein et al., 2010).

Promising findings are emerging using a technique in which the self-affirmation itself is formulated as an implementation intention, or if-then plan (e.g., "If I feel threatened … then I will think about the things I value about myself"). This technique has been shown to be effective at promoting openness to health risk information (e.g., Armitage et al., 2011), buffering stress (e.g., Morgan & Harris, 2015), and protecting well-being (e.g., Armitage, 2016). However, little is known about its mechanism of action.

There have also been attempts to incorporate more standard self-affirmation manipulations into health warnings and leaflets. Dillard et al. (2005) embedded a positive self-statement ("You are a kind person") in health-warning messages about smoking, but found no effects, whereas Jessop et al. (2009) found that a positive traits affirmation incorporated into a leaflet about the health risks of sunbathing led to more positive cognitions regarding sunscreen use and more requests for a free sample of sunscreen.

Research by Walter and colleagues suggests that it might be possible to vicariously affirm participants, which may have practical potential. In an initial study, participants who read a text-based narrative in which the main character received an award before being told about the dangers of e-cigarette use were more receptive to this information, as reflected in greater perceptions of risk and intentions to stop using e-cigarettes (Walter, Demetriades et al., 2019). In a subsequent study, they demonstrated similar findings when the narrative was presented as a short film (Walter, Saucier et al., 2019).

Other interesting approaches to self-affirming—such as the use of Facebook profiles (Toma & Hancock, 2013) or product choice (Townsend & Sood, 2012)—have also been developed. However, these have yet to be applied to health threats.

Research attention has also been paid to the possibility of combining self-affirmation with other interventions to optimise its efficacy. In particular, several studies have examined the potential for self-affirmation to promote behaviour change when combined with implementation intentions formulated as if-then plans to promote spotting and acting upon occasions to implement the targeted behaviour (Gollwitzer & Sheeran, 2006). These studies have produced some positive results, although findings are mixed (e.g., Ehret & Sherman, 2018; Harris et al., 2014; Jessop et al., 2014).

Research in patient groups has also tested an intervention in which self-affirmation is combined with a positive-affect induction (Peterson et al., 2013). The resultant intervention has been shown to promote health behaviour change (e.g., Ogedegbe et al., 2012). However, it is not clear whether the combined intervention is more effective than would be self-affirmation alone.

Finally, there are other practical issues and considerations that need to be borne in mind when investigating the potential use of self-affirmation in health interventions. For instance, we should not assume that self-affirmation manipulations—and any associated outcomes—will translate across cultures; indeed, Ma and Nan (2019) highlighted how the efficacy of a self-affirmation manipulation may depend on whether its focus (on independent or interdependent values) is well-matched to the dominant self-construal of the recipient. In another vein, Sherman, Cohen et al. (2009) showed that being aware of the effects of self-affirmation can reduce its benefits. It may prove challenging to justify the intervention to prospective participants without informing them of the intended benefits. However, Silverman et al. (2013) have shown that when participants freely choose to self-affirm, the effect of awareness is eradicated, which may prove useful in interventions.

Individual Differences in Self-Affirmation

Recent research suggests that there may be individual differences in the propensity to self-affirm that may have important implications for health. In the context of defensive resistance to health-related information, Harris et al. (2019) demonstrated that their Spontaneous Self-Affirmation Measure (SSAM) predicted less defensive responses to both a novel and a familiar health message (see also Persoskie et al., 2015; Pietersma & Dijkstra, 2012). Although Harris et al. (2019) reported no relationship between SSAM and perceived stress, Taber et al. (2016) found that SSAM items were associated with less cognitive impairment and more positive affect among cancer survivors, raising the possibility that spontaneous self-affirmation may buffer the negative impacts of a stressor. With regard to well-being, Jessop et al. (2023) showed in three studies that spontaneous self-affirmation consistently predicted hedonic and eudaimonic well-being outcomes, both cross-sectionally and longitudinally (see also Emanuel et al., 2016). In the context of self-weighing, Webb et al. (2020) found that people who were preoccupied with their weight anticipated and reported feeling less negatively about weighing themselves if they also reported on the SSAM that they tended to affirm themselves spontaneously and do so by reflecting on their strengths.

Further exploration of the associations between individual differences in self-affirmation and defensive resistance, stress reactivity, and well-being represent profitable avenues for future research. It also seems plausible that individual differences in the propensity to self-affirm spontaneously might provide an important moderator of the effectiveness of self-affirmation manipulations in these domains (see Harris et al., 2023; Jessop et al., 2023). Given the apparent benefits of spontaneous self-affirmation, it would also be informative to establish whether interventions can be developed to encourage individuals to self-affirm automatically in the face of psychological threats (see e.g., Morgan & Harris, 2015).

Self-Affirmation Theory Developments

In terms of theory, the principal developments since Steele (1988) have involved elucidating the processes by which self-affirming renders the individual less defensive (e.g., by influencing the contents of the working self-concept and disconnecting the self from the threat) and clarifying the conditions under which a small intervention can have such big effects (e.g., by inducing a cycle of supportive changes in external circumstances). These are well summarised in Cohen and Sherman's (2014) Annual Review article. The principal challenge to Steele's original interpretation in terms of self-integrity has come from Crocker and colleagues, who have argued for an interpretation instead in terms of self-transcendence (e.g., Crocker et al., 2008).

In relation to health, Harris (2011) has outlined various points in the behaviour change process at which self-affirmation could prove influential and Ferrer and Cohen (2019) have developed a "Trigger and Channel" framework for explaining the conditions under which self-affirmation may facilitate health behaviour change that emphasises the conditionality of self-affirmation effects.

Harris et al. (2020) have also recently outlined some outstanding practical and theoretical issues that future research might usefully address. Practically, these include broadening the range of manipulations employed and populations sampled, including "no task" control conditions, and increasing the sample sizes routinely used. Theoretically, these include integration with theories of persuasion of health-behaviour change, and with other theories of self and identity.

Summary

There is evidence that self-affirmation, typically by affirming personal values or strengths, can reduce information resistance and avoidance, foster health-behaviour change, mitigate negative responses to stressors and also, potentially, bolster well-being. Future research should be directed at establishing mediators and moderators of effects and improving aspects of study design. It could also profitably address the development of brief, accessible self-affirmation manipulations that can be easily implemented, either alongside health promotion materials or as a means of buffering stress and fostering well-being, and integration with other relevant theoretical frameworks. Research attention should also be paid to the role of individual differences in self-affirmation and health and, ultimately, to exploring ways of boosting this potentially valuable resource.

References

Armitage, C. J. (2016). A brief psychological intervention to protect subjective well-being in a community sample. *Quality of Life Research, 25*, 385–391. https://doi.org/10.1007/s11136-015-1076-6

Armitage, C. J., Harris, P. R., & Arden, M. A. (2011). Evidence that self-affirmation reduces alcohol consumption: Randomized exploratory trial with a new, brief means of self-affirming. *Health Psychology, 30*, 633–641. https://doi.org/10.1037/a0023738

Armitage, C. J., Harris, P. R., Hepton, G., & Napper, L. (2008). Self-affirmation increases acceptance of health-risk information among UK adult smokers with low socioeconomic status. *Psychology of Addictive Behaviors, 22*, 88–95. https://doi.org/10.1037/0893-164X.22.1.88

Arpan, L. M., Lee, Y. S., & Wang, Z. (2016). Integrating self-affirmation with health risk messages: Effects on message evaluation and response. *Health Communication*. Advance online publication. https://doi.org/10.1080/10410236.2015.1113483

Churchill, S., Jessop, D. C., Green, R., & Harris, P. R. (2018). Self-affirmation improves self-control over snacking among participants low in eating self-efficacy. *Appetite, 123*, 264–268. https://doi.org/10.1016/j.appet.2017.12.028

Cohen, G. L., & Sherman, D. K. (2014). The psychology of change: Self-affirmation and social psychological intervention. *Annual Review of Psychology, 65*, 333–371. https://doi.org/10.1146/annurev-psych-010213-115137

Cooke, R., Trebaczyk, H., Harris, P., & Wright, A. J. (2014). Self-affirmation promotes physical activity. *Journal of Sport and Exercise Psychology, 36*, 217–223. https://doi.org/10.1123/jsep.2013-0041

Correll, J., Spencer, S. J., & Zanna, M. P. (2004). An affirmed self and an open mind: Self-affirmation and sensitivity to argument strength. *Journal of Experimental Social Psychology, 40*, 350–356. https://doi.org/10.1016/j.jesp.2003.07.001

Creswell, J. D., Dutcher, J. M., Klein, W. M., Harris, P. R., & Levine, J. M. (2013). Self-affirmation improves problem-solving under stress. *PLoS ONE, 8*, e62593. https://doi.org/10.1371/journal.pone.0062593

Creswell, J. D., Lam, S., Stanton, A. L., Taylor, S. E., Bower, J. E., & Sherman, D. K. (2007). Does self-affirmation, cognitive processing, or discovery of meaning explain cancer-related health benefits of expressive writing? *Personality and Social Psychology Bulletin, 33*, 238–250. https://doi.org/10.1177/0146167206294412

Creswell, J. D., Welch, W. T., Taylor, S. E., Sherman, D. K., Gruenewald, T. L., & Mann, T. (2005). Affirmation of personal values buffers neuroendocrine and psychological stress responses. *Psychological Science, 16*, 846–851. https://doi.org/10.1111/j.1467-9280.2005.01624.x

Critcher, C. R., & Dunning, D. (2015). Self-affirmations provide a broader perspective on self-threat. *Personality and Social Psychology Bulletin, 41*, 3–18. https://doi.org/10.1177/0146167214554956

Crocker, J., Niiya, Y., & Mischkowski, D. (2008). Why does writing about important values reduce defensiveness? Self-affirmation and the role of positive other-directed feelings. *Psychological Science, 19*, 740–747. https://doi.org/10.1111/j.1467-9280.2008.02150.x

Dillard, A. J., McCaul, K. D., & Magnan, R. E. (2005). Why is such a smart person like you smoking? Using self-affirmation to reduce defensiveness to cigarette warning labels1. *Journal of Applied Biobehavioral Research, 10*, 165–182. https://doi.org/10.1111/j.1751-9861.2005.tb00010.x

Dutcher, J. M., Eisenberger, N. I., Woo, H., Klein, W. M., Harris, P. R., Levine, J. M., & Creswell, J. D. (2020). Neural mechanisms of self-affirmation's stress buffering effects. *Social Cognitive and Affective Neuroscience, 15*, 1086–1096.

Ehret, P. J., & Sherman, D. K. (2018). Integrating self-affirmation and implementation intentions: Effects on college student drinking. *Annals of Behavioral Medicine, 52*, 633–644. https://doi.org/10.1093/abm/kax032

Emanuel, A. S., Howell, J. L., Taber, J. M., Ferrer, R. A., Klein, W. M., & Harris, P. R. (2016). Spontaneous self-affirmation is associated with psychological well-being: Evidence from a US national adult survey sample. *Journal of Health Psychology*, Advance online publication. https://doi.org/10.1177/1359105316643595

Epton, T., & Harris, P. R. (2008). Self-affirmation promotes health behavior change. *Health Psychology, 27*, 746–752. https://doi.org/10.1037/0278-6133.27.6.746

Epton, T., Harris, P. R., Kane, R., van Koningsbruggen, G. M., & Sheeran, P. (2015). The impact of self-affirmation on health-behavior change: A meta-analysis. *Health Psychology, 34*, 187–196. https://doi.org/10.1037/hea0000116

Falk, E. B., O'Donnell, M. B., Cascio, C. N., Tinney, F., Kang, Y., Lieberman, M. D., Taylor, S. E., An, L., Resnicow, K., & Strecher, V. J. (2015). Self-affirmation alters the brain's response to health messages and subsequent behavior change.

Proceedings of the National Academy of Sciences, 112, 1977–1982. https://doi.org/10.1073/pnas.1500247112

Ferrer, R. A., & Cohen, G. L. (2019). Reconceptualizing self-affirmation with the trigger and channel framework: Lessons from the health domain. *Personality and Social Psychology Review, 23*, 285–304. https://doi.org/10.1177/1088868318797036

Gollwitzer, P. M., & Sheeran, P. (2006). Implementation intentions and goal achievement: A meta-analysis of effects and processes. In M. P. Zanna (Ed.), *Advances in experimental social psychology* (Vol. 38, pp. 69–119). Elsevier Academic Press. https://doi.org/10.1016/S0065-2601(06)38002-1

Good, A., & Abraham, C. (2011). Can the effectiveness of health promotion campaigns be improved using self-efficacy and self-affirmation interventions? An analysis of sun protection messages. *Psychology & Health, 26*, 799–818. https://doi.org/10.1080/08870446.2010.495157

Good, A., Harris, P. R., Jessop, D. C., & Abraham, C. (2015). Open-mindedness can decrease persuasion amongst adolescents: The role of self-affirmation. *British Journal of Health Psychology, 20*, 228–242. https://doi.org/10.1111/bjhp.12090

Griffin, D. W., & Harris, P. R. (2011). Calibrating the response to health warnings limiting both overreaction and underreaction with self-affirmation. *Psychological Science, 22*, 572–578. https://doi.org/10.1177/0956797611405678

Harris, P. R. (2011). Self-affirmation and the self-regulation of health behavior change. *Self and Identity, 10*(3), 304–314. https://doi.org/10.1080/15298868.2010.517963

Harris, P. R., Brearley, I., Sheeran, P., Barker, M., Klein, W. M., Creswell, J. D., Levine, J. M., & Bond, R. (2014). Combining self-affirmation with implementation intentions to promote fruit and vegetable consumption. *Health Psychology, 33*, 729–736. https://doi.org/10.1037/hea0000065

Harris, P. R., Griffin, D. W., Napper, L. E., Bond, R., Schüz, B., Stride, C., & Brearley, I. (2019). Individual differences in self-affirmation: Distinguishing self-affirmation from positive self-regard. *Self and Identity, 18*, 589–630. https://doi.org/10.1080/15298868.2018.1504819

Harris, P. R., Jessop, D., & Harris, P. S. (2020). Self-affirmation and health. In L. Cohen (Ed.), *The encyclopedia of health psychology*. John Wiley & Sons Ltd.

Harris, P. R., Mayle, K., Mabbott, L., & Napper, L. (2007). Self-affirmation reduces smokers' defensiveness to graphic on-pack cigarette warning labels. *Health Psychology, 26*, 437–446. https://doi.org/10.1037/0278-6133.26.4.437

Harris, P. R., & Napper, L. (2005). Self-affirmation and the biased processing of threatening health-risk information. *Personality and Social Psychology Bulletin, 31*, 1250–1263. https://doi.org/10.1177/0146167205274694

Harris, P. R., Richards, A., & Bond, R. (2023). Individual differences in spontaneous self-affirmation and mental health: Relationships with self-esteem, dispositional optimism and coping. *Self and Identity, 22*, 351–378. https://doi.org/10.1080/15298868.2022.2099455

Harris, P. S., Harris, P. R., & Miles, E. (2017). Self-affirmation improves performance on tasks related to executive functioning. *Journal of Experimental Social Psychology, 70*, 281–285. https://doi.org/10.1016/j.jesp.2016.11.011

Howell, A. J. (2016). Self-affirmation theory and the science of well-being. *Journal of Happiness Studies*. Advance online publication. https://doi.org/10.1007/s10902-016-9713-5

Jessop, D. C., Ayers, S., Burn, F., & Ryda, C. (2018). Can self-affirmation exacerbate adverse reactions to stress under certain conditions? *Psychology and Health, 33*, 827–845. https://doi.org/10.1080/08870446.2017.1421187

Jessop, D. C., Simmonds, L. V., & Sparks, P. (2009). Motivational and behavioural consequences of self-affirmation interventions: A study of sunscreen use among women. *Psychology and Health, 24*, 529–544. https://doi.org/10.1080/08870440801930320

Jessop, D. C., Sparks, P., Buckland, N., Harris, P. R., & Churchill, S. (2014). Combining self-affirmation and implementation intentions: Evidence of detrimental effects on behavioral outcomes. *Annals of Behavioral Medicine, 47*, 137–147. https://doi.org/10.1007/s12160-013-9536-0

Jessop, D. J., Harris, P. R., & Gibbons, T. (2023). Individual differences in spontaneous self-affirmation predict well-being and mediate associations between socioeconomic status and well-being. *Self and Identity, 22*, 247–275. https://doi.org/10.1080/15298868.2022.2079711

Klein, W. M., & Harris, P. R. (2009). Self-affirmation enhances attentional bias toward threatening components of a persuasive message. *Psychological Science, 20*, 1463–1467. https://doi.org/10.1111/j.1467-9280.2009.02467.x

Klein, W. M., Harris, P. R., Ferrer, R. A., & Zajac, L. E. (2011). Feelings of vulnerability in response to threatening messages: Effects of self-affirmation. *Journal of Experimental Social Psychology, 47*, 1237–1242. https://doi.org/10.1016/j.jesp.2011.05.005

Klein, W. M., Lipkus, I. M., Scholl, S. M., McQueen, A., Cerully, J. L., & Harris, P. R. (2010). Self-affirmation moderates effects of unrealistic optimism and pessimism on reactions to tailored risk feedback. *Psychology and Health, 25*, 1195–1208. https://doi.org/10.1080/08870440903261970

Klein, W. M., Shepperd, J. A., Suls, J., Rothman, A. J., & Croyle, R. T. (2015). Realizing the promise of social psychology in improving public health. *Personality and Social Psychology Review, 19*, 77–92. https://doi.org/10.1177/1088868314539852

Knight, R., & Norman, P. (2016). Impact of brief self-affirmation manipulations on university students' reactions to risk information about binge drinking. *British Journal of Health Psychology, 21*, 570–583. https://doi.org/10.1111/bjhp.12186

Koole, S. L., Smeets, K., Van Knippenberg, A., & Dijksterhuis, A. (1999). The cessation of rumination through self-affirmation. *Journal of Personality and Social Psychology, 77*, 111–125. https://doi.org/10.1037/0022-3514.77.1.111

Lannin, D. G., Vogel, D. L., Kahn, J. H., Brenner, R. E., Heath, P. J., & Guyll, M. (2018). A multi-wave test of self-affirmation versus emotionally expressive writing. *Counselling Psychology Quarterly*. https://doi.org/10.1080/09515070.2018.1553144

Logel, C., & Cohen, G. L. (2012). The role of the self in physical health testing the effect of a values-affirmation intervention on weight loss. *Psychological Science, 23*, 53–55. https://doi.org/10.1177/0956797611421936

Ma, Z., & Nan, X. (2019). Investigating the interplay of self-construal and independent vs. interdependent self-affirmation. *Journal of Health Communication, 24*, 293–302. https://doi.org/10.1080/10810730.2019.1601300

Morgan, J. I., & Atkin, L. (2016). Expelling stress for primary school teachers: Self-affirmation increases positive emotions in teaching and emotion reappraisal. *International Journal of Environmental Research and Public Health, 13*, 500–510. https://doi.org/10.3390/ijerph13050500

Morgan, J. I., & Harris, P. R. (2015). Evidence that brief self-affirming implementation intentions can reduce work-related anxiety in downsize survivors. *Anxiety, Stress, & Coping, 28*, 563–575. https://doi.org/10.1080/10615806.2015.1004665

Napper, L., Harris, P. R., & Epton, T. (2009). Developing and testing a self-affirmation manipulation. *Self and Identity, 8*, 45–62. https://doi.org/10.1080/15298860802079786

Nelson, S. K., Fuller, J. A., Choi, I., & Lyubomirsky, S. (2014). Beyond self-protection: Self-affirmation benefits hedonic and eudaimonic well-being. *Personality and Social Psychology Bulletin, 40*, 998–1011. https://doi.org/10.1177/0146167214533389

Niles, A. N., Byrne Haltom, K. E., Lieberman, M. D., Hur, C., & Stanton, A. L. (2016). Writing content predicts benefit from written expressive disclosure: Evidence for repeated exposure and self-affirmation. *Cognition and Emotion, 30*, 258–274. https://doi.org/10.1080/02699931.2014.995598

Ogedegbe, G. O., Boutin-Foster, C., Wells, M. T., Allegrante, J. P., Isen, A. M., Jobe, J. B., & Charlson, M. E. (2012). A randomized controlled trial of positive-affect intervention and medication adherence in hypertensive African Americans. *Archives of Internal Medicine, 172*, 322–326. https://doi.org/10.1001/archinternmed.2011.1307

Persoskie, A., Ferrer, R. A., Taber, J. M., Klein, W. M., Parascandola, M., & Harris, P. R. (2015). Smoke-free air laws and quit attempts: Evidence for a moderating role of spontaneous self-affirmation. *Social Science & Medicine, 141*, 46–55. https://doi.org/10.1016/j.socscimed.2015.07.015

Peterson, J. C., Czajkowski, S., Charlson, M. E., Link, A. R., Wells, M. T., Isen, A. M., Mancuso, C. A., Allegrante, J. P., Boutin-Foster, C., Ogedegbe, G., & Jobe, J. B. (2013). Translating basic behavioral and social science research to clinical application: The EVOLVE mixed methods approach. *Journal of Consulting and Clinical Psychology, 8*, 217–230. https://doi.org/10.1037/a0029909

Pietersma, S., & Dijkstra, A. (2012). Cognitive self-affirmation inclination: An individual difference in dealing with self-threats. *British Journal of Social Psychology, 51*, 33–51. https://doi.org/10.1348/014466610X533768

Schmeichel, B. J., & Vohs, K. (2009). Self-affirmation and self-control: Affirming core values counteracts ego depletion. *Journal of Personality and Social Psychology, 96*, 770–782. https://doi.org/10.1037/a0014635

Schüz, B., Cooke, R., Schüz, N., & Van Koningsbruggen, G. M. (2017). Self-affirmation interventions to change health behaviors. In L. Little, E. Sillence, & A. Joinson (Eds.), *Behavior change research and theory: Psychological and technological perspectives* (pp. 87–114). Elsevier. https://doi.org/10.1016/B978-0-12-802690-8.00006-2

Schüz, N., & Schüz, B. (2017). Self-affirmation: Protecting the self and protecting subjective well-being. In M. D. Robinson & M. Eid (Eds.), *The happy mind: Cognitive contributions to well-being* (pp. 291–308). Springer International Publishing. https://doi.org/10.1007/978-3-319-58763-9_16

Schüz, N., Schüz, B., & Eid, M. (2013). When risk communication backfires: Randomized controlled trial on self-affirmation and reactance to personalized risk feedback in high-risk individuals. *Health Psychology, 32*, 561–570. https://doi.org/10.1037/a0029887

Sherman, D. A., Nelson, L. D., & Steele, C. M. (2000). Do messages about health risks threaten the self? Increasing the acceptance of threatening health messages via self-affirmation. *Personality and Social Psychology Bulletin, 2*, 1046–1058. https://doi.org/10.1177/01461672002611003

Sherman, D. K., Bunyan, D. P., Creswell, J. D., & Jaremka, L. M. (2009). Psychological vulnerability and stress: The effects of self-affirmation on sympathetic nervous system responses to naturalistic stressors. *Health Psychology, 28*, 554–562. https://doi.org/10.1037/a0014663

Sherman, D. K., & Cohen, G. L. (2006). The psychology of self-defense: Self-affirmation theory. In M. P. Zanna (Ed.), *Advances in experimental social psychology* (Vol. 38, pp. 183–242). Elsevier Academic Press. https://doi.org/10.1016/S0065-2601(06)38004-5

Sherman, D. K., Cohen, G. L., Nelson, L. D., Nussbaum, A. D., Bunyan, D. P., & Garcia, J. (2009). Affirmed yet unaware: Exploring the role of awareness in the process of self-affirmation. *Journal of Personality and Social Psychology, 97*, 745–764. https://doi.org/10.1037/a0015451

Silverman, A., Logel, C., & Cohen, G. L. (2013). Self-affirmation as a deliberate coping strategy: The moderating role of choice. *Journal of Experimental Social Psychology, 49*, 93–98. https://doi.org/10.1016/j.jesp.2012.08.005

Springer, A., Venkatakrishnan, A., Mohan, S., Nelson, L., Silva, M., & Pirolli, P. (2018). Leveraging self-affirmation to improve behavior change: A mobile health app experiment. *JMIR mHealth and uHealth, 6*, 1. https://doi.org/10.2196/mhealth.9151

Steele, C. M. (1988). The psychology of self-affirmation: Sustaining the integrity of the self. In L. Berkowitz (Ed.), *Advances in experimental social psychology* (Vol. 21, pp. 261–302). Academic Press.

Sweeney, A. M., & Moyer, A. (2015). Self-affirmation and responses to health messages: A meta-analysis on intentions and behavior. *Health Psychology, 34*, 149–159. https://doi.org/10.1037/hea0000110

Taber, J. M., Klein, W. M., Ferrer, R. A., Kent, E. E., & Harris, P. R. (2016). Optimism and spontaneous self-affirmation are associated with lower likelihood of cognitive impairment and greater positive affect among cancer survivors. *Annals of Behavioral Medicine, 50*, 198–209. https://doi.org/10.1007/s12160-015-9745-9

Taber, J. M., McQueen, A., Simonovic, N., & Waters, E. A. (2019). Adapting a self-affirmation intervention for use in a mobile application for smokers. *Journal of Behavioral Medicine, 42*, 1050–1061. https://doi.org/10.1007/s10865-019-00028-1

Tang, D., & Schmeichel, B. J. (2015). Self-affirmation facilitates cardiovascular recovery following interpersonal evaluation. *Biological Psychology, 104*, 108–115. https://doi.org/10.1016/j.biopsycho.2014.11.011

Toma, C. L., & Hancock, J. T. (2013). Self-affirmation underlies Facebook use. *Personality and Social Psychology Bulletin, 39*, 321–331. https://doi.org/10.1177/0146167212474694

Townsend, C., & Sood, S. (2012). Self-affirmation through the choice of highly aesthetic products. *Journal of Consumer Research, 39*, 415–428. https://doi.org/10.1086/663775

van Koningsbruggen, G. M., & Das, E. (2009). Don't derogate this message! Self-affirmation promotes online type 2 diabetes risk test taking. *Psychology and Health, 24*, 635–649. https://doi.org/10.1080/08870440802340156

van Koningsbruggen, G. M., Harris, P. R., Smits, A. J., Schüz, B., Scholz, U., & Cooke, R. (2014). Self-affirmation before exposure to health communications promotes intentions and health behavior change by increasing anticipated regret. *Communication Research, 43*, 1027–1044. https://doi.org/10.1177/0093650214555180

van Koningsbruggen, G. M., Miles, E., & Harris, P. (2016). Self-affirmation and self-control: Counteracting defensive processing of health information and facilitating health behavior change. In D. Ridder, M. Adriaanse, & K. Fujita (Eds.), *Handbook of self-control in health and wellbeing*. Routledge.

van't Riet, J., & Ruiter, R. A. (2013). Defensive reactions to health-promoting information: An overview and implications for future research. *Health Psychology Review, 7*(sup1), S104–S136. https://doi.org/10.1080/17437199.2011.606782

Walter, N., Demetriades, S. Z., & Murphy, S. T. (2019). Just a spoonful of sugar helps the messages go down: Using stories and vicarious self-affirmation to reduce e-cigarette use. *Health Communication, 34*, 352–360. https://doi.org/10.1080/10410236.2017.1407275

Walter, N., Saucier, C. J., & Murphy, S. T. (2019). Increasing receptivity to messages about e-cigarette risk using vicarious-affirmation. *Journal of Health Communication, 24*, 226–235. https://doi.org/10.1080/10810730.2019.1597951

Webb, T. L., Benn, Y., Chang, B. P. I., Reynolds, J. P., Sirois, F. M., Assinari, A., & Harris, P. R. (2020). The relationship between individual differences in spontaneous self-affirmation and affect associated with self-weighing. *Journal of Research in Personality, 89*, 104020. https://doi.org/10.1016/j.jrp.2020.104020

Wileman, V., Farrington, K., Chilcot, J., Norton, S., Wellsted, D. M., Almond, M. K., Davenport, A., Franklin, G., Gane, M. D. S., & Armitage, C. J. (2014). Evidence that self-affirmation improves phosphate control in hemodialysis patients: A pilot cluster randomized controlled trial. *Annals of Behavioral Medicine, 48*, 275–281. https://doi.org/10.1007/s12160-014-9597-8

Zhao, X., Peterson, E. B., Kim, W., & Rolfe-Redding, J. (2014). Effects of self-affirmation on daily versus occasional smokers' responses to graphic warning labels. *Communication Research, 41*, 1137–1158. https://doi.org/10.1177/0093650212465433

Zhu, X., & Yzer, M. (2019). Testing a brief scale format self-affirmation induction for use in health communication research and practice. *Communication Methods and Measures, 13*, 178–197. https://doi.org/10.1080/19312458.2019.1572084

10

Posttraumatic Growth and Physical Health

Ana I. Orejuela Dávila and Richard G. Tedeschi

Introduction

At some point in their lives, most human beings will encounter adverse experiences involving pain, suffering, grief, or loss. Although these experiences may be negative, they can also paradoxically create fertile ground for positive changes to bloom. This idea of growth through adversity (or, more simply, that something good can come out of something bad) is ancient and widespread. One can find examples of it in religious texts (such as the Bible and Quran) as well as in the hero's journey found in works of literature such as *The Iliad* and *The Odyssey*. However, the systematic and empirical study of this idea is a relatively new endeavor. Using the tools of quantitative and qualitative research from the social and behavioral sciences, researchers for the past 25 years have studied the phenomenon that has been termed Posttraumatic Growth (PTG; Tedeschi & Calhoun, 1996).

PTG is the positive psychological change that can occur as a result of struggling with highly stressful and challenging circumstances. According to Tedeschi and Calhoun (1996), this change can unfold across five domains: personal strength, appreciation for life, new possibilities, relating to others, and spiritual change. The domain of *personal strength* consists of the

A. I. Orejuela Dávila (✉)
James A. Haley Veterans' Hospital, Tampa, FL, USA

R. G. Tedeschi
Boulder Crest Institute for Posttraumatic Growth, Bluemont, VA, USA

F. M. Sirois (ed.), *The Palgrave Handbook of Positive Psychology and Health*,
https://doi.org/10.1007/978-3-031-89095-6_10

recognition that one is capable of handling whatever happens in life. This is because the encounter with a highly stressful event can induce the sense that one has been tested and survived the worst, thus producing a feeling of increased strength and confidence that one can handle future challenges. The domain of *appreciation for life* entails an increased awareness of the value of one's life as well as changed priorities. This can include some things receding in importance, while others attain greater significance (for example, a person with an established career might stop chronically working over time in favor of spending more time with one's family). The domain of *new possibilities* consists of identifying new opportunities for oneself that were not previously available, or that one may not have been able to recognize beforehand. For example, an individual who struggled with cancer as a child may later on decide to become an oncologist as a result of their experience. The domain of *relating to others* consists of having more meaningful and emotionally intimate relationships with others. It can also include having a greater sense of compassion for other people (especially those who are suffering), which can then lead to acts of altruism. And lastly, the domain of *spiritual and existential change* includes experiencing a stronger religious faith or a deepening of spirituality. This domain can also simply reflect a greater sense of purpose and meaning in one's life as well as achieving greater clarity regarding existential questions.

The theoretical model of PTG (Tedeschi et al., 2018) outlines how this process unfolds. The model first takes into account the person's pre-trauma, given that several pre-existing characteristics may influence how they respond to a traumatic event, including developmental stage, personality characteristics, coping styles, mental health history, prior stress exposure, and core beliefs. Core beliefs are fundamental beliefs about oneself, others, and the world in general (Cann et al., 2010). They also serve as schematic structures that help individuals navigate the world and make sense of it. For PTG to occur, a person's core beliefs must be challenged by the traumatic event. This might occur to varying degrees, depending on the strength of those beliefs and the impact of the traumatic event. To exemplify this, it is helpful to think of a traumatic event as an earthquake that can produce minor tremors that slightly shake one's core beliefs, or it can be a major seismic event that completely shatters those beliefs (Cann et al., 2010). In the aftermath of this earthquake, the disruption to core beliefs can lead to emotional distress and also initiate intrusive rumination (Cann et al., 2011), which consists of repetitive and unwanted thoughts about the traumatic event. To manage this distress, individuals may seek social support and engage in self-disclosure about the traumatic event, either by talking about it with others; writing about it in journals, blog posts, social media; or expressing it in other ways such as artistic creations. This self-disclosure helps to not only alleviate emotional distress but also facilitate cognitive processing of the event. Over time, intrusive rumination may shift into deliberate rumination, which is when a person thinks about the traumatic event in a conscious and effortful manner, with the intent of trying to make sense of it (Cann et al., 2011). It is through this process of deliberate rumination that core beliefs are re-examined and rebuilt, which then leads to the acceptance of the changed world and allows for the traumatic event to be integrated into one's life narrative.

It is important to emphasize that PTG is the result of the *struggle* with the aftermath of a traumatic event and not an immediate, direct product of the event itself (Tedeschi & Calhoun, 1996). This is a struggle to cope and survive and not a conscious struggle to grow or change. In fact, the growth that may occur as a result of this struggle tends to be unplanned and unexpected. It should also be noted that PTG is not the opposite of posttraumatic stress disorder (PTSD), and to place these two constructs on opposite ends of a continuum would be to reduce the complexity of human responses to trauma. In fact, the model posits that both PTG and posttraumatic stress (PTS) can co-exist, which has also been confirmed by a recent meta-analysis (Liu et al., 2017). Further, another meta-analysis (Shakespeare-Finch & Lurie-Beck, 2014) revealed a curvilinear relationship between PTSD symptoms and PTG, with PTG being higher when moderate levels of PTSD are present. This suggests that a certain amount of posttraumatic stress is necessary in order for PTG to unfold.

PTG has been associated with a variety of positive psychological outcomes, including greater wisdom (Webster & Deng, 2015), psychological preparedness (Janoff-Bulman, 2004), and altruism (Tsai et al., 2016). In addition to enhancing psychological well-being, PTG can also impact physical health, which will be the focus of this chapter. However, it is helpful to first contextualize research on the relationship between PTG and physical health within the wider umbrella of the meaning-making literature, which has established that the act of deriving meaning from our lived experiences is essential to overall well-being (Roepke et al., 2014). This includes finding purpose and generating a sense of coherence by determining why events occurred and what they imply about the future (Thompson & Janigian, 1988). Overall, research has shown that higher levels of meaning are associated with better physical health, as well as with factors that help decrease negative health outcomes and increase health-promoting behaviors (Roepke et al., 2014), such as physical activity, healthy diet, and lack of substance use. Further, this association exists for both subjective (e.g., health-related quality of life, self-reported health) and objective (e.g., biological measurements, mortality rates) indices of health

(Roepke et al., 2014), with recent research suggesting that the relationship is stronger for subjective measures (Czekierda et al., 2017). However, longitudinal studies are still needed to establish direction and causality between meaning and physical health (e.g., does meaning improve physical health, or does better physical health allow individuals to attain greater meaning in life?). It is likely that the relationship between meaning and physical health is bidirectional, with many moderators and mediators that play key roles depending on the health indices being examined (Czekierda et al., 2017).

Within the meaning-making literature, a narrower area of focus is meaning-making through the lens of a traumatic event. Similar to the research on meaning and physical health, studies on PTG and physical health have begun to elucidate a significant and positive relationship between these two variables. This chapter will explore this relationship within the context of brain function and chronic conditions, such as cancer, human immunodeficiency virus (HIV), cardiovascular disease (CVD), and spinal cord injury (SCI). Although this chapter is not a comprehensive review of each of these areas, it will still highlight key research findings that exemplify how PTG can impact physical health.

PTG and Life-Threatening Illness

A chronic illness is stressful not just because of the illness itself but also because it can entail a loss of identity, changes in daily activities and the structure of everyday life, disrupt social relationships and social roles, and create uncertainty about the future (Bury, 1991). In addition, studies have also shown that chronic and life-threatening illnesses have the potential to be traumatic and induce PTSD (Sommer et al., 2018). In fact, the diagnosis of a life-threatening illness meets the criterion of a traumatic event necessary for the development of PTSD according to the DSM-IV. However, there is a key difference between illness-related trauma and non-medical trauma. Whereas other forms of trauma may consist of one single event with a definite beginning and end, illness-related trauma consists not just of the moment of diagnosis but also of ongoing treatment and the continuous potential threat of death. In other words, while non-medical trauma often consists of an external event in the past, illness-related trauma consists of an ongoing internal event unfolding in one's body.

It should also be noted that PTG that arises from coping with a life-threatening illness is different from the concept of illness adjustment, which refers to psychologically adapting to a disease, regaining control over the disease, and returning to a level of pre-disease equilibrium (de Ridder et al., 2008). In contrast, PTG involves transformational changes that go beyond adapting to a disease and do not entail a return to a baseline level of functioning. Therefore, it is important to establish this conceptual distinction and apply it when discussing patients' experiences with chronic and life-threatening illnesses.

PTG and Cancer

Cancer diagnosis and treatment can be an extremely stressful and even traumatic experience (Gurevich et al., 2002), as evidenced by an extensive body of literature documenting cancer-related PTSD symptoms (Kangas et al., 2002; Neel, 2000). Increased acknowledgment of the potentially traumatic nature of cancer has also encouraged research on PTG within the context of this disease. To date, a growing body of literature continues to examine PTG among cancer patients (Cordova et al., 2007; Shand et al., 2015), showing that it is possible for these patients to experience PTG as a result of coping with their cancer experience.

It should also be noted that both PTG and PTS can co-occur within the context of cancer, as is also often the case with other forms of trauma. For example, Cordova et al. (2007) found that PTG and PTSD symptoms coexisted in a sample of women with breast cancer. Further, both PTG and PTSD symptoms were higher in patients who explicitly perceived their event as a traumatic stressor, relative to those who did not. Interestingly, although PTG and PTSD symptoms co-occurred in this sample, they were not significantly associated with each other, which is a finding that was also observed by Widows et al. (2005) among a sample of bone marrow transplant recipients. Still, other studies have shown significant relationships between the two (see meta-analysis by Shand et al., 2015), thus highlighting the variability of responses to trauma.

Although stress, PTS, and PTG can all co-occur within the context of cancer, they have been associated with different predictors and disease-related outcomes. For example, Shand et al. (2015) conducted a meta-analysis to examine psychosocial correlates of posttraumatic stress (PTS) and PTG in oncology populations. Results showed that PTS was positively associated with distress and depression, while PTG had a negative association with those two variables. PTS was also associated with greater anxiety and poorer quality of life, while PTG did not have a significant association with these two variables.

Additionally, PTG was associated with social support, optimism, positive reappraisal, and adaptive coping styles, while PTS was not.

In addition to the positive associations with psychological variables, longitudinal studies have also indicated that PTG may be active in decreasing cancer-related stress in the long run. For example, Groarke et al. (2017) did a longitudinal study across five time points over an 18-month period (which included stages of diagnosis, treatment, and transition to survivorship) to examine the relationship between distress and PTG among women with breast cancer. Results showed that, as expected, greater cancer-specific stress at diagnosis predicted greater PTG six months later. PTG was then, in turn, associated with subsequent reductions in cancer-specific stress at the 12-month follow-up, and global stress at the 18-month follow-up. These results suggest that PTG can improve stress management and adjustment to cancer over the long term by altering how one views and deals with stressors. Another longitudinal study of breast cancer patients by Wang et al. (2017a) yielded similar results, showing that increased levels of PTG predicted lower levels of distress over a 24-month period. This study also showed that for women who had undergone a mastectomy, PTG buffered the effects of cancer recurrence fear and perceived physical vulnerability on distress. Together, these findings highlight how PTG can be an important factor in managing stress over time within the context of this physical illness.

PTG and Physical Correlates Among Cancer Patients

While many studies have explored the relationships between PTG and psychosocial variables among cancer patients, there has been comparatively less research focusing on the relationship between PTG and cancer-related variables. A meta-analysis (Casellas et al., 2017) found no relationship between PTG and cancer site, cancer surgery, or cancer recurrence; however, some small correlations were found between PTG, cancer stage, and time elapsed since the diagnosis. Although more research is needed regarding illness-related variables, some studies have shown positive associations between PTG, survival rates, and immunity. For example, Dougall et al. (2017) conducted a longitudinal study to examine the relationship between PTG, PTS, mental and physical health quality of life (QoL), and survival among patients with lung cancer. Results revealed that although PTS and PTG co-occurred among patients, they had different effects on self-reported QoL and survival. Specifically, PTS symptoms predicted poorer mental QoL, but did not predict physical QoL or survival. Conversely, PTG predicted better physical health QoL and longer survival, even after accounting for disease variables (i.e., cancer stage, time since diagnosis), PTS symptoms, and attrition. The fact that the significant relationship between PTG and physical health QoL persisted in spite of these control variables suggests that PTG can have a unique protective effect on health outcomes.

Another study by Dunigan et al. (2007) also suggested that PTG can aid with survival. These authors examined the relationship between PTG, immunity, and survival in patients with hepatoma by measuring peripheral blood leukocytes (PBL) at baseline, as well as at three- and six-month follow-ups. PBLs (also known as white blood cells) are cells of the immune system that protect the body against disease, such that a higher PBL count indicates a better responsiveness of the immune system (Carrick & Begg, 2008). Dunigan et al. (2007) found that patients with higher PTG scores (especially in the domains of personal strength, relating to others, and spirituality) had higher PBL counts, and they also survived longer than patients with lower PTG scores. The authors suggested that the positive emotional and cognitive changes associated with PTG may help reduce stress levels, and thus help the endocrine and immune system return to a homeostatic (or balanced) state over time. Overall, these findings suggest that patients with higher PTG may recover more rapidly from chemotherapy, as indicated by PBL counts.

Lastly, there is one study that examined the relationship between PTG and cortisol, a hormone that helps regulate the immune response and how the body responds to stress. Diaz et al. (2014) examined the relationship between PTG and cortisol levels among patients with metastatic breast cancer. Previous studies have already demonstrated that cancer can produce negative psychological outcomes that can disrupt cortisol levels in breast cancer patients (Giese-Davis et al., 2006). Specifically, flatter diurnal cortisol levels tend to predict worse survival in breast cancer patients (Sephton et al., 2000), while a steeper decline (i.e., negative slope) throughout the day is indicative of healthier endocrine function. In their study, Diaz et al. (2014) found a significant negative correlation between PTG and diurnal cortisol levels, such that higher PTG was significantly associated with more negative cortisol slopes. This suggests that there is a positive link between PTG and healthier endocrine functioning in patients with cancer. However, this was a cross-sectional study, and longitudinal studies would be needed to determine if the presence of PTG leads to a better stress response, or if stabilization of the HPA axis helps to facilitate PTG.

PTG and Heart Health

PTG and Cardiovascular Disease

Cardiovascular disease (CVD) is one of the leading causes of death worldwide (Heron, 2019), and there is evidence that suggests that PTSD can arise from struggling with CVD due to its potentially life-threatening nature (Vilchinsky et al., 2017). In fact, a meta-analysis (Gander & von Känel, 2006) found that, on average, PTS symptoms can occur in 14% of patients who suffer a myocardial infarction (colloquially known as a "heart attack"). Conversely, a diagnosis of PTSD has been associated with increased CVD risk (Edmondson & von Känel, 2017) because exposure to trauma has the potential to dysregulate the hypothalamic-pituitary-adrenal (HPA) axis, increase inflammation, lower HRV, and increase blood pressure (Edmondson & von Känel, 2017). In addition, CVD can also be stressful in general due, in part, to the possibility of having to take medications for the rest of one's life, and to the fact that the occurrence of one heart attack increases the likelihood of having others in the future (Gander & von Känel, 2006).

Studies have also shown that it is possible for PTG to arise from the struggle with CVD. For example, Bluvstein et al. (2013) examined the impact of PTG and PTSS on mental health outcomes among patients who experienced myocardial infarction and acute coronary artery bypass graft. Results showed that PTG buffered the effect of PTSS on psychological distress. Results also showed that PTG had a protective effect on the relationship between PTSS and psychological well-being. Specifically, for patients with high PTSS, psychological well-being was higher if greater PTG was present, but lower if there was less PTG. Taken together, these findings suggest that PTG can help attenuate the negative effects of PTSS on mental health outcomes following a cardiac event.

PTG, CVD, and Personality. Recall that the PTG model states that an individual's personality pre-trauma affects how they respond to and cope with a traumatic event, which then ultimately affects PTG (Tedeschi et al., 2018). Studies have indicated that, among patients who have suffered a myocardial infarction, PTG is positively associated with extraversion, conscientiousness, and openness (Garnefski et al., 2008; Javed & Dawood, 2016; Sheikh, 2004), and negatively associated with neuroticism (Garnefski et al., 2008; Javed & Dawood, 2016). Studies on PTG within the context of non-medical trauma have also yielded similar findings (Karanci et al., 2012; Tedeschi & Calhoun, 1996). However, research has also suggested that the relationship between personality and PTG is mediated by coping strategies (Shakespeare-Finch et al., 2005). So, in the context of CVD, someone who is extraverted may be more likely to seek out social support and engage in self-disclosure regarding their CVD experience or use active coping strategies while someone with openness to experience may be more amenable to seeing things from a different perspective and revising life goals.

PTG, CVD, Coping, and Social Support. Studies have also indicated that how patients cope with CVD can also impact PTG. For example, Javed and Dawood (2016) found that among patients who recently experienced MI, PTG was positively associated with problem-focused coping, but negatively associated with avoidant emotional coping. Similarly, Garnefski et al. (2008) found that cognitive coping (consisting of the ability to put things into perspective, positive refocusing, and positive reappraisal) was positively associated with PTG, even after controlling for age, gender, and time since the MI. Together, these results suggest that interventions for heart attack recovery should teach patients how to utilize cognitive and problem-focused coping strategies that allow them to fully embrace the reality of their illness, rather than avoid it.

Coping with heart disease can also be affected by a patient's perceived social support. In fact, studies have shown that the interactions between coping styles and perceived social support can have an impact on PTG. For example, Senol-Durak and Ayvasik (2010) examined the impact of perceived social support, overall coping (which consisted of problem-focused, emotion-focused, and indirect coping), and perception of the cardiac event (which consisted of subjective perceived prognosis of health and threat to life) on PTG among Turkish patients who have had a myocardial infarction. Results revealed that coping was significantly related to PTG, and that it mediated the relationship between perceived social support and PTG. Interestingly, perception of the event was not related to PTG, nor did it mediate the relationship between perceived social support and PTG. These findings suggest that perceived social support affects the development of PTG by enhancing an individual's appropriate use of coping strategies, and by changing (or in this case, not changing) how an individual perceives their traumatic event. Sheikh (2004) also arrived at a similar conclusion, given that their study found that social support was not significantly correlated with PTG among patients with heart disease. However, they also found that PTG was positively correlated with problem-focused coping. To explain this finding, Sheikh (2004) suggested that for social support to affect PTG, it is necessary for social support to help foster cognitive processing and reappraisal of the event (and not consist of mere companionship).

PTG, CVD, and Spirituality. In addition to social support and coping, religion and spirituality can also impact PTG within the context of CVD. For example, Ai et al. (2013) examined the influence of pre-operative faith-based factors on PTG among patients at 30 months post-cardiac surgery. In particular, the faith-based factors that this study examined were positive religious coping (which consists of strategies such as focusing on religion and utilizing prayer during difficult times) and perceived spiritual support (which is the extent to which an individual feels supported by and connected to a higher spiritual power). Results revealed that pre-operative positive religious coping was significantly related to post-operative PTG, even after controlling for demographic and cardiac-related variables. Further, the influence of religious coping on PTG was mediated by perceived spiritual support, thus suggesting that a profound relationship with a spiritual force may be necessary for religious coping to impact PTG. Together, these findings suggest that for cardiac patients who value a particular faith or religion, it may be important to enhance their pre-operative use of religious coping strategies in order to facilitate long-term growth.

PTG, CVD, and Healthcare Utilization. Studies have also shown that for patients with CVD, PTG may impact the extent to which they utilize healthcare services. For example, Leung et al. (2012) explored the relationships between PTG, cardiac threat, and healthcare utilization among cardiac patients one year post hospitalization. Interestingly, PTG was related to a greater predicted risk of current cardiac events (which was calculated based on variables related to clinical risk). However, PTG was not related to the actual rate of recurrent cardiac events. When explaining this finding, the authors suggested that perhaps patients with greater cardiac risk may have perceived that they had survived a dangerous event, which then caused them to contemplate their own mortality and engage in the cognitive processes that lead to PTG. Growth, in turn, could then hypothetically motivate patients to improve their health, thus resulting in a reduced probability of having another cardiac event. Further, this study also found that PTG was significantly related to more physician visits and cardiac rehabilitation program enrollment (but not urgent healthcare), thus providing support for the idea that PTG may inspire patients to engage in healthy behaviors, such as preventative healthcare. However, it should be noted that this study by Leung et al. (2012) was cross-sectional, and longitudinal designs would be needed to establish causality between these variables.

PTG and Heart Rate Variability

Heart rate variability (HRV) is an objective physiological measure of autonomic nervous system activity, with higher resting levels of HRV indicating greater levels of flexibility for responding to stressors. As such, HRV can be used to assess links between the stress response and various indices of mental health (Appelhans & Luecken, 2006). In the context of trauma, reduced levels of HRV have been linked with PTSD (Nagpal et al., 2013), and recent research has begun to explore how HRV may be associated with PTG. Greenblatt Kimron et al. (2019) examined the relationship between PTS symptoms, PTG, and HRV among elderly Holocaust survivors and a matched control group with no Holocaust experience. Results showed that PTS and PTG co-existed among the Holocaust survivors and that lower PTS symptoms and higher PTG were related to healthier HRV. The authors also examined whether PTS and PTG mediated the relationship between Holocaust experience and HRV. Initially, belonging to the Holocaust group was associated with better HRV, but not when PTS symptoms were accounted for. However, when PTG was also accounted for, HRV was found to be better once again. This suggests that PTG may be a pathway to improved physical health among individuals with childhood trauma who also experience PTS symptoms in adulthood.

PTG and HIV

Historically, psychological research on people living with HIV has focused on the negative consequences of the disease (Ciesla & Roberts, 2001). However, progress in the treatment of HIV has changed it from a fatal disease to a chronic medical condition that can be managed (Deeks et al., 2013), thus extending the life expectancy of patients (Samji et al., 2013). This change also allowed for a shift in research, whereby scholars have begun to focus on potential positive psychological correlates among patients with HIV (Ironson & Hayward, 2008), including PTG (Rzeszutek & Gruszczyńska, 2018). For example, an HIV diagnosis can often serve as a motivating factor to engage in health behavior change (Siegel & Schrimshaw, 2000), and studies have found significant relationships between PTG and decreased substance use, a healthier diet, and utilization of safe sex practices (Milam, 2004; Siegel & Schrimshaw, 2000).

PTG, HIV, and Social Support

Similar to patients with cancer and CVD, studies have shown a significant positive relationship between social support and PTG among people living with HIV, as demonstrated by three cross-sectional studies (Cieślak et al., 2009; Kamen et al., 2016; Zeligman et al., 2016) and two longitudinal studies (Rzeszutek et al., 2017; Rzeszutek, 2017). In particular, emotional social support (e.g., providing empathy, demonstrating love, and caring) seems to be key, compared to tangible (e.g., assistance with tasks) or informational (e.g., providing advice) social support (Kamen et al., 2016). This is because emotional social support may help facilitate the emotional processing and distress management that is required to engage in deliberate rumination and ultimately experience PTG.

PTG and HIV-Related Stigma

In addition to social support, studies have also suggested that internalized HIV-related stigma (IHRS) is an important factor to address when it comes to promoting PTG among people living with HIV. IHRS occurs when a person living with HIV accepts negative societal views of HIV and applies them to the self (Murphy & Hevey, 2013). Research has shown that this stigma is associated with poorer adherence to HIV treatment (Sayles et al., 2009) and faster disease progression (Leserman, 2008). Cross-sectional studies have found a negative relationship between HIV-related stigma and PTG (Kamen et al., 2016; Murphy & Hevey, 2013; Zeligman et al., 2016), which has led to the suggestion that psychological interventions for people living with HIV should aim to reduce IHRS in order to enhance health behaviors and possibly PTG (Murphy & Hevey, 2013).

However, one longitudinal study (Garrido-Hernansaiz et al., 2017) found a positive relationship between IHRS and PTG. Specifically, the authors found that higher levels of IHRS at the time of HIV diagnosis predicted greater PTG eight months later within the domains of relating to others, personal strength, and appreciation for life (which the authors referred to as "philosophy of life"). This is in contrast to the cross-sectional studies (e.g., Murphy & Hevey, 2013) that have found that lower IHRS is related to greater PTG. To explain this discrepancy in the literature, Garrido-Hernansaiz et al. (2017) suggested that perhaps for some individuals, an HIV diagnosis by itself is not traumatic enough to disrupt core beliefs, given that antiretroviral therapy is more readily available and the likelihood of a normal life expectancy is greater in today's society. It is possible that for some individuals, IHRS may be what causes core belief disruption, which would then open a pathway for PTG. To explore this hypothesis, future studies on IHRS and PTG should incorporate a measure of core belief disruption in relation to HIV diagnosis.

However, longitudinal studies are needed to determine if decreased stigma leads to greater PTG, or if greater PTG helps to reduce stigma over the long term. Regardless of the direction of this relationship, it has been suggested that psychological interventions for people living with HIV should aim to reduce IHRS to enhance health behaviors and possibly PTG (Murphy & Hevey, 2013).

PTG and HIV-Related Variables

Unlike psychosocial research on PTG and HIV, research on the relationship between PTG and biological HIV-related variables has been mixed. For example, when examining PTG and CD4 count (i.e., white blood cells that fight infection), some studies have found no relationship between these two variables (Milam, 2004; Rzeszutek et al., 2017; Rzeszutek et al., 2019), while one study found a positive relationship only among Hispanic patients and individuals with low levels of optimism (Milam, 2006). Similarly, studies have also yielded mixed findings in regard to the relationship between PTG and viral load, with one study finding no relationship between the two variables (Milam, 2004) and another finding a negative relationship among individuals with low levels of pessimism (Milam, 2006). These studies highlight the complexity of the relationship between PTG and biological markers of HIV, which is unlikely to be straightforward due to the influence of a variety of psychosocial variables (Milam, 2006).

PTG and Spinal Cord Injury

Spinal cord injury (SCI) is a leading cause of long-term severe disability in the United States (National Spinal Cord Injury Statistical Center, 2006). Patients with SCI must contend not only with the physical challenges associated with their injury but also with the loss of functional ability and limited mobility that may result in social isolation, potential job loss, and negative reactions from others (Bonanno et al., 2012). These sources of stress may then lead to negative mental health outcomes, such as depression, anxiety, and substance use (Migliorini et al., 2008). However, similar to the other chronic conditions that were just discussed, the struggle to cope with SCI has also been linked to positive outcomes, including PTG. For example, Chun and Lee (2008) conducted a qualitative thematic analysis to examine the life experiences of individuals before and after SCI and see how they might influence PTG. Among these individuals, the most salient themes of PTG were greater appreciation of life, relating to others (specifically, having more meaningful family relationships), and engaging in meaningful experiences. The theme of appreciation of life consisted of appreciating everyday life in general, as well as appreciating the physical abilities that participants were able to retain. With regard to more meaningful family relationships, participants described greater emotional intimacy, trust, and mutuality (consisting of a greater sense of commonality and shared understanding with family members). Lastly, the act of engaging in meaningful activities fostered the recognition of personal strengths, deepened social relationships, and promoted positive emotions.

Wang et al. (2017b) also explored themes that emerge from the process of PTG among patients with SCI in China. The authors conducted semi-structured interviews that revealed the following subjects: struggling with hopelessness (including loss of autonomy and isolation from society), disentangling from disability (including the reconstruction of a new sense of identity and belonging, as well as reintegration into the community), and facing challenges (associated with achieving goals, enjoying success, and developing wisdom). This suggests that navigating these themes over time is important for achieving growth among patients with SCI.

PTG, SCI, Sports, and Leisure

Studies have shown that individuals with SCI can derive physical health benefits from participation in sports and other forms of physical activity, such as improved physical fitness, prevention of chronic disease, and better pain management (Martin Ginis et al,. 2010). Similarly, physical activities can also produce psychological benefits for individuals with SCI, such as improved mood, increased self-esteem, and greater life satisfaction (Martin Ginis et al., 2010).

Given this association, Crawford et al. (2014) examined if participation in a sports program facilitated PTG for individuals with acquired SCI. Qualitative data revealed two PTG themes: a greater appreciation for life and relating to others. In line with the concept of appreciation for life, participants revealed that sports allowed them to be more fully present, not take things for granted, and appreciate their physical abilities. The physically demanding and competitive nature of sports also allowed participants to bond with their teammates. Participants also indicated that they met people they otherwise would not have met, and felt like they became part of a community. Additionally, the data also revealed that sports helped participants engage in injury-relevant processing, which aided the process of re-establishing a self-identity post-injury. For those who engaged in sports for the first time through this program, it could be argued that they experienced growth in the domain of new possibilities for themselves. Overall, Crawford et al. (2014) concluded that sports-related interventions may help facilitate PTG among patients with SCI.

A study by Day (2013) also highlighted the role that sports can play in promoting PTG. Specifically, she conducted a qualitative analysis of how initial physical activity influences the development of PTG among post-Paralympic athletes with an acquired injury. While participation in physical activities and sports enhanced overall health and well-being, participants emphasized how exercise settings provided opportunities for growth. These environments allowed participants to take risks and test their physical limitations, which then allowed them to recognize their own personal strengths and identify new possibilities for themselves. This, in turn, allowed participants to take responsibility for their own choices, gain a sense of personal control, and create meaning in their lives.

In addition to sports, research has shown that leisure time in general can enhance PTG within the context of SCI. Similar to the studies by Crawford et al. (2014) and Day (2013), Chun and Lee (2010) found that leisure activities (such as music and art) promote PTG among patients with SCI through the same mechanisms as sports (e.g., they provide opportunities to discover personal strength, develop new abilities, experience success, form new relationships, find meaning, and generate positive emotions). This is supported by other studies that have highlighted the role of leisure as a coping strategy that buffers stress (Iwasaki & Mannell, 2000) and supports PTG (Kleiber et al., 2002) in the context of non-medical trauma.

PTG and Brain Function

Posttraumatic stress can have lasting impacts on brain structures and processes, especially those that are implicated in the stress response. For example, a heightened fear response is associated with increased amygdala function, and emotion regulation difficulties are associated with decreased prefrontal cortex function (Bremner, 2006). These neurological effects of trauma and the stress response can then have an impact on overall physical health (Gianaros & Wager, 2015). For this reason, it is important to examine associations between PTG and brain functioning.

Currently, there are limited neuroscientific studies on the relationship between PTG and the human brain. However, there are a few studies that have highlighted the role of certain prefrontal brain regions in PTG. Previous studies have shown that activation of the left prefrontal regions of the brain is associated with adaptive emotion regulation (Jackson et al., 2003), a resilient affective style (Davidson, 2004), and overall psychological well-being (Urry et al., 2004), which includes engaging with challenges and pursuing meaningful goals. Given these associations, Rabe et al. (2006) conducted an electroencephalogram (EEG) study to examine potential associations between PTG, activation of the left prefrontal cortex, and positive emotions among survivors of motor vehicle accidents. The study consisted of collecting EEG data during an emotion induction experiment while participants were exposed to traumatic images. Results showed that greater left baseline prefrontal activation was indeed correlated with PTG (except for the spiritual domain), even after controlling for dispositional positive affect (Rabe et al., 2006). Given that prefrontal regions are associated with goal-directed approach behaviors (Urry et al., 2004), the results from Rabe et al. (2006) suggest that PTG is largely driven by approach-related tendencies, rather than positive affect. The authors also suggested that left prefrontal activity was not associated with spiritual change because this domain is unlikely to be related to approach tendencies, relative to other PTG domains (e.g., new possibilities). Overall, the results of this study suggest that for PTG to unfold, left prefrontal regions need to be activated in order to support approach-related tendencies and goal-directed behaviors that ultimately lead to growth.

Within prefrontal regions, studies have also specifically highlighted the role of the dorsolateral prefrontal cortex (DLPFC) in PTG. The DLPFC is a brain region that plays an important role in regulating emotional processing and HRV. Previous studies have shown that greater DLPFC activation is associated with lower PTSD symptoms (Aupperle et al., 2012). In relation to PTG, Wei et al. (2017) examined how emotions affected the DLPFC and HRV among adults exposed to an explosion incident in Tianjin, China. The adults were divided into three groups, based on cut-off scores for measures of PTSD and PTG: control group (low PTSD/low PTG), PTSD group (high PTSD/low PTG), and PTG group (low PTSD/high PTG). Participants were shown a series of negative, positive, and neutral pictures while their DLPFC and HRV activity were measured. Results showed that the PTG group had increased activation of the left DLPFC in the negative condition while the

PTSD group had increased activation of the right DLPFC in the positive condition. Results also showed that the PTG group had significantly greater HRV in the negative and positive picture conditions, relative to the control group (there were no significant differences between the PTSD and control groups). This suggests that for individuals exposed to trauma, PTG may help facilitate more efficient emotional processing. Overall, Wei et al. (2017) stated that these findings suggest that PTSD and PTG may differentially affect emotion regulation patterns.

In addition to the activation of the DLPFC, studies have also examined how its physical structure may be related to PTG. Greater thickness of the DLPFC has been previously associated with decreased PTSD symptoms (Lyoo et al., 2011) and greater resilience (van der Werff et al., 2013) following a traumatic event. Given this association, Nakagawa et al. (2016) conducted a magnetic resonance imaging (MRI) study to examine if PTG was associated with greater gray matter volume in the DLPFC among survivors of an earthquake in Japan. Results showed that PTG was indeed significantly associated with greater gray matter volume in the right DLPFC, further highlighting the role of this brain region in PTG.

Although still in its nascent stage, the current research on PTG and brain function suggests that PTG is associated with increased activity in prefrontal regions of the brain that support goal-directed behavior and emotional processing. Overall, these activities that are supported by the prefrontal regions of the brain will impact how individuals manage traumatic stress, which can then, in turn, impact overall health.

Conclusion

PTG is the experience of positive psychological change that may occur as a result of coping with the aftermath of a traumatic event. For PTG to occur, an individual's core beliefs must be disrupted and they must engage in deliberate rumination to make meaning out of their traumatic experience. Emerging bodies of literature have begun exploring the links between PTG and physical health within the context of brain function and chronic health conditions, such as cancer, CVD, HIV, and SCI. These studies have shown that similar to non-medical trauma, PTG and distress can co-exist when individuals are struggling with chronic physical conditions. However, PTG and distress tend to be differently associated with health outcomes, with PTG having more positive effects over the long term. Further, in many cases, PTG can help attenuate the effects of subsequent stress within the context of chronic illnesses. While there is extensive research on the associations between PTG and psychological outcomes, more research is needed to explore the links between PTG, biomarkers (e.g., HRV, blood pressure, cortisol levels, CD4 count, etc.), and other objective measures of physical health (e.g., mortality rates, healthcare utilization, remission rates, etc.). In addition, the studies discussed in this chapter only measured PTG and not the associated cognitive processes leading up to it (e.g., core belief disruption, intrusive and deliberate rumination); therefore, future studies should incorporate measures of core belief disruption and rumination to further elucidate the impact that PTG can have on physical health. Lastly, many of these studies were cross-sectional, and more longitudinal designs are needed to establish causality between variables.

References

Ai, A. L., Hall, D., Pargament, K., & Tice, T. N. (2013). Posttraumatic growth in patients who survived cardiac surgery: The predictive and mediating roles of faith-based factors. *Journal of Behavioral Medicine, 36*(2), 186–198. https://doi.org/10.1007/s10865-012-9412-6

Appelhans, B. M., & Luecken, L. J. (2006). Heart rate variability as an index of regulated emotional responding. *Review of General Psychology, 10*(3), 229–240. https://doi.org/10.1037/1089-2680.10.3.229

Aupperle, R. L., Allard, C. B., Grimes, E. M., Simmons, A. N., Flagan, T., Behrooznia, M., Cissell, S. H., Twamley, E. W., Thorp, S. R., Norman, S. B., Paulus, M. P., & Stein, M. B. (2012). Dorsolateral prefrontal cortex activation during emotional anticipation and neuropsychological performance in posttraumatic stress disorder. *Archives of general psychiatry, 69*(4), 360–371. https://doi.org/10.1001/archgenpsychiatry.2011.1539

Bluvstein, I., Moravchick, L., Sheps, D., Schreiber, S., & Bloch, M. (2013). Posttraumatic growth, posttraumatic stress symptoms and mental health among coronary heart disease survivors. *Journal of Clinical Psychology in Medical Settings, 20*(2), 164–172. https://doi.org/10.1007/s10880-012-9318-z

Bonanno, G. A., Kennedy, P., Galatzer-Levy, I. R., & Lude, P. (2012). Trajectories of resilience, depression, and anxiety following spinal cord injury. *Rehabilitation Psychology, 57*(3), 236–247. https://doi.org/10.1037/a0029256

Bremner, J. D. (2006). Traumatic stress: Effects on the brain. *Dialogues in Clinical Neuroscience, 8*(4), 445–461. https://doi.org/10.31887/DCNS.2006.8.4/jbremner

Bury, M. R. (1991). The sociology of chronic illness: A review of research and prospects. *Sociology of Health and Illness, 13*(4), 451–468.

Cann, A., Calhoun, L. G., Tedeschi, R. G., Kilmer, R. P., Gil-Rivas, V., Vishnevsky, T., & Danhauer, S. C. (2010). The Core Beliefs Inventory: A brief measure of disruption in the assumptive world. *Anxiety, Stress & Coping: An International Journal, 23*(1), 19–34. https://doi.org/10.1080/10615800802573013

Cann, A., Calhoun, L. G., Tedeschi, R. G., Triplett, K. N., Vishnevsky, T., & Lindstrom, C. M. (2011). Assessing posttraumatic cognitive processes: The event related rumination inventory. *Anxiety, Stress & Coping: An International Journal, 24*(2), 137–156. https://doi.org/10.1080/10615806.2010.529901

Carrick, J. B., & Begg, A. P. (2008). Peripheral blood leukocytes. *The Veterinary clinics of North America. Equine practice, 24*(2), 239–23v. https://doi.org/10.1016/j.cveq.2008.05.003

Casellas, G. A., Ochoa, C., & Ruini, C. (2017). Psychological and clinical correlates of posttraumatic growth in cancer: A systematic and critical review. *Psycho-Oncology, 26*(12), 2007–2018. https://doi.org/10.1002/pon.4426

Chun, S., & Lee, Y. (2008). The experience of posttraumatic growth for people with spinal cord injury. *Qualitative Health Research, 18*(7), 877–890. https://doi.org/10.1177/1049732308318028

Chun, S., & Lee, Y. (2010). The role of leisure in the experience of posttraumatic growth for people with spinal cord injury. *Journal of Leisure Research, 42*(3), 393–415.

Ciesla, J. A., & Roberts, J. E. (2001). Meta-analysis of the relationship between HIV infection and risk for depressive disorders. *The American Journal of Psychiatry, 158*(5), 725–730. https://doi.org/10.1176/appi.ajp.158.5.725

Cieslak, R., Benight, C., Schmidt, N., Luszczynska, A., Curtin, E., Clark, R. A., & Kissinger, P. (2009). Predicting posttraumatic growth among Hurricane Katrina survivors living with HIV: The role of self-efficacy, social support, and PTSD symptoms. *Anxiety, Stress, and Coping, 22*, 449–463. https://doi.org/10.1080/10615800802403815

Cordova, M. J., Giese-Davis, J., Golant, M., Kronenwetter, C., Chang, V., & Spiegel, D. (2007). Breast cancer as trauma: Posttraumatic stress and posttraumatic growth. *Journal of Clinical Psychology in Medical Settings, 14*(4), 308–319. https://doi.org/10.1007/s10880-007-9083-6

Crawford, J. J., Gayman, A. M., & Tracey, J. (2014). An examination of post-traumatic growth in Canadian and American ParaSport athletes with acquired spinal cord injury. *Psychology of Sport and Exercise, 15*(4), 399–406. https://doi.org/10.1016/j.psychsport.2014.03.008

Czekierda, K., Banik, A., Park, C. L., & Luszczynska, A. (2017). Meaning in life and physical health: systematic review and meta-analysis. *Health Psychology Review, 11*(4), 387–418. https://doi.org/10.1080/17437199.2017.1327325

Davidson, R. J. (2004). Well-being and affective style: neural substrates and biobehavioural correlates. *Philosophical Transactions of the Royal Society of London. Series B: Biological Sciences, 359*(1449), 1395–1411. https://doi.org/10.1098/rstb.2004.1510

Day, M. C. (2013). The role of initial physical activity experiences in promoting posttraumatic growth in Paralympic athletes with an acquired disability. *Disability and Rehabilitation: An International, Multidisciplinary Journal, 35*(24), 2064–2072. https://doi.org/10.3109/09638288.2013.805822

de Ridder, D., Geenen, R., Kuijer, R., & van Middendorp, H. (2008). Psychological adjustment to chronic disease. *The Lancet, 372*(9634), 246–255. https://doi.org/10.1016/S0140-6736(08)61078-8

Deeks, S. G., Lewin, S. R., & Havlir, D. V. (2013). The end of AIDS: HIV infection as a chronic disease. *Lancet (London, England), 382*(9903), 1525–1533. https://doi.org/10.1016/S0140-6736(13)61809-7

Diaz, M., Aldridge-Gerry, A., & Spiegel, D. (2014). Posttraumatic growth and diurnal cortisol slope among women with metastatic breast cancer. *Psychoneuroendocrinology, 44*, 83–87. https://doi.org/10.1016/j.psyneuen.2014.03.001

Dougall, A. L., Swanson, J., Kyutoku, Y., Belani, C. P., & Baum, A. (2017). Posttraumatic symptoms, quality of life, and survival among lung cancer patients. *Journal of Applied Biobehavioral Research, 22*(3), 1–23. https://doi.org/10.1111/jabr.12065

Dunigan, J. T., Carr, B. I., & Steel, J. L. (2007). Posttraumatic growth, immunity and survival in patients with hepatoma. *Digestive Diseases and Sciences, 52*(9), 2452–2459. https://doi.org/10.1007/s10620-006-9477-6

Edmondson, D., & von Känel, R. (2017). Post-traumatic stress disorder and cardiovascular disease. *The Lancet Psychiatry, 4*(4), 320–329. https://doi.org/10.1016/S2215-0366(16)30377-7

Gander, M., & von Känel, R. (2006). Myocardial infarction and post-traumatic stress disorder: Frequency, outcome, and atherosclerotic mechanisms. *European Journal of Cardiovascular Prevention and Rehabilitation, 13*(2), 165–172. https://doi.org/10.1097/01.hjr.0000214606.60995.46

Garnefski, N., Kraaij, V., Schroevers, M. J., & Somsen, G. A. (2008). Posttraumatic growth after a myocardial infarction: A matter of personality, psychological health, or cognitive coping? *Journal of Clinical Psychology in Medical Settings, 15*, 270–277. https://doi.org/10.1007/s10880-008-9136-5

Garrido-Hernansaiz, H., Murphy, P. J., & Alonso-Tapia, J. (2017). Predictors of resilience and posttraumatic growth among people living with HIV: A longitudinal study. *AIDS and Behavior, 21*(11), 3260–3270. https://doi.org/10.1007/s10461-017-1870-y

Gianaros, P. J., & Wager, T. D. (2015). Brain-body pathways linking psychological stress and physical health. *Current Directions in Psychological Science, 24*(4), 313–321. https://doi.org/10.1177/0963721415581476

Giese-Davis, J., Wilhelm, F. H., Conrad, A., Abercrombie, H. C., Sephton, S., Yutsis, M., Neri, E., Taylor, C. B., Kraemer, H. C., & Spiegel, D. (2006). Depression and stress reactivity in metastatic breast cancer. *Psychosomatic Medicine, 68*(5), 675–683. https://doi.org/10.1097/01.psy.0000238216.88515.e5

Greenblatt Kimron, L., Marai, I., Lorber, A., & Cohen, M. (2019). The long-term effects of early-life trauma on psychological, physical and physiological health among the elderly: The study of Holocaust survivors. *Aging & Mental Health, 23*(10), 1340–1349. https://doi.org/10.1080/13607863.2018.1523880

Groarke, A., Curtis, R., Groarke, J. M., Hogan, M. J., Gibbons, A., & Kerin, M. (2017). Post-traumatic growth in breast cancer: How and when do distress and stress contribute? *Psycho-oncology, 26*(7), 967–974. https://doi.org/10.1002/pon.4243

Gurevich, M., Devins, G. M., & Rodin, G. M. (2002). Stress response syndromes and cancer: Conceptual and assessment issues. *Psychosomatics, 43*, 259–281.

Heron M. (2019). Deaths: Leading causes for 2017. *National Vital Statistics Reports: from the Centers for Disease Control and Prevention, National Center for Health Statistics, National Vital Statistics System, 68*(6), 1–77. PMID: 32501203.

Ironson, G., & Hayward, H. (2008). Do positive psychosocial factors predict disease progression in HIV-1? A review of the evidence. *Psychosomatic medicine, 70*(5), 546–554. https://doi.org/10.1097/PSY.0b013e318177216c

Iwasaki, Y., & Mannell, R. C. (2000). Hierarchical dimensions of leisure stress coping. *Leisure Sciences, 22*, 163–181.

Jackson, D. C., Mueller, C. J., Dolski, I., Dalton, K. M., Nitschke, J. B., Urry, H. L., et al. (2003). Now you feel it, now you don't: Frontal brain electrical asymmetry and individual differences in emotion regulation. *Psychological Science, 14*, 612–617.

Janoff-Bulman, R. (2004). Posttraumatic growth: Three explanatory models. *Psychological Inquiry, 15*(1), 30–34.

Javed, A., & Dawood, S. (2016). Psychosocial predictors of post-traumatic growth in patients after myocardial infarction. *Pakistan Journal of Psychological Research, 31*(2), 365–381.

Kamen, C., Vorasarun, C., Canning, T., Kienitz, E., Weiss, C., Flores, S., Etter, D., Lee, S., & Gore-Felton, C. (2016). The impact of stigma and social support on development of post-traumatic growth among persons living with HIV. *Journal of Clinical Psychology in Medical Settings, 23*(2), 126–134. https://doi.org/10.1007/s10880-015-9447-2

Kangas, M., Henry, J. L., & Bryant, R. A. (2002). Posttraumatic stress disorder following cancer: A conceptual and empirical review. *Clinical Psychology Review, 22*, 499–524.

Karanci, A. N., Isikli, S., Aker, A. T., Gul, E., Erkan, B. B., Ozkol, H., & Guzel, H. Y. (2012). Personality, post-traumatic stress and trauma type: Factors contributing to post-traumatic growth and its domains in a Turkish community sample. *European Journal of Psychotraumatology, 3*. https://doi.org/10.3402/ejpt.v3i0.17303

Kleiber, D. A., Hutchinson, S. L., & Williams, R. (2002). Leisure as a resource in transcending negative life events: Self-protection, self-restoration, and personal transformation. *Leisure Sciences, 24*, 219–235.

Leserman, J. (2008). Role of depression, stress, and trauma in HIV disease progression. *Psychosomatic Medicine, 70*(5), 539–545. https://doi.org/10.1097/PSY.0b013e3181777a5f

Leung, Y. W., Alter, D. A., Prior, P. L., Stewart, D. E., Irvine, J., & Grace, S. L. (2012). Posttraumatic growth in coronary artery disease outpatients: Relationship to degree of trauma and health service use. *Journal of Psychosomatic Research, 72*(4), 293–299. https://doi.org/10.1016/j.jpsychores.2011.12.011

Liu, A. N., Wang, L. L., Li, H. P., Gong, J., & Liu, X. H. (2017). Correlation between posttraumatic growth and posttraumatic stress disorder symptoms based on Pearson correlation coefficient: A meta-analysis. *The Journal of Nervous and Mental Disease, 205*(5), 380–389. https://doi.org/10.1097/NMD.0000000000000605

Lyoo, I. K., Kim, J. E., Yoon, S. J., Hwang, J., Bae, S., & Kim, D. J. (2011). The neurobiological role of the dorsolateral prefrontal cortex in recovery from trauma: Longitudinal brain imaging study among survivors of the South Korean subway disaster. *Archives of General Psychiatry, 68*(7), 701–713. https://doi.org/10.1001/archgenpsychiatry.2011.70

Martin Ginis, K. A., Jetha, A., Mack, D. E., & Hetz, S. (2010). Physical activity and subjective well-being among people with spinal cord injury: A meta-analysis. *Spinal Cord, 48*(1), 65e72. https://doi.org/10.1038/sc.2009.87

Migliorini, C., Tonge, B., & Taleporos, G. (2008). Spinal cord injury and mental health. *Australian and New Zealand Journal of Psychiatry, 42*(2), 309e314. https://doi.org/10.1080/00048670801886080

Milam, J. (2006). Posttraumatic growth and HIV disease progression. *Journal of Consulting and Clinical Psychology, 74*(5), 817–827. https://doi.org/10.1037/0022-006X.74.5.817

Milam, J. E. (2004). Posttraumatic Growth among HIV/AIDS Patients. *Journal of Applied Social Psychology, 34*(11), 2353–2376. https://doi.org/10.1111/j.1559-1816.2004.tb01981.x

Murphy, P. J., & Hevey, D. (2013). The relationship between internalised HIV-related stigma and posttraumatic growth. *AIDS and Behavior, 17*(5), 1809–1818. https://doi.org/10.1007/s10461-013-0482-4

Nagpal, M. L., Gleichauf, K., & Ginsberg, J. P. (2013). Meta-analysis of heart rate variability as a psychophysiological indicator of posttraumatic stress disorder. *Journal of Trauma & Treatment, 3*(182), 2167–1222.

Nakagawa, S., Sugiura, M., Sekiguchi, A., Kotozaki, Y., Miyauchi, C. M., Hanawa, S., ... & Kawashima, R. (2016). Effects of post-traumatic growth on the dorsolateral prefrontal cortex after a disaster. *Scientific Reports, 6*(1), 34364. https://doi.org/10.1038/srep34364

National Spinal Cord Injury Statistical Center. (2006). *Spinal cord injury: Facts and figures at a glance*. Author.

Neel, M. L. (2000). Posttraumatic stress symptomatology and cancer. *International Journal of Emergency Mental Health, 2*, 85–94.

Rabe, S., Zöllner, T., Maercker, A., & Karl, A. (2006). Neural correlates of posttraumatic growth after severe motor vehicle accidents. *Journal of Consulting and Clinical Psychology, 74*(5), 880–886. https://doi.org/10.1037/0022-006X.74.5.880

Roepke, A. M., Jayawickreme, E., & Riffle, O. M. (2014). Meaning and health: A systematic review. *Applied Research in Quality of Life, 9*(4), 1055–1079. https://doi.org/10.1007/s11482-013-9288-9

Rzeszutek, M. (2017). Social support and posttraumatic growth in a longitudinal study of people living with HIV: The mediating role of positive affect. *European Journal of Psychotraumatology, 8*(1). https://doi.org/10.1080/20008198.2017.1412225

Rzeszutek, M., & Gruszczyńska, E. (2018). Posttraumatic growth among people living with HIV: A systematic review. *Journal of Psychosomatic Research, 114*, 81–91. https://doi.org/10.1016/j.jpsychores.2018.09.006

Rzeszutek, M., Oniszczenko, W., & Firląg-Burkacka, E. (2017). Social support, stress coping strategies, resilience and posttraumatic growth in a Polish sample of HIV-infected individuals: Results of a 1 year longitudinal study. *Journal of Behavioral Medicine, 40*(6), 942–954. https://doi.org/10.1007/s10865-017-9861-z

Rzeszutek, M., Oniszczenko, W., & Gruszczyńska, E. (2019). Satisfaction with life, big-five personality traits and posttraumatic growth among people living with HIV. *Journal of Happiness Studies: An Interdisciplinary Forum on Subjective Well-Being, 20*(1), 35–50. https://doi.org/10.1007/s10902-017-9925-3

Samji, H., Cescon, A., Hogg, R. S., Modur, S. P., Althoff, K. N., Buchacz, K., Burchell, A. N., Cohen, M., Gebo, K. A., Gill, M. J., Justice, A., Kirk, G., Klein, M. B., Korthuis, P. T., Martin, J., Napravnik, S., Rourke, S. B., Sterling, T. R., Silverberg, M. J., et al. (2013). Closing the gap: Increases in life expectancy among treated HIV-positive individuals in the United States and Canada. *PloS one, 8*(12), e81355. https://doi.org/10.1371/journal.pone.0081355

Sayles, J. N., Wong, M. D., Kinsler, J. J., Martins, D., & Cunningham, W. E. (2009). The association of stigma with self-reported access to medical care and antiretroviral therapy adherence in persons living with HIV/AIDS. *Journal of General Internal Medicine, 24*(10), 1101–1108. https://doi.org/10.1007/s11606-009-1068-8

Senol-Durak, E., & Ayvasik, H. B. (2010). Factors associated with posttraumatic growth among myocardial infarction patients: Perceived social support, perception of the event and coping. *Journal of Clinical Psychology in Medical Settings, 17*, 150–158. https://doi.org/10.1007/s10880-010-9192-5

Sephton, S. E., Sapolsky, R. M., Kraemer, H. C., & Spiegel, D. (2000). Diurnal cortisol rhythm as a predictor of breast cancer survival. *Journal of the National Cancer Institute, 92*, 994–1000.

Shakespeare-Finch, J., Gow, K., & Smith, S. (2005). Personality, coping and posttraumatic growth in emergency ambulance personnel. *Traumatology, 11*(4), 325–334. https://doi.org/10.1177/153476560501100410

Shakespeare-Finch, J., & Lurie-Beck, J. (2014). A meta-analytic clarification of the relationship between posttraumatic growth and symptoms of posttraumatic distress disorder. *Journal of Anxiety Disorders, 28*(2), 223–229. https://doi.org/10.1016/j.janxdis.2013.10.005

Shand, L. K., Cowlishaw, S., Brooker, J. E., Burney, S., & Ricciardelli, L. A. (2015). Correlates of post-traumatic stress symptoms and growth in cancer patients: A systematic review and meta-analysis. *Psycho-oncology, 24*(6), 624–634. https://doi.org/10.1002/pon.3719

Sheikh, A. I. (2004). Posttraumatic growth in the context of heart disease. *Journal of Clinical Psychology in Medical Settings, 11*(4), 265–273. https://doi.org/10.1023/B:JOCS.0000045346.76242.73

Siegel, K., & Schrimshaw, E. W. (2000). Perceiving benefits in adversity: Stress-related growth in women living with HIV/AIDS. *Social Science & Medicine, 51*(10), 1543–1554. https://doi.org/10.1016/S0277-9536(00)00144-1

Sommer, J. L., Mota, N., Edmondson, D., & El-Gabalawy, R. (2018). Comorbidity in illness-induced posttraumatic stress disorder versus posttraumatic stress disorder due to external events in a nationally representative study. *General Hospital Psychiatry, 53*, 88–94. https://doi.org/10.1016/j.genhosppsych.2018.02.004

Tedeschi, R. G., & Calhoun, L. G. (1996). The Posttraumatic Growth Inventory: Measuring the positive legacy of trauma. *Journal of Traumatic Stress, 9*(3), 455–471. https://doi.org/10.1007/BF02103658

Tedeschi, R. G., Shakespeare-Finch, J., Taku, K., & Calhoun, L. G. (2018). Posttraumatic Growth: Theory, Research, and Applications (1st ed.). Routledge. https://doi.org/10.4324/9781315527451

Thompson, S. C., & Janigian, A. S. (1988). Life schemes: A framework for understanding the search for meaning. *Journal of Social and Clinical Psychology, 7*(2–3), 260–280.

Tsai, J., Sippel, L. M., Mota, N., Southwick, S. M., & Pietrzak, R. H. (2016). Longitudinal course of posttraumatic growth among US military veterans: Results from the National Health and Resilience in Veterans Study. *Depression and Anxiety, 33*(1), 9–18. https://doi.org/10.1002/da.22371

Urry, H. L., Nitschke, J. B., Dolski, I., Jackson, D. C., Dalton, K. M., Mueller, C. J., Rosenkranz, M. A., Ryff, C. D., Singer, B. H., & Davidson, R. J. (2004). Making a life worth living: Neural Correlates of Well-Being. *Psychological Science, 15*(6), 367–372. https://doi.org/10.1111/j.0956-7976.2004.00686.x

van der Werff, S. J., Pannekoek, J. N., Stein, D. J., & van der Wee, N. J. (2013). Neuroimaging of resilience to stress: Current state of affairs. *Human Psychopharmacology, 28*(5), 529–532. https://doi.org/10.1002/hup.2336

Vilchinsky, N., Ginzburg, K., Fait, K., & Foa, E. B. (2017). Cardiac-disease-induced PTSD (CDI-PTSD): A systematic review. *Clinical Psychology Review, 55*, 92–106. https://doi.org/10.1016/j.cpr.2017.04.009

Wang, A. W.-T., Chang, C.-S., Chen, S.-T., Chen, D.-R., Fan, F., Carver, C. S., & Hsu, W.-Y. (2017a). Buffering and direct effect of posttraumatic growth in predicting distress following cancer. *Health Psychology, 36*(6), 549–559. https://doi.org/10.1037/hea0000490

Wang, Y., Wang, H., Wang, Z., Xie, H., Shi, J., & Zhao, X. (2017b). The process of posttraumatic growth in individuals with traumatic spinal cord injury in Mainland China: An interpretative phenomenological analysis. *Journal of Health Psychology, 22*(5), 637–649. https://doi.org/10.1177/1359105315610812

Webster, J. D., & Deng, X. C. (2015). Paths from trauma to intrapersonal strength: Worldview, posttraumatic growth, and wisdom. *Journal of Loss and Trauma, 20*(3), 253–266. https://doi.org/10.1080/15325024.2014.932207

Wei, C., Han, J., Zhang, Y., Hannak, W., Dai, Y., & Liu, Z. (2017). Affective emotion increases heart rate variability and activates left dorsolateral prefrontal cortex in post-traumatic growth. *Scientific Reports, 7*(1), 1–10. https://doi.org/10.1038/s41598-017-16890-5

Widows, M. R., Jacobsen, P. B., Booth-Jones, M., & Fields, K. K. (2005). Predictors of posttraumatic growth following bone marrow transplantation for cancer. *Health Psychology, 24*, 266–273.

Zeligman, M., Barden, S. M., & Hagedorn, W. B. (2016). Posttraumatic growth and HIV: A study on associations of stigma and social support. *Journal of Counseling & Development, 94*(2), 141–149. https://doi.org/10.1002/jcad.12071

Part III

Preface: Character Strengths and Health (Forgiveness, Hope, and Optimism)

Fuschia M. Sirois

Character strengths, or positive traits, is the second key area within positive psychology that shifts the focus from the subjective level to the individual level. In short, the focus moves from momentary experiences of well-being to more enduring tendencies and strengths that exemplify the best of human nature. Importantly, these positive qualities can be cultivated and learned, and accordingly can be targeted with positive psychology interventions to enhance these strengths and maximize their potential health benefits.

This third section of the handbook presents three key character strengths and their role in health-related outcomes and contexts, namely, forgiveness, hope, and optimism. Each of these character strengths have figured prominently as key explanatory factors within the health domain over the past two decades. As evidence on their general benefits for health has continued to amass, research has turned to understanding the potential benefits of these strengths for specific populations and health outcomes, as well considering developmental perspectives. The chapters included in this section provide new perspectives on how these character strengths relate to a broad array of health topics including health behaviours, health states, and adjustment to chronic health conditions.

Chapter 11 provides a comprehensive overview of how forgiveness of self and forgiveness of others are linked to a range of key health outcomes. In reviewing different conceptualizations of forgiveness, Toussaint and colleagues suggest multiple routes through which forgiveness may benefit health. Their systematic review of 73 studies provides compelling evidence that forgiveness, in whichever form it takes, has clear and robust linkages to physical health, and self-rated health in particular.

Chapters 12 and 13 examine how hope and hopefulness can have positive impacts on health outcomes including health promotion, symptom management, health behaviours, and immune functioning. Hope is a character strength that holds particular importance during times of crisis and uncertainty as it helps individuals focus not only on their goals, but also on the pathways towards attaining these goals despite challenging circumstances. In Chap. 12, Altier and Hirsch argue that hopefulness is a valuable internal resource for people dealing with chronic and life-threatening health conditions as it helps to reduce stress and pain, and supports treatment adherence and adaptive coping with illness-related challenges. Chapter 12 reviews the evidence supporting this view of hope and further outlines how both hope-focused and general positive psychological interventions may be effective for fostering hope in patients with chronic health conditions.

In Chap. 13, Scioli takes a deep dive into the different ways in which hope has been conceptualized and measured, and the implications of these diverse views for understanding how hope relates to health outcomes across diverse populations. This comprehensive review of the research highlights the limitations of certain models for understanding hope in medical populations, and notes the conceptual challenges that need to be overcome to better understand the hope–health dynamic. To this end, Scioli proposes a new science-based model of hope–health interactions that provides insights into the multiple levels and pathways through which hope may exert its positive effects on health.

Chapter 14 concludes this section on character strengths by examining the role of dispositional optimism in health and well-being. Specifically, Wrosch and colleagues highlight how optimism contributes to the self-regulation of goals by providing positive expectations that can help individuals cope with stressful challenges and goal constraints and thus reduce physiological reactivity to stress. The enhanced self-regulation capabilities linked to optimism can also support the practice of health-promoting behaviours, a key pathway for maintaining and improving health. Importantly, they highlight the potential changing nature of optimism and that adopting a lifespan developmental approach is therefore critical for gaining a more nuanced view of the benefits of optimism for health.

11

Forgiveness and Physical Health: A Review of Theory and Evidence

Loren L. Toussaint, Jon R. Webb, Jameson K. Hirsch, Niko Kohls, Martin Offenbaecher, Jessie Dezutter, Quang Anh Nguyen, Miguel A. Vallejo, and Fuschia M. Sirois

This chapter will review the concepts of forgiveness of others and self-forgiveness and consider theoretical and empirical connections between these two constructs and physical health. An important starting place in any discussion of forgiveness is to be clear how the constructs are being conceptualized. Therefore, we will begin by considering how both forgiveness of others and self-forgiveness are defined. Notably, forgiveness of others and self-forgiveness have long and storied traditions in religion and philosophy but a much shorter existence in the field of psychology. Once defined, it is important to examine

L. L. Toussaint (✉) • Q. A. Nguyen
Department of Psychology, Luther College, Decorah, IA, USA
e-mail: tousl001@luther.edu

J. R. Webb
Department of Community, Family, and Addiction Sciences, Texas Tech University, Lubbock, TX, USA

J. K. Hirsch
Department of Psychiatry and Behavioral Sciences, East Tennessee State University, Johnson City, TN, USA

N. Kohls
Faculty of Natural Sciences and Health, Coburg University of Applied Sciences, Coburg, Germany

F. M. Sirois (ed.), *The Palgrave Handbook of Positive Psychology and Health*,
https://doi.org/10.1007/978-3-031-89095-6_11

the reasons why forgiveness of others and self-forgiveness might be related to physical health. Numerous theories support mind–body connections in modern-day psychology, but two key and relatively recent models outline the theoretical propositions supporting connections between forgiveness of others, self-forgiveness, and physical health. This chapter will then discuss the empirical literature supporting these models and offer a qualitative review of research examining forgiveness of others and self-forgiveness and their relationships to physical health in student, community, and patient populations. The chapter will conclude with a summary and general conclusion, followed by a discussion of limitations, and an agenda for future research.

Definitions

Forgiveness of Others

Peterson and Seligman (2004) situate forgiveness of others in the category of temperance virtues. As a member of the family of temperance virtues, forgiveness protects individuals from excess—specifically excess hate. Forgiveness, like other temperance virtues, is notable as it is most clearly evidenced in what an individual refrains from doing (Peterson & Seligman, 2004). In short, forgiveness requires not only the absence of negative thoughts, feelings, and motivations directed at an offender, as suggested by Peterson and Seligman (2004), but also many would agree that the void left by reduced negative thoughts, feelings, and motivations ought to be replaced by positive thoughts, feelings, and motivations for complete forgiveness to occur (McCullough et al., 1997). For example, one cannot only fail to hate one's spouse for a wrongdoing but hopefully will return to having loving and benevolent

M. Offenbaecher
Institute of Ecomedicine, Paracelsus Medical University, Salzburg, Austria

Gasteiner Heilstollen Clinic, Bad Gastein, Austria

J. Dezutter
School Psychology and Development in Context, KU Leuven, Leuven, Belgium

M. A. Vallejo
Department of Clinical Psychology, National Distance Education University, Madrid, Spain

F. M. Sirois
Department of Psychology, Durham University, Durham, UK

thoughts, feelings, and motives toward the spousal offender. Of course, in some situations perhaps with strangers, reductions of the negative thoughts, feelings, and motivations would be sufficient.

Motivational and emotional changes in forgiveness are closely linked (Exline et al., 2003). Often a decision to forgive either precedes or follows motivational and emotional changes. The decision to forgive is important to the process of forgiving an offender, but as forgiveness of others is related to physical health, it is likely the emotional component of the process that is most relevant (Worthington et al., 2007). Hence, it is important to consider whether forgiveness is defined as "emotional forgiveness" or "decisional forgiveness" (Worthington et al., 2007) when examining its association with physical health.

A final note on forgiveness of others regards the importance of understanding what forgiveness is and is not (Luskin, 2002). Forgiveness of others does not mean that the victim reconciles with the offender. Reconciliation is a social phenomenon whereby a broken relationship is restored and two parties may again regain each other's trust to the extent that they desire to be in one another's company. Often victims should not reconcile with offenders, and this is especially the case in situations of abuse or neglect. But, not reconciling does not prevent individuals from forgiving their offender. Forgiveness of others also does not mean that the victim forgoes a quest for justice (Luskin, 2002). Justice is served through a community, state, or national legal system and is handed down from judges in positions of authority. Victims do not have to give up seeking justice to forgive (Worthington, 2009). Justice and forgiveness exist on independent continuums. Justice may support the forgiveness process, especially if it ensure some measure of safety, but it is not required (Toussaint & Waldman, 2017). While forgiveness is certainly not to be confused with reconciliation or justice, what exactly it is remains to be defined. In short, forgiveness is a transformation, intraindividual in nature, whereby an individual releases or lets go of negative thoughts, feelings, and motivations directed at an offender and replaces them with positive, love-based thoughts, feelings, and motivations. It is a personal choice, and an expression of self-love and power.

Self-Forgiveness

Self-forgiveness can in many ways be similarly defined, like forgiveness of others, as the removal of negative and replacement with positive thoughts, feelings, and motivations directed at oneself (Hall & Fincham, 2005; Toussaint et al., 2014; Worthington, 2013; Worthington & Langberg, 2012). The main difference between forgiveness of others and self-forgiveness is that the offender is another person(s) in forgiveness of others and oneself in self-forgiveness. This is a distinction that is both obvious at some level and exceedingly important and critical at another level. Perhaps most importantly, self-forgiveness is something that the self as offender engages in as a means of dealing with self-condemnation (Worthington, 2013). Self-condemnation may be the result of guilt, shame, self-blame, or self-loathing resulting from a perceived offensive act that has hurt another or oneself. As both the offender and the granter of self-forgiveness, an individual must be primarily tasked with understanding the morality of the circumstance. Offering oneself "cheap grace" or easy self-forgiveness is merely an engagement in narcissistic thinking or feeding an overly inflated ego or sense of self-esteem (Fisher & Exline, 2010; Murphy, 2003; Wohl & Thompson, 2011). The moral weight of the decision to forgive oneself must only be made in light of the significance of the wrongdoing and the desire to want to not only feel better but be a better person (Woodyatt et al., 2017).

Self-forgiveness entails recognizing one's own wrongdoing, accepting it as such, attempting to make amends, and reconciliation and acceptance of oneself in light of a commitment to change (Webb et al., 2016). Self-forgiveness may indeed result in changed thoughts, feelings, and motivations directed toward oneself after a wrongdoing, but the emotions of self-condemnation are distinctly different from those aroused by being hurt by someone else. In the case of self-forgiveness the individual must confront guilt, shame, self-blame and the like directed toward oneself. In the case of being hurt by another individual, one must contend with anger, hatred, resentment, and revenge directed toward another. Furthermore, the emotions of forgiveness of others and self-forgiveness are elicited via different routes. For instance, in the case of anger and hatred toward another person this emotional reaction may be most salient and impactful when reminded of or when actually interacting personally with the offender. Quite often the victim may not be reminded of or interact with the offender all that often resulting in fewer intensely emotional experiences. Contrast this with the emotions of self-forgiveness. Because in self-forgiveness the offender is oneself, the experiences of guilt, self-blame, and self-loathing may be a virtual constant in one's life (Worthington, 2013).

Finally, the distinction between self-forgiveness and self-compassion is important to make. Self-compassion involves taking a kind, connected, and mindful stance toward oneself in instances of difficulty and failure (Neff, 2003). In short, self-compassion is often referred to as treating yourself with gentleness and understanding, the way you might treat a good friend who is suffering or struggling. Self-compassion might be a healthy response to all too common feelings of self-criticism or overly perfectionistic tendencies (Ferrari et al., 2018); however, self-compassion need not require a prior wrongdoing. Self-forgiveness does. Self-compassion can be a productive and healthy attitude to take after a rough day when your performance wasn't what you had hoped it would be and you are starting to get down on yourself, but no objective harm was done. Self-forgiveness is called for when, for example, at the end of the day one realizes that the exceptionally rude behavior that was exhibited in dealing with one's coworkers caused them great distress and offense. Self-compassion might help a person cope with a rough day, whereas, self-forgiveness might help a person cope with wrongful actions committed during a rough day.

Conceptual Models of Forgiveness and Health

Two separate models have been proposed to draw the theoretical and empirical connections between forgiveness of others and self-forgiveness with physical health (Toussaint et al., 2017; Worthington, 2003; Worthington & Scherer, 2004). In both cases, the models are built on the theory of stress and coping developed by Lazarus and his colleagues (Lazarus & Folkman, 1984). In Lazarus' theory, for an event to be consider stressful it must be appraised as such. Primary appraisals determine whether an event is benign, threatening, or challenging. Secondary appraisals evaluate the coping resources that are available, and in turn, those coping resources are deployed to manage the stressful event. Coping responses can be categorized at the broadest level as being of one of two types. Coping can be problem-focused—aimed directly at reducing the impact of or eliminating the sources of the stressful event. Alternatively, coping can be emotion-focused—aimed at managing the emotional upset and distress in response to the stressful event.

According to Lazarus' theory of stress, events that are appraised as harmful or threatening result in the activation of several coping mechanisms meant to contend with the stressor. The attempt to cope with stressful events involves emotional, behavioral, and physiological sequalae, and hence, ineffective coping, prolonged chronic demands on coping resources, or dramatically intense and traumatic events have the potential for reducing mental and physical health and well-being and impairing health-related quality of life, and even increasing the likelihood of untimely death. Knowing this, it remains imperative to the field to identify efficacious coping resources that assist individuals in coping with stressful events.

Forgiveness of others and self-forgiveness have both been characterized as emotion-focused coping responses that are well-suited to ameliorate stress arising from interpersonal conflict, family disharmony, and social, community, national, and international strife. Following an intrapersonal or interpersonal transgression it is entirely possible, and in fact, probable that many individuals will engage in forms of coping that do not include forgiveness. For instance, when being hurt by another a victim might immediately seek revenge. Conversely, as the perpetrator of an offense, an individual might blame the victim or deny wrongdoing. While these responses might be common and may sometimes reduce stress, they come with additional negative social side effects. The stress-and-coping models of forgiveness of others and self-forgiveness both contend that forgiveness-based coping may offer a healthy and productive response.

According to the stress-and-coping theory of forgiveness of others (Worthington, 2003; Worthington & Scherer, 2004), a transgression results in unforgiveness. Unforgiveness arises following an appraisal of the situation that deems the event as harmful or threatening. Worthington has deemed this appraisal as an evaluation of the "injustice-gap" (Worthington & Scherer, 2004). The injustice gap is the difference between what happened and what an individual wanted to happen. As the injustice-gap widens so too does the experience of unforgiveness and its associated stressful consequences. Although a variety of different responses to an appraised injustice-gap may indeed result in less stress and better health and well-being, it is hypothesized that forgiveness might be an ideally suited coping response in these situations. It is proposed that forgiveness might act through both direct and indirect mechanisms to achieve its benefits. Direct mechanisms involve the activation or modulation of neurological, neuro-endocrine, and immune system responses to stress, as well as health-promoting stimulation of motivational and emotional systems. Indirect mechanisms are thought to be through the reduction of unhealthy personality traits such as hostility and neuroticism, and improvements in marital relations, social skills, and social support.

In the case of the stress-and-coping theory of self-forgiveness (Toussaint et al., 2017), the process again begins with a transgression. But in the case of self-forgiveness, it is important to remember that the transgressor, who is oneself, may commit a transgression against oneself or others. Falling short of one's ideals, failing to follow through on a commitment to self-improvement, or simply underperforming might be good examples of intrapersonal transgressions, whereas, an insult, rude gesture, or ignoring a friend could be interpersonal transgressions. In either case, an individual appraises their own behavior as offensive and this becomes intrapersonally stressful. Again, the notion of injustice gap might apply here, as self-forgiveness is called for when one recognizes that one's thoughts, behaviors, or feelings are incongruent with how one would wish them to be—a state of cognitive dissonance. The plethora of thoughts and feelings associated with this injustice gap appraisal has been termed "self-condemnation" and consists of guilt, shame, anger, regret, disappointment, and despair all directed toward oneself. This self-condemnation is quite similar to the notion of unforgiveness and in itself is quite stressful (Griffin et al., 2015; McConnell, 2015). The stress of self-condemnation might act to impair health and well-being through direct and indirect mechanisms. Direct connections might involve the activation of similar neurological, neuro-endocrine, immune, and motivational systems to those involved in connections between forgiveness of others and health. Indirect mechanisms might well involve reductions in self-blame, hopelessness, and pessimism and enhancements in hopefulness, health behavior, and social support.

In regards to both forgiveness of others and self-forgiveness and relations with physical health, key propositions can be garnered from both of the stress-and-coping theories. First, a perceived injustice-gap resulting in unforgiveness toward others or condemnation of oneself can directly and negatively impact physical health and well-being. Second, both forgiveness of others and self-forgiveness can be directly related to physical health and well-being. Third, forgiveness of others could mediate and/or moderate the association of unforgiveness with poorer physical health. Fourth, self-forgiveness could mediate and/or moderate the association of self-condemnation with poorer physical health. To highlight where there is support for these propositions, and identify where further work might need to be done, we conducted a literature review on forgiveness and health.

Literature Review of Forgiveness and Health

Psychological and medical literatures were searched on November 23, 2020, using title, keyword, and abstract searches of the databases PsycINFO, PubMed, and Google Scholar. PsycINFO was searched with the term, "forg*v* and physical health," PubMed was searched with "forgiv* and physical health" (searching "forgav* and physical health" resulted in zero articles), and Google

Scholar was searched with the term "forgiveness and physical health." No publication-year restrictions were specified. Inclusion criteria were: (a) a measure of forgiveness, and (b) a measure of physical health. Exclusion criteria were: (a) experiments or trials that involved eclectic interventions including forgiveness with, for example, gratitude or mindfulness; and (b) studies whose exclusive focus was on outcomes such as mental health, happiness, suicide, global non-health-related quality of life, neurological or physiological parameters or biomarkers, or combined mental and physical health composites.

The PsycINFO search turned up 124 articles, and the PubMed search added another 45 articles. Google Scholar added no non-redundant articles. The reference sections of recent reviews (Cheadle & Toussaint, 2015; Davis et al., 2015) and meta-analyses were examined (Lee & Enright, 2019; Rasmussen et al., 2019). Twenty-three non-redundant articles were added. Thus, the total number of articles was 192. The titles, keywords, and abstracts of these articles were reviewed by the first author for relevance and 78 articles were retained. After reviewing the text of the 78 articles, 5 articles were eliminated because they did not meet inclusion/exclusion criteria. Although summary statistics for the review will include all 73 studies spanning 2000 to 2020, a couple of examples will be reviewed to highlight more current work. A summary of the results are provided in Table 11.1.

Table 11.1 Literature review summary of research on forgiveness and health

Content area of review	*N* (%) of studies	*N* (%) evidence of benefit
Total studies	73 (100%)	55 (75%)
Forgiveness		
Forgiveness of others	57 (78%)	41 (72%)
Self-forgiveness	34 (47%)	24 (71%)
Other forgiveness dimensions	23 (32%)	19 (83%)
Health		
Self-rated health	19 (26%)	16 (84%)
Health-related quality of life	25 (34%)	14 (56%)
Symptoms	21 (28%)	14 (67%)
Other (e.g., BMI, glucose)	22 (30%)	14 (64%)
Sample characteristics		
Undergraduate	14 (19%)	9 (64%)
Community	42 (58%)	33 (79%)
Patient	13 (18%)	6 (46%)
Mixed/other sample	4 (5%)	2 (50%)
Design		
Cross-sectional	61 (84%)	40 (66%)
Longitudinal	8 (11%)	7 (88%)
Experimental/intervention	4 (5%)	3 (75%)

Note. Content areas are not mutually exclusive

Dimensions of Forgiveness

Forgiveness of Others

The study of forgiveness of others began earlier than the study of other dimensions of forgiveness, and as such, the literature is more developed here. Seventy-eight percent (n = 57) of studies examining forgiveness and health have included a measure of forgiveness of others. Of the studies examining forgiveness of others, 72 percent (n = 41) have demonstrated at least one beneficial connection between forgiveness of others and some physical health outcome. A nice example of this type of study is the work of Derdaele et al. (2019). In this study, 329 elderly residents of nursing homes in the Flanders region of Belgium were given assessments of forgiveness of others, self-reported health, mental health, and well-being. Results showed that forgiveness of others had a direct association with self-reported physical health, but associations with mental health and well-being were indirect and acted through mechanisms of integrity and despair—two key psychosocial processes proposed by Erik Erikson (Erikson, 1982).

Another example of work examining forgiveness of others and health outcomes is the research conducted by Long et al. (2020b). In this study of over 50,000 female nurses assessed over a seven-year time span, forgiveness of others was examined to determine if it was associated with a number of physical health outcomes including: all-cause mortality, type 2 diabetes, stroke, heart diseases, cancer, overweight/obesity, and total number of physical health problems. Mental health and health behavior outcomes were also included in this study. Findings revealed that forgiveness of others was beneficially associated with a number of mental health and health behavior outcomes, but no robust associations were found between forgiveness of others and physical health outcomes.

Self-Forgiveness

Forty-seven percent (n = 34) of studies of forgiveness and health included a measure of self-forgiveness. Of these studies, 71 percent showed an association between self-forgiveness and at least one physical health outcome. A nice illustration of this type of study comes from work done in Chengdu city, Sichuan province, China (Ye et al., 2019). In this study, 457 hemodialysis patients completed measures of self-forgiveness (forgiveness of others and forgiveness of situations were also included) and measures of physical symptoms and kidney-disease-related quality of life. Self-forgiveness, as well as the other dimensions of forgiveness, was inversely related with physical symptoms and positively related to kidney-disease-related quality of life.

Another example of research examining connections between self-forgiveness and physical health is the work of Long et al. (2020a). In this study, over 50,000 female nurses followed for eight years (same dataset as Long et al., 2020b) were assessed on self-forgiveness, divine forgiveness, and several health outcomes. Results showed that neither self-forgiveness nor divine forgiveness showed consistent associations with physical health outcomes, but associations with mental health outcomes were much more consistent.

Other Forgiveness Dimensions

Thirty-two percent of studies (n = 23) of forgiveness and health included a measure of forgiveness that was not forgiveness of others and self-forgiveness. Of these studies, 83 percent (n = 19) showed at least one beneficial association between these other dimensions of forgiveness and physical health outcomes. In 48 percent of these studies (n = 11), the other dimension that was assessed was feeling forgiven by God. In 22 percent of these studies (n = 5), the other dimension assessed was forgiveness of a situation. Although these other dimensions of forgiveness are important to understand, rarely are they the sole focus of study. An interesting and enlightening exception is the work done by Krause and Ironson (2017). In this study of nearly 2500 US adults of all ages, the investigators found that feeling forgiven by God was associated with a more favorable waist–hip ratio for those individuals that were highly committed to their religion. For those individuals with less religious commitment, however, the association was reversed, showing that the more an individual felt forgiven by God, the more unfavorable their waist–hip ratio was. The authors of this study offered some interesting observations on this pattern of findings and suggested that low religious commitment may reflect poor human–divine relationship quality and a sense of unearned divine forgiveness that may prompt stress or other unhealthy obesogenic behaviors. Although this is an interesting possibility, the ability of theories of forgiveness to explain a finding of this nature is quite limited, and perhaps this is why the focus of few studies is on feeling forgiven by God or forgiveness of situations. In both cases, theory is being outpaced by measurement and design.

Physical Health

Self-Reported Health

Self-reported health, often assessed using a single item, is one of the most common methods of assessing one's perceptions of health status, and it has been shown to be an important and independent predictor of objective physical health outcomes (Jylhä, 2009). Not surprisingly then, the investigation of forgiveness and physical health relies heavily on self-reported health with 26 percent of forgiveness and health studies using this assessment. Of those studies, 84 percent (n =16) showed at least one beneficial association between some dimension of forgiveness and self-reported physical health. No doubt, the use of self-reported physical health will continue to be a staple in studies seeking to understand forgiveness–health connections because of its brevity and validity.

Health-Related Quality of Life

Another common means of assessing physical health is through measures of health-related quality of life. These are notably different from broader measures of quality of life that often include measures of educational attainment, economic indicators, and family and social well-being. Measures of health-related quality of life, such as the SF-36 (Ware & Sherbourne, 1992), include dimensions such as: (a) limitations in physical functioning, (b) physical health-related social limitations, (c) physical health-related interference with important roles held by an individual, (d) pain, (e) mental health, (f) interference with important roles resulting from health-related emotional problems, (g) energy and fatigue, and (h) global health perceptions. Health-related quality of life is a common means of measurement in studies examining forgiveness and health and represents 34 percent of the studies (n = 25). Of those studies, 56 percent (n = 14) showed at least one beneficial association between some dimension of forgiveness and a dimension of health-related quality of life.

Physical Health Symptoms

Physical health symptoms include such things as a headache, neck ache, runny or stuffy nose, irritated eyes, or nagging cough. It could also include any symptom that is specifically related to a particular chronic illness or disease category, for instance, tingling in extremities, unusual taste in one's mouth, or loss of smell or other senses. In the studies included in our review most studies included measures of broad symptoms, but a couple studies did include measures of specific disease symptoms such as fibromyalgia or HIV. Twenty-eight percent of studies (n = 21) of forgiveness and health included a measure of physical symptoms. Of these studies, 67 percent (n = 14) showed at least one beneficial association between some dimension of forgiveness and physical health symptoms.

Other Physical Health Measures

In addition to the self-rated health, health-related quality of life, and physical health symptom measures used in the majority of the studies of forgiveness and health, other chronic illness and disease specific measures were included in a few studies. These measures included such things as specific infection symptoms, counts of physical health conditions (e.g., heart disease, diabetes, etc.), cortisol, glucose tolerance, and body mass index. Although this review is not intended to encompass biomarkers of health, some studies included both measures of physical health and biomarkers. Thirty percent of studies (n = 22) of forgiveness and health included a measure of physical health other than self-reported health, health-related quality of life, or physical symptoms. Of these studies, 64 percent (n = 14) showed at least one beneficial association between forgiveness and other dimensions of physical health.

Sample Characteristics

The characteristics of the samples used in the study of the relationship between forgiveness and physical health have been diverse. Generally speaking, the samples can be broken down into four categories. Community samples represent over half of the studies accounting for 58 percent (n = 42). Surprisingly, undergraduate samples amount to just 19 percent (n = 14) of the total and an almost equal amount are patient samples with 18 percent of the total (n = 13). Mixed or other (e.g., high school) samples represent only 5 percent (n = 4) of the total. Evidence of beneficial associations between forgiveness and physical health have been most consistently found in community samples (79%, n = 33), followed by samples of undergraduates (64%, n = 9), and then mixed/other samples (50%, n = 2) and patient samples (46%, n = 6). Within community samples there has been wide variability in the types of participants. Some include adults of all ages, other examine only elderly, while others are exclusive to females nurses, Seventh-Day Adventists, male prisoners, Iraqi refugees, Chilean elders, and religious adherents of five different world religions. Patients samples range from individuals with HIV, traumatic brain injury, spinal cord injury, stroke, breast cancer, chronic pain, heart failure, arthritis, COPD, and diabetes. There is also a wide range of sample sizes. Community samples range in size from N = 20 to N =54,703 with an average sample size of 2500, but a median sample size of 340. Undergraduate samples range in size from N = 39 to N = 721 with an average sample size of 291, but a median sample size of 227. Patient samples range in size from N = 11 to N = 678 with an average sample size of 212, but a median sample size of 150. Mixed/other samples range in size from N = 36 to N = 541 with an average sample size of 291, but a median sample size of 293. In looking at the samples and the dispersion of the distributions with standard deviations within each content category ranging from almost 200 to nearly 9000, two things are quite clear. One, the sample size distributions are most often positively skewed. Two, community samples tend to be similar in size to mixed/other samples, but tend to be larger than undergraduate, and especially patient samples.

Research Design

The designs employed to examine connections between forgiveness and physical health fall into three different categories. Most studies are cross-sectional in nature (84%, n = 61), some are longitudinal (11%, n = 8), and only a handful are experimental/interventional (5%, n = 4). Within each of these categories of design, there are several studies showing at least one beneficial connection between forgiveness and physical health. Evidence of beneficial associations between forgiveness and physical health has been found in cross-sectional (66%, n = 40), longitudinal (88%, n = 7), and experimental/interventional (75%, n = 3) studies.

What This Research Tells Us About Forgiveness and Health

Just 30 years ago the study of forgiveness in scientific disciplines was virtually unheard of, and barely 20 years ago some of the first studies examining connections between forgiveness and physical health started to emerge. In just two decades there has been consistent growth in interest in the scientific study of forgiveness in general and in particular the intersection between forgiveness and physical health. This could be for several reasons such as increased divisiveness both at national and global levels, growing levels of individual stress and difficulties coping, increasing levels of loneliness, and the emergence of moral outrage and cancel culture in social media environments. Whatever the driver of this interest, we now have over 70 scientific investigations of forgiveness and physical health in a variety of samples.

A couple of broad conclusions can be gleaned from this body of work. First, considering all of the studies reviewed herein, there are a majority (75%) that find some evidence of a healthy connection between forgiveness and physical health. Second, though the proportion of studies examining forgiveness of others remains the dominant focus, the evidence of an important health connection appears to be equally in favor of all types of forgiveness including forgiveness of others, self-forgiveness, and other forms of forgiveness such as feeling forgiven by God and forgiveness of situations. Third, studies of forgiveness and physical health have been evenly spread across multiple physical health outcomes. Evidence weighs more heavily in favor of a beneficial association between forgiveness and self-rated health than it does in other categories, but that should not diminish the observations that show that forgiveness is beneficially related to health-related quality of life and physical symptoms as these are important aspects of healthy and chronically ill persons' lives. And, a subset of studies do show that forgiveness is related to objective measures of physical health including, for example, body mass index.

Finally, it is clear that the most common type of study is the cross-sectional study done in a community sample. Given the convenience of undergraduate samples, it is surprising that a larger number of studies are not based on those participants. But, it may also prompt one to ask if there is some type of implicit bias against these types of studies in college and university settings. There could be some hesitancy on the part of faculty and students to conduct or participate in studies of forgiveness. Perhaps this might arise out of concern that forgiveness is a religious and possibly taboo topic (Monahan et al., 2020). If this were found to be so, then perhaps we should consider whether studies that have been done in college students might be influenced by selection bias. Might this also be true in medical settings? It is a bit surprising that there are not more studies of forgiveness and health in patient samples. Longitudinal studies and experimental/interventional studies are only a small fraction of the studies in this area, but until stronger support from federal funding agencies or private foundations becomes available, this might continue to be the case.

Caveats and Limitations

There are several areas of limitation in this research literature including sample types and size, measurement, and theoretical and empirical modeling. While it is refreshing to see a literature dominated by community samples, it could also be of some concern. Community samples provide a rich array of diverse participants and allow for the investigation of factors such as age, race, education, and income and offer insights often not available in other samples. However, in this particular instance where we have so many cross-sectional studies, the focus on community samples may become a hindrance to progress. This might be because in order to utilize community-based samples and do longitudinal designs there is considerable labor and cost. As in most things, there are trade-offs. Community samples offer diversity but college student samples offer the necessary convenience and affordability to do longitudinal work.

Given that both community and patient samples involve greater logistics and potentially greater cost, the utility of college student samples should not be overlooked. Of course, it would be ideal to have community and patient samples that use longitudinal or experimental/interventional designs, but these are a distinct minority of the studies at the moment. It would be all too easy to simply recommend that studies in this area focus on more community or patient longitudinal studies, but the crucial question is how feasible is that? At the moment it might be possible for a few well-funded investigators, but until it is more widely manageable, it might be worthwhile to prioritize understanding the causal connections in forgiveness and physical health and in so doing utilize the most readily available resources—college students—for accomplishing that task. Of course there are limits to what can be examined in college student samples largely because individuals of this age group tend to be quite physically robust and healthy and physical health conditions take more than a couple of years to change or develop. At the moment, it would appear that prudent advice would be to focus more on understanding the causal relationships between forgiveness and health, but inasmuch as it is possible, continue to use community and patient samples. Investigators would be wise to also turn attention to gathering samples that are not WEIRD (Henrich et al., 2010), that is, those that are not from populations that are white, educated, industrialized, rich, and democratic.

Measurement concerns exist within this literature. Early on in the development of this area, a couple of key measures were developed. The Brief Multidimensional Measure of Religiousness and Spirituality (BMMRS) (Idler et al., 2003) forgiveness subscale is a commonly used measure. So too are the Trait Forgiveness Scale (Berry et al., 2005), Transgression-Related Interpersonal Motivations Inventory (TRIM) (McCullough et al., 2006), and the Heartland Forgiveness Scale (HFS) (Thompson et al., 2005). The TFS and HFS are both dispositional measures and in terms of examining connections to health are good choices. The TRIM is an event- or person-specific measure that focuses feelings of forgiveness on a single wrongdoing, and hence, depending on the timing and context of this event is may or may not still have effects that would impact on physical health. The TRIM might also better be thought of as a measure of "unforgiveness" instead of forgiveness as it has subscales that focus on revenge, avoidance, and benevolence (reverse coded) motivations. Much discussion has focused on how forgiveness and unforgiveness are independent constructs (Wade & Worthington, 2003; Worthington & Wade, 1999) and one should not be mistaken for the other.

Last, the BMMRS measure is the most popular measure by far for physical health-related studies. The BMMRS is a very brief three-item scale that is reliable and valid. But due to its brevity, the comprehensiveness with which it covers the construct is limited. Add to this that the BMMRS actually has single-item measures of self-forgiveness, forgiveness of others, and feeling forgiven by God. Given the distinctiveness of these different types of forgiveness and the different psychology and theology that underlies them (Enright, 1996; McConnell & Dixon, 2012), it would be wise to use these as separate indicators. Often however these three items are combined to form an overall forgiveness scale. The motivation in doing so, of course, is that the three items can form a scale that offers the ability to evaluate reliability and reduce measurement error, but the total construct might be so diverse as to call into question what such a score might actually mean.

Although there are certainly other limiting factors present in this literature, the last one that will be discussed here is the theoretical and empirical modeling that has been accomplished in this area. Although stress-and-coping theories of forgiveness of others (Worthington, 2003; Worthington & Scherer, 2004) and self-forgiveness (Toussaint et al., 2017) have been offered and, in both cases, offer sound theoretical predictions and explanations for how forgiveness might relate to physical health, the number of studies that make specific tests of these models remains quite low. As the stress-and-coping models of forgiveness of others and self-forgiveness are reviewed above, it should be noted that there are a number of useful predictions about how forgiveness might serve as a mediator or moderator of relationships between unforgiveness and other negative emotions, thoughts, and motivations and physical health, as well as, a number of predictions for how other psychosocial variables might be involved in mediating or moderating the association between forgiveness and physical health. Unfortunately, at present, most studies continue to examine forgiveness main effects and while some studies do possess greater theoretical and empirical model elaboration these are quite varied in nature and in the types and number of constructs involved. Additional theoretical elaboration might be useful to help guide this work, but so too would empirical work that maps statistical models more closely onto proposed theories.

Research Agenda

Given the findings of this review and the limitations of this literature, we end this chapter with some suggestions for future research examining the connections between forgiveness and physical health. Continued time and attention should be given to developing and refining our theoretical understanding of how forgiveness is related to physical health. Stress-and-coping theories suggest that forgiveness is key in assuaging the effects of stress, which arise from unforgiveness, on physical health. Lazarus and his colleagues long ago established that stress, at its core, is a negative emotional experience (Lazarus, 1999). This is key to the role of stress in physical health. Negative emotions, through several psychoneuroimmunological pathways, impact normal biological functioning which when experienced chronically result in deterioration of physical health and the development of chronic illnesses and diseases (McEwen, 2005; McEwen et al., 2004). Knowing this, it would be important for forgiveness studies to focus on the ability of forgiveness to douse negative emotional flare-ups and replace these with emotional reactions that either have limited untoward effects or even evoke the healing relaxation response. Regrettably, at the present moment, we know more about how the broad disposition of forgiveness is related to physical health than we do about how emotional forgiveness is involved. Importantly, this isn't for lack of measurement. The emotional forgiveness scale has been available for use for years

(Worthington et al., 2007), but seems to get less traction in studies focusing on health than it does in other non-health-related studies (Mróz et al., 2020).

Stress-and-coping theories are not the only theories that are relevant to the question of forgiveness and health connections. Developmental theories such as Erik Erikson's psychosocial stages of development (Erikson, 1982), Martin Seligman's theory of learned helplessness (Seligman, 1972), Julian Rotter's theory of locus of control (Rotter, 1966), Aton Antonevsky's theory of sense of coherence (Antonovsky, 1979) could all be applied to forgiveness of oneself and others and help in predicting and explaining why forgiveness might be related to physical health outcomes. Forgiveness may well be a means of facilitating integrity, as opposed to despair, as individuals age. Forgiveness might help individuals reorient or reframe seemingly uncontrollable circumstances. Or, perhaps it could help individuals, especially those experiencing traumatic events, make sense and regain focus and control over one's life. With additional theoretical work and guidance, the meaning and utility of forthcoming data will be enhanced and we will be better able to understand the how, when, why, and where of the association between forgiveness and health.

In the name of comprehensiveness studies often measure multiple dimensions of forgiveness, but we might recommend that this practice be eschewed in favor of studies that focus more specifically on one particular type of forgiveness. We say this because often studies are not designed to meaningfully compare and contrast forgiveness of others and self-forgiveness and their predictors, correlates, and outcomes against each other. Rather, forgiveness of others and self-forgiveness are commonly entered simultaneously into the same analytic model. This removes considerable covariance between the two constructs and makes it difficult to then examine their relationship with physical health outcomes because of limited unique variance.

Furthermore, when forgiveness of others and self-forgiveness are simultaneously tested, it is rare to see differing moderators/mediators included in the study and in analytical models that preferentially act on one or the other forgiveness dimension. That is, variables such as self-blame and guilt would be important in the self-forgiveness equation, but variables such as hostility, empathy, and rumination might be more relevant to forgiveness of others, but too often only one set of additional psychosocial variables is available for analysis. Including both forgiveness of others and self-forgiveness in the same study and analytic model then might also require inclusion of separate sets of unique and appropriate mediators/moderators, and as such, the comprehensive structural model that might be required becomes potentially untenable from an analytic and interpretive stand point. It might be more effective to focus exclusively on forgiveness of others and its associated mediators/

moderators, and in a separate study, similarly focus exclusively on self-forgiveness and associated necessary variables for inclusion. All too often forgiveness of others and self-forgiveness are used in the same breath and it is implicitly assumed that they are merely two different shades of the same overall construct with similar predictors and mediators/moderators. This is not the case. Forgiveness of others and self-forgiveness are two different constructs with considerably different antecedents, processes, and outcomes.

Our final suggestion again relates to how we conceptualize and design our studies of forgiveness and physical health. Though a number of studies contain both mental and physical health outcomes, few examine potential indirect effects of forgiveness on physical health through mental health. Most often studies simply use mental and physical health as parallel outcomes predicted by forgiveness. While this is a useful approach and certainly informs us of the connections between forgiveness and mental and physical health, it stops short of modeling potentially more sophisticated and meaningful relationships among these variables. For instance, it may be that forgiveness has its effects on cardiovascular health through its impact on depression. Studies show that forgiveness training has a beneficial impact on depressive symptoms (Wade et al., 2014), but to our knowledge, no studies have examined the impact of forgiveness on cardiovascular health that results from its beneficial impact on depression. Likewise, forgiveness may act in a serial mediation fashion mediating the effects of interpersonal stress on depression, hope, anxiety, etc. whose collective effects are then transmitted to physical health (stress → forgiveness → depression/hope/anxiety → physical health). Further still, forgiveness might act to moderate the effects of mental health variables such as anger and depression on self-harm or suicidal intent, both of which have direct impact on physical health. In short, forgiveness appears to have direct connections to physical health, but some investigators have suggested that its effects on mental health may be larger (Long et al., 2020). We believe it is important to note that if this pattern bears out, it is critically important to understand if mental health benefits of forgiveness are transmitted to benefits in physical health.

Conclusion

We reviewed 73 empirical studies in this chapter that examine the connections between multiple dimensions of forgiveness and multiple dimensions of physical health in a diverse array of samples using mostly, but by no means exclusively, cross-sectional community studies. The majority of these studies offer evidence of a beneficial relationship between forgiveness and physical health. This relationship takes many different forms, but at its core, there appears to be a real and meaningful connection between our ability to forgive others, forgive ourselves, feel forgiven by God, or forgive situations and the state of our physical health. A number of limitations exist and we outlined some of those key issues above, but these limits are not unique to this area of science and offer several opportunities for improvement in studies yet to come.

We urge investigators to draw on diverse theoretical models to motivate the study of forgiveness and physical health, design community- or patient-based, longitudinal studies as is feasible, and rely on undergraduate samples when other designs are not financially or logistically manageable. We should aim to refine our understanding of forgiveness of others and self-forgiveness, among other forgiveness dimensions, as important predictors of physical health with unique mediators/moderators that should be considered. This review represents a collection of work that has developed over approximately 20 years and has led us from our earliest and most rudimentary understanding to our current, more refined, understanding of forgiveness as a multidimensional, potentially salutagenic trait and process in physical health. We look forward to equally invigorating and enlightening work in the decades ahead.

References

Antonovsky, A. (1979). *Health, stress and coping*. Jossey-Bass.

Berry, J. W., Worthington, E. L., Jr., O'Connor, L. E., Parrott, L., III, & Wade, N. G. (2005). Forgivingness, vengeful rumination, and affective traits. *Journal of Personality, 73*(1), 183–226. https://doi.org/10.1111/j.1467-6494.2004.00308.x

Cheadle, A. C. D., & Toussaint, L. L. (2015). Forgiveness and physical health in healthy populations. In L. L. Toussaint, E. L. Worthington Jr., & D. R. Williams (Eds.), *Forgiveness and health: Scientific evidence and theories relating forgiveness to better health* (pp. 91–106). Springer.

Davis, D. E., Ho, M. Y., Griffin, B. J., Bell, C., Hook, J. N., Van Tongeren, D. R., DeBlaere, C., Worthington, E. L., Jr., & Westbrook, C. J. (2015). Forgiving the self and physical and mental health correlates: A meta-analytic review. *Journal of Counseling Psychology, 62*(2), 329–335. https://doi.org/10.1037/cou0000063

Derdaele, E., Toussaint, L., Thauvoye, E., & Dezutter, J. (2019). Forgiveness and late life functioning: The mediating role of finding ego-integrity. *Aging & Mental Health, 23*(2), 238–245. https://doi.org/10.1080/13607863.2017.1399346

Enright, R. D. (1996). Counseling within the forgiveness triad: On forgiving, receiving, forgiveness, and self-forgiveness. *Counseling & Values, 40*(2), 107–126. https://doi.org/10.1002/j.2161-007X.1996.tb00844.x

Erikson, E. H. (1982). *The life cycle completed: A review*. W. W. Norton.

Exline, J. J., Worthington, E. L., Jr., Hill, P., & McCullough, M. E. (2003). Forgiveness and justice: A research agenda for social and personality psychology. *Personality and Social Psychology Review, 7*(4), 337–348. https://doi.org/10.1207/S15327957PSPR0704_06

Ferrari, M., Yap, K., Scott, N., Einstein, D. A., & Ciarrochi, J. (2018). Self-compassion moderates the perfectionism and depression link in both adolescence and adulthood. *PloS one, 13*(2), e0192022–e0192022. https://doi.org/10.1371/journal.pone.0192022

Fisher, M. L., & Exline, J. J. (2010). Moving toward self-forgiveness: Removing barriers related to shame, guilt, and regret. *Social and Personality Psychology Compass, 4*(8), 548–558.

Griffin, B. J., Worthington, E. L., Jr., Lavelock, C. R., Greer, C. L., Lin, Y., Davis, D. E., & Hook, J. N. (2015). Efficacy of a self-forgiveness workbook: A randomized controlled trial with interpersonal offenders. *Journal of Counseling Psychology, 62*(2), 124–136. https://doi.org/10.1037/cou0000060

Hall, J. H., & Fincham, F. D. (2005). Self-forgiveness: The stepchild of forgiveness research. *Journal of Social and Clinical Psychology, 24*(5), 621–637.

Henrich, J., Heine, S. J., & Norenzayan, A. (2010). Most people are not WEIRD. *Nature, 466*(7302), 29–29. https://doi.org/10.1038/466029a

Idler, E. L., Musick, M. A., Ellison, C. G., George, L. K., Krause, N., Ory, M. G., Pargament, K. I., Powell, L. H., Underwood, L. G., & Williams, D. R. (2003). Measuring multiple dimensions of religion and spirituality for health research: Conceptual background and findings from the 1998 General Social Survey. *Research on Aging, 25*(4), 327–365.

Jylhä, M. (2009). What is self-rated health and why does it predict mortality? Towards a unified conceptual model. *Social Science & Medicine, 69*(3), 307–316. https://doi.org/10.1016/j.socscimed.2009.05.013

Krause, N., & Ironson, G. (2017). Forgiveness by God, religious commitment, and waist/hip ratios. *Journal of Applied Biobehavioral Research, 22*(4), 1–12. https://doi.org/10.1111/jabr.12104

Lazarus, R. S. (1999). *Stress and emotion*. Springer Publishing Company.

Lazarus, R. S., & Folkman, S. (1984). *Stress, appraisal, and coping*. Springer Publishing Company.

Lee, Y.-R., & Enright, R. (2019). A meta-analysis of the association between forgiveness of others and physical health. *Psychology and Health*. https://doi.org/10.1080/08870446.2018.1554185

Long, K. N., Worthington, E. L., VanderWeele, T. J., & Chen, Y. (2020b). Forgiveness of others and subsequent health and well-being in mid-life: A longitudinal study on female nurses. *BMC psychology, 8*(1), 1–11.

Long, K. N. G., Chen, Y., Potts, M., Hanson, J., & VanderWeele, T. J. (2020a). Spiritually motivated self-forgiveness and divine forgiveness, and subsequent health and well-being among middle-aged female nurses: An outcome-wide longitudinal approach. *Frontiers in Psychology, 11*, 1337. https://doi.org/10.3389/fpsyg.2020.01337

Luskin, F. (2002). *Forgive for Good: A Proven Prescription for Health and Happiness.* HarperCollins.

McConnell, J. M. (2015). A conceptual-theoretical-empirical framework for self-forgiveness: Implications for research and practice. *Basic and Applied Social Psychology, 37*(3), 143–164. https://doi.org/10.1080/01973533.2015.1016160

McConnell, J. M., & Dixon, D. N. (2012). Perceived forgiveness from god and self-forgiveness. *Journal of Psychology and Christianity, 31*, 31–39.

McCullough, M. E., Root, L. M., & Cohen, A. D. (2006). Writing about the benefits of an interpersonal transgression facilitates forgiveness. *Journal of Consulting and Clinical Psychology, 74*(5), 887–897. https://doi.org/10.1037/0022-006X.74.5.887

McCullough, M. E., Worthington, E. L. J., & Rachal, K. C. (1997). Interpersonal forgiving in close relationships. *Journal of Personality & Social Psychology, 73*(2), 321–336. https://doi.org/10.1037/0022-3514.73.2.321

McEwen, B. S. (2005). Stressed or stressed out: what is the difference? *Journal of Psychiatry & Neuroscience, 30*(5), 315–318.

McEwen, B. S., Cacioppo, J. T., & Berntson, G. G. (2004). Protective and damaging effects of stress mediators. *New England Journal of Medicine, 338*(3), 171–179. https://doi.org/10.1056/NEJM199801153380307

Monahan, A., Jacobo, A., & Nguyen, A.-M. (2020). Interview with Dr. Neal Krause. *Public Health, Religion, and Spirituality Bulletin, 3*(Fall), 4–9.

Mróz, J., Kaleta, K., & Sołtys, E. (2020). Decision to forgive scale and emotional forgiveness scale in a polish sample. *Current Psychology*. https://doi.org/10.1007/s12144-020-00838-6

Murphy, J. G. (2003). *Self forgiveness. In Getting even: Forgiveness and its limits.* Oxford University Press.

Neff, K. (2003). Self-compassion: An alternative conceptualization of a healthy attitude toward oneself. *Self and Identity, 2*(2), 85–101.

Peterson, C., & Seligman, M. E. (2004). *Character strengths and virtues: A handbook and classification* (Vol. 1). Oxford University Press.

Rasmussen, K. R., Stackhouse, M., Boon, S. D., Comstock, K., & Ross, R. (2019). Meta-analytic connections between forgiveness and health: The moderating effects of forgiveness-related distinctions. *Psychology and Health*. https://doi.org/10.1080/08870446.2018.1545906

Rotter, J. B. (1966). Generalized expectancies for internal versus external control of reinforcement. *Psychological Monographs: General and Applied, 80*(1), 1–28.

Seligman, M. E. P. (1972). Learned helplessness. *Annual review of medicine, 23*(1), 407–412.

Thompson, L. Y., Snyder, C. R., Hoffman, L., Michael, S. T., Rasmussen, H. N., Billings, L. S., Heinze, L., Neufeld, J. E., Shorey, H. S., Roberts, J. C., & Roberts, D. E. (2005). Dispositional forgiveness of self, others, and situations. *Journal of Personality, 73*(2), 313–359. https://doi.org/10.1111/j.1467-6494.2005.00311.x

Toussaint, L., Barry, M., Bornfriend, L., & Markman, M. (2014). Restore: The journey toward self-forgiveness: A randomized trial of patient education on self-forgiveness in cancer patients and caregivers. *Journal of Healthcare Chaplaincy, 20*(2), 54–74.

Toussaint, L., & Waldman, E. (2017). Forgiveness & reconciliation: Processes and outcomes. In A. K. Schneider & C. Honeyman (Eds.), *The negotiators desk reference*. American Bar Association.

Toussaint, L. L., Webb, J. R., & Hirsch, J. K. (2017). Self-forgiveness and health: A stress-and-coping model. In L. Woodyat, E. L. Worthington Jr., M. Wenzel, & B. J. Griffin (Eds.), *Handbook of the psychology of self-forgiveness* (pp. 87–99). Springer International Publishing.

Wade, N. G., Hoyt, W. T., Kidwell, J. E. M., & Worthington, E. L. (2014). Efficacy of psychotherapeutic interventions to promote forgiveness: A meta-analysis. *Journal of Consulting and Clinical Psychology, 82*(1), 154–170. https://doi.org/10.1037/a0035268

Wade, N. G., & Worthington, E. L., Jr. (2003). Overcoming interpersonal offenses: Is forgiveness the only way to deal with unforgiveness? *Journal of Counseling & Development, 81*(3), 343–353. https://doi.org/10.1002/j.1556-6678.2003.tb00261.x

Ware, J. E., Jr., & Sherbourne, C. D. (1992). The MOS 36-item short-form health survey (SF-36). I. Conceptual framework and item selection. *Medical Care, 30*(6), 473–483.

Webb, J. R., Bumgarner, D., Conway-Williams, E., & Dangel, T. J. (2016). A consensus definition of self-forgiveness: Implications for assessment and treatment. *Spirituality in Clinical Practice, 4*(3), 216–227. https://doi.org/10.1037/scp0000138

Wohl, M. J. A., & Thompson, A. (2011). A dark side to self-forgiveness: Forgiving the self and its association with chronic unhealthy behaviour. *British Journal of Social Psychology, 50*(2), 354–364.

Woodyatt, L., Wenzel, M., & de Vel-Palumbo, M. (2017). Working through psychological needs following transgressions to arrive at self-forgiveness. In *Handbook of the Psychology of Self-Forgiveness* (pp. 43–58). Springer.

Worthington, E. L., Jr. (2003). *Forgiving and reconciling: Bridges to wholeness and hope*. InterVarsity Press.

Worthington, E. L., Jr. (2009). *A just forgiveness: Responsible healing without excusing injustice*. IVP Books.

Worthington, E. L., Jr. (2013). *Moving forward: Six steps to forgiving yourself and breaking free from the past*. Waterbrook Press.

Worthington, E. L., Jr., Hook, J. N., Utsey, S. O., Williams, J. K., & Neil, R. L. (2007). *Decisional and emotional forgiveness*. Paper presented at the International Positive Psychology Summit Washington.

Worthington, E. L., Jr., & Langberg, D. (2012). Religious considerations and self-forgiveness in treating complex trauma and moral injury in present and former soldiers. *Journal of Psychology & Theology, 40*(4), 274–288.

Worthington, E. L., Jr., & Scherer, M. (2004). Forgiveness is an emotion-focused coping strategy that can reduce health risks and promote health resilience: Theory, review, and hypotheses. *Psychology & Health, 19*(3), 385–405. https://doi.org/10.1080/0887044042000196674

Worthington, E. L., Jr., & Wade, N. G. (1999). The psychology of unforgiveness and forgiveness and implications for clinical practice. *Journal of Social & Clinical Psychology, 18*(4), 385–418. https://doi.org/10.1521/jscp.1999.18.4.385

Ye, Y., Ma, D., Yuan, H., Chen, L., Wang, G., Shi, J., Yu, Y., Guo, Y., & Jiang, X. (2019). Moderating effects of forgiveness on relationship between empathy and health-related quality of life in hemodialysis patients: A structural equation modeling approach. *Journal of Pain and Symptom Management, 57*(2), 224–232.

12

Hopefulness in the Context of Chronic Illness: Theory, Research, and Practice

Heather R. Altier and Jameson K. Hirsch

The investigation of hopefulness as a beneficial character strength and source of resilience has existed for more than a millennium. In Greek philosophy, Hesiod's myth of Pandora's box is one of the earliest and best-known references to hope. Zeus, seeking revenge on Prometheus for stealing fire, purposely gave a box containing mental (e.g., envy, ignorance) and physical evils (e.g., disease, death), and virtues (e.g., harmony, happiness), to Pandora to bring to Earth, knowing that she would open it and release them despite Zeus's instructions to leave it closed (Snyder et al., 1991b). Hope, commonly interpreted as a consolation for the evils that were released, was all that remained inside the box when Pandora closed it (Gravlee, 2020). It must also be noted that other Greek philosophers, including Solon and Thucydides, viewed hope negatively, as wishful thinking occurring in the absence of adequate problem-solving ability (Vogt, 2017).

The assumption that hope is beneficially linked to well-being has endured, however, including in the Judeo-Christian belief system (e.g., hope for

H. R. Altier (✉)
Department of Psychiatry and Behavioral Sciences, Johns Hopkins University School of Medicine, Baltimore, MD, USA
e-mail: haltier1@jh.edu

J. K. Hirsch
Department of Psychiatry and Behavioral Sciences, Quillen College of Medicine, East Tennessee State University, Johnson City, TN, USA
e-mail: hirsch@etsu.edu

F. M. Sirois (ed.), *The Palgrave Handbook of Positive Psychology and Health*,
https://doi.org/10.1007/978-3-031-89095-6_12

eternity or healing) and in modern psychosocial conceptualizations, such as Viktor Frankl's (2004) description of hope during the Holocaust (Feldman & von Garnier, 2018; Vogt, 2017). Yet, empirical investigation of the construct as a contributor to mental health did not occur until the mid-1900s, when Karl Menninger identified hopefulness as an imperative for scientific study, and when Ezra Stotland operationalized hope as a positive expectancy for achieving an important goal (Rasmussen et al., 2018). In the 1980s, the study of hopefulness gained momentum, including application to the experience of physical health problems and chronic illness. For example, Nowotny (1989) developed a hope scale for use with individuals with cancer, conceptualizing hopefulness as encompassing the belief that a future is possible, confidence in an outcome, interpersonal relationships, and spirituality. Similarly, a hope measure developed by Miller and Powers (1988), for use with persons with chronic illness, characterized hope as the expectation of a positive future and a good prognostic outcome, and purpose and meaning in life. Although these early endeavors to operationalize and investigate hope were often disparate, sometimes based on anecdotal reports from patients and caregivers, and lacked rigor, they paved the way for the development of the science of hope and the evolution of our understanding of the role of hopefulness for the lived experience and well-being of persons with chronic illness. What follows is a discussion of the primary conceptualizations of hope as they relate to the experience of chronic illness, and a delineation of hope from other future-oriented protective characteristics. We then review the extant literature on hopefulness in the context of chronic illness, including its beneficial effect on the development, maintenance, and recovery from disease.

Conceptualization and Assessment of Hopefulness

Broadly, hopefulness appears to exert a wide array of benefits for persons with chronic illness, including across cardiovascular, metabolic, and respiratory systems (Richman et al., 2005). Such salubrious effects may occur because hope contributes to the facilitation of coping and adjustment, quality of life, purposefulness, self-esteem, and resilience (Griggs & Walker, 2016). More recently, hope has been posited as a sense of determination for patients to attain their health goals, including for rehabilitation patients (Kortte et al., 2012), and is proposed to encompass personal (e.g., meaningfulness), situational (e.g., risk, confidence), and interpersonal (e.g., trust, support) realms (Nekolaichuk et al., 1999).

Although theoretical interpretations of hope abound, three conceptualizations recur frequently in the health psychology and medical literature and appear to align with health and well-being most closely. Their associated measures, with accompanying theoretical underpinnings and evidence of research usage, are outlined in the following sections.

Herth Hope Index (HHI)

The Herth Hope Index (HHI) was developed for use in nursing and has been widely utilized to evaluate hope among individuals with physical disease and disability. Herth (1990) defined hope as "an inner power that facilitates the transcendence of the present situation and movement toward new awareness and enrichment of being" (p. 1256), and emphasized its cognitive-behavioral, emotional, and social elements. The HHI measures three dimensions of hope: positive readiness and expectancy (i.e., affective-behavioral; confidence in ability to implement plans to achieve the outcome), interconnectedness (i.e., affiliative-contextual; recognizing the connection between self and spirit, and self and others), and temporality and future (i.e., cognitive-temporal; perceived high likelihood of achieving a desired outcome) (Herth, 1992). Such characteristics are well-established contributors to health and wellness, including during the experience of illness. For example, social support and interpersonal well-being are strongly linked to physical health, including in patients with comorbid chronic conditions, multiple sclerosis, and cardiac disease (De Maria et al., 2020; Kaiser et al., 2020; Koutsogeorgou et al., 2020).

To develop the 12-item HHI, items were extracted from the Herth Hope Scale (HHS; Herth, 1991), a 30-item scale. This briefer version was considered more clinically useful and was designed to be completed by adults experiencing alterations in mental status (Herth, 1992). The HHI has been utilized to measure hopefulness across numerous medical populations; for example, greater scores on the HHI have been linked to less depression in stroke patients (Tantisuvanitchkul et al., 2020) and, in a sample of nursing home patients, to better physical functioning and less pain intensity (Marcus et al., 2017). However, factor analyses of the HHI in medical samples have yielded between one and three factors across at least nine studies, including in patients with cardiac conditions, cancer, and other chronic and terminal illnesses (Rustøen et al., 2018), calling into question its ability to measure the construct of hope in a reliable and valid manner across different settings, disease groups, and cultures.

Trait Hope Scale and State Hope Scale

While the HHI was under development, Snyder et al. (1991a) devised the State Hope Scale and Trait Hope Scale based on their own hope theory. Expanding unidimensional goal models that solely emphasized positive goal attainment (e.g., Stotland, 1969), Snyder proposed a multidimensional model of hopefulness comprised of the elements of goals, agency, and pathways. Broadly, goals are conceptualized as the targets of cognitive sequences that facilitate actions toward a desired outcome (Snyder et al., 1997). Goal pursuits can be long or short term, must be attainable with a degree of uncertainty, must be valuable enough to necessitate sustained attention, and center on either negative goal outcomes, in which the detrimental outcome never appears or is delayed, or positive goal outcomes, in which the outcome is either reached, sustained, or increased (Snyder et al., 2000). Pathways reflects the ability to plan multiple, realistic routes toward goal attainment and involves active problem-solving to produce additional routes when barriers are encountered, whereas agency reflects motivation, or the perceived capability to initiate and sustain movement toward desired outcomes, particularly when initial paths are obstructed (Snyder et al., 1998). Pathways and agency cognitions are synergistic; an increase in one generates an increase in the other (Snyder et al., 1991a). One's level of hope over time is influenced by the emotions generated in response to perceived successes or failures and the resultant perceptions regarding one's general and situational agentic and pathway-related aptitudes (Snyder et al., 2000).

Snyder's Hope Scale consists of 12 items, including four filler items, that assess the two primary factors comprising hope, including agency (e.g., "I energetically pursue my goals") and pathways (e.g., "There are lots of ways around any problem"). Response anchors range from 1 (definitely false) to 8 (definitely true), and the items for the agency and pathways subscales are summed to generate a total hope score (range = 8 to 64), with greater scores indicating higher levels of hopefulness. Across chronic illness samples, internal consistency is good to excellent, including in cancer patients (Cronbach's $\alpha = 0.92$; Mazzotti et al., 2020) and breast cancer survivors ($\alpha = 0.82$; Rashidi et al., 2019).

Numerous theoretical and empirical efforts have been made to link Snyder's formulation of hope to mental and physical health, including in persons with chronic illness. Indeed, Snyder suggested that, in the context of the pain, loss, and suffering that often accompanies chronic illness or impairment, blockages of goal visualization and attainment may occur, resulting in hopelessness and a sense of loss that may lead to increased suffering. Whether it is the loss of previous good health, or the perceived loss of future possibilities, chronic illness and pain may erode confidence in abilities and the future (Snyder, 1998). Of note, when such an action crisis occurs (e.g., when setbacks and goal frustration are experienced), deleterious affective, cognitive, and physiological consequences often result, including goal discounting, psychosocial distress, and increased stress reactivity (Brandstätter et al., 2013). Yet, through the processes of goal disengagement (i.e., relinquishing unlikely or unattainable goals) and regoaling or goal reengagement (i.e., finding alternative health and personal goals), and taking into consideration affect and hope, the illness experience can be shifted toward a path of resilience (Hill et al., 2014).

Comprehensive Hope Scales

In their comprehensive model, which is detailed in their chapter of this volume, Scioli et al. (2011) posited that hope is a future-directed emotion network comprised of four channels, systems, or subnetworks: attachment (i.e., sense of continued connectedness, behaviors promoting openness and trust), survival (i.e., managing stress, escaping danger, belief in one's well-being), mastery (i.e., feeling and beliefs associated with empowerment, establishing and pursuing goals), and spiritual (i.e., belief in a higher power, transcendence, eternal truths). The hope network is regulated through feedback between these four channels, which are arranged into a foundational structure of five levels, including biological motives, nature and nurture, hope trait clusters, faith, and daily hope-related beliefs, feelings, and actions (Scioli et al., 2011).

Briefly, the Comprehensive Hope Scales comprise an item pool based on 16 conceptualizations of hope, arranged into state and trait hope items (Scioli et al., 2011). Across numerous analyses, Scioli identified a 4-factor structure for state hope, comprising the four channels, and a 6-factor structure for trait hope, including spirituality, basic trust, and further differentiation of mastery and survival into four distinct forms (i.e., personalized and attached mastery, self-generated and attached survival). Mastery and survival efforts can be either attachment-based or internalized and self-focused. Scioli et al. (2011) speculated that attachment may spawn all other configurations of hope, supporting the large body of research indicating a beneficial association between social support and psychosocial well-being, including in colorectal cancer survivors and among persons with HIV/AIDS (Asante, 2012; Haviland et al., 2017). Of note, the trait hope scales of the CHS (CHS-T) and Snyder's Hope

Scale (1991) are moderately correlated, with a shared variance of 20 percent (Scioli et al., 2016).

Scioli and colleagues have asserted that the Comprehensive Hope Scales (CHS) are relevant to health and, thus, to chronic illness, because hopefulness is partially predicated on psychosocial health and wellness factors, including social support (attachment), perceived control (mastery), self-regulation (coping and survival) and spirituality (Scioli et al., 2011). Indeed, these proposed underlying factors of hope have well-established associations with health and wellness in chronic illness samples. For example, in a sample of patients with inflammatory bowel disease, mastery was associated with disease self-efficacy and current health status (Donnelley, 2019) and, in a review of the literature, insecure attachment was related to poor health outcomes and mortality in persons with chronic illness (Jimenez, 2017). Finally, in a sample of cardiac patients, self-regulation was linked to better self-management of disease (Zaharova et al., 2021) and, across numerous chronic illness samples, spirituality was beneficially associated with reduced disease burden and psychopathology in patients with chronic obstructive pulmonary disease (COPD), and better quality of life in patients with kidney disease (Fradelos, 2020; Mendes et al., 2021).

Differentiating Hopefulness from Other Future-Oriented Constructs

For both research accuracy and clinical efficacy, it is important to differentiate between hopefulness and other future-oriented and goal-directed constructs. Prospective temporal factors, such as optimism, future orientation, and hopelessness, and cognitive-emotional characteristics, such as self-efficacy, may often be considered comparable to hopefulness, but each comprises unique elements distinguishable from hopefulness.

Optimism

Although hope and optimism are both future-directed constructs and frequently examined in health contexts, they are often conflated despite being theoretically differentiated (Bryant & Cvengros, 2004). Perhaps the most common theory of optimism is Scheier and Carver's (1985), which posits that optimism embodies a generalized expectation for positive outcomes or success. According to Scheier and Carver, optimism is goal-directed, like the agency component of Snyder's hope theory, although it lacks an explicit pathways component (Snyder et al., 1998).

Optimism has been defined as psychological distancing from previous negative outcomes, attributing them to external, specific, and transient factors instead of internal, global, and stable factors (Seligman, 1991). Hope, in contrast, involves the process of attempting to acquire desired outcomes (Snyder et al., 1998), and past failures and negative outcomes are considered only to the extent that such information can facilitate effective pursuit of future goals (Snyder et al., 2000). In two studies designed to discriminate between hope and optimism, Bury et al. (2016) determined that hope arises when probability of an outcome is low, but still possible, whereas optimism increases linearly with likelihood. Theoretically, optimism is predicated on a general confidence about future goals, whereas hope encompasses a sense of self-control and self-efficacy related to future goals (Krafft et al., 2021). Despite these differences, however, greater optimism and hope are both linked to increased engagement in health-promoting behaviors in individuals with chronic disease (Schiavon et al., 2017).

Self-Efficacy

Bandura's (1982) self-efficacy theory parallels hope theory, in that both constructs are goal-directed. For example, Bandura stated that cognitive processing must be assessed contextually; that is, an individual must evaluate their ability to perform the behaviors needed to achieve a goal (akin to agency) and the necessary circumstances that must exist to achieve a goal (akin to pathways) (Snyder et al., 2000). Whereas self-efficacy, conceptualized as the perceived ability to complete a behavior, occurs prior to initiating a behavior and does not encompass goal-directed planning, pathways and agency thoughts occur throughout the goal-directed cognitive process (Snyder et al., 2000). Further, although both self-efficacy and hope emphasize confident expectancies about goal-oriented actions, only hope also focuses on outcome expectancies, and these constructs are only moderately correlated, suggesting they are related but independent (Magaletta & Oliver, 1999).

Future Orientation

Although hopefulness encompasses an adaptive view of the future, the ability to engage in positive prospection, or future orientation, is somewhat broader in scope. Future orientation is conceptualized to encompass: (1) the expectation that life will improve despite the existence of current stressors; (2) confidence in the ability to make successful plans and reach goals in the future; and (3) confidence in the ability to overcome barriers to goal attainment (Hirsch et al., 2015; Lucas et al., 2019). To assess this construct, Hirsch et al. (2006) developed the Future Orientation Scale (FOS) by extracting six temporally relevant items from the Reasons for Living Inventory—Older Adult scale (RFL-OA; Linehan et al., 1983). Higher scores on the FOS have been linked to better quality of life in primary care patients and reduced pain severity in persons with fibromyalgia (Chang et al., 2019; Hirsch et al., 2015). Among primary care patients, hope and future orientation shared approximately 31 percent of common variance, suggesting their independence as constructs (Nsamenang & Hirsch, 2015).

Hopelessness

Often considered the antithesis of hopefulness, hopelessness is conceptualized as negative expectancies about oneself and one's future, including global and stable attributions for negative outcomes that make problems appear unresolvable (Beck et al., 1974). Yet, hope and hopelessness are considered theoretically distinct constructs (i.e., hopelessness does not encompass a pathways component), and have been empirically distinguished (Chang, 2017; Hirsch et al., 2012; Huen et al., 2015). For example, in the original psychometric study of Snyder's Hope Scale, hope and hopelessness were only moderately correlated ($r = -0.51$; Snyder et al., 1991a). In a sample of patients with terminal cancer, hope was described as having an active component that facilitates coping, whereas hopelessness was described as a passive construct comprised of cognitive, affective, and motivational components (Sachs et al., 2013).

Despite such differences, the detrimental impact of hopelessness on health is well-established. Across studies, hopelessness is related to risk for atherosclerosis (Do et al., 2010), mortality (Everson et al., 1996), cancer progression (Price et al., 2016), suicide (Hirsch et al., 2012), fatigue in patients with cardiac disease (Dunn et al., 2020), and flatter diurnal cortisol rhythm (i.e., indicative of hypothalamic–pituitary–adrenal axis dysfunction; Pössel et al., 2015).

Hope in the Context of Disease and Impairment

Given the empirical prominence of hopefulness in the fields of health psychology and positive psychology for over 30 years, there exists a vast literature examining its relation to physical well-being in the context of chronic illness, including health behaviors, functional impairment, and disease trajectory, among others. For example, broadly, hopefulness is associated with resilience in patients with hypertension (Namvar & Ghasedi, 2020), better adjustment to disease in patients with multiple sclerosis (Madan & Pakenham, 2014), reduced posttraumatic stress in oral cancer patients (Zhang et al., 2021a), posttraumatic growth and meaning in life in patients with COPD (Wang et al., 2021), quality of life in hemodialysis patients and patients with oral cancer and bleeding disorders (Alshraifeen et al., 2020; Klein et al., 2020; Zhang et al., 2020), lower death anxiety in patients with heart disease (Soleimani et al., 2020), less somatic symptom disturbance in hemodialysis patients (Yu et al., 2020), less depression in Jordanian cancer patients (Malak et al., 2021), and fewer effects and symptoms of kidney disease (Billington et al., 2008). In the following sections, we briefly outline consistent, yet recent, findings confirming these beneficial associations, across several chronic illness groups and pertaining to disease-related health behaviors.

Hope and Health-Related Functioning in Persons with Chronic Illness

Unlike most other future-oriented constructs, Snyder et al. (2000) posited that, as a motivational characteristic, hope can be harnessed to engage in health-directed goals through primary prevention, which involves using actions or thoughts to avert the development of chronic illness, and secondary prevention, or actions or thoughts that facilitate recovery from, or maintenance of, a chronic health condition once it has appeared. Hopeful thinkers tend to use both approach and avoidance schemes to promote health, generally being proactive in utilizing health information to engage in health-promoting behaviors while avoiding health risks (Snyder et al., 2000). As well, high-hope thinkers utilize information about previous obstacles to influence planning for pathways toward similar goals, which may allow them to cope more effectively with the demands of physical illness (Snyder, 2002), including perceptions of, and consequences from, disease-related stress. Finally, Snyder's theory (2000) asserts that it is the tendency of hopeful individuals to acknowledge, incorporate, and utilize past health-related experiences and knowledge to work toward wellness-focused goals, which contributes to engagement in health promotion and rehabilitative behaviors, including stress reduction, in persons with chronic illness.

Hope and Health Promotion in Persons with Chronic Illness. The beneficial effects of hopefulness in the context of chronic disease may manifest at all stages of disease and within all disease processes, including behavioral engagement and health promotion. For example, in a sample of obese primary care patients, individuals who were more hopeful had a greater likelihood of engaging in dietary planning strategies, self-monitoring, and portion-control, food buying and preparation behaviors that reduce fat intake, and social interactions that promote healthy eating and physical exercise (Nothwehr et al., 2013). Similarly, in a sample of children with pediatric obesity undergoing a weight management intervention, beneficial changes in hope scores were related to increased physical activity (Van Allen & Steele, 2012). In peritoneal dialysis patients, hopefulness was associated with volume management behaviors, including reduced salt intake (Miaomiao et al., 2020). Hope is also associated with a healthy diet and exercise among cancer survivors (Coleman et al., 2014), and smoking cessation in persons who have received a smoking-related cancer diagnosis (Berg et al., 2013). Such positive coping behaviors are linked to enhanced self-efficacy and hopefulness, for instance, in patients with gastric cancer (Wu et al., 2021).

Hopefulness also appears to promote adherence to physician recommendations, with consequent benefits for physical health, including less functional impairment and better quality of life (Perry et al., 2018; Souza et al., 2016). For instance, greater hope predicted adherence to metered-dose inhaler usage among children with asthma (Berg et al., 2007), to treatment for multidrug resistant tuberculosis in a qualitative study of adults (Horter et al., 2016), and to medication adherence in patients with Type II diabetes (Pazokian et al., 2020). In a longitudinal study of adolescents with type 1 diabetes, an elevation in hope scores, but not optimism scores, was associated with more favorable hemoglobin A1c levels and self-monitored blood glucose levels, and frequency of blood glucose monitoring mediated the linkage between hope and reduced hemoglobin A1c levels (Van Allen et al., 2016). Similarly, hope was related to lower hemoglobin A1c levels among a Brazilian sample of adolescents and young adults with type 1 diabetes (Santos et al., 2015). Higher health-related hope was also associated with less perceived treatment burden and lower systolic blood pressure, considered a manifestation of treatment adherence, among patients with chronic kidney disease (CKD; Kurita et al., 2020).

Hopefulness, Stress, and Health in Persons with Chronic Illness. Adaptive coping and problem-solving strategies arising from hopefulness may also help to mitigate the development and impact of stress on physical and psychological functioning for persons with chronic illness. For example, in patients with breast cancer, hopefulness was related to less perceived stress, and in individuals with fibromyalgia, arthritis, and inflammatory bowel disease, hope was associated with less perceived stress and, in turn, to less fatigue (Abdollahi et al., 2019; Hirsch & Sirois, 2016). The beneficial effects of hope may also help to reduce the impact of stress on immunological and inflammatory processes, perhaps by counteracting the well-established deleterious effects of negative affect on health, including exacerbated and/or prolonged inflammatory responses, increased HPA-axis and cortisol activation, and prefrontal cortex dysfunction that results in disrupted immune functioning (Corn et al., 2020; Lopez et al., 2018). In a study of persons with breast cancer, for instance, greater hopefulness was related to better immune functioning, including greater $CD8^{+}$ T-cell percentage and lower $CD4^{+}$ T-cell and $CD19^{+}$ B-cell percentage (Kim et al., 2011). In a prospective study of individuals with HIV, greater hope (CHS-T) was related to better self-reported health, fewer missed doses of HIV medications, and higher CD-4 levels, indicating healthier immunological status (Scioli et al., 2012). Similarly, in another sample of HIV patients ($N = 1702$), hope was related to better self-reported mental and physical health, and to enhanced T-cell counts (Coduti et al., 2018).

Hope, Functional Impairment, and Quality of Life in Persons with Chronic Illness. In addition to the benefits of hopefulness for health promotion and stress reduction, hope appears to salubriously impact functionality and perceived quality of life, which are often critical areas of concern for persons with chronic illness (Megari, 2013). To begin, hopefulness contributes to successful adjustment to, and resilience during the experience of, chronic illness and impairment, including in bladder cancer patients (Dong et al., 2021). In turn, in stomach cancer patients, greater acceptance of disease was related to more hope (Luo et al., 2018), suggesting a bidirectional linkage between hope and adjustment to illness. In a longitudinal study of patients in inpatient rehabilitation due to amputation, stroke, acute spinal cord dysfunction, or recovery from orthopedic surgery, hope predicted functional role abilities three months post discharge (Kortte et al., 2012). As well, hopefulness was related to higher levels of self-care (i.e., an intentional behavior aimed at mitigating threats to functional capacity or health) among patients with COPD (Alberto & Joyner, 2008). Finally, hope has a well-established link to health-related quality of life in persons with disease, including in breast cancer survivors (Shen et al., 2020), patients with bleeding disorders (Klein et al., 2020), head and neck cancer survivors (Tsan et al., 2021), patients with colorectal cancer (Sharour et al., 2020), and in adolescents with chronic illness and cancer (Mardhiyah et al., 2020; Xue et al., 2021).

Hope in Persons with Cancer

One of the most substantial topical areas of research linking hope to chronic illness is focused on persons experiencing and recovering from cancer. In a systematic review of studies of persons undergoing cancer treatment, hope was associated with better quality of life, perceived health, and life satisfaction, and less symptom burden (Nierop-van Baalen et al., 2020). Similarly, across several diary studies of individuals with lung cancer currently receiving treatment, patients endorsing greater hope reported higher same-day and next-day social, role, and physical functioning, and fewer symptoms, including less fatigue and pain (Steffen et al., 2018, 2020). Such benefits exist across the lifespan; for instance, in a sample of children and adolescents with cancer, the linkage between hope and health-related quality of life (HRQL) was mediated by a reduction in anxiety (Martins et al., 2018) and, in older adults with terminal cancer, hopefulness was associated with better HRQL (Duggleby et al., 2007). Hope also contributes to the decision, by patients with advanced cancer, to continue anticancer therapy and engage in clinical trials (Clarke et al., 2015; Todd et al., 2009).

Of note, according to Scioli et al. (2016), although hope as a contributor to survival is important, it is the interpersonal and spiritual components of hopefulness that are considered most valuable by cancer survivors, particularly in the early and late stages of cancer. Indeed, given its focus on resolving barriers to attainment of meaningful goals, hopefulness may be particularly salient in the context of advanced disease (Feldman et al., 2008). Indeed, prognostic factors may interact with emotional functioning to influence hope and its correlates. As an example, in a sample of terminally ill cancer patients, those with a positive mood were less impacted by emotional instability in the manifestation of hope, whereas patients with a negative mood were more susceptible to having emotion-based motivational processes that disrupt hopefulness (Baczewska et al., 2020). Similarly, in another sample of advanced cancer patients, those with a stronger sense of control over their disease reported greater hope, suggesting that illnesses which are manageable or survivable may allow greater opportunity for the manifestation of hopefulness (Brown et al., 2017).

Hope in Persons with Chronic Pain Diseases

Another group of chronic illness that are predominant in the extant hope-focused literature are pain-related diseases. For example, in a sample of individuals with chronic pain conditions, either fibromyalgia, inflammatory bowel disease, or arthritis, hope was related to less perceived stress, pain, and fatigue, and lower stress levels partially explained the relation between higher levels of hope and less fatigue (Hirsch & Sirois, 2016). Psoriasis patients with higher levels of hope reported better quality of life in all domains (i.e., physical, social, psychological, environmental, and global; Hawro et al., 2014). Similarly, in a meta-analysis of studies focused on chronic pain patients, hope was associated with less pain severity and better physical functioning (Shanahan, et al., 2021). From an experimental perspective, in a non-clinical sample, lower pain catastrophizing explained the beneficial effect of hope on pain during a cold pressor task (Hood et al., 2012), suggesting that hopefulness may contribute to the generation of alternate methods of exerting control over and coping with pain.

There is theoretical precedent for these effects, as posited by the BIS-BAS theory (i.e., Behavioral Inhibition System-Behavioral Activation System), which suggests that behavioral activation and inhibition underlie motivational processes, and that behavioral activation involves problem-solving efforts and agency toward desired outcomes, whereas the behavioral inhibition system is involved in avoidance of unpleasant outcomes (Bossola et al., 2020). For persons with chronic pain, the experience of pain may be so aversive as to activate the BIS system, resulting in the development of an array of negative reactions, including symptoms of psychopathology and functional impairment (Serrano-Ibáñez et al., 2019). For example, in patients with chronic pain, behavioral inhibition was related to greater pain catastrophizing and interference, and less pain self-efficacy and hope, and behavioral activation was associated with less pain catastrophizing, greater activity engagement, and increased hope (Sánchez-Rodríguez et al., 2021). Similar patterns are indicated across disease populations, including beneficial associations between the BAS system and fatigue, and deleterious associations between the BIS system and mental health, in stroke patients, persons with multiple sclerosis and Parkinson's disease, and patients undergoing hemodialysis, suggesting that approach/avoidance tendencies may be critical in understanding the motivational processes underlying hopefulness in the context of illness and impairment (Bossola et al., 2020; Oniszczenko et al., 2018).

Hopefulness: Examining Health Benefits across Medical Samples

Next, we shift our discussion to findings from our own chronic illness data, presented to substantiate the extant literature linking hopefulness to self-reported well-being. We investigated the relation of hope to an array of health constructs among three medical populations, including primary care patients ($N = 223$), fibromyalgia patients ($N = 508$), and cancer patients ($n = 235$) and caregivers ($n = 48$). All respondents provided informed consent, and all studies were approved by an Institutional Review Board. Data were collected in-person (primary care) and online (fibromyalgia and cancer). For each sample, the Trait Hope Scale was utilized (Snyder et al., 1991a), and all multivariate linear regression analyses covaried age, sex, and race.

In our primary care sample, greater hope was significantly related to less self-reported alcohol misuse and substance abuse, better treatment adherence ($p < 0.05$), less bodily pain, better general health and physical functioning, more vitality, and fewer role limitations due to physical and emotional difficulties (all $p < 0.001$, except treatment adherence). In fibromyalgia patients, hope was negatively related to fibromyalgia impact, depressive symptoms, and perceived stress, and positively related to treatment adherence, health self-efficacy, health vigilance, vitality, and the ability to complete activities of daily living and engage in physical self-maintenance (all $p < 0.001$). Finally, hope was negatively related to depressive symptoms and perceived stress, and positively related to wellness behaviors, treatment adherence, vitality, and physical functioning, among cancer patients and caregivers (all $p < 0.001$; See Tables 12.1, 12.2 and 12.3 for Results).

Our findings suggest that hope is a beneficial transdiagnostic characteristic that exerts a protective influence on an array of health-related variables, in patients with and without chronic illness, supporting previous research (Corn et al., 2020). Across our samples, hope had a consistent salubrious effect on vitality and treatment adherence, and on varied forms of perceived quality of life, including role limitations, physical functioning, and functional impairment, consistent with the extant literature documenting such effects with inpatient rehabilitation patients (Kortte et al., 2012), COPD patients (Alberto & Joyner, 2008), and diabetes patients (Pazokian et al., 2020). As well, hopefulness exhibited context-specific effects that may hold value for persons with specific diseases. For example, in persons with fibromyalgia, hope was related to reduced perceptions of stress and depression, which are common characteristics of the disease (Galvez-Sánchez et al., 2019), and to health vigilance and

Table 12.1 The effects of hope on health-related outcomes in a sample of primary care patients

	Hope coefficient	Full model (with covariates)						
Dependent variable	*B*	*SE*	*t*	*p*	R^2	*df*	*F*	*p*
Alcohol misuse	−0.28	0.10	−2.85	0.005	0.27	4, 189	6.13	0.000
Substance abuse	−0.21	0.05	−4.19	0.000	0.14	4, 192	7.57	0.000
Treatment adherence	0.11	0.04	2.51	0.013	0.06	4, 199	2.93	0.022
Bodily pain	−0.57	0.15	−3.66	0.000	0.10	4, 205	5.76	0.000
General health	0.98	0.14	6.99	0.000	0.28	4, 207	19.77	0.000
Physical functioning	0.78	0.15	5.28	0.000	0.26	4, 207	18.50	0.000
Vitality	0.87	0.13	.68	0.000	0.33	4, 207	25.57	0.000
Role limitations—emotional	1.41	0.17	8.23	0.000	0.30	4, 206	21.73	0.000
Role limitations—physical	0.80	0.14	5.60	0.000	0.26	4, 205	17.85	0.000

Note: Linear regression analyses examining the effect of hope on health-related outcomes. Regression coefficients are unstandardized. *df* = degrees of freedom for regression, degrees of freedom for residuals. Alcohol Misuse = Alcohol Use Disorders Identification Test (Bohn et al., 1995); Substance Abuse = Drug Abuse Screening Test (Skinner, 1982); Treatment Adherence = Medical Outcomes Study General Adherence Scale (Sherbourne et al., 1992); Bodily Pain, General Health, Physical Functioning, Vitality, Emotional and Physical Role Limitations = Subscales of 36-Item Short Form Survey (SF-36 - Version 2) (Ware et al., 1996)

self-efficacy, which may be critical skills for coping with the uncertainty of fibromyalgia (Rowe et al., 2019). Finally, in patients with or recovering from cancer, linkages existed between hopefulness and reduced stress and depression, consistent with Malak et al.'s (2021) research, and increased wellness behaviors, which are requisite for recovery from cancer (Weber & O'Brien, 2017). Our findings substantiate past work, for instance in cancer survivors (Coleman et al., 2014), linking hopefulness to enhanced engagement in health promoting activities, including exercise and a nutritious diet. Such patterns suggest that hopefulness may help to assuage the psychological distress inherent in the cancer treatment and recovery process and may stimulate motivation to engage in health promoting behaviors to thwart cancer recurrence.

Research Implications

Effects of Hope May Differ across Disease Groups. Although our review of the literature and our multi-sample study findings suggest that the construct of hope offers promise for the promotion of health in persons with chronic

Table 12.2 The effects of hope on health-related outcomes in a sample of fibromyalgia patients

	Hope coefficient				Full model (with covariates)			
Dependent variable	*B*	*SE*	*t*	*p*	R^2	*df*	*F*	*p*
FIQR	−0.45	0.08	−5.79	0.000	0.14	4, 298	12.19	0.000
Depression	−0.54	0.05	−11.38	0.000	0.33	4, 311	37.82	0.000
Treatment adherence	0.09	0.03	3.07	0.002	0.06	4, 298	4.84	0.001
Health self-efficacy	0.11	0.01	7.63	0.000	0.20	4, 305	19.57	0.000
Health vigilance	0.08	0.02	4.61	0.000	0.07	4, 301	5.32	0.000
Vitality	0.34	0.03	12.04	0.000	0.35	4, 306	40.50	0.000
Stress	−0.37	0.04	−8.78	0.000	0.29	4, 311	31.94	0.000
IADL	0.02	0.01	3.00	0.003	0.18	4, 310	17.51	0.000
PSMS	0.02	0.01	2.39	0.018	0.11	4, 310	9.13	0.000

Note: Linear regression analyses examining the effect of hope on health-related outcomes. Regression coefficients are unstandardized. *df* = degrees of freedom for regression, degrees of freedom for residuals. FIQR = Fibromyalgia Impact Questionnaire – Revised (Bennett et al., 2009). Depression, Stress = Depression, Anxiety and Stress Scale - Short Form (Henry & Crawford, 2005); Treatment Adherence = Medical Outcomes Study General Adherence Scale (Sherbourne et al., 1992); Health Self-efficacy, Health Vigilance = Multidimensional Health Profile - Health Functioning Index, Health Self-efficacy and Health Vigilance Subscales (Karoly et al., 2005); Vitality = Subjective Vitality Scale (Ryan & Frederick, 1997); IADL = Instrumental Activities of Daily Living Scale (Lawton & Brody, 1988a); PSMS = Physical Self-Maintenance Scale (Lawton & Brody, 1988b)

Table 12.3 The effects of hope on health-related outcomes in a sample of persons with active and remitted cancer

	Hope coefficient				Full model (with covariates)			
Dependent variable	*B*	*SE*	*t*	*p*	R^2	*df*	*F*	*p*
Wellness behaviors	0.02	0.01	4.48	0.000	0.12	4, 184	6.30	0.000
Depression	−0.15	0.02	−7.44	0.000	0.26	4, 186	16.63	0.000
Treatment adherence	0.03	0.01	4.06	0.000	0.10	4, 181	5.02	0.001
Vitality	0.64	0.06	10.40	0.000	0.39	4, 180	29.18	0.000
Stress	−0.16	0.02	−7.44	0.000	0.28	4, 186	18.32	0.000
Physical functioning	0.38	0.09	4.27	0.000	0.10	4, 186	5.06	0.001

Note: Linear regression analyses examining the effect of hope on health-related outcomes. Regression coefficients are unstandardized. *df* = degrees of freedom for regression, degrees of freedom for residuals. Wellness Behaviors = Wellness Behaviors Inventory (Sirois, 2001, 2019); Depression = Multidimensional Health Profile – Psychosocial Functioning Index, Depression Subscale (Ruehlman et al., 1999); Treatment Adherence = Medical Outcomes Study General Adherence Scale (Sherbourne et al., 1992); Vitality = Subjective Vitality Scale (Ryan & Frederick, 1997); Stress = Perceived Stress Scale 4 (Cohen et al., 1983); Physical Functioning = 12-Item Short Form Survey (Version 2) – Physical Functioning Domain (Ware et al., 1996) illness, some areas remain to be addressed sufficiently. To begin, despite hopefulness being investigated in the context of a wide array of chronic health conditions, little is known about how hope may manifest across types of illness, including its dependency on stage or severity of disease, or whether its influence on health differs based on such factors. Broadly, individuals without a chronic illness may have greater hope than persons with a chronic illness, suggesting that the presence of illness does, indeed, deleteriously impact hopefulness (Zhong et al., 2021). Similarly, in a cross-sample study, veterans with disabilities had greater hopefulness and meaning in life than cancer patients (Rahimi et al., 2021), perhaps due to differences in etiology and prognosis of their respective health conditions. Yet, in a study of patients with brain tumors, levels of hope and distress did not differ between individuals with high-grade versus low-grade tumors; that is, patients with advanced tumors maintained greater hope than expected, whereas those with lesser tumors experienced greater distress than expected, suggesting that hopefulness and its benefits are dependent on disease characteristics (Mayer et al., 2021). Similar patterns emerged in a sample of patients undergoing hemodialysis, who also reported high levels of hope (Alves Moreira & da Silva Borges, 2020), and in a sample of end-of-life oncology patients, who reported moderate to high hope, despite the presence of clinically significant psychopathology and demoralization, suggesting that hope remains a robust influence even when death is imminent (Bovero et al., 2021).

Effects of Hope May Differ across Health Outcomes. The target of hopefulness may also be critical for the manifestation of health benefits, though hope may sometimes be misdirected or futile. Few studies have examined targeted hope in the context of chronic illness, yet such inquiries are necessary to inform our understanding of the conditions under which hope may manifest, and how the manifestation and efficacy of hope may differ based on which health-related goals are being pursued. For instance, in a sample of advanced cancer patients with less than a year to live, greater hope was associated with increased odds of believing their disease was curable and that their chances of survival were greater than that of the average patient (Finkelstein et al., 2021). In a qualitative study of cancer patients, hope for survival and will to survive were common hopeful themes, which may be different than the target of hopefulness for a person with a nonterminal chronic condition (Nazam et al., 2021). Similarly, in another qualitative study of lung cancer patients, several themes of hopefulness emerged, including autonomy to make health decisions, building of relationships, usefulness to peer patients, and meaning-making during the illness experience (Ota et al., 2020). Finally, in a sample of hospice patients in the last six months of life, joyful memories and family relationships were the primary sources of hope (Byrne & Morgan, 2020). Such patterns suggest that hopefulness, and the likelihood of goal attainment, may be predicated on a behavior-specific, or disease-specific, vision of a desired outcome, and may manifest differentially based on disease parameters.

Indeed, across studies, the influence of hope on the health and well-being of persons who have a chronic illness appears to fluctuate contextually, based on life experiences and circumstances, including health. For example, in a 4-wave longitudinal study of patients who had suffered acute myocardial infarction, both health-related quality of life and hope increased over time, in parallel (Eriksson et al., 2013), suggesting that the recovery trajectory may instill motivation and a sense of well-being. Yet, for others, such as gastroparesis patients who received a gastric pacemaker, presurgery levels of hope did not predict physical HRQL at 3-month and 6-month follow-up (Parenteau et al., 2006). Such differential findings may indicate that hopefulness and HRQL are conditional upon the type and stage of disease, as well as likelihood of recovery and risk of mortality. This assertion has some precedent; for instance, in a sample of persons with chronic kidney disease, patients with Stage 4 and 5 CKD had lower levels of hope than patients in Stages 2 and 3 (Kurita et al., 2020). Importantly, however, hope can exist in the absence of perceptions of control over disease and can contribute to treatment compliance even when the prognostic outlook for disease is bleak (Makarem, 2016). Even in end-of-life situations, a strong sense of hopefulness may be present and can exert mental and physical benefits, but may be focused on dignity, building relationships, or meaning-making, rather than on a cure, symptom reduction, or the prolonging of life (Hill & Feudtner, 2018).

Effects of Hope and Health are Bidirectional. Of note, relatively few studies have examined the bidirectional association between hopefulness and health in persons with chronic illness. Instead, much of the extant research focuses on the benefits of hope for health, rather than on the impact of health, whether salubrious or deleterious, on hopefulness. Yet, it is clear, from both theory and past research, that one's personal experiences, including chronic illness, can shape the parameters of hopefulness. For example, in patients with breast cancer, poor quality of life and greater symptom burden were associated with less hope (Li et al., 2021; Moradi et al., 2020) and, in a sample of uninsured/underinsured adults, chronic illness was associated with reduced hope and, in turn, to lower health-related quality of life (Wippold & Roncoroni, 2020). Broadly, in a systematic review of literature on medical patients, Olsman (2020) noted that interpersonal well-being is associated with increased hope, that the loss of relationships and physical health are linked to reduced hope, and that hopefulness is linked to motivational processes and decision-making. Such patterns suggest a synergistic association between health and hope, perhaps throughout the lifespan, with cyclical influences as psychosocial and environmental experiences interact with biological and physiological processes across a lifetime.

It must be increasingly acknowledged that sociocultural and public health experiences can significantly impact goal-oriented and motivational well-being, and future research is needed to better understand the impact of such events on persons with chronic illness. Further, given that recent research has identified neurobiological correlates of hopefulness (e.g., cortical grey matter volume; amplitude of low-frequency fluctuations in left frontal pole cortex, which is responsible for directing cognitive resources toward new goal opportunities), future investigation of the neurodevelopmental interrelations between life experiences, positive psychological functioning, and chronic health conditions is a critical need (Wang et al., 2020; Xiang et al., 2021).

Clinical Implications

Hope-Focused Interventions. Previous research indicates that interventions designed to enhance hopefulness are successful and have beneficial downstream effects on health and well-being. For example, in a sample of rehabilitating adult cancer patients, a brief hope intervention designed to increase goal, pathway, and agency thoughts resulted in significant physical and psychological symptom improvement, including increased appetite and energy, and reduced pain (Chan et al., 2019). In patients with chronic pain, across two intervention studies, engagement in hope counseling resulted in increased hope and well-being and reduced pain catastrophizing (Howell et al., 2015). For patients with orofacial pain, participation in a hopefulness intervention resulted in increased hope, higher pain threshold, less heat pain sensitivity, and reduced pain catastrophizing (Bartley et al., 2019). Finally, in a sample of patients with metastatic breast cancer, participation in a hope-enhancement workshop resulted in increased hope scores (Shah et al., 2021).

Spiritual and Positive Psychological Interventions. Hope promotion also occurred after engagement in spiritual therapy, in a sample of Iranian patients with multiple sclerosis (Afshar et al., 2021), and in a sample of hemodialysis patients (Oshvandi et al., 2020). Similarly, engagement in Buddhist practice (e.g., meditation and observance of moral precepts) was related to increased hope in a sample of persons with HIV/AIDS (Rakhab et al., 2007). Using the PERMA model (i.e., a focus on positive emotion, engagement, relationships, meaning, and accomplishment), in a study of lung cancer patients undergoing chemotherapy, a positive psychological intervention resulted in increased hope, and decreased psychopathology and fatigue (Tu et al., 2021). Finally, a peer social support intervention resulted in increased hope in a sample of hemodialysis patients (Pasyar et al., 2020) and, in a randomized controlled trial (RCT), dignity therapy resulted in increased hope in patients with hematologic neoplasms (Chen et al., 2021).

Psychotherapeutic and Treatment-as-Usual Interventions. Mainstream therapies are also effective in promoting hopefulness, including in patients with chronic health conditions. For example, in samples of Iranian cardiovascular patients and adolescents with cancer in China, engagement in solution-focused therapy resulted in increased hopefulness (Abdollahi et al., 2020; Zhang et al., 2021b) and, in a sample of cancer patients, therapeutic training in cognitive-emotional regulation increased hopefulness (Abdollahi & Bardideh, 2020). Mindfulness-integrated cognitive-behavior therapy was effective in improving hope, and reducing depression and anxiety, in patients with multiple sclerosis (Pouyanfard et al., 2020), while positive behavior management resulted in increased hope and self-efficacy, better quality of life, and reduced psychopathology, in patients recovering from breast cancer (Hao et al., 2020).

Even routine treatment can promote hopefulness, making hope-based encouragement of treatment adherence a critical need. For example, for patients who experienced coronary artery bypass surgery, participation in a cardiac rehabilitation program involving education and counseling resulted in increased levels of hope (Rakhshan et al., 2020) and, in patients with venous leg ulcers, compression boot therapy improved hope (Faria et al., 2020). Hopefulness-based high-quality nursing, administered to patients undergoing surgical treatment for endometrial cancer, resulted in less fatigue, passive coping, and depression, and increased hopefulness, positive coping, self-efficacy, and health-related quality of life (Lei et al., 2021). Similarly, psychological intervention nursing care was associated with increased hope, and better general health and physical functioning, in patients undergoing knee arthroplasty (Yu & Liu, 2021), and with greater hope and treatment compliance in patients with rectal cancer (Sun et al., 2021). Passive efforts to promote hopefulness can also be effective; for example, in an RCT, the presence of a dedicated art gallery in the perioperative area for patients recovering from oncologic surgery resulted in less anxiety, and greater hope and well-being (Lone et al., 2021). Finally, although it seems intuitive that discussing end-of-life plans may erode hopefulness, a sample of terminally ill cancer patients reported greater hopefulness after receiving an end-of-life conversation, suggesting that it is never too late in the disease process to facilitate goal-directed thoughts and behaviors (Cohen et al., 2021).

Physiological Benefits of Hope Interventions. In addition to self-reported health functioning and quality of life, interventions that improve hopefulness also appear to beneficially impact physiological functioning, as assessed biometrically. For example, in an RCT of patients with temporomandibular disorder, a hope intervention was associated with increases in state and trait hope, and a reduction in cortisol levels (Hossain et al., 2018). Similarly, in an RCT with patients experiencing acute coronary syndrome, a spiritual intervention was associated with significant improvements in hope, which persisted at 3- and 6-month follow-up, and with improved stress, depression, and positive cardiovascular outcomes, including reductions in cholesterol, inflammatory biomarkers, and blood pressure (Warber et al., 2011). Finally, in a sample of cervical cancer patients, a psychological nursing intervention resulted in greater hope, less psychopathology, reduced cortisol, and increased interleukin-2, a marker of white blood cells that indicates greater immune function (Shi et al., 2021).

Conclusion

In sum, hopefulness is a positive psychological construct that is comprised of cognitive, emotional, motivational, and behavioral components, and which is focused on the identification and attainment of meaningful goals. Importantly, there is growing theoretical and empirical support for the role of hope in the context and trajectory of chronic illness, including salubrious effects on symptom management, treatment adherence, quality of life, immune functioning, and mortality. Across disease groups, including patients with fibromyalgia, chronic pain, cardiac disease, HIV/AIDS, and cancer, hope offers an adaptive and prospective view of the future that can facilitate coping and adjustment to illness. Indeed, in our original study of primary care patients, and persons with cancer and fibromyalgia, we found that hope was associated with an array of health-related benefits, including greater engagement in wellness behaviors, less stress and pain, and better physical functioning. Although rigorous, prospective research is needed, our findings and the extant literature may have implications for treatment, as they suggest that the therapeutic facilitation of hopefulness can contribute to the health and well-being of persons with chronic illness.

Sources of Funding There is no funding to report.

Conflict of Interest There are no conflicts of interest to report.

References

Abdollahi, A., Panahipour, H., Hosseinian, S., & Allen, K. A. (2019). The effects of perceived stress on hope in women with breast cancer and the role of psychological hardiness. *Psycho-Oncology, 28*(7), 1477–1482.

Abdollahi, S., & Bardideh, M. R. (2020). The effect of training emotional cognitive regulation on hopefulness and emotional well-being of cancer sufferers in Shiraz. *Journal of Advanced Pharmacy Education & Research, 10*(S4), 141.

Abdollahi, S. M., Rafiepoor, A., & Sabet, M. (2020). Effectiveness of solution-focused therapy in mental health and hopefulness among patients with cardiovascular diseases. *Avicenna Journal of Neuropsychophysiology, 7*(3), 145–150.

Afshar, M., Sadat, Z., & Bagheri, M. (2021). The effect of spiritual counseling on hope in patients with multiple sclerosis: A randomized clinical trial. *International Journal of Community Based Nursing & Midwifery, 9*(4), 313–324.

Alberto, J., & Joyner, B. (2008). Hope, optimism, and self-care among Better Breathers Support Group members with chronic obstructive pulmonary disease. *Applied Nursing Research, 21*(4), 212–217. https://doi.org/10.1016/j.apnr.2006.12.005

Alshraifeen, A., Al-Rawashdeh, S., Herth, K., Alnuaimi, K., Alzoubi, F., Khraim, F., & Ashour, A. (2020). The association between hope and quality of life in haemodialysis patients. *British Journal of Nursing, 29*(21), 1260–1265.

Alves Moreira, R., & da Silva Borges, M. (2020). Profile and level of hope in patients undergoing hemodialysis and peritoneal dialysis. *Cogitare Enfermagem, 25.*

Asante, K. O. (2012). Social support and the psychological wellbeing of people living with HIV/AIDS in Ghana. *African Journal of Psychiatry, 15*(5), 340–345.

Baczewska, B., Block, B., Kropornicka, B., Malm, M., Musiał, D., Makara-Studzińska, M., & Zwolak, A. (2020). Hope in advanced cancer patients in the terminal phase of neoplastic disease and stability of basic mood. *Journal of Clinical Medicine, 9*(11), 3550.

Bandura, A. (1982). Self-efficacy mechanism in human agency. *American Psychologist, 37*(2), 122–147. https://doi.org/10.1037/0003-066X.37.2.122

Bartley, E. J., LaGattuta, N. R., Robinson, M. E., & Fillingim, R. B. (2019). Optimizing resilience in orofacial pain: a randomized controlled pilot study on hope. *Pain Reports, 4*(2), e726.

Beck, A. T., Weissman, A., Lester, D., & Trexler, L. (1974). The measurement of pessimism: The Hopelessness Scale. *Journal of Consulting and Clinical Psychology, 42*(6), 861–865. https://doi.org/10.1037/h0037562

Bennett, R. M., Friend, R., Jones, K. D., Ward, R., Han, B. K., & Ross, R. L. (2009). The Revised Fibromyalgia Impact Questionnaire (FIQR): Validation and psychometric properties. *Arthritis Research & Therapy, 11*(4), R120. https://doi.org/10.1186/ar2783

Berg, C., Rapoff, M., Snyder, C., & Belmont, J. (2007). The relationship of children's hope to pediatric asthma treatment adherence. *The Journal of Positive Psychology, 2*(3), 176–184. https://doi.org/10.1080/17439760701409629

Berg, C. J., Thomas, A. N., Mertens, A. C., Schauer, G. L., Pinsker, E. A., Ahluwalia, J. S., & Khuri, F. R. (2013). Correlates of continued smoking versus cessation among survivors of smoking-related cancers: Smoking and cancer survivorship. *Psycho-Oncology, 22*(4), 799–806. https://doi.org/10.1002/pon.3077

Billington, E., Simpson, J., Unwin, J., Bray, D., & Giles, D. (2008). Does hope predict adjustment to end-stage renal failure and consequent dialysis? *British Journal of Health Psychology, 13*(4), 683–699.

Bohn, M. J., Babor, T. F., & Kranzler, H. R. (1995). The Alcohol Use Disorders Identification Test (AUDIT): Validation of a screening instrument for use in medical settings. *Journal of Studies on Alcohol, 56*(4), 423–432.

Bossola, M., Angioletti, L., Di Stasio, E., Vulpio, C., De Filippis, D., & Balconi, M. (2020). Reward (BIS/BAS) mechanisms and fatigue in patients on chronic hemodialysis. *Psychology, Health & Medicine, 25*(6), 710–718.

Bovero, A., Opezzo, M., Botto, R., Gottardo, F., & Torta, R. (2021). Hope in end-of-life cancer patients: A cross-sectional analysis. *Palliative & Supportive Care*, 1–7.

Brandstätter, V., Herrmann, M., & Schüler, J. (2013). The struggle of giving up personal goals: Affective, physiological, and cognitive consequences of an action crisis. *Personality and Social Psychology Bulletin, 39*(12), 1668–1682.

Brown, A. J., Thaker, P. H., Sun, C. C., Urbauer, D. L., Bruera, E., Bodurka, D. C., & Ramondetta, L. M. (2017). Nothing left to chance? The impact of locus of control on physical and mental quality of life in terminal cancer patients. *Supportive Care in Cancer, 25*(6), 1985–1991.

Bryant, F. B., & Cvengros, J. A. (2004). Distinguishing hope and optimism: Two sides of a coin, or two separate coins? *Journal of Social and Clinical Psychology, 23*(2), 273–302. https://doi.org/10.1521/jscp.23.2.273.31018

Bury, S. M., Wenzel, M., & Woodyatt, L. (2016). Giving hope a sporting chance: Hope as distinct from optimism when events are possible but not probable. *Motivation and Emotion, 40*(4), 588–601. https://doi.org/10.1007/s11031-016-9560-z

Byrne, C. M., & Morgan, D. D. (2020). Patterns of religiosity, death anxiety, and hope in a population of community-dwelling palliative care patients in new Zealand—What gives hope if religion can't? *American Journal of Hospice and Palliative Medicine, 37*(5), 377–384.

Chan, K., Wong, F. K. Y., & Lee, P. H. (2019). A brief hope intervention to increase hope level and improve well-being in rehabilitating cancer patients: A feasibility test. *SAGE Open Nursing, 5*, 1–13. https://doi.org/10.1177/2377960819844381

Chang, E. C. (2017). Hope and hopelessness as predictors of suicide ideation in Hungarian college students. *Death Studies, 41*(7), 455–460. https://doi.org/10.1080/07481187.2017.1299255

Chang, E. C., Lucas, A. G., Chang, O. D., Angoff, H. D., Li, M., Duong, A. H., et al. (2019). Relationship between future orientation and pain severity in fibromyalgia patients: Self-compassion as a coping mechanism. *Social Work, 64*(3), 253–258.

Chen, J., Yan, J., Wang, C., Wang, Y., Wu, Y., & Hu, R. (2021). Effects and satisfaction of dignity therapy among patients with hematologic neoplasms in the Chinese cultural context: a randomized controlled trial. *Supportive Care in Cancer*, 1–11.

Clarke, G., Johnston, S., Corrie, P., Kuhn, I., & Barclay, S. (2015). Withdrawal of anticancer therapy in advanced disease: A systematic literature review. *BMC Cancer, 15*, 892. https://doi.org/10.1186/s12885-015-1862-0

Coduti, W. A., Eissenstat, S. J., & Conyers, L. M. (2018). Linking hope factors, barriers to employment and health outcomes for individuals living with Human Immunodeficiency Virus (HIV). *Work, 61*(2), 225–236. https://doi.org/10.3233/WOR-182794

Cohen, M., Althouse, A., Chu, E., Arnold, R. M., White, D. B., Rosenzweig, M. Q., Bulls, H. W., Smith, K., & Schenker, Y. (2021). The impact of advance care planning on hope among patients with advanced cancer. *Journal of Clinical Oncology, 39*(15), 12029–12029.

Cohen, S., Kamarck, T., & Mermelstein, R. (1983). A global measure of perceived stress. *Journal of Health and Social Behavior, 24*, 385–396. https://doi.org/10.2307/2136404

Coleman, S., Berg, C. J., & Thompson, N. J. (2014). Social support, nutrition intake, and physical activity in cancer survivors. *American Journal of Health Behavior, 38*(3), 414–419. https://doi.org/10.5993/AJHB.38.3.10

Corn, B. W., Feldman, D. B., & Wexler, I. (2020). The science of hope. *The Lancet Oncology, 21*(9), e452–e459.

De Maria, M., Tagliabue, S., Ausili, D., Vellone, E., & Matarese, M. (2020). Perceived social support and health-related quality of life in older adults who have multiple chronic conditions and their caregivers: A dyadic analysis. *Social Science & Medicine, 262*, 113193.

Do, D. P., Beam Dowd, J., Ranjit, N., House, J. S., & Kaplan, G. A. (2010). Hopelessness, depression, and early markers of endothelial dysfunction in U.S. adults. *Psychosomatic Medicine, 72*(7), 613–619. https://doi.org/10.1097/PSY.0b013e3181e2cca5

Dong, M., Nie, A., Liu, C., & Zheng, J. (2021). Psychological resilience of patients with bladder cancer after radical cystectomy and urinary diversion: A cross-sectional study. *Psycho-Oncology, 31*(1), 21–29. https://doi.org/10.1002/pon.5770

Donnelley, M. (2019). Functional mastery in patients with inflammatory bowel disease. *Research and Theory for Nursing Practice, 33*(4), 410–427.

Duggleby, W. D., Degner, L., Williams, A., Wright, K., Cooper, D., Popkin, D., & Holtslander, L. (2007). Living with hope: Initial evaluation of a psychosocial hope intervention for older palliative home care patients. *Journal of Pain and Symptom*

Management, 33(3), 247–257. https://doi.org/10.1016/j.jpainsymman.2006.09.013

Dunn, S. L., DeVon, H. A., Buursma, M. P., Boven, E., & Tintle, N. L. (2020). Reliability and validity of the State-Trait Hopelessness Scale in patients with heart disease and moderate to severe hopelessness. *Journal of Cardiovascular Nursing, 35*(2), 126–130.

Eriksson, M., Asplund, K., Hochwälder, J., & Svedlund, M. (2013). Changes in hope and health-related quality of life in couples following acute myocardial infarction: A quantitative longitudinal study. *Scandinavian Journal of Caring Sciences, 27*(2), 295–302. https://doi.org/10.1111/j.1471-6712.2012.01032.x

Everson, S. A., Goldberg, D. E., Kaplan, G. A., Cohen, R. D., Pukkala, E., Tuomilehto, J., & Salonen, J. T. (1996). Hopelessness and risk of mortality and incidence of myocardial infarction and cancer. *Psychosomatic Medicine, 58*(2), 113–121. https://doi.org/10.1097/00006842-199603000-00003

Faria, E. C., Loiola, T., Salomé, G. M., & Ferreira, L. M. (2020). Unna boot therapy impact on wellbeing, hope and spirituality in venous leg ulcer patients: A prospective clinical trial. *Journal of Wound Care, 29*(4), 214–220.

Feldman, D. B., Kasl-Godley, J., Khouzam, A., Pisca, N. E., Cabrera, A. P., & Donboli, M. (2008). In W. Bauman (Ed.), *From cure to quality of life: The shifting meaning of hope at the end of life* (pp. 133–146). Inter-Disciplinary Press.

Feldman, D. B., & von Garnier, S. (2018). Nurturing hope: Tools for cultivating hopeful thinking and a meaningful life. In T. Plante (Ed.), *Healing with spiritual practices: Proven techniques for disorders from addictions and anxiety to cancer and chronic pain* (pp. 14–26). ABC-Clio.

Finkelstein, E. A., Baid, D., Cheung, Y. B., Schweitzer, M. E., Malhotra, C., Volpp, K., et al. (2021). Hope, bias and survival expectations of advanced cancer patients: A cross-sectional study. *Psycho-Oncology, 30*(5), 780–788.

Fradelos, E. (2020). Predictors of quality of life in chronic kidney disease: The contribution of spirituality. *Archives of Hellenic Medicine, 37*(2), 227–236.

Frankl, V. E. (2004). *Man's search for meaning: The classic tribute to hope from the Holocaust.* Random House.

Galvez-Sánchez, C. M., Duschek, S., & Del Paso, G. A. R. (2019). Psychological impact of fibromyalgia: Current perspectives. *Psychology Research and Behavior Management, 12*, 117.

Gravlee, G. S. (2020). Hope in ancient Greek philosophy. In S. C. van den Heuvel (Ed.), *Historical and multidisciplinary perspectives on hope* (pp. 3–23). Springer International Publishing. https://doi.org/10.1007/978-3-030-46489-9_1

Griggs, S., & Walker, R. K. (2016). The role of hope for adolescents with a chronic illness: An integrative review. *Journal of Pediatric Nursing, 31*(4), 404–421.

Hao, Y. J., Sun, H. B., Li, H. W., Chen, B. J., Chen, X. L., Ma, L., & Li, Y. L. (2020). Application of positive behavior management in patients after breast cancer surgery. *World Journal of Clinical Cases, 8*(4), 689.

Haviland, J., Sodergren, S., Calman, L., Corner, J., Din, A., Fenlon, D., et al. (2017). Social support following diagnosis and treatment for colorectal cancer and associations with health-related quality of life: Results from the UK ColoREctal Wellbeing (CREW) cohort study. *Psycho-Oncology, 26*(12), 2276–2284.

Hawro, T., Maurer, M., Hawro, M., Kaszuba, A., Cierpiałkowska, L., Królikowska, M., & Zalewska, A. (2014). In psoriasis, levels of hope and quality of life are linked. *Archives of Dermatological Research, 306*(7), 661–666. https://doi.org/10.1007/s00403-014-1455-9

Henry, J. D., & Crawford, J. R. (2005). The short-form version of the Depression Anxiety Stress Scales (DASS-21): Construct validity and normative data in a large non-clinical sample. *The British Journal of Clinical Psychology, 44*(Pt 2), 227–239. https://doi.org/10.1348/014466505X29657

Herth, K. (1990). Fostering hope in terminally-ill people. *Journal of Advanced Nursing, 15*(11), 1250–1259. https://doi.org/10.1111/j.1365-2648.1990.tb01740.x

Herth, K. (1991). Development and refinement of an instrument to measure hope. *Scholarly Inquiry for Nursing Practice, 5*(1), 39–56.

Herth, K. (1992). Abbreviated instrument to measure hope: Development and psychometric evaluation. *Journal of Advanced Nursing, 17*(10), 1251–1259. https://doi.org/10.1111/j.1365-2648.1992.tb01843.x

Hill, D. L., & Feudnter, C. (2018). Hope in the midst of terminal illness. In M. Gallagher & S. Lopez (Eds.), *The Oxford handbook of hope*. Oxford University Press.

Hill, D. L., Miller, V., Walter, J. K., Carroll, K. W., Morrison, W. E., Munson, D. A., et al. (2014). Regoaling: A conceptual model of how parents of children with serious illness change medical care goals. *BMC Palliative Care, 13*(1), 1–8.

Hirsch, J. K., Duberstein, P., Conner, K. R., Heisel, M. J., Beckman, A., & Conwell, Y. (2006). Future orientation and suicide ideation and attempts in depressed adults ages 50 and over. *American Journal of Geriatric Psychiatry, 14*, 752–757. https://doi.org/10.1097/01.JGP.0000209219.06017.62

Hirsch, J. K., Molnar, D., Chang, E. C., & Sirois, F. M. (2015). Future orientation and health quality of life in primary care: Vitality as a mediator. *Quality of Life Research, 24*(7), 1653–1659. https://doi.org/10.1007/s11136-014-0901-7

Hirsch, J. K., & Sirois, F. M. (2016). Hope and fatigue in chronic illness: The role of perceived stress. *Journal of Health Psychology, 21*(4), 451–456. https://doi.org/10.1177/1359105314527142

Hirsch, J. K., Visser, P. L., Chang, E. C., & Jeglic, E. L. (2012). Race and ethnic differences in hope and hopelessness as moderators of the association between depressive symptoms and suicidal behavior. *Journal of American College Health, 60*(2), 115–125. https://doi.org/10.1080/07448481.2011.567402

Hood, A., Pulvers, K., Carrillo, J., Merchant, G., & Thomas, M. D. (2012). Positive traits linked to less pain through lower pain catastrophizing. *Personality and*

Individual Differences, 52(3), 401–405. https://doi.org/10.1016/j.paid.2011.10.040

Horter, S., Stringer, B., Greig, J., Amangeldiev, A., Tillashaikhov, M. N., Parpieva, N., Tigay, Z., & du Cros, P. (2016). Where there is hope: A qualitative study examining patients' adherence to multi-drug resistant tuberculosis treatment in Karakalpakstan, Uzbekistan. *BMC Infectious Diseases, 16*, 362. https://doi.org/10.1186/s12879-016-1723-8

Hossain, N. I., Robinson, M. E., Fillingim, R. B., & Bartley, E. J. (2018). Examining the impact of a resilience-based hope intervention on pain-evoked cortisol response. *Journal of Undergraduate Research (Gainesville, Fla.), 19*(2) https://ufdc.ufl.edu/UF00091523/00858

Howell, A. J., Jacobson, R. M., & Larsen, D. J. (2015). Enhanced psychological health among chronic pain clients engaged in hope-focused group counseling. *The Counseling Psychologist, 43*(4), 586–613. https://doi.org/10.1177/0011000014551421

Huen, J. M. Y., Ip, B. Y. T., Ho, S. M. Y., & Yip, P. S. F. (2015). Hope and hopelessness: The role of hope in buffering the impact of hopelessness on suicidal ideation. *PLOS ONE, 10*(6), e0130073. https://doi.org/10.1371/journal.pone.0130073

Jimenez, X. F. (2017). Attachment in medical care: A review of the interpersonal model in chronic disease management. *Chronic Illness, 13*(1), 14–27.

Kaiser, P., Allen, N., Delaney, J. A., Hirsch, C. H., Carnethon, M., Arnold, A. M., & Odden, M. C. (2020). The association of prediagnosis social support with survival after heart failure in the Cardiovascular Health Study. *Annals of Epidemiology, 42*, 73–77.

Karoly, P., Ruehlman, L. S., & Lanyon, R. I. (2005). The assessment of adult health care orientations: Development and preliminary validation of the Multidimensional Health Profile-Health Functioning Index (MHP-H) in a national sample. *Journal of Clinical Psychology in Medical Settings, 12*(1), 79–91. https://doi.org/10.1007/s10880-005-0915-y

Kim, S. W., Kim, S. Y., Kim, J. M., Park, M. H., Yoon, J. H., Shin, M. G., et al. (2011). Relationship between a hopeful attitude and cellular immunity in patients with breast cancer. *General Hospital Psychiatry, 33*(4), 371–376.

Klein, D. E., Winterowd, C. L., Ehrhardt, M. D., Carter, J. C., Khan, O., & Mayes, S. (2020). The relationship of self-compassion and hope with quality of life for individuals with bleeding disorders. *Haemophilia, 26*(3), e66–e73.

Kortte, K. B., Stevenson, J. E., Hosey, M. M., Castillo, R., & Wegener, S. T. (2012). Hope predicts positive functional role outcomes in acute rehabilitation populations. *Rehabilitation Psychology, 57*(3), 248–255. https://doi.org/10.1037/a0029004

Koutsogeorgou, E., Chiesi, A. M., & Leonardi, M. (2020). Social capital components and social support of persons with multiple sclerosis: A systematic review of the literature from 2000 to 2018. *Disability and Rehabilitation, 42*(24), 3437–3449.

Krafft, A. M., Guse, T., & Maree, D. (2021). Distinguishing perceived hope and dispositional optimism: Theoretical foundations and empirical findings beyond future expectancies and cognition. *Journal of Well-Being Assessment*, 1–27.

Kurita, N., Wakita, T., Ishibashi, Y., Fujimoto, S., Yazawa, M., Suzuki, T., Koitabashi, K., Yanagi, M., Kawarazaki, H., Green, J., Fukuhara, S., & Shibagaki, Y. (2020). Association between health-related hope and adherence to prescribed treatment in CKD patients: Multicenter cross-sectional study. *BMC Nephrology, 21*(1), 453. https://doi.org/10.1186/s12882-020-02120-0

Lawton, M. P., & Brody, E. M. (1988a). Instrumental activities of daily living (IADL): Original observer-rated version. *Psychopharmacology Bulletin, 24*, 785–791.

Lawton, M. P., & Brody, E. M. (1988b). Physical self-maintenance scale (PSMS): Original observer- related version. *Psychopharmacology Bulletin, 24*, 793–797.

Lei, R., Cao, H., Rao, A., & Zhang, H. (2021). Application effect of high-quality nursing model based on hope theory in endometrial cancer patients. *Clinical and Experimental Obstetrics & Gynecology, 48*(3), 691–696.

Li, Y., Ni, N., Zhou, Z., Dong, J., Fu, Y., Li, J., et al. (2021). Hope and symptom burden of women with breast cancer undergoing chemotherapy: A cross-sectional study. *Journal of Clinical Nursing, 30*, 2293–2300.

Linehan, M. M., Goodstein, L. J., Nielsen, S. L., & Chiles, J. A. (1983). Reasons for staying alive when you are thinking of killing yourself: The reasons for living inventory. *Journal of Consulting and Clinical Psychology, 51*, 276–286.

Lone, Z., Hussein, A. A., Khan, H., Steele, M., Jing, Z., Attwood, K., et al. (2021). Art heals: Randomized controlled study investigating the effect of a dedicated in-house art gallery on the recovery of patients after major oncologic surgery. *Annals of Surgery, 274*(2), 264–270.

Lopez, R. B., Denny, B. T., & Fagundes, C. P. (2018). Neural mechanisms of emotion regulation and their role in endocrine and immune functioning: A review with implications for treatment of affective disorders. *Neuroscience & Biobehavioral Reviews, 95*, 508–514.

Lucas, A. G., Chang, E. C., Morris, L. E., Angoff, H. D., Chang, O. D., Duong, A. H., Li, M., & Hirsch, J. K. (2019). Relationship between hope and quality of life in primary care patients: Vitality as a mechanism. *Social Work, 64*(3), 233–241. https://doi.org/10.1093/sw/swz014

Luo, B. J., Zheng, M. C., Zhang, J. E., Jiang, M. X., Pan, Z. Z., Wan, D. S., et al. (2018). Stoma self-efficacy, hope and social relationships among patients with permanent colostomy. *World Council of Enterostomal Therapists Journal, 38*(1), 12–20.

Madan, S., & Pakenham, K. I. (2014). The stress-buffering effects of hope on adjustment to multiple sclerosis. *International Journal of Behavioral Medicine, 21*(6), 877–890.

Magaletta, P. R., & Oliver, J. M. (1999). The hope construct, will, and ways: Their relations with self-efficacy, optimism, and general well-being. *Journal of Clinical Psychology, 55*(5), 539–551.

Makarem, S. C. (2016). Emotions and cognitions in consumer health behaviors: Insights from chronically ill patients into the effects of hope and control perceptions. *Journal of Consumer Behaviour, 15*(3), 208–215.

Malak, M. Z., Tawalbeh, L. I., & Al-Amer, R. M. (2021). Depressive symptoms among older Jordanian patients with cancer undergoing treatment. *Clinical Gerontologist, 44*(2), 133–142.

Marcus, E., Turchinsky, A., Naydich, A., Cohen-Goichman, P., & Adler, E. (2017). Hope in the nursing home: Relation with quality of life, function, pain, social support, religiosity. *Innovation in Aging, 1*(Suppl 1), 854.

Mardhiyah, A., Philip, K., Mediani, H. S., & Yosep, I. (2020). The association between hope and quality of life among adolescents with chronic diseases: A systematic review. *Child Health Nursing Research, 26*(3), 323–328.

Martins, A. R., Crespo, C., Salvador, Á., Santos, S., Carona, C., & Canavarro, M. C. (2018). Does hope matter? Associations among self-reported hope, anxiety, and health-related quality of life in children and adolescents with cancer. *Journal of Clinical Psychology in Medical Settings, 25*(1), 93–103. https://doi.org/10.1007/s10880-018-9547-x

Mayer, S., Fuchs, S., Fink, M., Schäffeler, N., Zipfel, S., Geiser, F., et al. (2021). Hope and distress are not associated with the brain tumor stage. *Frontiers in Psychology, 12*, 1844.

Mazzotti, E., Costantini, A., & Lamacchia, L. (2020). Reliability and validity of the Italian version of the HOPE scale in a sample of cancer patients. *Journal of Cancer Research and Therapeutics, 1*, 1–6.

Megari, K. (2013). Quality of life in chronic disease patients. *Health Psychology Research, 1*(3), e27. https://doi.org/10.4081/hpr.2013.e27

Mendes, N. S., Malaguti, C., dos Anjos Sena, L., Lucchetti, G., de Jesus, L. A. S., Vitorino, L. M., et al. (2021). Spirituality and religiosity are associated with physical and psychological status in patients with chronic obstructive pulmonary disease. *Journal of Clinical Nursing, 31*, 669–678.

Miaomiao, L. I., Pengfei, X. U., & Wei, L. U. (2020). Correlation between volume-management behaviors, illness perception and hope level of peritoneal dialysis patients. *Chinese Journal of Integrative Nursing, 6*(10), 53.

Miller, J. F., & Powers, M. J. (1988). Development of an instrument to measure hope. *Nursing Research, 37*(1), 6–10. https://doi.org/10.1097/00006199-198801000-00002

Moradi, F., Salehi, M., Kochak Entezar, R., & Ezanloo, B. (2020). Hopefulness prediction modeling based on resilience and cognitive emotional regulation considering the mediating of quality of life in women with breast cancer. *Scientific Journal of Social Psychology, 8*(56), 45–56.

Namvar, H., & Ghasedi, M. (2020). Interpersonal dependency and social support as the predictors of resilience among hypertensive patients with the mediating role of hope. *Qom University of Medical Sciences Journal, 14*(7), 31–39.

Nazam, F., Husain, A., Devi, S., & Singh, R. K. (2021). An interpretive phenomenological analysis of hope in cancer patients: A qualitative study. *Indian Journal of Cancer, 60*(1), 32–36.

Nekolaichuk, C. L., Jevne, R. F., & Maguire, T. O. (1999). Structuring the meaning of hope in health and illness. *Social Science & Medicine, 48*(5), 591–605.

Nierop-van Baalen, C., Grypdonck, M., Hecke, A., & Verhaeghe, S. (2020). Associated factors of hope in cancer patients during treatment: A systematic literature review. *Journal of Advanced Nursing, 76*(7), 1520–1537. https://doi.org/10.1111/jan.14344

Nothwehr, F., Clark, D. O., & Perkins, A. (2013). Hope and the use of behavioural strategies related to diet and physical activity. *Journal of Human Nutrition and Dietetics, 26*, 159–163. https://doi.org/10.1111/jhn.12057

Nowotny, M. L. (1989). Assessment of hope in patients with cancer: Development of an instrument. *Oncology Nursing Forum, 16*(1), 57–61.

Nsamenang, S. A., & Hirsch, J. K. (2015). Positive psychological determinants of treatment adherence among primary care patients. *Primary Health Care Research & Development, 16*(04), 398–406. https://doi.org/10.1017/S1463423614000292

Olsman, E. (2020). Hope in health care: A synthesis of review studies. In S. C. van den Heuvel (Ed.), *Historical and multidisciplinary perspectives on hope* (pp. 197–214). Springer Open.

Oniszczenko, W., Bitner-Szulc, J., Szylberg, A., Kuczko-Piekarska, E., Zaborowska, M., & Wawrzyniak, S. (2018). Mental health and BIS/BAS dimensions in Parkinson's disease and multiple sclerosis patients and in stroke survivors. *Personality and Individual Differences, 132*, 1–5.

Oshvandi, K., Amini, S., Moghimbeigi, A., & Sadeghian, E. (2020). The effect of a spiritual care on hope in patients undergoing hemodialysis: A randomized controlled trial. *Current Psychiatry Research and Reviews Formerly: Current Psychiatry Reviews, 16*(1), 68–75.

Ota, H., Ueta, I., & Ono, M. (2020). The hopes of lung cancer patients receiving chemotherapy. *Kawasaki Journal of Medical Welfare, 26*(1), 9–21.

Parenteau, S. C., Gallant, S., Sarosiek, I., & McCallum, R. W. (2006). The role of hope in the psychological adjustment of gastropareutic patients receiving the gastric pacemaker: A longitudinal study. *Journal of Clinical Psychology in Medical Settings, 13*(1), 46–53. https://doi.org/10.1007/s10880-005-9005-4

Pasyar, N., Rambod, M., & Jowkar, M. (2020). The effect of peer support on hope among patients under hemodialysis. *International Journal of Nephrology and Renovascular Disease, 13*, 37.

Pazokian, M., Beigmoradi, S., Movafegh, F., & Akbarzadeh, S. (2020). Correlation between social support and hope with medication adherence in Type II diabetic patients. *Archives of Pharmacy Practice, 1*, 130.

Perry, J., Chen, A., Kariyawasam, V., Collins, G., Choong, C., Teh, W. L., Mitrev, N., Kohler, F., & Leong, R. (2018). Medication non-adherence in inflammatory bowel diseases is associated with disability. *Intestinal Research, 16*(4), 571–578. https://doi.org/10.5217/ir.2018.00033

Pössel, P., Mitchell, A. M., Sjögren, E., & Kristenson, M. (2015). Do depressive symptoms mediate the relationship between hopelessness and diurnal cortisol rhythm? *International Journal of Behavioral Medicine, 22*(2), 251–257. https://doi.org/10.1007/s12529-014-9422-6

Pouyanfard, S., Mohammadpour, M., ParviziFard, A. A., & Sadeghi, K. (2020). Effectiveness of mindfulness-integrated cognitive behavior therapy on anxiety, depression and hope in multiple sclerosis patients: a randomized clinical trial. *Trends in Psychiatry and Psychotherapy, 42*, 55–63.

Price, M. A., Butow, P. N., Bell, M. L., de Fazio, A., Friedlander, M., Fardell, J. E., Protani, M. M., Webb, P. M., & AOCS—Quality of Life Study Investigators on behalf of the Australian Ovarian Cancer Study Group. (2016). Helplessness/hopelessness, minimization and optimism predict survival in women with invasive ovarian cancer: A role for targeted support during initial treatment decision-making? *Supportive Care in Cancer, 24*(6), 2627–2634. https://doi.org/10.1007/s00520-015-3070-5

Rahimi, H., Ebrahimi, S., & Baseri, A. (2021). The relationship between the meaning of life and hope with mental health and its comparison in disabled veterans and patients suffering from cancer. *Military Psychology, 11*(42), 31–41.

Rakhab, A., Thaniwattananon, P., Nilmanut, K., & Apichato, A. (2007). Buddhist practice, health perception and hope in persons with HIV infection/AIDS. *Songklanagarind Medical Journal, 25*(4), 259–271.

Rakhshan, M., Toufigh, A., Dehghani-Firouzabadi, A., & Yektatalab, S. (2020). Effect of cardiac rehabilitation on hope among cardiac patients after coronary artery bypass graft surgery. *Risk Management and Healthcare Policy, 13*, 1319.

Rashidi, M., Khodabakhshi-koolaee, A., & Vahedian Ardakani, H. (2019). Comparison of spiritual experiences and hope between breast cancer survivors and healthy counterparts. *Journal of Clinical and Basic Research, 3*(2), 21–26.

Rasmussen, H. N., O'Byrne, K. K., Vandament, M., & Cole, B. P. (2018). Hope and physical health. In M. W. Gallagher & S. J. Lopez (Eds.), *Oxford library of psychology. The Oxford handbook of hope* (pp. 159–168). Oxford University Press.

Richman, L. S., Kubzansky, L., Maselko, J., Kawachi, I., Choo, P., & Bauer, M. (2005). Positive emotion and health: Going beyond the negative. *Health Psychology, 24*(4), 422.

Rowe, C. A., Sirois, F. M., Toussaint, L., Kohls, N., Nöfer, E., Offenbächer, M., & Hirsch, J. K. (2019). Health beliefs, attitudes, and health-related quality of life in persons with fibromyalgia: Mediating role of treatment adherence. *Psychology, Health & Medicine, 24*(8), 962–977.

Ruehlman, L. S., Lanyon, R. I., & Karoly, P. (1999). Development and validation of the Multidimensional Health Profile, Part I: Psychosocial functioning. *Psychological Assessment, 11*(2), 166–176. https://doi.org/10.1037/1040-3590.11.2.166

Rustøen, T., Lerdal, A., Gay, C., & Kottorp, A. (2018). Rasch analysis of the Herth Hope Index in cancer patients. *Health and Quality of Life Outcomes, 16*(1). https://doi.org/10.1186/s12955-018-1025-5

Ryan, R. M., & Frederick, C. M. (1997). On energy, personality and health: Subjective vitality as a dynamic reflection of well-being. *Journal of Personality, 65*, 529–565. https://doi.org/10.1111/j.1467-6494.1997.tb00326.x

Sachs, E., Kolva, E., Pessin, H., Rosenfeld, B., & Breitbart, W. (2013). On sinking and swimming: The dialectic of hope, hopelessness, and acceptance in terminal cancer. *American Journal of Hospice and Palliative Medicine, 30*(2), 121–127.

Sánchez-Rodríguez, E., Racine, M., Castarlenas, E., Tomé-Pires, C., Galán, S., Jensen, M. P., & Miró, J. (2021). Behavioral activation and inhibition systems: Further evaluation of a BIS-BAS model of chronic pain. *Pain Medicine, 22*(4), 848–860.

Santos, F. R., Sigulem, D., Areco, K. C., Gabbay, M. A., Dib, S. A., & Bernardo, V. (2015). Hope matters to the glycemic control of adolescents and young adults with type 1 diabetes. *Journal of Health Psychology, 20*(5), 681–689. https://doi.org/10.1177/1359105315573429

Scheier, M. F., & Carver, C. S. (1985). Optimism, coping, and health: Assessment and implications of generalized outcome expectancies. *Health Psychology, 4*(3), 219–247. https://doi.org/10.1037/0278-6133.4.3.219

Schiavon, C. C., Marchetti, E., Gurgel, L. G., Busnello, F. M., & Reppold, C. T. (2017). Optimism and hope in chronic disease: A systematic review. *Frontiers in Psychology, 7*. https://doi.org/10.3389/fpsyg.2016.02022

Scioli, A., MacNeil, S., Partridge, V., Tinker, E., & Hawkins, E. (2012). Hope, HIV and health: A prospective study. *AIDS Care, 24*(2), 149–156. https://doi.org/10.1080/09540121.2011.597943

Scioli, A., Ricci, M., Nyugen, T., & Scioli, E. R. (2011). Hope: Its nature and measurement. *Psychology of Religion and Spirituality, 3*(2), 78–97. https://doi.org/10.1037/a0020903

Scioli, A., Scioli-Salter, E. R., Sykes, K., Anderson, C., & Fedele, M. (2016). The positive contributions of hope to maintaining and restoring health: An integrative, mixed-method approach. *The Journal of Positive Psychology, 11*(2), 135–148. https://doi.org/10.1080/17439760.2015.1037858

Seligman, M. E. P. (1991). *Optimism*. Knopf.

Serrano-Ibáñez, E. R., López-Martínez, A. E., Ramírez-Maestre, C., Esteve, R., & Jensen, M. P. (2019). The behavioral inhibition and activation systems and function in patients with chronic pain. *Personality and Individual Differences, 138*, 56–62.

Shah, M., Ferguson, A., Corn, P. D., Varadhan, R., Ariely, D., Stearns, V., et al. (2021). Developing workshops to enhance hope among patients with metastatic breast cancer and oncologists: A pilot study. *JCO Oncology Practice, 17*(6), e785–e793.

Shanahan, M. L., Fischer, I. C., Hirsh, A. T., Stewart, J. C., & Rand, K. L. (2021). Hope, optimism, and clinical pain: A meta-analysis. *Annals of Behavioral Medicine, 55*(9), 815–832.

Sharour, L. A., Omari, O. A., Salameh, A. B., & Yehia, D. (2020). Health-related quality of life among patients with colorectal cancer. *Journal of Research in Nursing, 25*(2), 114–125.

Shen, A., Qiang, W., Wang, Y., & Chen, Y. (2020). Quality of life among breast cancer survivors with triple negative breast cancer—Role of hope, self-efficacy and social support. *European Journal of Oncology Nursing, 46*, 101771.

Sherbourne, C. D., Hays, R. D., Ordway, L., DiMatteo, M. R., & Kravitz, R. L. (1992). Antecedents of adherence to medical recommendations: Results from the Medical Outcomes Study. *Journal of Behavioral Medicine, 15*(5), 447–468. https://doi.org/10.1007/BF00844941

Shi, X., Ma, L., Hao, J., & Yan, W. (2021). Regulatory effects of comprehensive psychological intervention on adverse emotions and immune status of cervical cancer patients during the perioperative period. *American Journal of Translational Research, 13*(6), 6362.

Sirois, F. M. (2001). *The wellness behaviors inventory.* Unpublished manual. Psychology. University of Sheffield, UK.

Sirois, F. M. (2019). *The wellness behaviors inventory.* Unpublished manual. Psychology. University of Sheffield, UK.

Skinner, H. A. (1982). The Drug Abuse Screening Test. *Addictive Behaviors, 7*(4), 363–371.

Snyder, C. R. (1998). A case for hope in pain, loss and suffering. In J. Harvey (Ed.), *Perspectives on loss: A sourcebook* (pp. 63–80), (5427), 63. Brunner / Mazel.

Snyder, C. R. (2002). Hope theory: Rainbows in the mind. *Psychological Inquiry, 13*(4), 249–275. https://doi.org/10.1207/S15327965PLI1304_01

Snyder, C. R., Cheavens, J., & Sympson, S. C. (1997). Hope: An individual motive for social commerce. *Group Dynamics: Theory, Research, and Practice, 1*(2), 107–118. https://doi.org/10.1037/1089-2699.1.2.107

Snyder, C. R., Feldman, D. B., Taylor, J. D., Schroeder, L. L., & Adams, V. H. (2000). The roles of hopeful thinking in preventing problems and enhancing strengths. *Applied and Preventive Psychology, 9*(4), 249–269. https://doi.org/10.1016/S0962-1849(00)80003-7

Snyder, C. R., Harris, C., Anderson, J. R., Holleran, S. A., Irving, L. M., Sigmon, S. T., Yoshinobu, L., Gibb, J., Langelle, C., & Harney, P. (1991a). The will and the ways: Development and validation of an individual-differences measure of hope. *Journal of Personality and Social Psychology, 60*(4), 570–585. https://doi.org/10.1037/0022-3514.60.4.570

Snyder, C. R., Irving, L. M., & Anderson, J. R. (1991b). Hope and health. In C. R. Snyder & D. R. Forsyth (Eds.), *Pergamon general psychology series, Vol. 162. Handbook of social and clinical psychology: The health perspective* (pp. 285–305). Pergamon Press.

Snyder, C. R., LaPointe, A. B., Crowson, J. J., & Early, S. (1998). Preferences of high- and low-hope people for self-referential input. *Cognition and Emotion, 12*(6), 807–823. https://doi.org/10.1080/026999398379448

Soleimani, M. A., Bahrami, N., Zarabadi-Pour, S., Motalebi, S. A., Parker, A., & Chan, Y. H. (2020). Predictors of death anxiety among patients with heart disease. *Death Studies, 44*(3), 160–167.

Souza, A. C. C. d., Borges, J. W. P., & Moreira, T. M. M. (2016). Quality of life and treatment adherence in hypertensive patients: Systematic review with meta-analysis. *Revista de Saúde Pública, 50*, 71–71. https://doi.org/10.1590/s1518-8787.2016050006415

Steffen, L. E., Cheavens, J. S., Vowles, K. E., Gabbard, J., Nguyen, H., Gan, G. N., et al. (2020). Hope-related goal cognitions and daily experiences of fatigue, pain, and functional concern among lung cancer patients. *Supportive Care in Cancer, 28*(2), 827–835.

Steffen, L. E., Vowles, K. E., Smith, B. W., Gan, G. N., & Edelman, M. J. (2018). Daily diary study of hope, stigma, and functioning in lung cancer patients. *Health Psychology, 37*(3), 218–227. https://doi.org/10.1037/hea0000570

Stotland, E. (1969). *The psychology of hope*. Jossey-Bass.

Sun, X., Zhong, W., Lu, J., & Zhuang, W. (2021). Influence of psychological nursing intervention on psychological state, treatment compliance, and immune function of postoperative patients with rectal cancer. *Journal of Oncology, 2021*.

Tantisuvanitchkul, P., Thanakiatpinyo, T., & Kuptniratsaikul, V. (2020). Psychometric properties of the Thai Herth Hope Index in stroke patients. *ASEAN J Rehabil Medicine, 30*(1), 15–20.

Todd, A. M. H., Laird, B. J. A., Boyle, D., Boyd, A. C., Colvin, L. A., & Fallon, M. T. (2009). A systematic review examining the literature on attitudes of patients with advanced cancer toward research. *Journal of Pain and Symptom Management, 37*(6), 1078–1085. https://doi.org/10.1016/j.jpainsymman.2008.07.009

Tsan, Y. H., Wung, S. H., Lin, M. W., Lo, W. L., & Wang, Y. J. (2021). Predictors of quality of life change in head-and-neck cancer survivors during concurrent chemo-radiotherapy: A prospective study. *Asia-Pacific Journal of Oncology Nursing, 8*(3), 237.

Tu, M., Wang, F., Shen, S., Wang, H., & Feng, J. (2021). Influences of psychological intervention on negative emotion, cancer-related fatigue and level of hope in lung cancer chemotherapy patients based on the PERMA framework. *Iranian Journal of Public Health, 50*(4), 728.

Van Allen, J., & Steele, R. G. (2012). Associations between change in hope and change in physical activity in a pediatric weight management program. *Children's Health Care, 41*(4), 344–359. https://doi.org/10.1080/02739615.2012.721724

Van Allen, J., Steele, R. G., Nelson, M. B., Peugh, J., Egan, A., Clements, M., & Patton, S. R. (2016). A longitudinal examination of hope and optimism and their role in type 1 diabetes in youths. *Journal of Pediatric Psychology, 41*(7), 741–749. https://doi.org/10.1093/jpepsy/jsv113

Vogt, K. M. (2017). Imagining good future states. In R. Seaford, J. Wilkins, & M. Wright (Eds.), *Selfhood and the soul: Essays on ancient thought and literature in honour of Christopher Gill* (pp. 33–48). Oxford University Press.

Wang, J., She, Y., Wang, M., Zhang, Y., Lin, Y., & Zhu, X. (2021). Relationships among hope, meaning in life, and post-traumatic growth in patients with chronic obstructive pulmonary disease: A cross-sectional study. *Journal of Advanced Nursing, 77*(1), 244–254.

Wang, S., Zhao, Y., Li, J., Lai, H., Qiu, C., Pan, N., & Gong, Q. (2020). Neurostructural correlates of hope: Dispositional hope mediates the impact of the SMA gray matter volume on subjective well-being in late adolescence. *Social Cognitive and Affective Neuroscience, 15*(4), 395–404.

Warber, S. L., Ingerman, S., Moura, V. L., Wunder, J., Northrop, A., Gillespie, B. W., Durda, K., Smith, K., Rhodes, K. S., & Rubenfire, M. (2011). Healing the Heart: A randomized pilot study of a spiritual retreat for depression in acute coronary syndrome patients. *EXPLORE, 7*(4), 222–233. https://doi.org/10.1016/j.explore.2011.04.002

Ware, J., Kosinski, M., & Keller, S. D. (1996). A 12-Item Short-Form Health Survey: Construction of scales and preliminary tests of reliability and validity. *Medical Care, 34*(3), 220–233. https://doi.org/10.1097/00005650-199603000-00003

Weber, D., & O'Brien, K. (2017). Cancer and cancer-related fatigue and the inter-relationships with depression, stress, and inflammation. *Journal of Evidence-Based Complementary & Alternative Medicine, 22*(3), 502–512.

Wippold, G. M., & Roncoroni, J. (2020). Hope and health-related quality of life among chronically ill uninsured/underinsured adults. *Journal of Community Psychology, 48*(2), 576–589.

Wu, X., Xu, H., Zhang, X., Han, S., Ge, L., Li, X., & Zhang, X. (2021). Self-efficacy, hope as mediators between positive coping and resilience among patients with gastric cancer before the first chemotherapy. *Cancer Nursing, 44*(*1*), 79–85.

Xiang, G., Li, Q., Xiao, M., He, L., Chen, X., Du, X., et al. (2021). Goal setting and attaining: Neural correlates of positive coping style and hope. *Psychophysiology, e13887.*

Xue, S., Cao, B., & Liu, X. (2021). Investigation on quality of life and its influencing factors in young cancer patients. *International Journal of Clinical and Experimental Medicine Research, 5*(2), 208–213.

Yu, I. C., Fang, J. T., & Tsai, Y. F. (2020). Exploring demands of hemodialysis patients in Taiwan: A two-step cluster analysis. *PloS One, 15*(2), e0228259.

Yu, J., & Liu, X. (2021). Effect of psychological intervention care on the negative mood and hope level of elderly patients undergoing knee arthroplasty. *American Journal of Translational Research, 13*(6), 6584.

Zaharova, S., Litwack, K., Gopalakrishnan, S., Ellis, J., & Saltzberg, M. T. (2021). Self-management in heart failure: The importance of self-regulation but not complexity of condition. *Western Journal of Nursing Research*, 0193945921997428.

Zhang, Y., Cui, C., Wang, L., Yu, X., Wang, Y., & Wang, X. (2021a). The mediating role of hope in the relationship between perceived stress and post-traumatic stress disorder among Chinese patients with oral cancer: A cross-sectional study. *Cancer Management and Research, 13*, 393.

Zhang, A., Ji, Q., Zhang, K., Cao, Q., Chen, Y., Chen, J., & DuVall, A. (2021b). Solution-focused brief therapy for adolescent and young adult cancer patients in China: A pilot randomized controlled trial. *Journal of Psychosocial Oncology*, 1–18.

Zhang, Y., Cui, C., Wang, Y., & Wang, L. (2020). Effects of stigma, hope and social support on quality of life among Chinese patients diagnosed with oral cancer: A cross-sectional study. *Health and Quality of Life Outcomes, 18*(1), 1–8.

Zhong, G. Q., Lin, B. H., & Xiao, C. X. (2021). Hope levels and resilience in patients with severe novel coronavirus pneumonia: The current situation and a correlation analysis. *International Journal of General Medicine, 14*, 1959.

13

Hope and Health: Challenges and Opportunities

Anthony Scioli

The best physician is also a philosopher
– Galen of Pergamon

In his treatise on healing, Galen lamented the state of "modern medicine." He asked his contemporaries to follow Hippocrates, to resist haste … [for] if we practice philosophy … it is open to us to learn everything" (Singer, 1997, pp. 30–34). In this chapter, I examine the hope–health interaction. Following Galen, I suggest that a deeper understanding of this relationship must incorporate conceptual issues as well as empirical evidence. I begin with a review of health conditions that have been studied in relation to hope, then transition to interventions designed to increase hope. I conclude with several higher-level conceptual challenges and a proposed working model of the hope–health dynamic.

A. Scioli (✉)
Psychology Department, Keene State College, University System of New Hampshire, Keene, NH, USA
e-mail: tscioli@keene.edu

F. M. Sirois (ed.), *The Palgrave Handbook of Positive Psychology and Health*,
https://doi.org/10.1007/978-3-031-89095-6_13

Models and Methods

The scientific literature on hope is dwarfed by scholarship emanating from the humanities. Important insights appear in the philosophical and theological literature (e.g., Bloch, 1959/1986; Godfrey, 1987: Lynch, 1965, Marcel, 1951; Moltmann, 1967). Only a few of these ideas have found their way into the science of hope. Much of the empirical evidence can be viewed from the perspective of three leading approaches. Within psychology, Snyder's model is most frequently employed (Snyder et al., 1991; Gallagher & Lopez, 2009). The most complex model is that of Scioli and his colleagues (Scioli & Biller, 2009; Scioli et al., 2011). Within nursing, the best developed measure is Herth's (1991) Hope Index. Following a review of studies utilizing these measures, I briefly consider other models and measures.

Herth Hope Index (H-Hope)

The Herth (1991) Hope Index was inspired by the theoretical insights of Dufault and Martocchio (1985). Herth validated her scale on four samples: cancer patients, healthy adults, the elderly, and bereaved elderly. Three factors emerged: temporality and the future; positive readiness and expectancy; and interconnectedness.

Herth H-Hope and Mental Health

The Herth Hope Index (also "H-Hope") has been used in studies of recovery, and to assess links with trauma, depression, and suicide risk. Among individuals attending AA meetings, Wnuk (2017) found that H-Hope scores were positively correlated with lower perceived stress and greater life satisfaction. Hope was not correlated with duration of abstinence or time spent attending meetings. Lim et al. (2019) collected reports of personal recovery from psychosis in 115 adults in Singapore. At baseline, the strongest correlate of perceived recovery was H-Hope, followed by internalized stigma. However, two weeks later, baseline depression, not hope, was the strongest predictor of recovery.

Wang et al. (2019) found that H-Hope scores were associated with reduced PTSD symptoms in childless couples who had lost a child, and the mother was no longer able to conceive (Chinese "Shidu" parents). The strength of the hope-PTSD association was comparable for mothers and fathers. Perceived stress was a partial mediator of the relationship between hope and PTSD.

Morote et al. (2017) compared H-Hope with a 6-factor resilience construct (RSA; Hjemdal, 2007) to assess their respective protective effects against depression and anxiety in Peruvian adults. Both H-Hope and resilience were linked to reduced depression and anxiety. However, the RSA measure demonstrated greater incremental validity. Goodman et al. (2017) surveyed adult males in Kenya who reported suicidal ideation. The data outlined a path, originating with (lower) collective self-esteem, leading to reduced H-Hope, which then precipitated suicidal thoughts.

Hutchison et al. (2017) examined both behavioral and physical health outcomes among adults enrolled in a midwestern US psychiatric rehabilitation service, using a single-item version of the Hope Herth Index. After 12 months, more hopeful individuals reported higher wellness scores (diet, nutrition, physical activity, sleep, and medication management).

Herth H-Hope and Physical Health

H-Hope studies have also included individuals with diabetes, stroke, and ALS, as well as cancer. Makarem et al. (2014) focused on treatment adherence among type-2 diabetics. Perceived self-efficacy for diabetes management was assessed along with H-Hope and health-related locus of control. Hope demonstrated significant incremental validity in predicting adherence, beyond self-efficacy and locus of control.

Cross and Schneider (2010) examined hope in women recovering from stroke. Participants completed the H-Hope scale and a series of open-ended questions. Most of the participants appeared "very hopeful," and a majority "believed that hope played an integral role in their recovery" (p. 493), which they attributed to support systems, receiving information, inspiration from other survivors, goal setting, and spirituality. Hirano et al. (2006) assessed ALS patients in Japan who were ventilator-dependent for an average of six years. Lower hope scores were associated with emotional distress, social difficulties, and physical pain. Higher hope scores were found among individuals who reported a larger support network.

The H-Hope studies of cancer have addressed adjustment and the impact of diagnostic disclosure, as well as conceptions of hope. Rustøen et al.'s (2010) investigation in Norwegian cancer patients revealed that H-Hope scores mediated both perceived psychological distress, and life satisfaction. Lin and Tsay (2005) explored the impact of diagnostic disclosure on H-Hope and health-related locus of control in Taiwanese cancer patients. The disclosure group reported higher H-Hope scores, a finding consistent with perspectives on hope that highlight openness, and an enlarged perspective on reality (Breznitz, 1986; Marcel, 1951; Folkman, 2010). Gibson and Gorman (2012) interviewed long-term care residents with cancer and administered the H-Hope measure. Greater variability was found for subscales related to future outlook and positive affect. Less variability (primarily higher scores) was found for items related to interconnectedness, faith, and inner strength.

Snyder's Wills and Ways (S-Hope)

The most widely used measure of hope in psychology is the Snyder et al. (1991) Hope Scale, sometimes called the Goals Scale. Snyder and his colleagues view hope in terms of perceived agency and pathways for achieving goals, a continuation of the Stotland (1969) tradition (abbreviated as S-Hope, or S-Agency and S-Pathways).

Snyder S-Hope and Adult Mental Health

Many S-Hope studies involve college students. Liu et al. (2017) found that higher S-Hope scores were associated with less depression and PTSD symptoms in a cohort that experienced a mass school shooting. Chang et al. (2021) reported greater life satisfaction and reasons for living in students with higher S-Hope. Hirsch et al.'s (2012) study with college students suggested that S-Hope scores might be suicide-protective for Caucasians and Hispanics but not African Americans. Geiger and Kwon (2010) reported that S-Hope scores reduced the negative impact of rumination on depression in college students.

Gallagher and Lopez (2009) assessed S-Hope and Optimism (LOT; Scheier et al., 1994) in nearly 600 college students, as well as levels of eudemonic, social, and hedonic well-being. The H-Hope scores showed a stronger connection with mastery-related constructs (autonomy, purpose, personal growth, and social impact). Optimism was linked to a greater degree with social adjustment (positive relations, social coherence, social integration, and faith in society). Additionally, hope scores showed a stronger connection with positive affect but optimism demonstrated a greater association with less negative affect, and higher life satisfaction.

The data on S-Hope obtained from older adults reveals more complex interactions. Ociskova et al. (2015) found that S-Hope scores were significantly correlated with a global assessment of relative change (but not self-rated improvement) in adult Czech Republic patients with neurotic disorders. Among residents in a substance abuse facility, May et al.'s (2015) investigation showed that S-Agency scores were "marginally significant" predictors of lower depression and anxiety. In veterans exposed to trauma, S-Hope scores were related to reduced depression but not the degree of PTSD symptomatology (Hassija et al., 2012). Trezise et al. (2018) detected interaction effects that were limited to low hope individuals with insomnia, who reported greater depression. In a sample of older adults (Mean = 70.4 yrs.), Cheavens et al. (2016) reported that self-forgiveness but not S-Hope moderated the relationship between thwarted attachment needs and suicidal ideation.

Snyder S-Hope and Child Mental Health

Snyder et al. (1997) introduced a parallel six-item Children's Hope Scale (agency and pathways items). Higher scores were correlated with reductions in depressive symptoms and a more optimistic attributional style in 8–16-year-olds. The strongest correlate of hope was scholastic self-confidence. Fite et al. (2017) reported lower scores on measures of depression and suicidal behaviors as well as reactive and proactive aggression for youth (6–17 years) with higher Child S-Hope scores.

Jiang et al. (2018) reviewed research on children and adolescents, primarily involving the Child S-Hope Scale. Studies with adolescents indicate an association with positive affect, optimism, and life satisfaction, as well as fewer behavior problems (e.g., Edwards et al., 2007; Valle et al., 2006). However, this review combined research derived from other approaches to the hope construct (e.g., Mahat & Scoloveno, 2001). Also, a number of studies involved adults rather than children.

Marques (2016) explored Child S-Hope, stress, and mental health in Portuguese public-school children. Data were collected when the children were approximately 11–12 years of age, then again in five years. While T1 and T2 levels of mental health were strongly correlated, T1 hope demonstrated incremental predictive validity beyond T1 stress levels.

Zhang et al. (2019a) assessed bullying victimization, Child S-Hope, self-compassion, and depression in a large sample of middle-school children living in rural China, separated from parents. The impact of bullying victimization on depression was partially mediated by both hope and self-compassion but more so by the latter.

Snyder S-Hope and Physical Health

Snyder et al. (2005) observed higher levels of pain tolerance in college students with higher S-Hope scores. However, Hood et al. (2012) detected a stronger relationship between (LOT) optimism and pain variables, as compared to S-Hope scores. Berg et al. (2011) reported higher S-Hope scores among college nonsmokers, and a modest correlation with more exercise and reduced intake of dietary fat.

Wlodarczyk (2017) studied post-myocardial infarction patients. Hope and Optimism (LOT) were assessed, along with coping strategies, and subjective health. After controlling for the shared variance between hope and optimism, indirect effects were found for LOT scores but not S-Hope.

Several studies have been done with spinal cord-injured patients (SCI). During the course of an acute rehabilitation stay, Kortte et al. (2012) discovered that greater S-Hope was correlated with life satisfaction at admission and 3 months after discharge. In an investigation by Kennedy et al. (2009), higher S-hope scores were associated with greater fighting spirit and acceptance.

Research with SCI patients by Smedema et al. (2014) revealed a direct effect on life satisfaction for S-Agency whereas S-Pathways was indirectly linked to life satisfaction via an association with self-reported community participation. Phillips et al. (2016) also detected interactions, whereby proactive coping, self-esteem, and perceived social support mediated the relationship between SCI functional disability and S-Hope.

The majority of S-Hope studies on cancer have been retrospective. Yuen et al. (2014) found that adult childhood cancer survivors, higher in S-Hope, reported fewer negative ruminations about the disease and more positive thoughts about their experience with the illness. Stanton et al. (2002) focused on women with early-stage breast cancer. Women high in hope reported less fear of recurrence if they coped by engaging in positive reinterpretations. Women low in hope who turned to religion for coping, reported less fear of recurrence.

Ho et al. (2011) compared hope and optimism, in relation to anxiety and depression, in oral cancer patients, diagnosed between six months and ten years prior to the study. Both higher S-Hope (particularly S-Pathways) and LOT optimism were associated with greater posttraumatic growth. Hasson-Ohayon et al. (2009) studied long-term breast cancer survivors (median 11.0 years). Hope scores were correlated with greater fighting spirit and reductions in fatalistic acceptance.

Blank and Bellizzi (2006) assessed six facets of well-being in male, long-term (prostate) cancer survivors (median survival time = 42 months). S-Agency scores were correlated with greater positive affect and happiness as well as less negative affect and depression. In a prospective study, Ho et al. (2010) reported fewer symptoms of anxiety and depression for higher S-Hope individuals after colorectal cancer genetic testing in individuals with a positive family history.

There is scant data on child S-Hope and physical health. In Jiang et al.'s (2018) review one study is reported by Barnum et al. (1998) utilizing the adult S-Hope scale with adolescents (13–19) who were burn survivors, treated 8–23 years prior to the study. The sample was relatively small and data from burn patients and controls were combined.

Scioli Integrative Model of Hope (I-Hope)

Scioli and colleagues developed an integrative model of hope (Scioli & Biller, 2009; Scioli et al., 2011). Hope is conceptualized as a four-dimensional network, derived from attachment, survival, and mastery needs. The proposed function of hope is to address inevitable gaps in meeting humanity's basic needs. Spirituality is a fourth component, operating as an additional-support network for the first three needs (i.e., providing: "presence" (attachment), "salvation" (survival), and "empowerment" (mastery). A variety of hope assessment tools have been derived from this model, including adult trait and state scales, a child hope scale, a Rorschach Hope Index, and a coding system for content analysis.

Scioli I-Hope and Mental Health

Scioli et al. (2011) reported significant relationships between a variety of mental health variables and theoretically related state and trait I-Hope Scales. Higher mastery state hope was associated with greater meaning in life; attachment hope was related to reduced feelings of loneliness; and survival hope was linked to lower anxiety. Structural modeling of the trait version of the I-Hope Scale revealed a six-factor profile. The strongest relationships were found between "personalized mastery hope" and NEO Achievement, and both "attached survival" (supported coping) and "self-generated survival" (personal coping) with lower NEO Vulnerability. The "spirituality" factor was correlated with transcendent experiences of universality and connectedness (Piedmont, 1999).

Scioli et al. (2018) developed a Rorschach Hope Index to derive attachment, survival, and mastery components from the Exner (2003) Comprehensive System. The Hope Index was applied retrospectively to a case of completed suicide. The individual was not considered a high risk according to the Exner Suicide Constellation. In contrast, the Hope Index revealed adequate levels of mastery hope but very low levels of attachment and survival/coping hope.

Scioli I-Hope and Child Mental Health

Several studies have been done with a parallel (four-factor) I-Hope Child Scale (Scioli et al., 2013). Attachment, survival, and mastery hope scores were positively associated (respectively) with self-reported popularity among schoolmates, freedom from anxiety, and school-related self-esteem. Higher hope scores were also related to parental reports of fewer symptoms of both anxious and withdrawn depression subtypes. A strong association was reported for the three spiritual subscales, and a modified version of the Children's Religious Coping Scale (Ezop, 2002). In Rwanda, the I-Hope Child Scale was administered to adolescents, ages 17–18. Higher hope scores were associated with fewer symptoms of depression, fewer thoughts of death or suicide, and less anger (Scioli et al., 2020).

Scioli I-Hope and Physical Health

Scioli et al. (2016) found significant correlations between trait hope factor scores and health habits, including: increased exercise, adequate sleep, safer sex practices, and reduced substance use. A second investigation focused on diet and exercise, incorporating the transtheoretical model (Prochaska et al., 2009). With regards to diet (fruits and vegetable consumption), greater hope scores were found among individuals in the Action stage as compared to Pre-Contemplation. However, for exercise, greater hope scores distinguished Pre-Contemplators from Contemplators.

In a four-year, prospective study of HIV+ individuals, Scioli et al. (2012) reported a significant correlation between greater dispositional I-Hope and increased blood levels of CD4 (immune proteins) at 8, 24, and 48 months. Hope scores were independent of case managers' blind ratings of illness acceptance or denial on the part of the infected individuals. Attachment hope demonstrated the strongest association with self-reported physical or psychological health. Additional statistical analyses confirmed that hope was the driving force of health and not vice versa.

Scioli et al. (2016) developed a coding system for extracting themes related to attachment, survival, mastery, and spiritual hope. Twenty female breast cancer survivors were randomly selected from testimonials on the Susan Komen foundation website (ww5.komen.org). Raters isolated content reflecting events, processes, etc. credited by the women with a role in their survival. Ten women were diagnosed at stage 0 or 1; the other ten were in stages 2 or 3. The early and late-stage groups were comparable in terms of: year diagnosed, age at diagnosis, years of survival, and years of survival post-testimony. The survivor testimonies suggested that attachment and spiritual hope were vital to recovery, particularly for the later-stage group. An emphasis on attachment and spirituality in coping with cancer has been highlighted in other studies (Bulkley et al., 2013; Epplein et al., 2011; Hsieh et al., 2014; Sachs et al., 2013; Salsman et al., 2015; Taleghani et al., 2008).

Other Models of Hope

Mental Health

The writings of Frank (1961), Lynch (1965), and Menninger (1959) should be required reading for serious students of the hope-health dynamic. In *Persuasion and Healing*, Frank (1961) stressed the shaman-like role of all healers, whose primary function is to arouse and inspire hope. In Lynch's (1965) *Images of Hope*, the author highlights collaborative relationships that nurture the imagination. In his address to medical students, Menninger (1959) offered an array of arguments for viewing hope as the ultimate expression of the life instinct.

Abu-Kaf and Braun-Lewensohn (2019) studied Bedouin Arab adolescents in southern Israel during stressful periods of escalating violence. Hope was assessed with the Staats (1989) Hope Index which defines the construct in terms of net expected positive affect over the next few weeks. During T1 (less violence), hope (but not sense of coherence) was associated with less distress. However, in T3 (most violent), only sense of coherence was associated reduced distress.

Gum and Ayalon (2018) accessed a large, nationally representative sample of Americans ages 50 and older. A measure of hopelessness was derived from four items in two different hopelessness scales (Beck et al., 1974; Everson et al., 1996). Three of the four items reference goal attainment while one addresses perceptions of the future. Self-perceptions of aging mediated the relationship between hopelessness and depressive symptoms, six years later.

Chen et al. (2018) developed a "Virtual Hope Box" (VHB), a smartphone app for high-risk veterans. A clinical trial was conducted with 58 veterans over a 12-week period. Modules were created to relax, distract, inspire, and remind (targeted coping strategies). The results were inconclusive. A small effect was detected. More frequent VHB users tended to demonstrate an enhanced coping repertoire and reduced risk of suicidal ideation.

Krafft et al. (2019) propose a Perceived Hope Scale adapted from a hope and optimism subscale of the World Health Organization. The authors sought "to measure how people perceive hope in everyday life" (p. 1598). In addition to the WHO scale, other items were derived from various theoretical models, and language modifications were made to align with existing psychological scales. While the intent to capture everyday experiences of hope is commendable, a grounded theory approach (Walsh et al., 2015) may be better suited for this purpose.

Physical Health

Gottshalk (1974) created a hope scale using content analysis of prompted speech samples. In a subsequent article, Gottschalk (1985) cited two small-scale studies of cancer patients with metastatic cancers. In both studies, hope, measured through content analysis, was significantly correlated with survival time. Unfortunately, Gottschalk did not publish further details about these findings, and few studies have relied on this methodology (See Scioli et al., 1997).

Nowotny (1989) created a measure of hope (NHS) for cancer patients, encompassing future orientation, active involvement, an internal resource related to trust, possibility, others (humans and/or higher power), and importance of the object. Esbenson et al. (2007) incorporated the NHS in a six-month investigation of elderly cancer patients. A low level of hope was associated with a deterioration in perceived quality of life. Vellone et al. (2006) used the NHS to study Italian cancer patients. Higher levels of hope (NHS) were correlated with lower psychological distress, fewer physical symptoms, less pain, greater autonomy in daily living, and higher perceived quality of life.

Wright and Shontz's (1968) article, "Process and tasks in hoping," is an important contribution to the literature on hope and coping. Their work focused on the hopes of families with a severely disabled child. Wright and Shontz uncovered seven different "hope structures," two child forms and five adult versions. They also delineated 12 different reality grounding methods used by parents of the children.

Hinds (1984) has done the most research on hope in adolescents with cancer. Her interviews with adolescents revealed four dimensions: effort to adopt a positive view; possibilities of a second chance; generalized expectations of a better tomorrow; and anticipation of specific, personal possibilities. From this earlier work, Hinds and Gattuso (1991) developed a 24-item, visual-analog Hopefulness Scale for Adolescents (HSA). Few studies have utilized this measure. One exception is Cantrell et al. (2017) who observed greater self-esteem for female adolescent cancer patients (but not males) with higher HSA scores.

Section Summary

A summary of the empirical data suggests that the Snyder model may be more relevant for younger and healthier individuals. The focus is on goal-attainment rather than social integration or self-regulation. Higher S-Hope scores seem especially protective against depression, perhaps by offsetting potential goal frustrations. By comparison, the Herth scale was derived and validated with a special focus on older individuals with health problems. Higher Herth scores appear to protect against anxiety and emotional fallout from trauma. The Scioli model is an attempt to broaden the hope construct. Some compelling findings have emerged, particularly with respect to health habits and the immune system. However, the model and measure are newer additions to the hope literature and data from other labs will be helpful in evaluating the strength and range of this approach.

Taken together, the three primary approaches to hope, along with the insights of Frank (1961), Lynch (1965), and Menninger (1959), raise deeper issues. What is hope? How much conceptual and empirical space should the hope construct occupy relative to the concept (idea) that permeates lay discussions, manifests across various disciplines, or finds expression in the arts? To what extent is the current wave of interest in positive psychology as compared to clinical or health psychology a factor in the preference for a particular measure of hope? These and other meta-theoretical issues will be addressed in a later section. Nevertheless, at this juncture, readers may prime themselves for a deeper reflection by asking whether hope is always situation-bound, that is, should investigators abandon generalized models in favor of special populations or context-specific approaches? Note that Wright and Shontz (1968) interviewed parents of children with a limited set of life-threatening illnesses. For Nowotny, the focus was adult cancer. Hinds studied adolescents with cancer. Conversely, is a comprehensive approach to hope possible that "leaves nobody behind"?

Hope Interventions

In this section, I review interventions for increasing hope. To maintain the focus of this chapter, I limit my discussion to applications for individuals dealing with mental or physical health challenges.

Mental Health Interventions

McDermott and Snyder (1999) developed a "Making Hope Happen" (MHH) workbook for middle school students, focusing on personally relevant goals. Jiang et al. (2018) cited several investigations demonstrating significant increases in students' self-reported S-Hope. Buchanan (2008) found that MMH did not increase hope in students with educational disabilities.

Marques et al. (2011) describe a five-week, hope-based intervention (Building Hope for the Future) for Portuguese middle-school students. The program derives from the S-Hope model; "summoning mental energy to maintain goal pursuit" and reframing obstacles. S-Hope scores were significantly higher for the intervention group versus controls, at 3, 6, and 18 months. However, there was evidence of regression to the mean over time.

Clauss et al. (2018) used the Snyder Hope Scale to assess an intervention for reducing distress among caregivers via a positive work reflection exercise. Hope scores did not significantly increase in the intervention group. Ericson et al. (2018) introduced a six months' resistance training program for Swedish women, ages 65–70. Snyder hope scores were assessed but did not show a significant increase from pre- to post-intervention.

Barbic et al. (2009) evaluated the effectiveness of a group-based workbook (Spaniol et al., 1994) for individuals with a serious mental illness. Participation in the group was associated with slight increases in hope, as measured by the Herth Hope Index, as well as perceived empowerment and recovery (but not quality of life).

Eisen et al. (2018) evaluated the efficacy of a bibliotherapy program with respect to Herth hope scores. Participants read autobiographies of individuals confronting and managing mental illness and participated in group discussions led by a psychologist. A satisfaction survey revealed that approximately 60% felt more hopeful. The experimental and control groups showed a non-significant trend toward greater hope and recovery self-efficacy.

Scioli et al. (2017) assessed the feasibility and efficacy of a group intervention to instill hope in adolescents using paraprofessionals. Teens received a five-week workshop led by pairs of trained undergraduates. The treatment group but not controls reported increases in hope, utilization of social coping methods, and self-acceptance. Workshop participants (but not controls) also reported a significant reduction in depression. Participant engagement, SES, and preexisting health habits moderated a number of effect sizes.

Physical Health Interventions

Research on hope interventions for individuals with serious physical health problems is limited. Zhang et al. (2019b) developed an eight-module, video-based (WeChat) Life Review therapy for Chinese cancer patients (stages 3 or 4). Hope was assessed with the Herth Hope Index. A nonsignificant trend toward increased hope was found.

Rustøen et al. (2011) describe a Norwegian study of oncology patients. An eight-session, 16-hour HOPE-In intervention was developed using the six constructs underlying the Nowotny (1989) hope scale. The Herth Hope Index was selected to measure hope, pre and post-intervention. Hope scores increased immediately after the intervention but then decreased slightly at 3 months and again at 12 months.

Duggleby et al. (2007) describe a two-session, "Living with Hope Program" (LWHP) for older, terminally cancer patients in a community-living setting. After watching a film demonstrating ways that individuals in palliative care sustain hope, participants selected one of three activities: letter-writing, assembling a hope chest (box of mementos), or an autobiographical portfolio activity. The increase in Herth hope scores was statistically significant.

Shoshani et al. (2016) assessed the impact of a Make-a-Wish intervention on hope in Israeli children with life-threatening forms of cancer. Herth Hope items were read and explained to children. Hope scores increased significantly from 5 to 6 months prior to receiving the gift to 5 weeks after the reception.

Murdoch et al. (2020) designed a six-week, group-based hope intervention for individuals with Parkinson's disease. Activities included storytelling and discussions focusing on hope and personal strengths as well as arts-based expressions. Hope was assessed with the Herth Hope index. Hope scores did not increase from pretreatment to immediately post-intervention. However, scores were significantly higher at a six-week follow-up.

Bentley et al. (2014) implemented a dignity-focused therapy for Australians diagnosed with ALS. Hope was assessed via the Hope Herth Index. As a group, the treatment scores were not significantly different from pre- to post-intervention. However, individuals who demonstrated an increase in hope tended to identify as religious or spiritual and were diagnosed approximately four years earlier as compared to those who showed a decrease in hope.

Section Summary

The data regarding hope interventions is quite limited. With respect to mental health, interventions to increase S-Hope appear most promising in school settings with normative samples of children. Herth-based interventions for serious mental illness reveal a small effect size. Future work could focus on developing more robust interventions that parallel the specific factors in the Herth hope scale. Indeed, investigators should be intentional in whether they are crafting a generally "positive psychology" intervention that offers "hopeful" content in a pro forma sense or designing a true "hope-based" protocol. The strongest effects were observed by Scioli et al. (2017). However, this intervention needs to be replicated and evaluated with more diverse samples. The Herth hope scale emerged from the nursing literature, which may explain its use in studies directed at increasing hope in individuals with a serious physical illness. A different intervention was implemented in each of the reviewed studies, making it difficult to reach any firm conclusions about efficacy. It is also important to note the lack of research on hope interventions designed to directly impact physical health.

Conceptual Challenges

In this section, I discuss three conceptual challenges that must be addressed for investigators to achieve a better understanding of the hope–health dynamic: operationalizing hope, clarifying constituents of health and illness vis-à-vis hope, and incorporating the role of culture. I begin with the most critical issue, definitions of hope. This issue goes beyond the present focus on health. However, it is important to include some thoughts on this topic as it relates to health. For example, Olsman (2020) reviewed 73 studies of hope in the context of healthcare. His most important finding was that conceptualizations of hope tend to vary across different healthcare settings. Additionally, even within a particular setting, there is too often a lack of alignment in the meaning of hope for patients as compared to physicians or other medical care professionals.

Operationalizing Hope: From the Looking Glass to Wittgenstein's Warning

In Lewis Carroll's (1871/1917) *Through the looking glass*, Humpty Dumpty tells Alice, "When I use a word … it means just what I choose it to mean." Alice asks, "whether you can make words mean so many things." Humpty Dumpty replies, "The question is which is to be master – that's all" (p. 99). Within psychology, the dominant approach to hope is focused on goal estimations. Scioli et al. (2020) notes some of the limitations of this perspective, including confounding hope with self-efficacy and optimism. Moreover, the goal perspective ignores seminal writings on the attachment and coping elements of hope, as well as its spiritual dimensions (e.g., Erikson, 1950; Menninger, 1959; Marcel, 1951; Moltmann, 1967). Along these lines, Markus (2008) differentiates broader "concepts" (ideas) from narrower scientific "constructs" adapted for measurement, sample, or paradigm purposes. Beyond pragmatics, the preference for a narrow, Westernized construct in terms of goal attainment reveals hope as a "myth carrier" for beliefs about individualism, unending progress, and personal control (Scioli, 2020).

What Is Hope?

In psychology, many studies have employed the Snyder et al. (1991) Hope Scale. Relatively healthy, young college students constituted 95% of the data used to validate the measure. The Snyder et al. approach represents the continuation of a goal-oriented or instrumental hope that began with Stotland (1969). Wehmeyer and Shogren (2018) acknowledge overlaps between S-Hope and the "self-determination" construct. Bonfils et al. (2016) conducted a linguistic analysis of word use by individuals diagnosed with Schizophrenia-spectrum disorders. Higher S-hope scores were not linked to future, family, or friends but instead with greater use of first-person pronouns. When these findings are combined with classic literature in the psychology of stress and coping (e.g., Averill, 1973), it is reasonable to presume that control beliefs (rather than hope per se) may underlie the reported connection between S-Hope scores and greater pain tolerance (Snyder et al., 2005).

Li et al.'s (2021) assessment of American college student's beliefs about hope highlighted interpersonal relationships and spirituality. The authors noted, "beliefs associated with Snyder's theory of hope (agency and pathways) were rarely mentioned" (p. 249). Harley's (2015) interview of low-income, urban African American adolescents also evoked themes of caring connections and spirituality.

Hope is also viewed differently by non-college adults dealing with significant health concerns. Herbrand and Dimond (2018) interviewed women of reproductive age at risk of transmitting genetic disorders to their children. Multiple levels of hope emerged, including a more transcendent sense of trust that future generations may benefit from new technologies.

Duggleby and Wright's (2005) study of Canadian palliative care patients revealed a dynamic, transformative hope that included supportive relationships, as well as a spiritual framework that fostered understanding, acceptance, and meaning. Robieux et al. (2018) found that when individuals with a chronic disease are given open-ended questions about hope, coping is the dominant theme, not goals. Wolf et al. (2018) interviewed physicians, who described hope as "personal, philosophical, and abstract … shaping new meaning … with emotional and relational roots … a response to the existential inevitability of suffering and death" (p. 997).

Hope is complex. Unfortunately, it appears that many mind–body investigators have prematurely settled on narrowed conceptions of hope in response to a combination of philosophical biases and/or heuristic pressures. A procrustean bed has been propagated. This misstep would not have occurred if greater care was taken to conceptualize hope. Stated differently, investigators might reflect on how much of the hope concept remains to be incorporated in empirical research. In Table 13.1, I present a summary of thirteen major components of the hope construct that have been presented across disciplines. Due to space considerations, I abbreviate the descriptions. However, every component listed here is explicitly linked to hope by the authors, except for Kohut, whose ideas on mirroring and idealization are extended (to hope) by Randall (1984). To borrow a phrase from the film industry, science has left a great deal of hope on "the cutting room floor."

Table 13.1 Key elements of the hope construct

Need	Components	Contributors (discipline)
Attachment	Connection to a caring milieu	Erikson (1950) (Psychology): belief in another who desires to and can appear on one's behalf
	Trust	Erikson (1950) (Psychology): relationship fidelity
	Openness	Gabriel Marcel (1951) (Philosophy): creation of a phenomenal field conductive to presence, care, and support
Survival	Reality construction	Pettit (2004) (Philosophy): imagination used to craft a sanguine outlook; active mental self-regulation
	Reality surveillance	Wright and Shontz (1968) (Rehabilitation Psychology): the coordination of hope with reality
	Options	Godfrey (1987) (Philosophy): securing a margin or range
	Care recruitment	Capps (2001) (Theology): the capacity to access social or emotional support
Mastery	Validation	Kohut (1971) (Psychiatry): mirroring for strengths
	Inspiration	Kohut (1971) (Psychiatry): models for forming ideals
	Collaboration	Lynch (1965) (Philosophy): enhanced power via mutuality
Spirituality	Spiritual attachment	Pruyser (1986) (Pastoral Psychology): belief in a universe that includes a benevolent disposition toward the self
	Spiritual survival	Gabriel Marcel (1951) (Philosophy): a perceived presence that promises to be available in times of trouble
	Spiritual mastery	Marcel (1949) (Philosophy): a perceived "mysterious principle" in connivance with one's will

Triple "Bypass"

The diverse, yet typically limited representations of "hope" in empirical studies of health preclude a traditional meta-analysis. Indeed, it can be argued that in many studies, it is difficult to gauge if a "hope effect" occurred. Along these lines, Averill (1995) invoked Wittgenstein's (1973) critique of psychology when addressing a similar problem in the study of emotions. In paraphrasing Wittgenstein, Averill suggested there is often a bypass or disconnect between problems and methods in research. I suggest there is similarly a mind–body "bypass," resulting from under-defined conceptions of hope as well as health.

Consider three programs of research (see Table 13.2). In program one, "hope" is not identified but cardinal elements of this concept are employed, and significant links with health are reported (*false negative by substitution*). In

Table 13.2 Three potential hope-health bypasses

Research program 1	Hope is undefined	*False negative by substitution (proxy)* Cardinal elements of hope are employed but the term "hope" is not used. Links to health are found but hope is not given credit
Research program 2	Hope in under-defined	*False negative by omission* A partial hope construct is studied in relation to health. No health links are found. Investigators falsely assume hope is not a factor in health
Research program 3	Hope is over-defined	*False positive by addition* "Hope" is expanded to incorporate unrelated concepts. These extraneous elements link with health, and hope is falsely credited

program two, an under-defined hope is operationalized that does not yield a significant link with health (*false negative by omission*). In program three, an overly broad definition of hope results in erroneous hope–health conclusions (*false positive by addition*).

At this early stage of inquiry, investigators should be most concerned about false negatives. A broader, consensus definition of hope is needed. While it is reasonable to focus on just one or two elements of hope in a single study (e.g., attachment or coping), investigators should be intentional in their *construct* selection, and recognize that they are isolating only part of a larger *concept.*

Hope for an Embodied Health

Achieving conceptual clarity regarding hope is necessary but not sufficient. The "body" side of the equation, that is, emotional and physical health, must be mapped out with greater precision,

to incorporate the full spectrum of related psychosocial factors. Ghane and Sweeny (2013) clearly present the problem. "… many studies in health psychology reflect a more-narrow focus on the psychosocial influences of health, leaving out physical influences, while the majority of medical studies neglect the influence of psychosocial variables (p. 159). A 2021 Medline search shows 671, 241 publications under the subject term "illness." When hope is added as a subject term, there are just 207 publications (approx. 3 per every 10,000 studies). Stated differently, hope is a complex phenomenon requiring an interdisciplinary understanding. Most of the research has been drawn from one (cognitive) perspective, and a single discipline (psychology). Health is also complex. A broader and more interdisciplinary approach to both hope and health will undoubtedly reveal a greater array of interrelationships.

In Table 13.3 below, I summarize the results of a 2021 PsycInfo search across 12 health conditions. In column 2, I indicate the number of publications that include hope or hopelessness as a subject term. In columns 3 through 6, I list studies of health that incorporate a potential element of the hope concept (attachment, coping, etc.) but it (hope) is omitted as a subject term.

Interestingly, there are significantly more "non-hope" studies with the keywords: attachment, coping, or spirituality, and far fewer potential "misses" involving mastery. How many of these studies might have come under the umbrella of hope research if a broader construct (of hope) was adopted? How many more "hits" would result if medical research was more invested in psychosocial correlates of health and illness? For example, attachment may be the single most important factor in the development of hope as well as the most robust psychosocial variable in PNI research (Scioli & Biller, 2009). If the keyword "social" is added as a qualifier to the nearly 700,000 "illness" publications in Medline, less than 20,000 articles appear (2.9%).

Table 13.3 Room for hope: potential frame errors in conceptualizing hope and illness (2021 search)

	N. of PsycInfo hope publications	N. of PsycInfo publications with ostensibly related hope constructs in "non-hope" studies			
	Subject term: hope or hopelessness[a]	Attachment	Coping	Mastery	Spirituality
Narrow frames					
Depression	1226	1802	3676	128	596
Suicide	765	260	451	3	123
Trauma	125	1076	1268	21	296
Cancer	297	131	2204	15	586
Chronic illness[b]	43	43	525	5	101
Rehabilitation	85	45	416	14	107
Limited frames					
Child depression	2	12	9	0	0
Treatment adherence	5	4	37	1	11
Clinical trials	17	22	62	1	29
Assisted living	2	1	11	1	3
Nursing home	17	24	209	7	53
End of life	32	3	51	1	204

[a]Across all health conditions, the percentage of studies with keywords hope or hopelessness, relative to all publications on the topic, was consistent (approx. 0.03 percent)

[b]Sum of four leading chronic illnesses (heart disease, stroke, COPD, diabetes)

The disconnect between hope and coping is particularly surprising. One of the earliest definitions of hope is an island in the middle of a wasteland (Scioli & Biller, 2009). A number of classic writings on hope emphasize its role in dealing with adversity (Arnold, 1960; Breznitz, 1986; Menninger, 1959; Wright & Shontz, 1968). Few Medline "illness" publications include a reference to "coping" (one per thousand).

Spirituality is a third element in many "non-hope" health studies. For over two millennia, spiritual beliefs have been a primary source of hope (Scioli & Biller, 2009). Spirituality was referenced in the studies of Duggleby and Wright (2005), Harley (2015), Herbrand and Dimond (2018), as well as Li et al. (2021) and Scioli et al. (2016). However, Medline shows only 1 in 10,000 "illness" publications incorporate spirituality.

Conversely, hopelessness has been implicated in both *depression* and *suicide* (Abramson et al., 1989; Franklin et al., 2017). Medline includes nearly 140,000 publications on suicide but only 838 include hope or hopelessness (approximately 6 per 1000). Hope is also critical in healing from trauma. Herman (1992) highlighted safety, reconnection, and a renewed purpose as critical factors in recovery from PTSD. Hope has been described as an island, an anchor, and a vital principle (Scioli & Biller, 2009). With respect to cancer, only 1% of Medline publications on this topic include hope or hopelessness as subject terms. Nevertheless, in Scioli et al.'s (2016) study of long-term female breast *cancer* survivors, hope derived from quality relationships and spiritual beliefs was considered pivotal in the recovery process.

Robieux et al. (2018) asked adults dealing with *chronic illness* [what] "comes to mind when you think about hope." Rather than goals, hope was mainly described as a coping strategy.

Schiavon et al. (2017) searched the chronic illness literature for hope and confirmed a small number of articles. In 62% of the studies, the construct was assessed with the Snyder et al. scale.

De Ruysscher et al. (2017) reviewed the literature on *rehabilitation* for substance use. Hope was cited as a critical factor in nearly 70% of the studies. However, as Table 13.3 suggests, many substance use studies may allude to hope but stop short of making it a focus. Only 4% of Medline studies include hope as a keyword.

The bottom half of Table 13.3 highlights six health issues that have been relatively neglected in terms of hope research. In the case of *child depression*, the ratio of adult to youth hope studies is approximately 350:1. Only five publications were found relating hope to *treatment adherence*. An exception is a study by Makarem et al. (2014) who incorporated one of the broader measures of hope (Herth Scale) to study adherence among individuals with type-2 diabetes. Hope demonstrated incremental validity after accounting for self-efficacy and health-related locus of control. Mistrust of medical professionals often underlies treatment noncompliance, particularly in cases of vaccine hesitancy (Hornsey et al., 2020). Trust is a cornerstone of hope (Erikson, 1950).

A hallmark of hope is liberation; hopelessness involves a sense of entrapment (Breznitz, 1986). Natale et al. (2021) conducted a review of *clinical trials* from the patient's perspective. Barriers to participation included lacking awareness of opportunities, skepticism, or fear of being a guinea pig. As previously noted, hope encompasses perceived degrees of freedom, trust, and assurance as well as higher aims (Erikson, 1950; Pruyser, 1987; Marcel, 1949). Dellborg et al. (2016) studied participants in long-term cardiovascular trials. The two most important reasons for participation were: "I am able to see the same doctor and nurse at the visits," and "I want to promote science."

Holmberg et al.'s (2019) interviews with frail *nursing home* residents revealed an overall theme of "assent to exposedness" which included sub-themes of "having hope in hopelessness," existing "between power and powerlessness," and "oscillating" between acts of personal responsibility and care recruitment (p. 868). There are about 95,000 Medline studies on nursing home care. Hope or hopelessness is found in roughly 7 per 1000 studies.

Hope in *end-of-life* studies are equally rare (5% of all Medline studies on this topic). However, hope still matters. Duggleby and Wright's (2005) investigation of palliative care patients revealed a transformed hope that was spiritual and meaning-centered, not focused on either future gain or loss prevention but instead a deeper understanding of life and personal mortality.

The Role of Culture

Hope may be viewed as a network derived from "a soft, pliable initial assembly" of attachment, mastery, and survival circuits as well as personal and cultural experiences (Fogel et al., 1992, p. 127; Averill, 1997). Cultural differences have been reported regarding hope and health, particularly with respect to the role of self versus others, perceptions of control, and spirituality. Wang et al. (2019) studied childless Chinese couples ("Shidu parents"). Higher Herth hope scores were associated with fewer PTSD symptoms. The findings were interpreted in light of the importance of family and children among the Chinese. They offer a quote from a Shidu parent in Song (2014), "What we are afraid of is not death, but illness and having no one to rely on when we get old" (p. 28). Chen et al. (2015) explored hope in older Chinese with advanced cancer. "Hope work" was "tied to and driven by hope for interpersonal connectedness" (p. 166).

Lee and Gallagher (2018) compare Eastern and Western notions of well-being and the implications for hope. Self-acceptance and autonomy define wellness in the West; positive relations are the sine qua non of mental health in the East. Tsai et al. (2007) explored "ideal affect" preferences and found that European-Americans and Asian-American demonstrated a greater preference for influence-generating goals and high-arousal positive affect whereas Hong Kong Chinese favored adjustment goals and low-arousal positive affect.

Benzein and Berg (2003) adapted the Herth Hope Index for a study of Scandinavian palliative care patients. Several challenges emerged, including a different factor structure as well as difficulties translating notions of "faith," "value," and "worth." Hernandez et al. (2019) interviewed Latinos diagnosed with Schizophrenia and their caregivers regarding the meaning of hope, and how it is maintained and strengthened. Hope had strong religious, spiritual, and relational components which "may be more prominent in groups that share a collectivist culture" (p. 48).

Section Summary

Research on hope is at an important juncture. Over the past 30 years, psychology has begun to take the construct (of hope) seriously as a scientific topic. Between 1990 and 2021, approximately 4000 articles have appeared in PsycInfo under the subject term "hope." However, the literature contains a heterogenous set of constructs offered as proxies for the concept (idea) of hope. Ironically, this diversity of narrow hope constructs has created a mountain of "exclusive" data, with studies that cannot address differences in cultures and spiritual traditions, do not translate well across gender, age, or history, or speak with equal resonance to the healthy and the sick.

Clearly, a broader approach to hope is needed. A working group is needed to generate a consensus definition that will guide further scholarship and empirical research.

I favor a broader conceptualization that encompasses attachment, survival, mastery, and spiritual elements. With regard to health, it cannot be a mere coincidence that the PNI literature highlights the value of analogous concepts such as social support, emotional regulation, perceived control, as well as religious and spiritual involvement (cf. Scioli & Biller, 2009).

Equipped with an adequate hope construct, investigators will be able to move beyond descriptive and primarily correlation-based studies to model the dynamics of the hope–health interaction.

Hope for Today: From Definitions to Dynamics

There is enough evidence gathered from the kaleidoscope of hope research to suggest an impact on health. Eventually, science must address "how" hope impacts health. Along these lines, experimentalists invoke "mediators" and "moderators" in an effort to explain relationships among variables (Baron & Kenny, 1986). Mediators are posited as a critical link in a causal chain, an intervening variable or "go-between." A moderator changes the relationship between two other variables. Most of the studies reviewed in this chapter suggest a moderation of thoughts and feelings. Simply put, the strongest evidence suggests that hope may reduce (moderate) suffering in the context of health challenges.

More research is needed to assess the direct impact of hope on physical health. Hypothesized mind–body linkages can be tested with mediation or moderation studies as well as more sophisticated, mixed-causation inquiries. Indeed, Rychlak (1968) questioned psychology's narrow focus on mediation rather the full complement of Aristotelian causes: formal, final, material, and efficient. In Fig. 13.1, I present a working model of the hope–health interaction in terms of formal, final, and efficient causes that includes moderation and mediation effects. I include traits, states, and processes. I presuppose a four-component approach to hope as discussed above.

The proposed model incorporates Godfrey's (1987) philosophical distinction between fundamental and ultimate hope. The former (fundamental hope) was mentioned, albeit briefly, by Erikson (1950) who labeled it "basic hope." This "hope" refers to a capacity rather than a focus or aim (ultimate hope). In psychology, we might label this construct "dispositional hope." Ultimate hopes can be sorted into longer-lasting aspirations, and event-activated states. Folkman (2010) hypothesized that dispositional hope may serve as a reservoir that impacts one or more hopes activated by the event of an illness. We lack empirical research to verify this hypothesis. Consequently, I offer a working model for evaluation and refinement via further inquiry, and also provide a scenario for how it may manifest in a real-life situation (dynamics).

Dispositional hope likely operates at multiple levels, through various forms of moderation, shaping initial appraisals of a health challenge (A-Appraise),

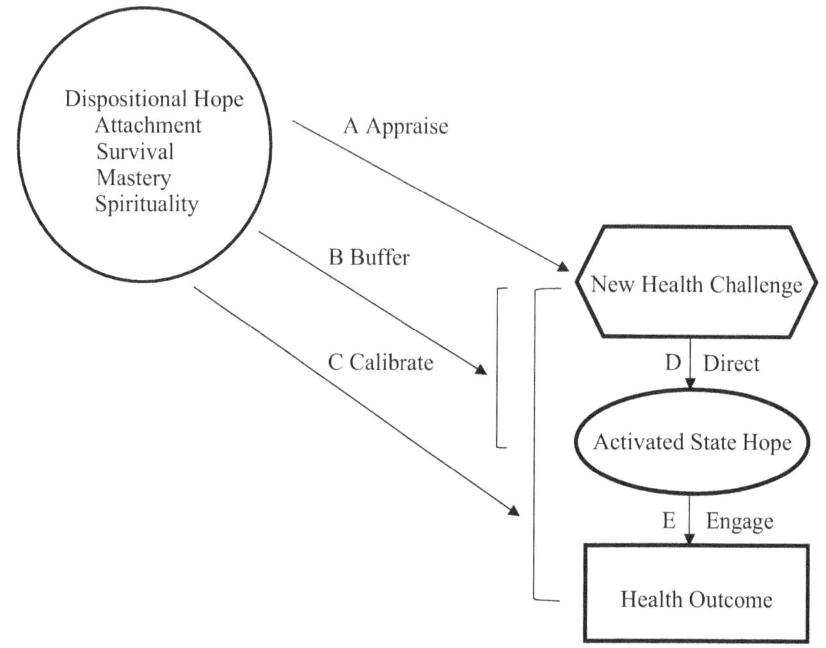

Levels	Type of Cause [Aristotelian]	Type of Cause [Psychological]	Process Metaphors
A	Formal Cause 1	Moderator	A Appraise (Framing)
B	Formal Cause 2	Moderator	B Buffer (Gap Closures)
C	Formal Cause 3	Moderator	C Calibrate
D	Final Cause 1	Mediator	D Direct
E	Efficient Cause 1	Mediator	E Engage

Fig. 13.1 Generalized working model of hope–health interactions

influencing the formation of a hoping process to close the perceived gap between desired health and a new reality (B-Buffer), and monitoring the hoping process to assure an outcome that is aligned with higher-order values and beliefs (C-Calibrate). The health challenge may be viewed as a final cause (mediator) to activate state hope, with the aim of restoring health (D-Direct).

The specific behaviors that derive from activated state hope may be conceptualized as mediators of the health-outcome (E-Engage). Of course, other mediators may be present at the point of engagement (e.g., surgery, pharmacology, or nutrition).

For example, consider a very hopeful woman. She is high in trust and openness (attachment). The bias in her imaginative process is in a positive direction and she is used to grounding fantasies with effective reality surveillance strategies (survival). She has internalized a sense of her own worth as well as the lessons of inspirational role models (mastery). She has transcendent beliefs which offer a bridge between reality-based access to attachment, survival, and mastery resources, and perceived, parallel, yet-to-be realized support for these needs (spirituality).

When this hopeful woman is confronted by a diagnosis of stage II breast cancer, she frames it as a challenge that will be met with her internal and external resources (*appraisal/framing*). It will not be a battle of ego or willpower, but a journey enabled by trust and support. *"Gap closure"* (buffering) comes next. She considers her relational needs in light of potential confidantes. Her imaginative process is a blend of healing options and the reality of the illness. She favorably evaluates her strength and the collective strength of other survivors vis-à-vis the illness. Her spiritual beliefs assure there is adequate "back-up power" to confront the cancer. She aims for health (directing). With the activation of state hope (engagement), she discloses to confidantes, consults with experts, exercises appropriate levels and types of control, and continues her spiritual practices. The health benefits of these behaviors are well-documented. However, as suggested earlier, additional evidence may be hidden in hope "bypasses." From the activation of hope to the resolution of the illness, she continuously reviews her progress in light of her core beliefs (work, home, relationships, notions about the afterlife, etc.) (calibration).

An additional comment on mediators and moderators is warranted. Given the limit explications of hope that have been employed to date, we cannot accurately gauge its potential for either moderating or mediating health outcomes. Ideally, a more complex rendering of hope is needed for studies of immunosurveillance (mediation) as well as inflammatory control (moderation). If science ultimately concludes that hope operates primarily as a moderator, its role in mind–body interactions should not be downplayed. To cite just one example, consider how initial COVID-19 vaccines reduced hospitalizations, respirator-dependence, and death by "moderating" the immune system.

Hope for Tomorrow

The most encouraging interpretation of the reviewed literature is that an under-defined hope construct nevertheless demonstrates compelling links with health. A more robust hope construct, along with more holistic models of health and illness is likely to reveal an even stronger and richer array of relationships. Mathematically oriented readers may wonder about effect sizes. To improve readability for this chapter, statistical outcomes were omitted. In general, the effect sizes are in the low to moderate range, with hope accounting for 10–20% of the variance in health. However, there is a huge caveat. Any attempt to provide a meta-analytic summary of the literature begs the question of which hope construct is to be evaluated.

I omitted Aristotle's "material causes" in the proposed working model. Would insights at this level provide a valuable link in the chain of events underlying the hope–health dynamic? Two intriguing research methods exist. In neuroscience, advances in fMRI technology may someday lead to the circuitry of hope and hopelessness. In philosophy of mind, emotion metaphors have been touted as a portal to the inner experience of otherwise ineffable experiences.

In closing, I reference Whitley's (2010) edict, aimed at his rehabilitation colleagues. His comments amplify the major challenge and opportunity suggested by this review; to operationalize the construct of hope in a more complex manner, in closer alignment with the rich concept that has long fascinated scientists and humanists. Whitley suggested looking "outside psychology" [for hope] … as something more profound than 'expectations." He identified theological and philosophical thinkers such as Tillich (1963) who viewed hope as an ethical reframing of the past; Moltmann (1964/1967), who understood hope in terms of spatial-temporal transcendence; and Kierkegaard (1849/1989), who highlighted release from despair via a realization of a benign presence.

References

Abramson, L. Y., Metalsky, G. I., & Alloy, L. B. (1989). Hopelessness depression: A theory-based subtype of depression. *Psychological Review, 96*(2), 358–372. https://doi-org.keenestate.idm.oclc.org/10.1037/0033-295X.96.2.358

Abu-Kaf, S., & Braun-Lewensohn, O. (2019). Coping resources and stress reactions among Bedouin Arab adolescents during three military operations. *Psychiatry Research, 273*, 559–566. https://doi.org/10.1016/j.psychres.2019.01.088

Arnold, M. B. (1960). *Emotion and personality, Vol I, psychological aspects*. Columbia University Press.

Averill, J. R. (1973). Personal control over aversive stimuli and its relationship to stress. *Psychological Bulletin, 80*(4), 286–303. https://doi.org/10.1037/h0034845

Averill, J. R. (1995). Passersby. *Psychological Inquiry, 6*(3), 204–208. https://doi.org/10.1207/s15327965pli0603_3

Averill, J. R. (1997). The emotions: An integrative approach. In R. Hogan, J. A. Johnson, & S. R. Briggs (Eds.), *Handbook of personality psychology* (pp. 513–541). Academic Press. https://doi.org/10.1016/B978-012134645-4/50022-6

Barbic, S., Krupa, T., & Armstrong, I. (2009). A randomized controlled trial of the effectiveness of a modified recovery workbook program: Preliminary findings. *Psychiatric Services, 60*(4), 491–497. https://doi.org/10.1176/ps.2009.60.4.491

Barnum, D. D., Snyder, C. R., Rapoff, M. A., Mani, M. M., & Thompson, R. (1998). Hope and social support in the psychological adjustment of children who have survived burn injuries and their matched controls. *Children's Health Care, 27*(1), 15–30. https://doi.org/10.1207/s15326888chc2701_2

Baron, R. M., & Kenny, D. A. (1986). The moderator–mediator variable distinction in social psychological research: Conceptual, strategic, and statistical considerations. *Journal of Personality and Social Psychology, 51*(6), 1173–1182. https://doi.org/10.1037/0022-3514.51.6.1173

Beck, A. T., Weissman, A., Lester, D., & Trexler, L. (1974). The measurement of pessimism: The hopelessness scale. *Journal of Consulting and Clinical Psychology, 42*(6), 861–865. https://doi.org/10.1037/h0037562

Bentley, B., O'Connor, M., Kane, R., & Breen, L. J. (2014). Feasibility, acceptability, and potential effectiveness of dignity therapy for people with motor neuron disease. *PLoS One, 9*(5).

Benzein, E., & Berg, A. (2003). The Swedish version of Herth Hope index: An instrument for palliative care. *Scandinavian Journal of Caring Sciences, 17*(4), 409–415. https://doi.org/10.1046/j.0283-9318.2003.00247.x

Berg, C. J., Ritschel, L. A., Swan, D. W., An, L. C., & Ahluwalia, J. S. (2011). The role of Hope in engaging in healthy behaviors among college students. *American Journal of Health Behavior, 35*(4), 402–415.

Blank, T. O., & Bellizzi, K. M. (2006). After prostate cancer: Predictors of well-being among Long-term prostate cancer survivors. *Cancer, 106*(10), 2128–2135. https://doi.org/10.1002/cncr.21865

Bloch, E. (1986). *The principle of hope* (N. Plaice, S. Plaice, & P. Knight, Trans., Vol. 1). MIT Press. (Original work published 1959).

Bonfils, K. A., Luther, L., Firmin, R. L., Lysaker, P. H., Minor, K. S., & Salyers, M. P. (2016). Language and hope in schizophrenia-spectrum disorders. *Psychiatry Research, 245*, 8–14. https://doi.org/10.1016/j.psychres.2016.08.013

Breznitz, S. (1986). The effect of hope on coping with stress. In M. H. Appley & R. Trumbull (Eds.), *Dynamics of stress: Physiological, psychological, and social perspectives* (pp. 295–306). Plenum Press.

Buchanan, C. L. (2008). *Making Hope Happen for students receiving special education services*. ProQuest Information & Learning. In Dissertation Abstracts International: Section B: The Sciences and Engineering (Vol. 69, Issue 3–B, p. 1943).

Bulkley, J., McMullen, C. K., Hornbrook, M. C., Grant, M., Altschuler, A., Wendel, C. S., & Krouse, R. S. (2013). Spiritual well-being in long-term colorectal cancer survivors with ostomies. *Psycho-Oncology, 22*(11), 2513–2521. https://doi.org/10.1002/pon.3318

Cantrell, M. A., Conte, T. M., Hudson, M. M., Ruble, K., Herth, K., Shad, A., & Canino, A. (2017). Developing the evidence base in pediatric oncology nursing practice for promoting health-related quality of life in pediatric oncology patients. *Journal of Pediatric Oncology Nursing, 34*(2), 90–97. https://doi.org/10.1177/1043454216669678

Capps, D. (2001). *Agents of hope: A pastoral psychology*. Wipf and Stock.

Carroll, L. (1917). *Through the looking glass: And what Alice found there*. Rand McNally. (Original work published 1871).

Chang, E. C., Jiang, X., Tian, W., Yi, S., Liu, J., Liang, P., Liang, Y., Lai, S., Shi, X., Li, M., Chang, O. D., & Hirsch, J. K. (2021). Hope as a process in understanding positive mood and suicide protection: A test of the broaden-and-build model. *Crisis: The Journal of Crisis Intervention and Suicide Prevention*. https://doi.org/10.1027/0227-5910/a000755

Cheavens, J. S., Cukrowicz, K. C., Hansen, R., & Mitchell, S. M. (2016). Incorporating resilience factors into the interpersonal theory of suicide: The role of hope and self-forgiveness in an older adult sample. *Journal of Clinical Psychology, 72*(1), 58–69. https://doi.org/10.1002/jclp.22230

Chen, H., Komaromy, C., & Valentine, C. (2015). From hope to hope: The experience of older Chinese people with advanced cancer. *Health: An Interdisciplinary Journal for the Social Study of Health, Illness and Medicine, 19*(2), 154–171. https://doi.org/10.1177/1363459314555238

Chen, J. I., Smolenski, D. J., Dobscha, S. K., Bush, N. E., & Denneson, L. M. (2018). Correlates of mental health smartphone application use among patients with suicidal ideation. *Journal of Technology in Human Services, 36*(4), 191–207. https://doi.org/10.1080/15228835.2018.1502119

Clauss, E., Hoppe, A., O'Shea, D., González Morales, M. G., Steidle, A., & Michel, A. (2018). Promoting personal resources and reducing exhaustion through positive work reflection among caregivers. *Journal of Occupational Health Psychology, 23*(1), 127–140. https://doi.org/10.1037/ocp0000063

Cross, A., & Schneider, M. (2010). A preliminary qualitative analysis of the impact of hope on stroke recovery in women. *Topics in Stroke Rehabilitation, 17*(6), 484–495. https://doi.org/10.1310/tsr1706-484

De Ruysscher, C., Vandevelde, S., Vanderplasschen, W., De Maeyer, J., & Vanheule, S. (2017). The concept of recovery as experienced by persons with dual diagnosis: A systematic review of qualitative research from a first-person perspective. *Journal of Dual Diagnosis, 13*(4), 264–279. https://doi.org/10.1080/15504263.2017.1349977

Dellborg, H., Hultsberg-Olsson, G., & Dellborg, M. (2016). Why do patients participate in long-term cardiovascular trials?--A questionnaire-based study. *Scandinavian Cardiovascular Journal, 50*(2), 83–87. https://doi.org/10.3109/14017431.2015.1133843

Dufault, K., & Martocchio, B. C. (1985). Hope: Its spheres and dimensions. *Nursing Clinics of North America, 20*(2), 379–391.

Duggleby, W., & Wright, K. (2005). Transforming hope: How elderly palliative patients live with hope. *Canadian Journal of Nursing Research, 37*(2), 71–84.

Duggleby, W., Wright, K., Williams, A., Degner, L., Cammer, A., & Holtslander, L. (2007). Developing a living with Hope program for caregivers of family members with advanced cancer. *Journal of Palliative Care, 23*(1), 24–31.

Edwards, L. M., Ong, A. D., & Lopez, S. J. (2007). Hope measurement in Mexican American youth. *Hispanic Journal of Behavioral Sciences, 29*(2), 225–241. https://doi.org/10.1177/0739986307299692

Eisen, K., Lawlor, C., Wu, C. D., & Mason, D. (2018). Reading and recovery expectations: Implementing a recovery-oriented bibliotherapy program in an acute inpatient psychiatric setting. *Psychiatric Rehabilitation Journal, 41*(3), 243–245. https://doi.org/10.1037/prj0000307

Epplein, M., Zheng, Y., Zheng, W., Chen, Z., Gu, K., Penson, D., Lu, W., Shu, X. O., Epplein, M., Zheng, Y., Zheng, W., Chen, Z., Gu, K., Penson, D., Lu, W., & Shu, X.-O. (2011). Quality of life after breast cancer diagnosis and survival. *Journal of Clinical Oncology, 29*(4), 406–412. https://doi.org/10.1200/JCO.2010.30.6951

Ericson, H., Skoog, T., Johansson, M., & Whahlin-Larsson, B. (2018). Resistance training is linked to heightened positive motivational state and lower negative affect among healthy women aged 65–70. *Journal of Women and Aging, 30*(5), 366–381.

Erikson, E. H. (1950). *Childhood and society*. Norton.

Esbenson, B. A., Osterlind, K., & Hallberg, I. R. (2007). Quality of life of elderly persons with cancer: A six-month follow-up. *Nordic College of Caring Science, 21*, 178–190.

Everson, S. A., Goldberg, D. E., Kaplan, G. A., Cohen, R. D., Pukkala, E., Tuomilehto, J., & Salonen, J. (1996). Hopelessness and risk of mortality and incidence of myocardial infarction and cancer. *Psychosomatic Medicine, 58*(2), 113–121. https://doi.org/10.1097/00006842-199603000-00003

Exner, J. E., Jr. (2003). *The Rorschach: A comprehensive system* (4th ed.). John Wiley & Sons Inc.

Ezop, S. J. (2002). *Religious and spiritual coping in children with chronic illness*. ProQuest Information & Learning. In Dissertation Abstracts International: Section B: The Sciences and Engineering (Vol. 63, Issue 5–B, p. 2580).

Fite, P. J., Poquiz, J., Frazer, A. L., & Reiter, N. (2017). Further evaluation of associations between reactive and proactive aggression and suicidal behavior in a treatment seeking sample of youth. *Child Psychiatry and Human Development, 48*(6), 903–910. https://doi.org/10.1007/s10578-017-0713-4

Fogel, A., Nwokah, E., Dedo, J. Y., Messinger, D., Dickson, K. L., Matusov, E., & Holt, S. A. (1992). Social process theory of emotion: A dynamic systems approach. *Social Development, 1*(2), 122–142. https://doi-org.keenestate.idm.oclc.org/10.1111/j.1467-9507.1992.tb00116.x

Folkman, S. (2010). Stress, coping, and hope. *Psycho-Oncology, 19*(9), 901–908. https://doi.org/10.1002/pon.1836

Frank, J. D. (1961). *Persuasion and healing: A comparative study of psychotherapy*. Johns Hopkins University Press.

Franklin, J. C., Ribeiro, J. D., Fox, K. R., Bentley, K. H., Kleiman, E. M., Huang, X., Musacchio, K. M., Jaroszewski, A. C., Chang, B. P., & Nock, M. K. (2017). Risk factors for suicidal thoughts and behaviors: A meta-analysis of 50 years of research. *Psychological Bulletin, 143*(2), 187–232. https://doi.org/10.1037/bul0000084

Galen (1997). *Selected works* (P.N. Singer, Trans.). Oxford University Press. (Original work published ca. 170 C.E.)

Gallagher, M. W., & Lopez, S. J. (2009). Positive expectancies and mental health: Identifying the unique contributions of hope and optimism. *The Journal of Positive Psychology, 4*(6), 548–556. https://doi.org/10.1080/17439760903157166

Geiger, K. A., & Kwon, P. (2010). Rumination and depressive symptoms: Evidence for the moderating role of hope. *Personality and Individual Differences, 49*(5), 391–395. https://doi.org/10.1016/j.paid.2010.04.004

Ghane, A., & Sweeny, K. (2013). Embodied health: A guiding perspective for research in health psychology. *Health Psychology Review, 7*(Suppl 1), S159–S184. https://doi.org/10.1080/17437199.2012.706988

Gibson, M., & Gorman, E. (2012). Long-term care residents with cancer and their health care providers reflect on hope. *Canadian Journal on Aging, 31*(3), 285–293. https://doi.org/10.1017/S0714980812000219

Godfrey, J. J. (1987). *A philosophy of human hope*. Martinus Nijhoff.

Goodman, M., Serag, H., Keiser, P., Gitari, S., Raimer, B., Goodman, M. L., Keiser, P. K., & Raimer, B. G. (2017). Relative social standing and suicide ideation among Kenyan males: The interpersonal theory of suicide in context. *Social Psychiatry & Psychiatric Epidemiology, 52*(10), 1307–1316. https://doi.org/10.1007/s00127-017-1427-4

Gottschalk, L. A. (1985). Hope and other deterrents to illness. *American Journal of Psychotherapy, 39*(4), 515–524.

Gottshalk, L. (1974). A hope scale applicable to verbal samples. *Archives of General Psychiatry, 30*, 779–785.

Gum, A. M., & Ayalon, L. (2018). Self-perceptions of aging mediate the longitudinal relationship of hopelessness and depressive symptoms. *International Journal of Geriatric Psychiatry, 33*(4), 591–597. https://doi.org/10.1002/gps.48

Harley, D. (2015). Reconceptualizing hope among urban African American adolescents through the lens of photovoice. *Journal of Ethnic & Cultural Diversity in Social Work: Innovation in Theory, Research & Practice, 24*(4), 280–299. https://doi.org/10.1080/15313204.2015.1028122

Hassija, C. M., Luterek, J. A., Naragon-Gainey, K., Moore, S. A., & Simpson, T. (2012). Impact of emotional approach coping and hope on PTSD and depression symptoms in a trauma exposed sample of veterans receiving outpatient VA mental health care services. *Anxiety, Stress & Coping: An International Journal, 25*(5), 559–573. https://doi.org/10.1080/10615806.2011.621948

Hasson-Ohayon, I., Braun, M., Galinsky, D., & Baider, L. (2009). Religiosity and hope: A path for women coping with a diagnosis of breast cancer. *Psychosomatics: Journal of Consultation and Liaison Psychiatry, 50*(5), 525–533. https://doi.org/10.1016/S0033-3182(09)70846-1

Herbrand, C., & Dimond, R. (2018). Mitochondrial donation, patient engagement and narratives of hope. *Sociology of Health & Illness, 40*(4), 623–638. https://doi.org/10.1111/1467-9566.12631

Herman, J. L. (1992). *Trauma and recovery*. Basic Books.

Hernandez, M., Barrio, C., Gaona, L., Helu-Brown, P., Hai, A., & Lim, C. (2019). Hope and schizophrenia in the Latino family context. *Community Mental Health Journal, 55*(1), 42–50. https://doi.org/10.1007/s10597-018-0354-5

Herth, K. (1991). Development and refinement of an instrument to measure hope. *Scholarly Inquiry for Nursing Practice, 5*(1), 39–51.

Hinds, P. S. (1984). Inducing a definition of hope through the use of grounded theory methodology... A study of adolescents. *Journal of Advanced Nursing, 9*(4), 357–362. https://doi.org/10.1111/j.1365-2648.1984.tb00384.x

Hinds, S., & Gattuso, J. S. (1991). Measuring hopefulness in adolescents. *Journal of Pediatric Oncology, 8*(2), 92–94.

Hirano, Y. M., Yamazaki, Y., Shimizu, J., Togari, T., & Bryce, T. J. (2006). Ventilator dependence and expressions of need: A study of patients with amyotrophic lateral sclerosis in Japan. *Social Science & Medicine, 62*(6), 1403–1413. https://doi.org/10.1016/j.socscimed.2005.08.015

Hirsch, J. K., Visser, P. L., Chang, E. C., & Jeglic, E. L. (2012). Race and ethnic differences in Hope and hopelessness as moderators of the association between depressive symptoms and suicidal behavior. *Journal of American College Health, 60*(2), 115–125.

Hjemdal, O. (2007). Measuring protective factors: The development of two resilience scales in Norway. *Child and Adolescent Psychiatric Clinics of North America, 16*(2), 303–321. https://doi.org/10.1016/j.chc.2006.12.003

Ho, S., Rajandram, R. K., Chan, N., Samman, N., McGrath, C., & Zwahlen, R. A. (2011). The roles of hope and optimism on posttraumatic growth in oral cavity cancer patients. *Oral Oncology, 47*(2), 121–124. https://doi.org/10.1016/j.oraloncology.2010.11.015

Ho, S. M., Ho, J. W., Bonanno, G. A., Chu, A. T., Chan, E. M., Ho, S. M. Y., Ho, J. W. C., Bonanno, G. A., Chu, A. T. W., & Chan, E. M. S. (2010). Hopefulness predicts resilience after hereditary colorectal cancer genetic testing: A prospective outcome trajectories study. *BMC Cancer, 10*, 279. https://doi.org/10.1186/1471-2407-10-279

Holmberg, B., Hellström, I., Norberg, A., & Österlind, J. (2019). Assenting to exposedness – Meanings of receiving assisted bodily care in a nursing home as narrated by older persons. *Scandinavian Journal of Caring Sciences, 33*(4), 868–877. https://doi.org/10.1111/scs.12683

Hood, A., Pulvers, K., Carrillo, J., Merchant, G., & Thomas, M. D. (2012). Positive traits linked to less pain through lower pain catastrophizing. *Personality and Individual Differences, 52*(3), 401–405. https://doi.org/10.1016/j.paid.2011.10.040

Hornsey, M. J., Lobera, J., & Díaz-Catalán, C. (2020). Vaccine hesitancy is strongly associated with distrust of conventional medicine, and only weakly associated with trust in alternative medicine. *Social Science & Medicine, 255*. https://doi.org/10.1016/j.socscimed.2020.113019

Hsieh, C., Chen, C., Hsiao, F., & Shun, S. (2014). The correlations of sexual activity, sleep problems, emotional distress, attachment styles with quality of life: Comparison between gynecological cancer survivors and noncancer women. *Journal of Clinical Nursing, 23*(7–8), 985–994. https://doi.org/10.1111/jocn.12232

Hutchison, S. L., MacDonald-Wilson, K. L., Karpov, I., Maise, A. M., Wasilchak, D., & Schuster, J. M. (2017). Value of psychiatric rehabilitation in a behavioral health Medicaid managed care system. *Psychiatric Rehabilitation Journal, 40*(2), 216–224. https://doi.org/10.1037/prj0000271

Jiang, X., Otis, K. L., Weber, M., & Huebner, E. S. (2018). Hope and adolescent mental health. In M. W. Gallagher & S. J. Lopez (Eds.), *The Oxford handbook of hope* (pp. 299–312). Oxford University Press.

Kennedy, P., Evans, M., & Sandhu, N. (2009). Psychological adjustment to spinal cord injury: The contribution of coping, hope and cognitive appraisals. *Psychology, Health & Medicine, 14*(1), 17–33.

Kierkegaard, S. (1989). *The sickness unto death*. Penguin. (Original work published 1849).

Kohut, H. (1971). *The analysis of the self.* International Universities Press.

Komen Foundation. (n.d.). https://www.komen.org

Kortte, K. B., Stevenson, J. E., Hosey, M. M., Castillo, R., & Wegener, S. T. (2012). Hope predicts positive functional role outcomes in acute rehabilitation populations. *Rehabilitation Psychology, 57*(3), 248–255. https://doi.org/10.1037/a0029004

Krafft, A. M., Martin-Krumm, C., & Fenouillet, F. (2019). Adaptation, further elaboration, and validation of a scale to measure Hope as perceived by people: Discriminant value and predictive utility Vis-à-Vis dispositional Hope. *Assessment, 26*(8), 1594–1609. https://doi.org/10.1177/1073191117700724

Lee, J. Y., & Gallagher, M. W. (2018). Hope and well-being. In M. W. Gallagher & S. J. Lopez (Eds.), *The Oxford handbook of hope* (pp. 287–298). Oxford University Press.

Li, P. F. J., Wong, Y. J., McDermott, R. C., Cheng, H.-L., & Ruser, J. B. (2021). U.S. college students' lay beliefs about hope: A mixed-methods study. *Journal of Positive Psychology, 16*(2), 249–262. https://doi.org/10.1080/17439760.2019.1689420

Lim, M., Li, Z., Xie, H., Tan, B. L., & Lee, J. (2019). An Asian study on clinical and psychological factors associated with personal recovery in people with psychosis. *BMC Psychiatry, 19*. https://doi.org/10.1186/s12888-019-2238-9

Lin, C.-C., & Tsay, H.-F. (2005). Relationships among perceived diagnostic disclosure, health locus of control, and levels of Hope in Taiwanese cancer patients. *Psycho-Oncology, 14*(5), 376–385. https://doi.org/10.1002/pon.854

Liu, S. R., Kia-Keating, M., & Modir, S. (2017). Hope and adjustment to college in the context of collective trauma. *Journal of American College Health, 65*(5), 323–330. https://doi.org/10.1080/07448481.2017.1312412

Lynch, W. F. (1965). *Images of hope: Imagination as healer of the hopeless*. Helicon Press.

Mahat, G., & Scoloveno, M. A. (2001). Factors influencing health practices of Nepalese adolescent girls. *Journal of Pediatric Healthcare, 15*(5), 251–255.

Makarem, S. C., Smith, M. F., Mudambi, S. M., & Hunt, J. M. (2014). Why people do not always follow the Doctor's orders: The role of Hope and perceived control. *Journal of Consumer Affairs, 48*(3), 457–485.

Marcel, G. (1949). *The philosophy of existentialism* (M. Harari Trans.). Philosophical Library.

Marcel, G. (1951). *Homo Viator: Introduction to the metaphysic of hope* (E. Craufurd, Trans.). Henry Regnery.

Markus, K. A. (2008). Constructs, concepts and the worlds of possibility: Connecting the measurement, manipulation, and meaning of variables. *Measurement: Interdisciplinary Research and Perspectives, 6*(1–2), 54–77.

Marques, S. C. (2016). Psychological strengths in childhood as predictors of longitudinal outcomes. *School Mental Health: A Multidisciplinary Research and Practice Journal, 8*(3), 377–385. https://doi.org/10.1007/s12310-016-9195-y

Marques, S. C., Lopez, S. J., & Pais-Ribeiro, J. L. (2011). "Building hope for the future": A program to foster strengths in middle-school students. *Journal of Happiness Studies: An Interdisciplinary Forum on Subjective Well-Being, 12*(1), 139–152. https://doi.org/10.1007/s10902-009-9180-3

May, E., Hunter, B., Ferrari, J., Noel, N., & Jason, L. (2015). Hope and abstinence self-efficacy: Positive predictors of negative affect in substance abuse recovery. *Community Mental Health Journal, 51*(6), 695–700. https://doi.org/10.1007/s10597-015-9888-y

McDermott, D., & Snyder, C. R. (1999). *Making hope happen*. New Harbinger.

Menninger, K. (1959). The academic lecture: Hope. *The American Journal of Psychiatry, 116*, 481–491. https://doi.org/10.1176/ajp.116.6.481

Moltmann, J. (1967). *Theology of hope* (J.W. Leitch Trans.). Harper and Row. (Original work published 1964).

Morote, R., Hjemdal, O., Krysinska, K., Martinez Uribe, P., & Corveleyn, J. (2017). Resilience or hope? Incremental and convergent validity of the resilience scale for adults (RSA) and the Herth hope scale (HHS) in the prediction of anxiety and depression. *BMC Psychology, 5*(1), 36. https://doi.org/10.1186/s40359-017-0205-0

Murdoch, K. C., Larsen, D., Edey, W., Arsenault, C., Howell, A., Joyce, A., Sandham, T., & Miyasaki, J. M. (2020). The efficacy of the strength, Hope and resourcefulness program for people with Parkinson's disease (SHARP-PWP): A mixed methods study. *Parkinsonism and Related Disorders, 70*, 7–12. https://doi.org/10.1016/j.parkreldis.2019.11.010

Natale, P., Saglimbene, V., Ruospo, M., Gonzalez, A. M., Strippoli, G. F., Scholes-Robertson, N., Guha, C., Craig, J. C., Teixeira-Pinto, A., Snelling, T., & Tong, A. (2021). Transparency, trust and minimizing burden to increase recruitment and retention in trials: A systematic review. *Journal of Clinical Epidemiology, 134*, 35–51. https://doi.org/10.1016/j.jclinepi.2021.01.014

Nowotny, M. (1989). Assessment of hope in patients with cancer: Development of an instrument. *Oncology Nursing Forum, 16*(1), 57–61.

Ociskova, M., Prasko, J., Kamaradova, D., Grambal, A., Kasalova, P., Sigmundova, Z., Latalova, K., & Vrbova, K. (2015). Coping strategies, hope, and treatment efficacy in pharmaco-resistant inpatients with neurotic spectrum disorders. *Neuropsychiatric Disease & Treatment, 11*, 1191–1201. https://doi.org/10.2147/NDT.S80325

Olsman, E. (2020). Hope in healthcare: A synthesis of review studies. In S. C. van den Heuvel (Ed.), *Historical and multidisciplinary perspectives on hope* (pp. 197–214). https://doi.org/10.1007/978-3-030-46489-9_14

Pettit, P. (2004). Hope and its place in mind. *Annals of the American Academy of Political and Social Science, 592*, 152–165. https://doi.org/10.1177/0002716203261798

Phillips, B. N., Smedema, S. M., Fleming, A. R., Sung, C., & Allen, M. G. (2016). Mediators of disability and hope for people with spinal cord injury. *Disability & Rehabilitation, 38*(17), 1672–1683.

Piedmont, R. L. (1999). Does spirituality represent the sixth factor of personality? Spiritual transcendence and the five-factor model. *Journal of Personality, 67*(6), 985–1013. https://doi.org/10.1111/1467-6494.00080

Prochaska, J. O., Johnson, S., & Lee, P. (2009). The Transtheoretical model of behavior change. In S. A. Shumaker, J. K. Ockene, & K. A. Riekert (Eds.), *The handbook of health behavior change* (3rd ed., pp. 59–83). Springer Publishing Company.

Pruyser, P. W. (1987). Maintaining hope in adversity. *Bulletin of the Menninger Clinic, 51*(5), 463–474.

Randall, R. L. (1984). The legacy of Kohut for religion and psychology. *Journal of Religion and Health, 23*(2), 106–114. https://doi.org/10.1007/BF00996153

Robieux, L., Zenasni, F., Flahault, C., & Tavani, J.-L. (2018). L'espoir dans la maladie chronique: Représentations sociales de l'espoir chez les patients et soignants =

Hope in chronic diseases: Social representations of patients' and caregivers' hope. *Psychologie Française, 63*(1), 37–50. https://doi.org/10.1016/j.psfr.2016.12.003
Rustøen, T., Cooper, B. A., & Miaskowski, C. (2010). The importance of hope as a mediator of psychological distress and life satisfaction in a community sample of cancer patients. *Cancer Nursing, 33*(4), 258–267. https://doi.org/10.1097/NCC.0b013e3181d6fb61
Rustøen, T., Cooper, B. A., & Miaskowski, C. (2011). A longitudinal study of the effects of a hope intervention on levels of hope and psychological distress in a community-based sample of oncology patients. *European Journal of Oncology Nursing, 15*(4), 351–357. https://doi.org/10.1016/j.ejon.2010.09.001
Rychlak, J. F. (1968). *A philosophy of science for personality theory*. Houghton Mifflin.
Sachs, E., Kolva, E., Pessin, H., Rosenfeld, B., & Breitbart, W. (2013). On sinking and swimming: The dialectic of hope, hopelessness, and acceptance in terminal cancer. *The American Journal of Hospice & Palliative Care, 30*(2), 121–127. https://doi.org/10.1177/1049909112445371
Salsman, J. M., Pustejovsky, J. E., Jim, H. S. L., Munoz, A. R., Merluzzi, T. V., George, L., Park, C. L., Danhauer, S. C., Sherman, A. C., Snyder, M. A., & Fitchett, G. (2015). A meta-analytic approach to examining the correlation between religion/spirituality and mental health in cancer. *Cancer, 121*(21), 3769–3778.
Scheier, M. F., Carver, C. S., & Bridges, M. W. (1994). Distinguishing optimism from neuroticism (and trait anxiety, self-mastery, and self-esteem): A re-evaluation of the life orientation test. *Journal of Personality & Social Psychology, 67*(6), 1063–1078. https://doi.org/10.1037/0022-3514.67.6.1063
Schiavon, C. C., Marchetti, E., Gurgel, L. G., Busnello, F. M., & Reppold, C. T. (2017). Optimism and hope in chronic disease: A systematic review. *Frontiers in Psychology, 7*. https://doi.org/10.3389/fpsyg.2016.02022
Scioli, A. (2020). The psychology of hope: A diagnostic and prescriptive account. In S. C. van den Heuvel (Ed.), *Historical and multidisciplinary perspectives on hope* (pp. 137–164). https://doi.org/10.1007/978-3-030-46489-9_14
Scioli, A., & Biller, H. B. (2009). *Hope in the age of anxiety*. Oxford University Press.
Scioli, A., Chamberlin, C. M., Samor, C. M., Lapointe, A. B., Campbell, T. L., Macleod, A. R., & McLenon, J. (1997). A prospective study of hope, optimism, and health. *Psychological Reports, 81*(3, Pt 1), 723–733. https://doi.org/10.2466/pr0.1997.81.3.723
Scioli, A., Cofrin, M., Aceto, F., & Martin, T. (2018). *Toward a Rorschach hope index. Rorschachiana, 39*(2), 157–179. https://doi.org/10.1027/1192-5604/a000110
Scioli, A., MacNeil, S., Partridge, V., Tinker, E., & Hawkins, E. (2012). Hope, HIV and health: A prospective study. *AIDS Care, 24*(2), 149–156.
Scioli, A., MacPherson, N., Murphy, R., Gooding, T., Love, M., Adachi-Mejia, A., & Lyons, K. (2017, August). *A feasibility and efficacy study of a hope-centered intervention*. Poster Presentation. American Psychological Association 125th Annual Convention.

Scioli, A., Ricci, M., Nyugen, T., & Scioli, E. R. (2011). Hope: Its nature and measurement. *Psychology of Religion and Spirituality, 3*(2), 78–97. https://doi.org/10.1037/a0020903

Scioli, A., Scioli-Salter, E. R., Sykes, K., Anderson, C., & Fedele, M. (2016). The positive contributions of hope to maintaining and restoring health: An integrative, mixed-method approach. *Journal of Positive Psychology, 11*(2), 135–148. https://doi.org/10.1080/17439760.2015.1037858

Scioli, A. Seibert, T., Karemera, D., Jacobi, M., Nkurunziza, J, & Nsengiyumva, C. (2020, August). *Hope, depression, and trauma in Rwandan youth*. Poster presentation. American Psychological Association 128th Annual Convention.

Scioli, A., Sykes, K., Harriman, C., & Heon, T. (2013, March 1–3). *Assessment of hope in children and teens* [Poster Presentation]. Eastern Psychological Association 84th Annual Convention, New York.

Shoshani, A., Mifano, K., & Czamanski-Cohen, J. (2016). The effects of the make a wish intervention on psychiatric symptoms and health-related quality of life of children with cancer: A randomized controlled trial. *Quality of Life Research : An International Journal of Quality of Life Aspects of Treatment, Care and Rehabilitation, 25*(5), 1209–1218. https://doi.org/10.1007/s11136-015-1148-7

Smedema, S. M., Chan, J. Y., & Phillips, B. N. (2014). Core self-evaluations and Snyder's hope theory in persons with spinal cord injuries. *Rehabilitation Psychology, 59*(4), 399–406. https://doi.org/10.1037/rep0000015

Snyder, C. R., Berg, C., Woodward, J. T., Gum, A., Rand, K. L., Wrobleski, K. K., Brown, J., & Hackman, A. (2005). Hope against the cold: Individual differences in trait Hope and acute pain tolerance on the cold pressor task. *Journal of Personality, 73*(2), 287–312. https://doi.org/10.1111/j.1467-6494.2005.00318.x

Snyder, C. R., Harris, C., Anderson, J. R., Holleran, S. A., Irving, L. M., Sigmon, S. T., Yoshinobu, L., Gibb, J., Langelle, C., & Harney, P. (1991). The will and the ways: Development and validation of an individual differences measure of hope. *Journal of Personality and Social Psychology, 60*(4), 570–585. https://doi.org/10.1037/0022-3514.60.4.570

Snyder, C. R., Hoza, B., Pelham, W. E., Rapoff, M., Ware, L., Danovsky, M., Highberger, L., Ribinstein, H., & Stahl, K. J. (1997). The development and validation of the Children's Hope scale. *Journal of Pediatric Psychology, 22*(3), 399–421. https://doi.org/10.1093/jpepsy/22.3.399

Song, Y. (2014). Losing an only child: The one-child policy and elderly care in China. *Reproductive Health Matters, 22*(43), 113–124. https://doi.org/10.1016/S0968-8080(14)43755-8

Spaniol, L., Koehler, M., & Hutchinson, D. (1994). *Recovery workbook: Practical coping and empowerment strategies for people with psychiatric disability*. Unpublished Manuscript. Center for Psychiatric Rehabilitation, Boston University.

Staats, S. (1989). Hope: A comparison of two self-report measures for adults. *Journal of Personality Assessment, 53*(2), 366–375. https://doi.org/10.1207/s15327752jpa5302_13

Stanton, A. L., Danoff-Burg, S., & Huggins, M. E. (2002). The first year after breast cancer diagnosis: Hope and coping strategies as predictors of adjustment. *Psycho-Oncology, 11*(2), 93–102. https://doi.org/10.1002/pon.574

Stotland, E. (1969). *The psychology of Hope*. Jossey-Bass.

Taleghani, F., Yekta, Z. P., Nasrabadi, A. N., & Käppeli, S. (2008). Adjustment process in Iranian women with breast cancer. *Cancer Nursing, 31*(3), E32–E41. https://doi.org/10.1097/01.NCC.0000305720.98518.35

Tillich, P. (1963). *The eternal now*. Charles Scribner.

Trezise, A., McLaren, S., Gomez, R., Bice, B., & Hodgetts, J. (2018). Resiliency among older adults: Dispositional hope as a protective factor in the insomnia-depressive symptoms relation. *Aging & Mental Health, 22*(8), 1088–1096. https://doi.org/10.1080/13607863.2017.1334191

Tsai, J. L., Miao, F. F., Seppala, E., Fung, H. H., & Yeung, D. Y. (2007). Influence and adjustment goals: Sources of cultural differences in ideal affect. *Journal of Personality and Social Psychology, 92*(6), 1102–1117. https://doi.org/10.1037/0022-3514.92.6.1102

Valle, M. F., Huebner, E. S., & Suldo, S. M. (2006). An analysis of hope as a psychological strength. *Journal of School Psychology, 44*(5), 393–406. https://doi.org/10.1016/j.jsp.2006.03.005

Vellone, E., Rega, M. L., Galletti, C., & Cohen, M. Z. (2006). Hope and related variables in Italian cancer patients. *Cancer Nursing, 29*(5), 356–366. https://doi.org/10.1097/00002820-200609000-00002

Walsh, I., Holton, J. A., Bailyn, L., Fernandez, W., Levina, N., & Glaser, B. (2015). What grounded theory is … a critically reflective conversation among scholars. *Organizational Research Methods, 18*(4), 581–599. https://doi.org/10.1177/1094428114565028

Wang, Q., Xu, W., Ren, L., Wang, W., & Wang, Y. (2019). The relationship between hope and post-traumatic stress disorder in Chinese shidu parents: The mediating role of perceived stress. *Journal of Affective Disorders, 251*, 23–30. https://doi.org/10.1016/j.jad.2019.03.049

Wehmeyer, M. L., & Shogren, K. A. (2018). Self-determination and hope. In M. W. Gallagher & S. J. Lopez (Eds.), *The Oxford handbook of hope* (pp. 59–68). Oxford University Press.

Whitley, R. (2010). Rediscovering hope. *Psychiatric Rehabilitation Journal, 33*(3), 239–241. https://doi.org/10.2975/33.3.2010.239.241

Wittgenstein, L. (1973). *Philosophical investigations* (G. Anscombe, Trans.). Pearson. (Original work published 1953).

Wlodarczyk, D. (2017). Optimism and hope as predictors of subjective health in post–myocardial infarction patients: A comparison of the role of coping strategies. *Journal of Health Psychology, 22*(3), 336–346. https://doi.org/10.1177/1359105315603470

Wnuk, M. (2017). Hope as an important factor for mental health in alcohol-dependent subjects attending alcoholics anonymous. *Journal of Substance Use, 22*(2), 182–186. https://doi.org/10.1080/14659891.2016.1177612

Wolf, A., Garlid, C. F., & Hyrkas, K. (2018). Physicians' perceptions of hope and how hope informs interactions with patients: A qualitative, exploratory study. *American Journal of Hospice & Palliative Medicine, 35*(7), 993–999. https://doi.org/10.1177/1049909117751877

Wright, B. A., & Shontz, F. C. (1968). Process and tasks in hoping. *Rehabilitation Literature, 29*(11), 322–333.

Yuen, A. N. Y., Ho, S. M. Y., & Chan, C. K. Y. (2014). The mediating roles of cancer-related rumination in the relationship between dispositional hope and psychological outcomes among childhood cancer survivors. *Psycho-Oncology, 23*(4), 412–419. https://doi.org/10.1002/pon.3433

Zhang, H., Chi, P., Long, H., & Ren, X. (2019a). Bullying victimization and depression among left-behind children in rural China: Roles of self-compassion and hope. *Child Abuse & Neglect, 96*. https://doi.org/10.1016/j.chiabu.2019.104072

Zhang, X., Xiao, H., & Chen, Y. (2019b). Evaluation of a WeChat-based life review programme for cancer patients: A quasi-experimental study. *Journal of Advanced Nursing, 75*(7), 1563–1574. https://doi.org/10.1111/jan.14018

14

The Importance of Optimism for Adaptive Self-Regulation: Associations with Subjective Well-Being and Physical Health

Carsten Wrosch, James Borenstein-Laurie, Meaghan A. Barlow, and Jesse Renaud

Dispositional optimism is considered a relatively stable personality construct, reflecting individual differences in generalized positive versus negative expectancies about future outcomes across life domains (Scheier & Carver, 1985). Optimists generally expect good outcomes to occur in their lives, while

We thank Michael F. Scheier for his continued discussion on the self-regulation of behavior and for his comments on an earlier draft of this chapter. It was further supported by grants and fellowships from Social Sciences and Humanities Research Council of Canada. Correspondence should be sent to Carsten Wrosch, Concordia University, Department of Psychology, Montreal, Canada; carsten.wrosch@concordia.ca.

C. Wrosch (✉) • J. Borenstein-Laurie
Department of Psychology, Concordia University, Montreal, QC, Canada
e-mail: carsten.wrosch@concordia.ca; james.borenstein-laurie@mail.concordia.ca

M. A. Barlow
Wilfred Laurier University, Waterloo, ON, Canada
e-mail: mbarlow@wlu.ca

J. Renaud
Department of Psychiatry, McGill University and McGill University Health Centre, Montreal, QC, Canada
e-mail: jesse.renaud@mail.mcgill.ca

F. M. Sirois (ed.), *The Palgrave Handbook of Positive Psychology and Health*,
https://doi.org/10.1007/978-3-031-89095-6_14

pessimists expect their endeavors to fail.[1] Optimism has been considered a construct relevant for the area of positive psychology (e.g., Dunn, 2018). In particular, the presence of optimism can be considered an important personal strength that fosters quality of life. This notion is supported by a wealth of research, associating dispositional optimism with a wide range of beneficial outcomes of psychological well-being and physical health (for quantitative and qualitative reviews, see Rasmussen et al., 2006; Scheier et al., 2021a).

This chapter addresses the importance of dispositional optimism beginning with a consideration of self-regulation principles that provide a framework for understanding how dispositional optimism contributes to a person's quality of life. Subsequently, we discuss the operationalization of dispositional optimism and review key findings from the literature describing associations of optimism with subjective well-being and physical health. To this end, we further address how coping and social resources may play a role in explaining the beneficial effects of optimism. The chapter closes with addressing different issues that inform researchers and practitioners about how optimism could be enhanced across the life course as well as the circumstances and aspects of optimism that make it particularly effective for improving psychological well-being and physical health.

Self-Regulatory Benefits of Optimism

Optimism can confer benefits for well-being and health because it supports the pursuit of personal goals (Carver et al., 2010; Wrosch & Scheier, 2003). Therefore, to understand the mechanisms that are related to its adaptive consequences, it is useful to consider theories of self-regulation that point to the importance of personal goals. A central aspect of these theories relates to the goals themselves that are being pursued. Typically, people pursue goals that they value highly and that they expect to attain (see expectancy-value models, Atkinson & Birch, 1978; Feather, 1982). In this regard, optimism reflects a broad, generalized aspect of the expectancy component of these models, enhancing the likelihood that valued goals are being pursued (Carver et al., 2010).

---

[1] We use the terms 'optimists' and 'pessimists' to describe people who fall on different ends of the continuous distribution of dispositional optimism. These terms are used to facilitate communication of theoretical propositions and empirical research. In addition, we note that the concept of dispositional optimism needs to be distinguished from other, related constructs, which do not target outcome expectancies directly (e.g., learned optimism, Scheier & Carver, 2018; Seligman, 1991, for further discussion, see also section on measurement provided later in this chapter).

The pursuit of valued goals can serve adaptive functions. Several theories of self-regulation support this idea by postulating that goals promote subjective well-being and physical health across the lifespan (e.g., Carver & Scheier, 1998; Emmons, 1986; Freund & Baltes, 2002; Heckhausen et al., 2010, 2019). Goals may confer benefits by providing purpose for living (Ryff & Keyes, 1995; Scheier et al., 2006) and directing specific behaviors toward the achievement of desired outcomes (Carver & Scheier, 1998; Heckhausen, 1999). These behaviors play important roles in the moment-to-moment regulation of action (e.g., buying groceries to cook a meal) and the achievement of longer-term developmental tasks (e.g., graduating from university). As such, the adoption of goals can promote planning, effort, and time investment into valued projects (Emmons, 1986; Gollwitzer, 1999; Heckhausen, 1999). In addition, goals become important if people confront severe, but potentially manageable, stressors or constraints. In such circumstances, goals may contribute to effective coping and overcoming goal-related barriers (Carver et al., 1989; Lazarus & Folkman, 1984).

The latter propositions are consistent with control theory, conceptualizing how a person's goals facilitate adaptive behaviors (Carver & Scheier, 1981, 2001). This approach assumes that goals can form negative feedback loops, in which a person compares her or his perception of goal-related circumstances to a reference value (i.e., a goal, Miller et al., 1960). If this comparison process detects a difference between where a person is and where the person wants to be with respect to the goal (i.e., the comparison yields a negative discrepancy), the person typically engages in proactive behaviors to reduce the goal-related discrepancy. The consequences of these behaviors are subsequently reevaluated, launching a new comparison process and promoting continuous cycles of goal regulation that move the person closer to the achievement of the desired outcome (Carver & Scheier, 1981).

People also differ in the extent to which they attain their goals. From a personality perspective, these differences are meaningful and may relate to individual difference variables that determine the type, intensity, and duration of goal-related behaviors. We think that optimism also facilitates such goal regulation processes. Consistent with this assumption, different research groups have identified a number of individual difference variables that support the attainment of goals, including optimism (Scheier & Carver, 1985, for other constructs, see research on self-efficacy, perceived control, control strategies, or grit, Bandura, 1997; Duckworth et al., 2007; Heckhausen et al., 2010; Pearlin & Schooler, 1978). Although all these individual differences seem to play an important role in the self-regulation of behavior, we focus here on the importance of dispositional optimism for subjective well-being and physical health. Our interest in optimism stems from its theoretical foundation in expectancy-value models and theories of self-regulation, which assume that optimistic, as compared to pessimistic, outcome expectancies foster the adoption and regulation of valued goals. These motivational processes may become paramount when goal-related obstacles are encountered by ensuring that people continue to invest time and effort in attaining threatened goals (Carver & Scheier, 1981).

The link between optimism and effective goal regulation may further explain how dispositional optimism can contribute to both subjective well-being and physical health. Although successful goal pursuits typically enhance people's well-being, goal failure and insufficient progress toward desired goals have been considered a source of emotional distress (Carver & Scheier, 1990; Emmons, 1986; Wrosch & Scheier, 2020). Emotional distress and low subjective well-being, in turn, are important contributors to the emergence of physical health problems (Diener & Chan, 2011), likely related to maladaptive health behaviors or a dysregulation of health-relevant physiological systems (e.g., endocrine or immune systems, Cohen et al., 2007). Since optimism is supposed to promote the pursuit of valued goals (Scheier & Carver, 1985), optimists should be less likely than pessimists to experience continued goal failure and insufficient progress, and consequently more likely to protect their well-being and physical health. Note that certain goals can also protect physical health directly, in particular if they target specific health outcomes (e.g., following the advice of a physician or starting to exercise), and if the pursuit of these goals promotes recovery from a health problem or prevents prospective health issues (e.g., Gollwitzer & Oettingen, 1998; Wrosch & Sabiston, 2013).

Measuring Optimism

The gold standard for measuring dispositional optimism is the Life Orientation Test-Revised (LOT-R, Scheier et al., 1994). This self-report instrument asks people to respond to six different statements, reflecting their general agreement on 5-point Likert-type scales. Three of the items reflect optimism (e.g., I'm always optimistic about my future), and three items reflect pessimism (e.g., If something can go wrong for me, it will). The two sets of items are typically combined, after reverse-coding of the pessimism items. Note that this operationalization of optimism assumes a unidimensional and bipolar construct, ranging from high optimism to high pessimism (for further consideration of dimensionality, see discussion provided later in this chapter). In addition, it assesses a person's outcome expectancies directly, which makes it different from other approaches to optimism that infer optimism by measuring people's attributions of failure events (Peterson et al., 1982; Seligman, 1991).

The LOT-R has shown appropriate reliability estimates across studies. For example, a recent meta-analysis on research of dispositional optimism and physical health obtained an average Cronbach's alpha of 0.75 for the LOT-R (Scheier et al., 2021a). In addition, longitudinal studies on optimism suggest that it can be stable over time, frequently as stable as other personality constructs such as the Big 5 personality factors (for development and change in optimism, see discussion provided later in this chapter). For example, stability estimates over a few weeks to 3 years ranged from 0.58 to 0.79 (Scheier & Carver, 2018). Even over longer periods, such as 10 years, dispositional optimism has been found to be quite stable (Matthews et al., 2004). These psychometric characteristics of the LOT-R suggest that it is well-suited for examining psychological and physical health consequences of dispositional optimism.

Optimism and Subjective Well-Being

Research has shown that dispositional optimism can predict high levels of subjective well-being across a wide variety of samples and stressful circumstances (for a review, see Scheier et al., 2001). Such an association has been reported, for example, in college students (Aspinwall & Taylor, 1992; Chang, 1998), caregivers of Alzheimer patients (Shifren & Hooker, 1995), cancer and coronary artery bypass patients (Carver et al., 1993; Scheier et al., 1989), and women after childbirth (Carver & Gaines, 1987). The beneficial association between optimism and subjective well-being is also reflected in the results from different meta-analyses. In a study evaluating 280 samples, Alarcon et al. (2013) showed reliable and positive associations between optimism and different indicators of subjective well-being, such as high life satisfaction, low depressive symptoms, and low anxiety. Similar conclusions were drawn by Andersson (1996), showing in 56 samples that dispositional optimism was inversely associated with the experience of negative affect. Together, these findings provide robust evidence for an association between greater dispositional optimism and subjective well-being.

Adaptive effects of optimism on subjective well-being have been found in both cross-sectional and longitudinal research. Longitudinal studies are important as they shed light on the associations between variables over time. In this regard, a study by Carver and Gaines (1987) examined postpartum depression by assessing depressive symptoms in a sample of women before childbirth and three weeks postpartum. The results of the study showed that those women who were more optimistic before childbirth were less likely to develop increases in depressive symptoms than their counterparts who were more pessimistic (Carver & Gaines, 1987). These findings document that dispositional optimism can produce longitudinal effects in the context of stressful life circumstances and benefit people's subjective well-being over time.

Optimism and Physical Health

There is ample evidence that dispositional optimism can be associated with physical health. Studies have linked dispositional optimism with a myriad of health outcomes, including better cardiovascular health (Boehm & Kubzansky, 2012), reduced disease progression (Matthews et al., 2004), and lower overall mortality (Kim et al., 2017). Dispositional optimism has also been associated with greater subjective health in normative populations (Achat et al., 2000) and at-risk populations (e.g., patients with myocardial infarction, Wlodarczyk, 2015).

The effects of optimism on physical health could be related to people's health behaviors and physiological functioning (Cohen et al., 2007). Consistent with this possibility, research has documented that dispositional optimism can predict health-relevant behaviors (e.g., improved sleep, Uchino et al., 2017). In addition, greater optimism has been shown to buffer a dysregulation of health-relevant physiological processes in the context of stress (e.g., cortisol output or immune responses; Jobin et al., 2014; Segerstrom et al., 1998).

To provide comprehensive evidence for the health effects of optimism, research findings have been subjected to different meta-analytic reviews (for a qualitative review, see also Boehm & Kubzansky, 2012). An earlier meta-analysis examined effect sizes of optimism on subjective and objective physical health indicators from 83 different samples (Rasmussen et al., 2009). In this study, the authors reported a reliable and positive association between dispositional optimism and physical health. This pattern of results was replicated in supplemental analyses for different groups of health outcomes, such as cardiovascular symptoms, biomarkers, cancer outcomes, or mortality (Rasmussen et al., 2009). A more recent study, using meta-analytic techniques, examined effects of optimism on objective health outcomes in 61 separate studies (Scheier et al., 2021a). Consistent with the former study, the later research confirmed a positive association between dispositional optimism and physical health. Importantly, these effects were consistent for cross-sectional, prospective, and longitudinal studies. In addition, 80% of samples in the latter study were not included in the earlier meta-analysis, bolstering confidence in the conclusion that optimism is associated with physical health benefits.

Research has also considered the role of subjective well-being in the association between dispositional optimism and physical health. One study examined sleep quality in a cross-sectional community sample. The study found that dispositional optimism predicted better sleep quality, and that this effect was mediated by low levels of depressive symptoms and high levels of life satisfaction (Uchino et al., 2017). Another study, consisting of a group of patients receiving cardiac rehabilitation, examined the role of optimism and depressive symptoms on physical functioning over time. The study's results showed that optimism was longitudinally associated with an improvement in physical functioning and that this effect was mediated by lower levels of depressive symptoms (Shen et al., 2004). Together, the mediation effects obtained in these studies suggest that the beneficial effects that optimism exerts on subjective well-being may have important downstream implications for people's physical health.

The Role of Coping

Although the previous discussion documents reliable associations between dispositional optimism, subjective well-being, and physical health, it did not address some of the specific psychological processes that could contribute to these associations. To shed light on this issue, a number of researchers have examined how optimists and pessimists cope with stress and goal constraints. This work is important as it reveals the behavioral and cognitive mechanisms that could explain the beneficial effects of dispositional optimism on subjective well-being and physical health.

The literature on coping suggests that optimists and pessimists react differently to stressful encounters. If they confront adversity or goal constraints, optimists tend to face the stressor head-on and engage in coping tactics aimed at resolving the stressful situation. Pessimists, by contrast, are more likely to engage in avoidant coping tactics. The latter conclusion is supported by a meta-analysis examining the association between dispositional optimism and coping in 50 independent samples (Nes & Segerstrom, 2006). The coping tactics that were used more frequently by optimists, as compared to pessimists, involved (among others) planning, active coping, seeking instrumental support, or positive reinterpretation. By contrast, pessimists used coping tactics that reflect denial or mental and behavioral disengagement more frequently than optimists (Nes & Segerstrom, 2006).

Interestingly, the same meta-analysis concluded that optimists may also be more likely than pessimists to adjust their coping strategies to the contextual demands of a stressor (Nes & Segerstrom, 2006). This assumption is consistent with earlier work on optimism and coping, examining how optimists and pessimists react to controllable versus uncontrollable situations (Scheier et al., 1986). For example, results from a study of college students showed that if a situation was controllable, optimists were more likely than pessimists to engage in problem-focused coping and positive reinterpretation. In uncontrollable circumstances, however, optimism predicted the acceptance of the intractable situation (Scheier et al., 1986). Thus, optimism seems to be associated with two different kinds of coping responses. It can help promote successful goal attainment, in contexts where it seems difficult to attain a goal, and it can promote acceptance, in contexts in which goal attainment seems impossible. Perhaps, if people generally expect positive outcomes to occur in their future, they feel that their life will be purposeful and satisfying even if they cannot resolve a current, uncontrollable problem. This positive outlook, in turn, could facilitate the acceptance of a specific problem or make it easier to abandon a goal that is not attainable (for optimism and disengagement from unsolvable tasks, see also Aspinwall & Richter, 1999).

There is also research examining whether the use of different coping tactics can mediate the effects of optimism on subjective well-being and physical health. A longitudinal study by Scheier et al. (1989) examined a sample of coronary artery bypass patients over time. Their study found that optimists engaged more frequently in recovery planning and focused less on the negative aspects of their health problem than their pessimistic counterparts. In addition, these coping tactics mediated the beneficial effects of dispositional optimism on patients' quality of life six months post-surgery (Scheier et al., 1989).

Another longitudinal study examined the mediating role of coping among breast cancer patients (Carver et al., 1993). The study's results suggested that dispositional optimism was associated with the use of active coping strategies and adaptive emotion-focused coping (e.g., positive reframing or acceptance of reality). In addition, the study obtained an effect of dispositional optimism on reduced levels of distress post-surgery, which was mediated by these coping tactics (Carver et al., 1993).

Conceptually similar findings were reported by Segerstrom et al. (1998), who examined prospectively associations between optimism and mood in a sample of law students. Results from this study showed that dispositional optimism predicted improved mood over time, and that this effect was partially mediated by less avoidant coping. Together, the reported evidence suggests that optimists use adaptive coping tactics in stressful circumstances more frequently than pessimists, and that these differences in coping can benefit their well-being and health.

The Role of Social Resources

Another line of work has examined whether optimism has beneficial consequences on people's social resources (for a review, see Carver et al., 2010). Supportive and satisfying social relations, for example, are essential resources that can contribute to subjective well-being and physical health (Cohen, 2004). These resources are important from a self-regulation perspective as they likely facilitate the attainment of important goals by promoting adaptive behaviors in stressful life circumstances, and helping people to overcome goal-related barriers (Brissette et al., 2002; Cohen & Wills, 1985).

One study engaged a community sample in thinking about positive future experiences (MacLeod & Conway, 2005). The study showed that to the extent participants thought about a greater number of positive future experiences, they also reported a larger social network. Another study examined social relations in a sample of university freshmen over the course of their first semester, a time when many people form new and important relationships (Brissette et al., 2002). Similar to the previous study, the researchers showed a positive association between dispositional optimism and social network size, although optimism did not predict an increase in social network size during the semester. Maybe more importantly, the study found that optimistic students perceived greater increases in social support and fewer increases in depressive symptoms and stress than their pessimistic counterparts. In addition, the analyses confirmed that the longitudinal effects of dispositional optimism on reduced levels of depressive symptoms and perceived stress were mediated by increases in perceived social support. Note that increased social support contributed to the optimism effects on subjective well-being even when relevant coping tactics were considered (Brissette et al., 2002). The latter result suggests that the effects of dispositional optimism on social relations and coping represent different pathways to subjective well-being.

We acknowledge that there appears to be a generally smaller body of research on the social effects of dispositional optimism than on optimism and coping. As a consequence, it is not entirely clear what drives the social benefits of optimism. One reason could be that people like optimists more than pessimists (Carver et al., 2010). In support of this possibility, research has shown that people are more willing to engage with others, when these others have an optimistic, rather than pessimistic, outlook (Carver et al., 1994). Another reason could be that optimists invest more time and energy into their social relations than pessimists, and thus may benefit to a greater extent from supportive relationships when they need them (Carver et al., 2010). The latter explanation would be consistent with research showing that, as compared with pessimists, optimists can be more satisfied with their relationships and perceive themselves (and their partners) as engaging more constructively during conflicts (Srivastava et al., 2006). Whatever the reason is, the extant research points to the conclusion that the social domain represents another important aspect of life that holds benefits for optimists. Clearly, more research is needed to understand the social consequences of optimism and the implications of those consequences for subjective well-being and physical health.

Developmental and Conceptual Issues

The previous discussion documents that dispositional optimism is an adaptive personality construct that fosters effective goal-related behaviors and social resources, and protects people's well-being and health. We think that this pattern of findings makes it relevant to address additional developmental and conceptual issues that could deepen our understanding of dispositional optimism research and provide useful information for colleagues who work on improving people's quality of life.

How Does Optimism Develop and Can it Change?

One issue relates to how dispositional optimism develops and changes during the lifespan. Understanding the mechanisms that contribute to changes in optimism may provide pathways toward increasing optimism and subsequently optimizing people's well-being and health. Despite the known benefits associated with greater optimism, the developmental pathways to becoming an optimist or a pessimist have not been fully elucidated. Both genetic and environmental factors have been implicated in the development of optimism. Twin studies show that optimism is partially inherited, with between 25 and 30% of the variability in optimism explained by genetic factors (Mosing et al., 2009, 2010; Plomin et al., 1992). With respect to environmental antecedents of optimism, our understanding is still in its infancy. Currently, the literature appears to implicate early exposure to supportive familial contexts in the development of optimism. In addition, life transitions and the experience of favorable opportunities for the successful pursuit of goals are promising factors that could contribute to optimism development.

Research on the early familial context points primarily to the role of positive parenting for promoting greater optimism. Results from retrospective studies show that optimistic adults recall having experienced greater warmth and more positive parent–child relationships compared to their pessimistic peers (Hjelle et al., 1996; Korkeila et al., 2004). In contrast, pessimism was linked to recollections of rejection and insecure attachment (Heinonen et al., 2004; Hjelle et al., 1996).

The importance of parent–child relationships for promoting optimism has also been demonstrated in prospective studies. In one study, mothers who rated their children as having a difficult temperament had more hostile child-rearing attitudes, which contributed to greater pessimism in their offspring 21 years later (Heinonen et al., 2005). More recently, a study found that greater maternal attachment security in childhood predicted higher levels of perceived control in adolescence, which contributed to higher levels of optimism and associated well-being in early adulthood. The authors concluded that successes may be experienced more frequently by people who perceive greater control, and that these people may thus be more likely to feel optimistic about their ability to secure successes in the future (Renaud et al., 2019). This possibility is consistent with research showing that higher levels of perceived control are associated with the use of adaptive behavioral strategies that contribute to increased opportunities for success (Lachman & Firth, 2004; Lang & Heckhausen, 2001).

Although optimism is relatively stable over time (Scheier & Carver, 2018), researchers are turning their attention to how personality constructs, like optimism, may be amenable to contextual factors beyond the early developmental years. In this regard, the available research on the malleability of personality constructs has shown that such changes are more likely to occur when people experience periods of important transitions or significant life events (Bleidorn et al., 2018; Schwaba & Bleidorn, 2018). Consistent with this idea, a study by Segerstrom (2007) showed in a sample of students who entered law school that they experienced considerable changes in optimism over ten years. The extent to which exposure to life transitions or changing contexts, such as entering university, may trigger changes in optimism may depend on whether self-regulation responses result in the repeated experience of success or failure

(Renaud et al., 2018). If individuals successfully negotiate transitions or environmental demands, they may be more likely to expect future successes and experience associated increases in optimism. However, failure to adaptively manage important transitions and life events may result in increased pessimism.

The possibility that optimism can change across the entire lifespan seems to be relevant for intervention research and clinical practice. In fact, results from a meta-analysis showed that even brief experimental interventions (e.g., writing about a best possible self) can promote short-term gains in optimism (Malouff & Schutte, 2017). Further evidence of the malleability of optimism stems from research showing that problem-solving therapy can promote adaptive psychological functioning, including optimism, that can help people overcome challenges by increasing effective coping with stressors (Nezu et al., 2015). Although less is known about the long-term effects of psychological interventions on optimism, these findings suggest that direct interventions to target optimism levels may be fruitful and may contribute to better well-being and health.

In sum, there are likely multiple pathways toward developing greater optimism across the lifespan. The current evidence suggests that individual differences in optimism during young adulthood emerge from a combination of genes and positive early parent–child relationships. However, research also suggests that personality constructs, including optimism, can change during subsequent periods of the lifespan, depending on a person's exposure to and management of significant life events and transitions. Although additional research is necessary to pinpoint the exact processes that facilitate naturally occurring and enduring personality changes, interventions that target self-regulation capacity appear to be effective for increasing optimistic outcome expectancies temporarily and may be an important step to promoting subjective well-being and physical health.

Do the Emotional Benefits of Optimism Vary across the Life Course?

Another issue pertains to the question of whether the emotional benefits of dispositional optimism are stable and consistent across different life circumstances. For example, some life circumstances may increase the adaptive consequences of optimism, while others could reduce them. Such effects could occur if some of the psychological mechanisms that link optimism with subjective well-being and physical health, such as coping, vary in their effectiveness for attaining important goals and managing stressors across life circumstances.

In this regard, the previously discussed research on coping suggests that optimists, more frequently than pessimists, approach stressors head-on by using problem-focused coping (Nes & Segerstrom, 2006). As such, it may be possible that the emotional benefits of optimism are particularly strong during life circumstances that involve favorable opportunities for attaining goals and overcoming goal-related barriers. This may be the case because optimists' greater use of problem-focused coping proves to be most effective in these life circumstances. By contrast, if life circumstances involve intractable stressors and the frequent experience of unattainable goals, optimists may not accrue the psychological benefits resulting from goal attainment, and similar to their pessimistic counterparts could encounter adverse emotional outcomes.

This possibility, however, may not imply that the benefits associated with greater optimism completely disappear, or are reversed, in contexts that involve intractable stressors. As discussed earlier, optimists also accept uncontrollable life circumstances more easily than pessimists, which could help them to psychologically adjust to the situation, thereby partially compensating for the inability to overcome certain stressors. Considering both the importance of attaining difficult goals and adjusting psychologically to intractable stressors, it seems likely that the capacity for goal attainment and resolving stressors takes precedence (cf. functional primacy of primary control for development and survival, Heckhausen & Schulz, 1999). As a consequence, there could be a net reduction in the effectiveness of optimism in life circumstances that involve intractable stressors (Wrosch et al., 2017).

To examine whether optimism is equally effective across life circumstances, it may be useful to adopt a lifespan developmental approach, which postulates that the effectiveness of self-regulation factors depends on an age-related configuration of opportunities and constraints for development. In particular, this approach assumes that an age-related increase in the experience of uncontrollable stressors can constrain people's opportunities for overcoming problems (Baltes & Baltes, 1990; Heckhausen et al., 2010). As a consequence, uncontrollable stressors and goal constraints are most likely to appear in advanced old age, a life phase that has been characterized by a reduction of personal resources, irreversible losses, and the experience of unattainable goals (Baltes & Smith, 2003; Smith et al., 2002; Wrosch & Scheier, 2020).

A corollary of the previous discussion is that the emotional benefits of dispositional optimism may become reduced toward the end of life. This prediction has been tested in a 6-year longitudinal study on optimism and depressive symptoms, examining a community sample of adults in early and advanced old age (Wrosch et al., 2017). The results showed that among participants in early old age, optimists experienced consistently low levels of depressive symptoms across the study period. Pessimists in early old age, by contrast, reported higher and linearly increasing levels of depressive symptoms. A different pattern was obtained among participants in advanced old age. Here, pessimists' high levels of depressive symptoms flattened, while optimists' level of depressive symptoms increased over time, inching closer to the levels of their pessimistic counterparts. Note, however, that even in advanced old age, after six years of study, optimists still held an emotional advantage over their pessimistic counterparts (Wrosch et al., 2017).

These findings suggest that dispositional optimism exerts a buffering effect on emotional well-being in early old age. In advanced old age, however, the benefits of optimism became increasingly reduced. We think that such a reduction in the effectiveness of optimism may be observed because, different from earlier periods of life, optimists in advanced old age are less likely to attain their goals and overcome intractable losses. In such circumstances, even optimists may experience a continuation of stress and associated depressive symptoms. However, optimists are still emotionally better adjusted than pessimists towards the end of life, which could relate to their greater capacity to accept and psychologically adjust to uncontrollable life circumstances (Scheier et al., 1986; Wrosch et al., 2017).

We feel it is important to further examine how the effects of optimism can vary across life circumstances because it may identify the contexts during which dispositional optimism is most effective. Such research may broaden its age-related scope by including young adult populations that often have abundant opportunities for their development. In addition, it may examine the influence of different coping strategies directly, and predict health-relevant physiological mediators and clinical end points.

Are Different Benefits Derived from Optimism and Pessimism?

A final issue relates to the question of whether the presence of optimism could be a stronger predictor of well-being and health than the absence of pessimism, or vice versa. This issue has important theoretical and practical implications. First, it addresses the fundamental question of how to best conceptualize dispositional optimism. Second, it may clarify whether it is more important to intervene by increasing optimism or reducing pessimism.

Although most research on dispositional optimism has combined the optimism and pessimism subscales of the LOT-R, there has been a decades-long debate in the literature about whether optimism and pessimism indeed reflect one unidimensional and bipolar construct, or two correlated, but partially independent constructs (e.g., Scheier & Carver, 2018; Kubzansky et al., 2004). Conceptually, it makes sense that a person who is not optimistic does not necessarily have to be pessimistic, and vice versa. Indeed, people could also score low on both optimism and pessimism (Scheier et al., 2021a). However, issues about the partial independence of optimism and pessimism have not been resolved. For example, different factor analytic studies showed that a 2-factor model of the optimism and pessimism subscales of the LOT-R fits the data best (Chang et al., 1994; Chang & McBride-Chang, 1996; Glaesmer et al., 2012). Other researchers, by contrast, have argued that a 2-factor solution is an artifact of response style (e.g., Monzani et al., 2014) and that analyses based on item response theory support a single-factor solution (e.g., Chiesi et al., 2013).

Nonetheless, the assumption of partial independence of optimism and pessimism would be consistent with research documenting relatively modest associations between the optimism and pessimism subscales of the LOT-R (average $r = -0.33$, Scheier et al., 2021a). Indeed, if crossing high/low optimism with high/low pessimism, there are people who fall in all four resulting quadrants. Importantly, this empirical reality also implies that there are people who can be characterized by both high optimism and high pessimism, which may not seem logical (see VanderWeele & Kubzanksy, 2021). These people, however, are more moderate and not at the extremes of the optimism and pessimism subscales (Benyamini, 2005), suggesting that it is unlikely that people generally expect the very best and the very worst at the same time (Scheier et al., 2021b). Still, research is needed to understand how moderate levels of optimism and pessimism can co-occur in people.

Another aspect that can shed light on the potential independence of optimism and pessimism relates to the predictive validity of the constructs. Stated differently, do the optimism and pessimism subscales predict the same outcomes to the same extent? In this regard, earlier research has shown that optimism and pessimism can relate differentially to physical health outcomes. For example, in one study the absence of optimism was a more important predictor for risk of stroke than the presence of pessimism (Kim et al., 2011). More frequently, however, studies have shown that pessimism is more strongly associated with physical health outcomes than optimism (e.g., inflammation, cardiovascular health, and successful in-vitro fertilization, Bleil et al., 2012; Ikeda et al., 2011; Serlachius et al., 2015).

Recent meta-analytic research supports the latter conclusion (Scheier et al., 2021a). This study involved a reanalysis of the extant research on dispositional optimism and objective physical health. The authors asked colleagues who had published data on dispositional optimism and physical health (e.g., immune function, disease progression, or mortality) to reanalyze their data by using either the optimism or the pessimism subscales as a predictor in separate analyses, obtaining data from 61 independent samples and 221,133 participants. The results of the study documented that both the presence of optimism and the absence of pessimism were associated with beneficial physical health outcomes. Importantly, however, the pessimism subscale was a significantly stronger predictor of physical health than the optimism subscale, with an almost three times larger effect size for pessimism (Scheier et al., 2021a).

The finding that the absence of pessimism is a stronger predictor of physical health than the presence of optimism makes it important to discuss potential reasons for such a differential effect. In this regard, one possibility would be that these differential effects are mediated by people's levels of subjective well-being (for well-being and health, see Diener & Chan, 2011). Findings from our current research are consistent with this possibility. In a longitudinal sample of romantic couples, Borenstein-Laurie et al. (2023) examined the independent effects of the optimism and pessimism subscales on both subjective well-being and physical health. This study found that the absence of pessimism was not only more strongly associated with a person's own (and their partner's) physical health than the presence of optimism, but also with several indicators of subjective well-being (e.g., low depressive symptoms or negative affect). In addition, these indicators of subjective well-being statistically mediated some of the effect of pessimism on levels (e.g., sleep or cold symptoms) and changes (e.g., chronic disease) in physical health (Borenstein-Laurie et al., 2023). Note that these findings are consistent with other research, suggesting stronger effects of pessimism on subjective well-being than optimism (e.g., Chang et al., 1997; Mahler & Kulik, 2000; Pinquart et al., 2007). In addition, they extend this line of work by documenting that stronger effects of pessimism on subjective well-being may have important implications for physical health.

Another potential mechanism linking optimism and pessimism differentially with well-being and health relates to coping. In this regard, preliminary findings from our research group suggest a pattern in which the optimism subscale was more closely related to certain approach-oriented coping strategies (e.g., active coping or acceptance), while the pessimism subscale was more frequently associated with avoidance coping (e.g., behavioral disengagement or self-blame, Borenstein-Laurie et al., 2021). Other research documents that such differences in coping may further predict subjective well-being. For example, studies of student and athlete samples showed that optimism promoted well-being via task-oriented coping, while pessimism was associated with reduced well-being via disengagement-oriented coping (Boileau et al., 2021; Gaudreau & Blondin, 2004; Gaudreau et al., 2015). Note that these results only provide preliminary evidence for the role of coping in the distinct health effects of optimism and pessimism. Research still needs to examine systematically the coping responses that could be elicited by either optimism or pessimism, and whether these responses mediate the differences that are observed in the associations between optimism and pessimism with physical health outcomes.

Together, it seems meaningful to distinguish optimism from pessimism (Scheier et al., 2021b). The two subscales of the LOT-R are only moderately correlated and can represent different factors (Chang et al., 1994; Scheier et al., 2021a). In addition, they show differential predictive validity, as indicated by stronger effects of pessimism, as compared to optimism, on subjective well-being and physical health (Borenstein-Laurie et al., 2023; Scheier et al., 2021a). We suggest that more research is needed to fully understand the mechanisms that contribute to such differential consequences of optimism and pessimism, including a comprehensive examination of coping responses and social aspects of life. Such research may provide useful information for identifying specific psychological variables that can be targeted in intervention to achieve the largest gains for a person's subjective well-being and physical health.

Conclusions

This chapter addressed the importance of dispositional optimism for subjective well-being and physical health. Based on theories of self-regulation, we discussed how optimism can promote the regulation of important and valued goals and people's quality of life. Current literature demonstrates the beneficial effects of optimism on subjective well-being and physical health. In addition, coping responses and social resources are identified as adaptive psychological mechanisms that can link dispositional optimism with outcomes of subjective well-being and physical health. The final part of the chapter addressed developmental and conceptual issues, suggesting that optimism can develop and change, and may elicit differential emotional consequences across the lifespan. In addition, it pointed to the possibility that optimism and pessimism may be correlated, but partially independent constructs that can predict well-being and health differently. We think that research on optimism will continue to thrive and has a potential to further illuminate the psychological pathways that contribute to people's well-being and health.

References

Achat, H., Kawachi, I., Spiro, A., DeMolles, D. A., & Sparrow, D. (2000). Optimism and depression as predictors of physical and mental health functioning: The normative aging study. *Annals of Behavioral Medicine, 22*(2), 127–130.

Alarcon, G. M., Bowling, N. A., & Khazon, S. (2013). Great expectations: A meta-analytic examination of optimism and hope. *Personality and Individual Differences, 54*(7), 821–827.

Andersson, G. (1996). The benefits of optimism: A meta-analytic review of the life orientation test. *Personality and Individual Differences, 21*(5), 719–725.

Aspinwall, L. G., & Richter, L. (1999). Optimism and self-mastery predict more rapid disengagement from unsolvable tasks in the presence of alternatives. *Motivation and Emotion, 23*, 221–245.

Aspinwall, L. G., & Taylor, S. E. (1992). Modeling cognitive adaptation: A longitudinal investigation of the impact of individual differences and coping on college adjustment and performance. *Journal of Personality and Social Psychology, 63*(6), 989–1003.

Atkinson, J. W., & Birch, D. (1978). The dynamics of achievement-oriented activity. In J. W. Atkinson & J. O. Raynor (Eds.), *Personality, motivation, and achievement* (pp. 143–197). Hemisphere.

Baltes, P. B., & Baltes, M. M. (1990). Psychological perspectives on successful aging: The model of selective optimization with compensation. In P. B. Baltes & M. M. Baltes (Eds.), *Successful aging: Perspectives from the behavioral sciences* (pp. 1–34). Cambridge University Press.

Baltes, P. B., & Smith, J. (2003). New frontiers in the future of aging: From successful aging of the young old to the dilemmas of the fourth age. *Gerontology, 49*(2), 123–135.

Bandura, A. (1997). *Self-efficacy: The exercise of control*. W.H. Freeman.

Benyamini, Y. (2005). Can high optimism and high pessimism co-exist? Findings from arthritis patients coping with pain. *Personality and Individual Differences, 38*, 1463–1473.

Bleidorn, W., Hopwood, C. J., & Lucas, R. E. (2018). Life events and personality trait change. *Journal of Personality, 86*(1), 83–96.

Bleil, M. E., Pasch, L. A., Gregorich, S. E., Millstein, S. G., Katz, P. P., Adler, N. E., & The Infertility Outcomes Program Project Group. (2012). Fertility treatment response: Is it better to be more optimistic or less pessimistic? *Psychosomatic Medicine, 74*(2), 193–199.

Boehm, J. K., & Kubzansky, L. D. (2012). The heart's content: The association between positive psychological well-being and cardiovascular health. *Psychological Bulletin, 138*(4), 655–691.

Boileau, L., Gaudreau, P., Gareau, A., & Chamandy, M. (2021). Some days are more satisfying than others: A daily-diary study on optimism, pessimism, coping, and academic satisfaction. *British Journal of Educational Psychology, 91*(1), 46–62.

Borenstein-Laurie, J., Barlow, M. A., Scheier, M. F., & Wrosch, C. (2023). Examining intra- and inter-personal health effects of optimism and pessimism: The role of subjective well-being in romantic couples. *Journal of Personality, 91*, 700–717

Borenstein-Laurie, J., Widmer, P., & Wrosch, C. (2021, May 26–27). *Optimism and pessimism differentially predict coping strategies among older adults: Implications for well-being*. Poster presentation. 2021 APS Virtual Convention.

Brissette, I., Scheier, M. F., & Carver, C. S. (2002). The role of optimism in social network development, coping, and psychological adjustment during a life transition. *Journal of Personality and Social Psychology, 82*(1), 102–111.

Carver, C. S., & Gaines, J. G. (1987). Optimism, pessimism, and postpartum depression. *Cognitive Therapy and Research, 11*, 449–462.

Carver, C. S., Kus, L. A., & Scheier, M. F. (1994). Effects of good versus bad mood and optimistic versus pessimistic outlook on social acceptance versus rejection. *Journal of Social and Clinical Psychology, 13*(2), 138–151.

Carver, C. S., Pozo, C., Harris, S. D., Noriega, V., Scheier, M. F., Robinson, D. S., Ketcham, A. S., Moffat, F. L., Jr., & Clark, K. C. (1993). How coping mediates the effect of optimism on distress: A study of women with early stage breast cancer. *Journal of Personality and Social Psychology, 65*(2), 375–390.

Carver, C. S., & Scheier, M. F. (1981). *Attention and self-regulation: A control-theory approach to human behavior*. Springer-Verlag.

Carver, C. S., & Scheier, M. F. (1990). Origins and functions of positive and negative affect: A control-process view. *Psychological Review, 97*(1), 19–35.

Carver, C. S., & Scheier, M. F. (1998). On the self-regulation of behavior. *Cambridge University Press.* https://doi.org/10.1017/cbo9781139174794

Carver, C. S., & Scheier, M. F. (2001). Optimism, pessimism, and self-regulation. In E. C. Chang (Ed.), *Optimism & pessimism: Implications for theory, research, and practice* (pp. 31–51). American Psychological Association.

Carver, C. S., Scheier, M. F., & Segerstrom, S. C. (2010). Optimism. *Clinical Psychology Review, 30*(7), 879–889.

Carver, C. S., Scheier, M. F., & Weintraub, J. K. (1989). Assessing coping strategies: A theoretically based approach. *Journal of Personality and Social Psychology, 56*(2), 267–283.

Chang, E. C. (1998). Dispositional optimism and primary and secondary appraisal of a stressor: Controlling for confounding influences and relations to coping and psychological and physical adjustment. *Journal of Personality and Social Psychology, 74*(4), 1109–1120.

Chang, E. C., D'Zurilla, T. J., & Maydeu-Olivares, A. (1994). Assessing the dimensionality of optimism and pessimism using a multi-measure approach. *Cognitive Therapy and Research, 18*(2), 143–160.

Chang, E. C., Maydeu-Olivares, A., & D'Zurilla, T. J. (1997). Optimism and pessimism as partially independent constructs: Relationship to positive and negative affectivity and psychological well-being. *Personality and Individual Differences, 23*(3), 433–440.

Chang, L., & McBride-Chang, C. (1996). The factor structure of the life orientation test. *Educational and Psychological Measurement, 56*(2), 325–329.

Chiesi, F., Galli, S., Primi, C., Borgi, P. I., & Bonacchi, A. (2013). The accuracy of the life orientation test-revised (LOT-R) in measuring dispositional optimism: Evidence from item response theory analyses. *Journal of Personality Assessment, 95*(5), 523–529.

Cohen, S. (2004). Social relationships and health. *American Psychologist, 59*(8), 676–684.

Cohen, S., Janicki-Deverts, D., & Miller, G. E. (2007). Psychological stress and disease. *JAMA, 298*(14), 1685–1687.

Cohen, S., & Wills, T. A. (1985). Stress, social support, and the buffering hypothesis. *Psychological Bulletin, 98*(2), 310–357.

Diener, E., & Chan, M. Y. (2011). Happy people live longer: Subjective well-being contributes to health and longevity. *Applied Psychology, 3*(1), 1–43.

Duckworth, A. L., Peterson, C., Matthews, M. D., & Kelly, D. R. (2007). Grit: Perseverance and passion for long-term goals. *Journal of Personality and Social Psychology, 92*(6), 1087–1101.

Dunn, D. S. (Ed.). (2018). *Positive psychology: Established and emerging issues.* Routledge.

Emmons, R. A. (1986). Personal strivings: An approach to personality and subjective well- being. *Journal of Personality and Social Psychology, 51*(1058), 1068.

Feather, N. T. (1982). *Expectations and actions: Expectancy-value models in psychology*. Erlbaum.

Freund, A. M., & Baltes, P. B. (2002). Life-management strategies of selection, optimization and compensation: Measurement by self-report and construct validity. *Journal of Personality and Social Psychology, 82*(4), 642–662.

Gaudreau, P., & Blondin, J.-P. (2004). Differential associations of dispositional optimism and pessimism with coping, goal attainment, and emotional adjustment during sport competition. *International Journal of Stress Management, 11*(3), 245–269.

Gaudreau, P., Gunnell, K. E., Hoar, S. D., Thompson, A., & Lelièvre, J. (2015). Optimism, pessimism, and coping in a dual-domain model of sport and school satisfaction. *Sport, Exercise, and Performance Psychology, 4*(2), 140–152.

Glaesmer, H., Rief, W., Martin, A., Mewes, R., Brähler, E., Zenger, M., & Hinz, A. (2012). Psychometric properties and population-based norms of the life orientation test revised (LOT-R). *British Journal of Health Psychology, 17*(2), 432–445.

Gollwitzer, P. M. (1999). Implementation intentions: Strong effects of simple plans. *American Psychologist, 54*(7), 493–503.

Gollwitzer, P. M., & Oettingen, G. (1998). The emergence and implementation of health goals. *Psychology and Health, 13*(4), 687–715.

Heckhausen, J. (1999). *Developmental regulation in adulthood.* Cambridge University Press.

Heckhausen, J., & Schulz, R. (1999). The primacy of primary control is a human universal: A reply to Gould's (1999) critique of the life-span theory of control. *Psychological Review, 106*(3), 605–609.

Heckhausen, J., Wrosch, C., & Schulz, R. (2010). A motivational theory of life-span development. *Psychological Review, 117*(1), 32–60.

Heckhausen, J., Wrosch, C., & Schulz, R. (2019). Agency and motivation in adulthood and old age. *Annual Review of Psychology, 70*(1), 191–217.

Heinonen, K., Raikkonen, K., & Keltikangas-Jarvinen, L. (2005). Dispositional optimism: Development over 21 years from the perspectives of perceived temperament and mothering. *Personality and Individual Differences, 38*, 425–435.

Heinonen, K., Raikkonen, K., Keltikangas-Jarvinen, L., & Strandberg, T. (2004). Adult attachment dimensions and recollections of childhood family context: Associations with dispositional optimism and pessimism. *European Journal of Personality, 18*, 193–207.

Hjelle, L. A., Busch, E. A., & Warren, J. E. (1996). Explanatory style, dispositional optimism and reported parental behaviours. *The Journal of Genetic Psychology: Research and Theory on Human Development, 157*, 489–499.

Ikeda, A., Schwartz, J., Peters, J. L., Fang, S., Spiro, A., Sparrow, D., Vokonas, P., & Kubzansky, L. D. (2011). Optimism in relation to inflammation and endothelial dysfunction in older men: The VA normative aging study. *Psychosomatic Medicine, 73*(8), 664–671.

Jobin, J., Wrosch, C., & Scheier, M. F. (2014). Associations between dispositional optimism and diurnal cortisol in a community sample: When stress is perceived as higher than normal. *Health Psychology, 33*(4), 382–391.

Kim, E. S., Hagan, K. A., Grodstein, F., DeMeo, D. L., De Vivo, I., & Kubzansky, L. D. (2017). Optimism and cause-specific mortality: A prospective cohort study. *American Journal of Epidemiology, 185*(1), 21–29.

Kim, E. S., Park, N., & Peterson, C. (2011). Dispositional optimism protects older adults from stroke: The health and retirement study. *Stroke, 42*(10), 2855–2859.

Korkeila, K., Kivela, S. L., Suominem, S., Vahtera, J., Kivimaki, M., Sundell, J., Helenius, H., & Koskenvuo, M. (2004). Childhood adversities, parent-child relationships and dispositional optimism in adulthood. *Social Psychiatry and Psychiatric Epidemiology, 39*, 286–292.

Kubzansky, L. D., Kubzansky, P. E., & Maselko, J. (2004). Optimism and pessimism in the context of health: Bipolar opposites or separate constructs? *Personality and Social Psychology Bulletin, 30*, 943–956.

Lachman, M. E., & Firth, K. M. (2004). The adaptive value of feeling in control during midlife. In O. G. Brim, C. D. Ryff, & R. C. Kessler (Eds.), *How healthy are we? A national study of well-being in midlife* (pp. 320–349). The University of Chicago Press.

Lang, F. R., & Heckhausen, J. (2001). Perceived control over development and psychological well-bring: Differential benefits across adulthood. *Journal of Personality and Social Psychology, 81*, 509–523.

Lazarus, R. S., & Folkman, S. (1984). *Stress, appraisal, and coping*. Springer Publishing.

MacLeod, A. K., & Conway, C. (2005). Well-being and the anticipation of future positive experiences: The role of income, social networks, and planning ability. *Cognition & Emotion, 19*(3), 357–374.

Mahler, H. I. M., & Kulik, J. A. (2000). Optimism, pessimism and recovery from coronary bypass surgery: Prediction of affect, pain and functional status. *Psychology, Health & Medicine, 5*(4), 347–358.

Malouff, J. M., & Schutte, N. S. (2017). Can psychological interventions increase optimism? A meta-analysis. *The Journal of Positive Psychology, 12*(6), 594–604.

Matthews, K. A., Räikkönen, K., Sutton-Tyrrell, K., & Kuller, L. H. (2004). Optimistic attitudes protect against progression of carotid atherosclerosis in healthy middle-aged women. *Psychosomatic Medicine, 66*(5), 640–644.

Miller, G. A., Galanter, E., & Pribram, K. H. (1960). *Plans and the structure of behavior*. Henry Holt and.

Monzani, D., Steca, P., & Greco, A. (2014). Brief report: Assessing dispositional optimism in adolescence—Factor structure and concurrent validity of the life orientation test-revised. *Journal of Adolescence, 37*(2), 97–101.

Mosing, M. A., Pederson, N. L., Martin, N. G., & Wright, M. J. (2010). Sex differences in the genetic architecture of optimism and health and their interrelation: A study of Australian and Swedish twins. *Twin Research in Human Genetics, 13*, 322–329.

Mosing, M. A., Zietsch, B. P., Shekar, S. N., Wright, M. J., & Martin, N. G. (2009). Genetic and environmental influences on optimism and its relationship to mental and self-rated health: A study of aging twins. *Behavioural Genetics, 39*, 597–604.

Nes, L. S., & Segerstrom, S. C. (2006). Dispositional optimism and coping: A meta-analytic review. *Personality and Social Psychology Review, 10*(3), 235–251.

Nezu, A. M., Greenfield, A. P., & Nezu, C. M. (2015). Contemporary problem-solving therapy: A Transdiagnostic intervention. *The Oxford handbook of cognitive and behavioral therapies*, 160–171.

Pearlin, L. I., & Schooler, C. (1978). The structure of coping. *Journal of Health and Social Behavior, 19*(1), 2–21.

Peterson, C., Semmel, A., von Baeyer, C., Abramson, L. Y., Metalsky, G. I., & Seligman, M. E. P. (1982). The attributional style questionnaire. *Cognitive Therapy and Research, 6*(3), 287–299.

Pinquart, M., Fröhlich, C., & Silbereisen, R. K. (2007). Optimism, pessimism, and change of psychological well-being in cancer patients. *Psychology, Health & Medicine, 12*(4), 421–432.

Plomin, R., Scheier, M. F., Bergeman, C. S., Pedersen, N. L., Nesselroade, J. R., & McClearn, G. E. (1992). Optimism, pessimism, and mental health: A twin/adoption analysis. *Personality and Individual Differences, 13*, 921–930.

Rasmussen, H. N., Wrosch, C., Scheier, M. F., & Carver, C. S. (2006). Self-regulation pro- cesses and health: The importance of optimism and goal adjustment. *Journal of Personality, 74*, 1721–1748.

Rasmussen, H. N., Scheier, M. F., & Greenhouse, J. B. (2009). Optimism and physical health: A meta-analytic review. *Annals of Behavioral Medicine, 37*(3), 239–256.

Renaud, J., Barker, E. T., Hendricks, C., Putnick, D. L., & Bornstein, M. H. (2019). The developmental origins and future implications of dispositional optimism in the transition to adulthood. *International Journal of Behavioral Development, 43*(3), 221–230.

Renaud, J., Wrosch, C., & Scheier, M. F. (2018). Optimism. In M. H. Bornstein (Ed.), *The SAGE encyclopedia of lifespan human development* (pp. 1550–1552). Sage Publications.

Ryff, C. D., & Keyes, C. L. (1995). The structure of psychological well-being revisited. *Journal of Personality and Social Psychology, 69*(4), 719–727.

Scheier, M. F., & Carver, C. S. (1985). Optimism, coping, and health: Assessment and implications of generalized outcome expectancies. *Health Psychology, 4*(3), 219–247.

Scheier, M. F., & Carver, C. S. (2018). Dispositional optimism and physical health: A long look back, a quick look forward. *American Psychologist, 73*(9), 1082–1094.

Scheier, M. F., Carver, C. S., & Bridges, M. W. (1994). Distinguishing optimism from neuroticism (and trait anxiety, self-mastery, and self-esteem): A re-evaluation of the life orientation test. *Journal of Personality and Social Psychology, 67*(6), 1063–1078.

Scheier, M. F., Carver, C. S., & Bridges, M. W. (2001). Optimism, pessimism, and psychological well-being. In E. C. Chang (Ed.), *Optimism & pessimism: Implications for theory, research, and practice* (pp. 189–216). American Psychological Association.

Scheier, M. F., Matthews, K. A., Owens, J. F., Magovern, G. J., Sr., Lefebvre, R. C., Abbott, R. A., & Carver, C. S. (1989). Dispositional optimism and recovery from coronary artery bypass surgery: The beneficial effects on physical and psychological well-being. *Journal of Personality and Social Psychology, 57*(6), 1024–1040.

Scheier, M. F., Swanson, J. D., Barlow, M. A., Greenhouse, J. B., Wrosch, C., & Tindle, H. A. (2021a). Optimism versus pessimism as predictors of physical health: A comprehensive reanalysis of dispositional optimism research. *American Psychologist, 76*(3), 529–548.

Scheier, M. F., Weintraub, J. K., & Carver, C. S. (1986). Coping with stress: Divergent strategies of optimists and pessimists. *Journal of Personality and Social Psychology, 51*(6), 1257–1264.

Scheier, M. F., Wrosch, C., Barlow, M. A., Swanson, J. D., & Tindle, H. A. (2021b). *It remains meaningful to distinguish optimism from pessimism: A reply to VanderWeele and Kubzansky (2021)*. Accepted for publication.
Scheier, M. F., Wrosch, C., Baum, A., Cohen, S., Martire, L. M., Matthews, K. A., Schulz, R., & Zdaniuk, B. (2006). The life engagement test: Assessing purpose in life. *Journal of Behavioral Medicine, 29*(3), 291–298.
Schwaba, T., & Bleidorn, W. (2018). Individual differences in personality change across the lifespan. *Journal of Personality, 86*, 450–464.
Segerstrom, S. C. (2007). Optimism and resources: Effects on each other and on health over 10 years. *Journal of Research in Personality, 41*(4), 772–786.
Segerstrom, S. C., Taylor, S. E., Kemeny, M. E., & Fahey, J. L. (1998). Optimism is associated with mood, coping, and immune change in response to stress. *Journal of Personality and Social Psychology, 74*(6), 1646–1655.
Seligman, M. (1991). *Learned optimism*. Knopf.
Serlachius, A., Pulkki-Råback, L., Elovainio, M., Hintsanen, M., Mikkilä, V., Laitinen, T. T., Jokela, M., Rosenström, T., Josefsson, K., Juonala, M., Lehtimäki, T., Raitakari, O., & Keltikangas-Järvinen, L. (2015). Is dispositional optimism or dispositional pessimism predictive of ideal cardiovascular health? The young Finns study. *Psychology & Health, 30*(10), 1221–1239.
Shen, B.-J., McCreary, C. P., & Myers, H. F. (2004). Independent and mediated contributions of personality, coping, social support, and depressive symptoms to physical functioning outcome among patients in cardiac rehabilitation. *Journal of Behavioral Medicine, 27*(1), 39–62.
Shifren, K., & Hooker, K. (1995). Stability and change in optimism: A study among spouse caregivers. *Experimental Aging Research, 21*(1), 59–76.
Smith, J., Borchelt, M., Maier, H., & Jopp, D. (2002). Health and well-being in the young old and oldest old. *The Journal of Social Issues, 58*(4), 715–732.
Srivastava, S., McGonigal, K. M., Richards, J. M., Butler, E. A., & Gross, J. J. (2006). Optimism in close relationships: How seeing things in a positive light makes them so. *Journal of Personality and Social Psychology, 91*(1), 143–153.
Uchino, B. N., Cribbet, M., de Grey, R. G. K., Cronan, S., Trettevik, R., & Smith, T. W. (2017). Dispositional optimism and sleep quality: A test of mediating pathways. *Journal of Behavioral Medicine, 40*(2), 360–365.
VanderWeele, T. J., & Kubzanksy, L. D. (2021). Facets of optimism: Comment on Scheier et al. 2021. *Accepted for publication, American Psychologist.*
Wlodarczyk, D. (2015). Optimism and hope as predictors of subjective health in post-myocardial infarction patients: A comparison of the role of coping strategies. *Journal of Health Psychology, 22*(3), 336–346.
Wrosch, C., Jobin, J., & Scheier, M. F. (2017). Do the emotional benefits of optimism vary across older adulthood? A life span perspective. *Journal of Personality, 85*(3), 388–397.

Wrosch, C., & Sabiston, C. M. (2013). Goal adjustment, physical and sedentary activity, and well-being and health among breast cancer survivors. *Psycho-Oncology, 22*, 581–589.

Wrosch, C., & Scheier, M. F. (2003). Personality and quality of life: The importance of optimism and goal adjustment. *Quality of Life Research, 12*, 59–72.

Wrosch, C., & Scheier, M. F. (2020). Adaptive self-regulation, subjective well-being, and physical health: The importance of goal adjustment capacities. In A. Elliot (Ed.), *Advances in motivation science, 7*, 199–238.

Part IV

Preface: Eastern Approaches to Positive States, Traits, and Health (Self-Compassion and Mindfulness)

Fuschia M. Sirois

Positive psychology has strong ties to the traditions of ancient Greek philosophies and their views on the nature of *The Good Life*. Yet recent years have seen the emergence of other, non-Western views of well-being that are rooted in Eastern thought, and specifically Buddhist philosophy. These Eastern approaches to well-being share many of the common goals of the more traditional views of positive psychology, including an emphasis on improving positive psychological states such as joy, awareness, and serenity, motivating self-improvement and flourishing, as well as the importance of remembering and fostering our connection with others. In this regard they have much in common with traditional positive psychological states and traits. Mindfulness and self-compassion are two qualities rooted in Buddhist traditions for which there is a rapidly growing evidence base demonstrating robust links to physical health outcomes, processes, and contexts.

One notable feature of Eastern views of well-being is an explicit recognition of the importance of positive practices for fostering the development of positive states and traits. This is not to say that the traditional positive psychological views of subjective and individual level qualities do not also acknowledge the role of positive interventions and even daily practice for developing positive qualities and mindsets. Indeed, gratitude diaries and lists, for example, are well-recognized as being central for promoting gratitude. However, engaging in practices that both develop and maintain positive qualities is a central and often essential component of the Eastern-based positive approaches, such as mindfulness.

With this in mind, this section of the handbook presents research focused on positive states and qualities not often considered under the umbrella of positive psychology but which nonetheless have clear relevance for understanding well-being, flourishing, and positive connectedness. The chapters in this section examine the relevance of mindfulness, self-compassion, and associated practices such as yoga, across different health-relevant contexts including chronic health conditions and body image, and for key health processes including health behaviours and stress. The chapters cover both momentary states and more enduring tendencies to be mindful and self-compassionate.

Chapters 15, 16 and 17 examine the potential role of mindfulness for two key areas of interest for health psychology: eating behaviours and adjustment to chronic health conditions. In Chap. 15, Mantzios presents a critical examination of the concept of mindful eating, identifying the theoretical gaps and issues that can make designing mindful eating interventions to improve healthy eating challenging at best. In Chap. 16, Schroevers highlights the value of mindfulness-based interventions to help people with cancer improve their health and well-being during their cancer journey. In Chap. 17, Hughes and Thompson continue the theme of mindfulness and adjustment to illness by outlining the role of mindfulness and mindfulness-based psychological investigations for addressing the psychosocial issues associated with skin conditions and contributing to positive adjustment.

With its roots dating back over 5000 years to ancient India and Vedic traditions, yoga has evolved into a diverse array of different styles, with many becoming mainstream practices for improving body and mind within modern Western culture. In Chap. 18, Park and Skoggard examine the benefits of yoga for managing stress from a positive psychological lens. From positive affect to social connection, to emotion regulation, mindfulness and other positive-psychology-related constructs, yoga's salutary effects on stress are proposed to be facilitated through its links to these constructs.

The final five chapters in this section focus on a construct that has seen a surge of interest in recent years with respect to health-related outcomes, namely, self-compassion. In Chap. 19, Biskas, Sirois, and Webb outline the potential benefits of responding to health behaviour goal lapses with self-compassion for supporting health-promoting behaviours, as well as the processes involved and the potential barriers to being self-compassionate that may interfere with health behaviour change. Troop and Beadle shift the focus to the role of self-compassion for addressing body image concerns in Chap. 20 and discuss the emerging concept of body compassion and its relevance for disordered eating and health behaviours. Chapters 21 and 22 explore the value of self-compassion for adjustment to challenging two chronic illnesses, inflammatory bowel disease (IBD) and cancer, respectively. Yeates and Rowse highlight the role of self-compassion for helping people with IBD trade avoidant coping for greater self-acceptance and more flexible coping to deal with the illness-related stressors and stigma. In Chap. 22, Trindade and colleagues explore the role of self-compassion for coping with psychological distress and behaviour management in the context of cancer, and further highlight the potential of compassion-based interventions for health-related improvements in diverse cancer populations. Although more evidence is needed, preliminary findings suggest self-compassion warrants further research in this domain.

In the final chapter in this section, Cha and Consedine address the issue of whether self-compassion can enhance other-focused care in health-care settings. They highlight the pathways that might explain why self-compassion is uniquely situated to address the challenges of health-care settings, and in doing so they propose a new model that captures the general and compassion-specific routes to enhancing other-focused care.

15

Mindful Eating: A Critical Assessment of the Literature

Michail Mantzios

Obesity—defined as an excess of body adiposity/body weight (Caballero, 2007)—continues to rise in developed countries, alongside associated risks to health (Public Health England, 2020; WHO, 1998). Excess adiposity is a leading cause of major health risks such as type 2 diabetes, cardiovascular disease and hypertension (Hossain et al., 2007; Ortega et al., 2016). A large proportion of the literature recommends specific eating behaviors to be responsible for an imbalance between energy intake and expenditure (e.g., French et al., 2012). For example, automatic and habitual eating behaviors (Cohen & Farley, 2008) are instances where people eat in response to the mere sight of food (e.g., Painter & Wansink, 2002) and overeat when presented with larger portions (Blass et al., 2006; McConahy et al., 2004; Nelson, 2017; Wansink & Kim, 2005). Such eating behaviors are considered instrumental in influencing excess intake but also propose ways of health behavior change.

A topic of discussion and research in contemporary literature and current clinical practice as a primary element of eating behavior change has been mindful eating. The term and practices of "mindful eating" were coined a couple of decades ago with the potential for healthier eating; mindful eating has been perceived as an instruction to reinstate a healthy relationship with

M. Mantzios (✉)
School of Life and Health Sciences, Department of Psychology,
Birmingham City University, Birmingham, UK
e-mail: michael.mantzios@bcu.ac.uk

F. M. Sirois (ed.), *The Palgrave Handbook of Positive Psychology and Health*,
https://doi.org/10.1007/978-3-031-89095-6_15

food. Descriptions propose that through the practices of mindful eating, people are aware of what they are eating, moment by moment (Kristeller, 2015), reversing the trend of habitual and automated consumption and overconsumption (Mantzios & Wilson, 2015). Mindful eating is derived from mindfulness—that is, being attentive and aware of the present moment, while maintaining a non-judgmental attitude (Kabat-Zinn, 2003). Mindfulness as a contemplative practice was found to be less relevant to eating behavior change but more useful in supporting emotion regulation and indirectly influencing weight regulation (Mantzios & Wilson, 2015; Marchiori & Papies, 2014). This chapter will provide a provisional definition of mindful eating and highlight differences in measuring mindful eating and differences between mindfulness and mindful eating, all in an attempt to present a new and concise direction for defining and conducting research directed toward healthier eating practices.

What Is Mindful Eating?

Before defining mindful eating, it is important to explore mindfulness, which allowed for the concept of mindful eating to emerge in contemporary research and practice. Defining mindful eating is straightforward when beholding definitions of mindfulness and foundational elements that can aid the portrayal of a clear definition. Kabat-Zinn (2003) suggested that mindfulness is "the awareness that emerges through paying attention on purpose, in the present moment, and nonjudgmentally to the unfolding of experience moment by moment" (p. 145). This definition puts forward two main components that should be present in any mindfulness practice: namely, present moment attention and non-judgmental (or non-evaluative) awareness, both supporting a cognitive and emotional self-regulatory system. Teasdale et al. (2000) discussed the non-judgmental awareness as an element that projects a meta-awareness, which offers quality guidelines and parameters of self-regulation to facilitate sustained attention to the present moment. Non-judgment supports people to circumvent the common experience of getting caught up in ruminative thoughts about the past or worries about the future. Non-judgment also shields people from elaborative perceptions of the present moment experience itself (e.g., "this is boring", "I am not doing a good job focusing") and empowers people to experience thoughts, emotions and physical sensations as passing events. Such non-judgmental attitude supports attempts for an easier enactment of the intention to return to what the practice states the focus should be on (e.g., the breath in mindfulness breathing meditation—see Teasdale et al., 1995).

Finding a definition of mindful eating that has met consensus has been proven to be quite problematic when exploring current and historic literature. Román and Urbán (2019) stated that "since there is no universally accepted definition of mindful eating, only its most commonly described features can be presented" (p. 2111), which is anticipated when conducting a literature review on the definitions within relevant academic writings. Taylor et al. (2015) proposed that "mindful eating is operationally defined as food consumption that is driven by appropriate cues for eating" (p. 229), which is a generic definition that is open-ended and lacks clarity. Framson et al. (2009) proposed a definition that has been widely repeated, whereby "mindful eating describes a non-judgmental awareness of physical and emotional sensations associated with eating" (p. 1439). Nevertheless, this definition is oblique in consideration of theory and past mindful eating literature. This definition neither considers the sustained attention on sensational elements of the eating experience (i.e., smell, taste, texture), nor does it account for earlier descriptions of mindful eating where physical cues, such as hunger and satiety cues (Kristeller, 2015) are used as features of decision-making (or judgment) as to whether to initiate or cease food consumption. Framson and colleagues proposed a definition where mindful eating is not associated with perceptions and thoughts, and emphasize on emotional experiences as a disjoined entity within mindful eating.

Meanwhile, Monroe (2015) proposed that "mindful eating is the enjoyment of food utilizing all of the senses without judgment" (p. 217), a substantially different definition that incorporates enjoyment, which is reported more of a consequence of eating mindfully (Hong et al., 2011), and importantly not a foundational element but rather an outcome of mindful eating. Overall, the loose and subjective way of defining mindful eating has led to corresponding methods of measuring and practicing mindful eating, which similarly present a challenging picture as to what mindful eating accurately embodies, especially when considering the development of an all-inclusive mindfulness-based practice.

Measuring Mindful Eating

Mindful eating measures represent an open-ended, vague and methodologically flawed notion of what is characteristic of mindful eating. Framson et al. (2009) proposed a mindful eating questionnaire (MEQ) that failed to adhere to any theory and concepts of mindfulness and was criticized for not being a valid measure (Hulbert-Williams et al., 2014). Furthermore, despite a clear association between mindful and emotional eating (Egan et al., 2020), emotional eating represents a completely separate scale, and its inclusion in this MEQ is misguiding. The inclusion of emotional eating inflates the overall association of mindful eating to other eating behaviors and constructs, projecting an inaccurate picture as to how mindful eating relates and influences other physiological and psychological outcomes. In other words, when a scale includes emotional eating as a subscale, the likelihood of predicting emotional eating is more probable, and the association to weight and obesity may be driven by emotional eating rather than mindful eating.

With an intention to enhance face validity, Hulbert-Williams et al. (2014) developed a mindful eating scale (MES). They suggested this to be more aligned to contemporary theories of mindfulness but included subscales measuring *routine* and *unstructured* eating, which again are unrelated to mindfulness theories and practices. Similarly, these elements are noted in the literature as independent and separate eating behaviors altogether (e.g., Carmel & Musante, 1980; Spamon, 1989; Wood et al., 2016). More recently, Winkens et al. (2018) proposed the Mindful Eating Behavior Scale (MEBS) that was guided by a recent review (Tapper, 2017) highlighting that attention (over non-judgment or acceptance) could promote changes in eating behaviors. Such evidence led Winkens and colleagues to justify the development of a scale that would not measure non-judgment or acceptance but only attention and awareness, adopted from a specific mindfulness theory (Brown & Ryan, 2003) that differs from traditional descriptions of mindfulness. Brown and Ryan's theory on mindfulness has been subjected to much criticism and controversy in the field of mindfulness (Grossman, 2011; Grossman, 2019; Grossman & Van Dam, 2011), which proposes that there may be problems with this MES as well. Winkens et al. (2018) proposed that the MEBS does not incorporate the foundational element of non-judgment that is observed across traditional and contemporary mindfulness literature.

Keyte et al. (2020) later argued the MEBS to inherently describe a scale that represents a notion that is more aligned to literature focusing on "attentive eating" (e.g., Higgs, 2015) rather than mindfulness or mindful eating. Nevertheless, items such as "My thoughts tend to wander while I am eating" propose a non-elaborative, non-ruminative, accepting and/or non-judgmental attitude in a more indirect way and imply non-judgment (or non-evaluative awareness). In other words, the indirect presence of "non-judgment" within MEBS items is something that requires more attention and further analyses, while Keyte and colleagues indicated that there was an association to mindfulness and non-judgment. When considering mindfulness in its entirety, consensus and further research is also needed to eradicate any subjectivity in labeling scales and questionnaires as mindful eating measures, when the reality may be that there is only an assumption of "non-judgment" being represented (implicitly or explicitly) within the psychometric tool. The aptitude of utilizing non-judgment to influence eating behaviors has been investigated in other scientific inquiries (Jenkins & Tapper, 2014; Keesman et al., 2017) and mandates recognition in mindful eating psychometric tools and practices to correspond to mindful eating and mindfulness theories.

Targeting Mindful Eating

By the same token, interventions that were formerly advocated as being "attentive eating" practices (Robinson et al., 2014) re-emerged in the literature as "mindful eating" practices (Tapper & Seguias, 2020), even though attentive eating interventions have been defined as being distinct from mindful eating practices (Robinson et al., 2014). Other literature exploring mindfulness-based interventions targeting healthier food choices utilized a "mindful attention" intervention (Papies et al., 2015), which the authors suggested was only one part of mindfulness meditation as participants observed thoughts and saw them as mere mental events—a process assimilating practices in acceptance and commitment therapy (ACT; Hayes et al., 2011), or, elsewhere identified as open monitoring (Malinowski, 2013)—which most definitely embraces acceptance and non-judgment. Papies et al. (2015) revised their views in the discussion of their initial conceptions, but the use of terminologies such as "mindfulness-based" or "mindfulness-derived" has been used across different projects where ACT (and other related, but essentially different discipline components) became vague descriptors of mindfulness (see also Tapper et al., 2009).

ACT shares origins and practices with mindfulness. However, they are separate entities and should be labeled accordingly. The field needs to come together before disseminating any further mindfulness and mindful eating research to meet consensus as to what mindful eating is, and what it is not, and respond by appropriately identifying ways to measure mindful eating and create corresponding practices. Earlier literature taking a more critical stance in response to the surge of mindfulness research has suggested that there is a necessity for enhancing methodological rigor (Van Dam et al., 2018), and an identical approach is needed for mindful eating, but this cannot take place without a consensus on the definition of mindful eating.

Mindful Eating Versus Mindfulness Practices

Cheung and Hanh (2010) recommended that mindful eating generally refers to the use of mindfulness practices in eating experiences (see also Allirot et al., 2018; Mantzios, Egan, Bahia et al., 2018; Mantzios, Egan, Hussain et al. 2018). There are two distinct differences between mindfulness and mindful eating practices that are significant in defining mindful eating.

First, mindful eating is an event-based practice that emerges when one is eating, whereas mindfulness practices do not require any other concurrent event. With mindfulness practices, for example, mindful breathing, the focus may be on the breath, observing every in-breath and every out-breath moment by moment. This focus on the breath serves as an attentional anchor to the present moment, while being aware of where the mind wanders during the meditation, with a non-judgmental or non-evaluative bearing on observed experiences that allow for an easier redirection of attention to the breath (Raes & Williams, 2010). With mindful eating practices, the focus is on the sensory experiences of eating (similar to mindful walking where the attention is placed on the physiological sensation of the body). Sensory experiences refer to the *smell*, *taste* or *texture* of the food (e.g., Mantzios et al., 2020; Mantzios & Wilson, 2014; Hussein et al., 2017), although focusing on one sense may simplify the practice and the experience, at least for beginners. When one remains attentive to only the *taste* (as one would focus on one aspect of the sensation of the breath in a mindfulness breathing practice), one can become aware of thoughts and feelings that may co-occur and respond non-judgmentally to bring about a quick reinstatement of attentional focus on the taste of the current eating experience. This can potentially assist with a smaller cognitive load for the person who is eating mindfully. Non-judgment may be more effective in tackling emotional and stress-related eating (e.g., Czepczor-Bernat et al., 2019; Egan et al., 2020), as well as respond more adaptively to cravings (Mason et al., 2018). Acknowledging and accepting emotions and cravings through a non-judgmental stance, rather than being carried away by thoughts, emotions or cravings, may exist concurrently and reinforce attention to be regulated and sustained on the sensory aspects of the eating experience.

Researchers have further proposed a theoretical mechanism that may explain the potential of mindful eating by exploring operant conditioning and craving (Brewer et al., 2018; Tapper & Turner, 2018). When eating becomes boring or a meal is plain and dull, the mind will wander away from the sensory experiences, and the ability or inability to shift attention back to the task may become a significant aspect of success in eating mindfully. Mindful eating may undeniably be more demanding without the aptitude to recognize, observe, acknowledge and accept what the mind does and where attention has shifted. Allowing non-judgmental to take its course during the practice (e.g., Jenkins & Tapper, 2014; Kristeller, 2015; Mantzios et al., 2019; Mantzios et al., 2020; Mantzios & Giannou, 2014; Papies et al., 2015) may reiterate the attentional focus on the experience of eating. Importantly, any non-eating experience does not constitute an opportunity to utilize a mindful eating practice, and any "mindfulness-based" practice incongruent to the eating experience itself is not a mindful eating practice, but more of a mindfulness practice that may indirectly influence eating behaviors.

Second, the way one responds to physiological cues in mindfulness practices is dissimilar to mindful eating, and aligning mindful eating more closely to mindfulness should be considered. Literature on the effectiveness of mindfulness practices has proposed that the observation of physiological signals (such as chronic pain) is another opportunity to decenter or detach non-judgmentally from the observation (e.g., "I am not my pain", i.e., not identifying with one's pain) and re-establish attention (e.g., by redirecting to the sensation of the breath) (Thompson, 2009). For mindful eating, however, physiological signals of hunger and satiety cannot be observed in a similar fashion, where one adopts a detached or non-judgmental stance of observing physiological cues, as common assumption dictates that there may be potential implications for overconsumption of food during eating. Furthermore, assessing, appraising, and/or estimating hunger and satiety, and responding by deciding as to when to cease food intake, is essentially a comparison, categorization, or evaluation (hungry vs. full). This connotes a judgment and has no place in mindful eating or any other mindfulness practice. Some researchers may be of a different opinion to the assertion of hunger and satiety being related to judgment, thus not purely representing corresponding theory, and they may argue that this proposition is based on semantics.

However, the reality is that considering hunger and satiety during the meal, and acting upon relevant cues, creates a conflicting feedback loop to the ability to upkeep a non-judgmental stance. *Decision-making for mindful eating* determines the nature of decisions prior to eating, such as judging hunger and satiety, but also decisions relevant to the environmental factors, such as finding a quiet place to eat, eating without the distraction of the TV, or anything that will drive and prepare the individual to eat more mindfully. *Decision-making for mindful eating* can also be an appraisal of emotional hunger or the presence of cravings, in addition to the potential of external factors influencing appetite, such as foods becoming available. *Mindful eating behavior* determines the nature of an eating behavior independently of decision-making. Such decision-making for mindful eating that is functioning outside the eating experience—in association with mindful eating behavior—could form a mindfulness-based eating program as observed in some literature, and present the closest description of mindful eating as a holistic structure (Kristeller, 2015).

Naturally, when someone adopts a mindfulness meditation practice, such as mindfulness breathing meditation, they are not calling on their motivation, the quiet environment to practice mindfulness meditation, the cushion they are sitting on and the dim lighting as "mindfulness meditation". These factors impact the practice separately from the foundational characteristics of the practice itself. In other words, the cushion someone is sitting on may influence the practice, but it is not part of the mindfulness practice. Mindfulness literature clearly outlines that paying more attention to behaviors offers an enhanced ability to initiate or cease a behavior. Developing mindfulness enables recollection of behavioral intentions (Chatzisarantis & Hagger, 2007) and safeguards decision-making (Black et al., 2012) to promote health and may substitute the need for instructions around hunger and satiety altogether when considering mindful eating. Within this context of not needing additional instructions and simply requiring the actual mindfulness practice for behavior change, measuring and exploring mindful eating behavior appears exact and significant in unfolding the potential of the eating behavior itself, rather than mindful eating as an abstract and diluted concept. Current literature and measurement tools of mindful eating, however, are assessing and evaluating both *mindful eating behavior* (i.e., present moment sensory experiences and non-judgmental attention and awareness) and *mindful decision-making around eating* (i.e., assessment of hunger and satiety, environmental factors, etc.). However, they do not assess mindful eating behavior segregated from non-eating-related behaviors, which weaken findings and potentially depict an imprecise impact of mindful eating behavior on health outcomes.

Furthermore, guidance on hunger and satiety is standardized care that is already present in nutritional counseling, observed in healthy or regulated eating across clinical and non-clinical settings. The merging of hunger and satiety with mindful eating is a topic area that should be tested in association and separately, to define optimal eating experiences and regulatory aptitudes; a similar proposition is true for the inclusion of ACT and self-compassion components in mindful eating interventions, discussed further below. Grossman and Van Dam (2011) stated that "many scientists with limited or no experience in mindfulness practice may confuse psychological and Buddhist characterizations of mindful awareness" (p. 227). This proposes yet another topic of discussion and debate in itself as to where Buddhist traditions become relevant in the discussion of mindful eating (e.g., see Kristeller & Jordan, 2018). It is not too late to create clarity in the field and advance the science behind mindful eating by separating *mindful eating behavior* (i.e., sensory experience of eating, non-judgmentally) from *decision-making for mindful eating* (i.e., "am I still hungry?" "I will not multitask while eating") in applied and experimental research.

A New Perspective on Mindful Eating

Defining mindful eating behavior may be a starting point to create more accurate and precise inquiries in future research. Therefore, mindful eating behavior is defined as *the sustained attention on a sensory element of the eating experience (e.g., the taste), and a non-judgmental (or non-evaluative) awareness of thoughts and feelings that are incongruent to the sensory elements of the present eating experience* (Mantzios, 2021). By removing decision-making from investigations of mindful eating behavior, this definition of mindful eating behavior may allow to advance research into more rigorous and precise testing environments, questionnaires and practices that build on empirical evidence able to be replicated. But it is not just a question of separating decision-making from behavior, but also ceasing the associations of mindful eating with other constructs that may blur the impact of mindful eating. For example, I propose the creation of separate interventions for mindful eating, as they may offer a more direct, evidence-based and methodologically rigorous body of literature.

Effectiveness of the Mindful Construal Diary/Reflection

Past research has attempted to associate mindful eating with self-compassion to develop a hybrid intervention targeting weight regulation but missed the opportunity to explore the potential of each intervention separately. Mantzios and Wilson (2014) developed a Mindful Construal Diary (MCD), which is a mindful eating tool that combines concepts of mindfulness, self-compassion and construal-level theory (CLT). CLT proposed that forming abstract (or high-level) mental construals acts as a barrier to experiencing the present moment, and those construals are populated within everyday self-perceptions of remembering and planning, which entail strong evaluative implications and questions around (non-)judgment (Trope & Liberman, 2010). Therefore, concrete (or low-level) construals were proposed to enhance the present moment attention and non-judgment that are fundamental to mindfulness practices (Mantzios & Wilson, 2014). Mantzios and Wilson (2014) proposed that such a model of reinforcing present moment attention and awareness, as well as non-judgment, was represented within CLT (e.g., Trope & Liberman, 2010), which suggests concepts can be identified on a close or distant continuum representing abstract or concrete understandings of one's reality (Freitas et al., 2004). Freitas et al. (2004) put forward an intervention, where abstract construals questioned *why* actions are being performed, whereas concrete construals drew participants' attention on *how* they carry out a behavior. Mantzios and Wilson (2014) considered how concrete construals could promote attention to the present moment, similar to mindfulness meditation by focusing on the *how* of eating, which they argued does not require any further judgmental interpretation as when asking *why* one is eating. Non-judgment, non-evaluation and acceptance have been driven and explained through self-compassion (e.g., Baer, 2010; Neff, 2009), and this healthier perception of oneself has shown to be particularly significant in determining health behaviors (Homan & Sirois, 2017; Sirois, 2015; Sirois & Hirsch, 2019). Importantly, Mantzios and Wilson (2014) incorporated self-compassion onto the practice and transformed a traditional meditation practice into an event-based diary (i.e., the MCD) that allowed people to step away from meditation, as research has indicated potential implications in inclusivity due to religious beliefs and skepticism (e.g., Mantzios & Wilson, 2015). The MCD simply requires participants to read the mindful and self-compassionate questions within the diary and write out the answers either whilst they are eating or immediately afterwards. This technique is considered to be much simpler to follow than meditation (Mantzios & Wilson, 2014).

Research has explored the effectiveness of the MCD as an alternative to mindful meditation. The findings from one study illustrated that those who used the MCD were able to maintain their weight significantly better than those participating in a mindful self-compassion contemplative program (Mantzios & Wilson, 2014). Later research utilized the MCD in a different way, renaming the tool to the Mindful Construal Reflection (MCR), where items of the diary were considered as a way of nudging participants in eating mindfully, rather than using the questions in a diary format and filling it in. Research proposed significant increases in mindfulness and self-compassion, and significant decreases in anxiety (Hussein et al., 2017), explaining potential mechanisms of previous findings around weight regulation (see also Hussain et al., 2021a, 2021b, 2021c). Other experimental research indicated that the raisin exercise (i.e., a traditional mindful eating practice—see

Kabat-Zinn, 2003) enabled participants to consume less chocolate when instructed to watch a video when compared to a control condition (Mantzios et al., 2019). Follow-up experimental research explored the MCR tool to find that it performed similarly to the raisin practice in eating less chocolate (Mantzios et al., 2020). Hussain et al. (2021c) recently attempted to enhance the performance of the MCR tool by infusing a more self-distanced perspective. Participants were randomly assigned to a self-immersed, self-distanced or control condition, where both experimental conditions received an adapted version of the original MCD (see Mantzios & Wilson, 2014). Participants in the self-immersed condition received an MCR tool that adapted questions to be in the first person, such as "How do I feel, and what passes through my mind now that I am eating this snack". Participants in the self-distanced condition received an MCR tool that was formatted in the third person, such as "How does Georgia feel and what passes through Georgia's mind now that she is eating this snack?". These adaptations were proposed to assist people to step away from emotional distress and overcome instances of emotional eating when in the distanced condition, and findings indicated that a self-distanced (over a self-immersed and control) condition assisted in eating less chocolate.

Further Issues in Research and Practice on Mindful Eating

While the research with the MCD/MCR continues, it does not offer much to the discussion on mindful eating, apart from some later research that omitted items of self-compassion and explored the benefits of using an MCR tool exclusively with mindful eating behavior items (e.g., Mantzios et al., 2020). Nevertheless, this research is receiving the same criticism as mindfulness-based programs (i.e., multiple practices that are taught and practiced over several days or weeks constituting a program). Despite the lack of an available evidence base for some practices, using evidence and non-evidence-based practices to constitute a program creates uncertainty on the contribution of practices to overall health outcomes and behavioral change. Questions that may add clarity and precision to the field of mindful eating are: is mindfulness meditation equally beneficial to mindful eating practices, are self-compassion and mindfulness interventions equally significant, and would mindful eating work equally well with and without hunger and satiety assessment to promote physical health and weight regulation? Packaging everything together, despite the theoretical and past research consolidation, allows for too many inaccuracies in signifying what works and what may be omitted in mindful eating interventions and programs. Mantzios et al. (2020) suggested that the use of priming or nudging people to eat more mindfully creates a more suitable practice to ease usage and adaptation in everyday life due to the sustainability, adherence and ease to use for a long-term constitution of healthier eating behaviors.

Future Directions and Implications

The capability to develop practices that could be utilized across the field of eating behaviors through habituation (Ouellette & Wood, 1998) and other psychological processes (see Mantzios & Giannou, 2019) provides an exceptional opportunity to delineate an affirmative transformation in health and eating behaviors. For example, as eating is a repetitive and automatic health-related action, which typically requires no forethought, the opportunity to adopt a simple and sustainable mindful eating behavior practice to create a habit of the practice itself may propose a lifestyle change (Mantzios & Giannou, 2019; Mantzios et al., 2020) that is less cognitively taxing and "second nature" (Lally et al., 2011). The (re)-introduction and reinstatement of pleasure and satisfaction that derives from every attentive meal (Hong et al., 2011) may enhance a *desirability* (Adriaanse et al., 2011) to engage with a mindful eating behavior practice. This could act as an *internal motivation* (Deci et al., 1999) to repeat a mindful eating practice, and without any removal or devaluation of the experienced reward when eating reinforces repetition (Wood & Neal, 2009). For habituation and other theories to tap into mindful eating, the central focus needs to rest on mindful eating behavior as previously described.

Overall, this chapter puts forward five points of action to rectify past drawbacks in mindful eating research. First, psychometric tools need reconsideration and clarity so that researchers and clinicians understand what is being measured. Second, and similar to the action with psychometric tools, mindful eating practices need clarity and reconsideration. The "mindfulness-based" umbrella allowed for past research to associate different practices (or select some mindfulness or mindful eating features), creating a vagueness as to what works and the objective relationship to mindful eating behaviors. Utilizing only the attentive aspects of mindful eating does not contribute to conclusions around mindful eating. Third, mindful eating is an event-based practice, and it should be investigated as such, allowing for in-depth investigations of the eating behavior itself, and the impact of attention and awareness during eating. Fourth, omitting elements that are associated with decision-making for mindful eating from psychometric tools and experimental research may offer further clarity on mindful eating behavior and practices. To reduce the likelihood of an enhanced cognitive load during mindful eating, observing and reacting to hunger or satiety needs separate consideration in both research and practice. Fifth, removing additional elements that are associated to other, potentially affiliated, but essentially different practices such as self-compassion, may offer clarity in investigating mindful eating behavior for what it actually is, an eating behavior. Utilizing this as a foundation and creating separate interventions of mindful eating and self-compassionate eating may offer a more direct, evidence-based and methodologically rigorous body of literature. Together, these action points may offer clarity and transparency to what mindful eating can offer to intervene for health and well-being.

To preserve transparency and precision, the way practices and psychometric tools are referred to needs further consideration. For example, when non-judgment is not included in a practice or measurement tool, we have a duty to refer to it as a *mindful attention eating* scale or practice, or *attentive eating* scale or practice. Similar to mindfulness meditation literature, the Five-Facet Mindfulness Questionnaire (FFMQ; Baer et al., 2006) proposes a more inclusive measure than the Mindful Attention and Awareness Scale (MAAS; Brown & Ryan, 2003), where the former explicitly measures non-judgment, while the latter does not, at least not explicitly. Meanwhile, *mindful eating behavior* should be preserved to describe the all-inclusive context that is aligned to mindfulness practices, and *mindful eating* should refer to mindfulness-based eating programs that train people in both decision-making for mindful eating and mindful eating behavior. The verdict to separate scales and practices by their actual name and tell apart the behavior from the decisions will create a framework for the field of mindful eating for the years to come. But advancing the field with a mentality of one term fits all, where anything remotely relevant to mindful eating is referred to as mindful eating, will do injustice to any potential for developing the science behind mindful eating behavior.

References

Adriaanse, M. A., Gollwitzer, P. M., de Ridder, D. T. D., de Wit, J. B. F., & Kroese, F. M. (2011). Breaking habits with implementation intentions: A test of underlying processes. *Personality and Social Psychology Bulletin, 37*, 502–513.

Allirot, X., Miragall, M., Perdices, I., Baños, R. M., Urdaneta, E., & Cebolla, A. (2018). Effects of a brief mindful eating induction on food choices and energy intake: External eating and mindfulness state as moderators. *Mindfulness, 9*(3), 750–760.

Baer, R. A. (2010). Self-compassion as a mechanism of change in mindfulness and acceptance-based treatments. In R. A. Baer (Ed.), *Assessing mindfulness & acceptance processes in clients: Illuminating the theory and practice of change* (pp. 135–153). Context Press.

Baer, R. A., Smith, G. T., Hopkins, J., Krietemeyer, J., & Toney, L. (2006). Using self-report assessment methods to explore facets of mindfulness. *Assessment, 13*(1), 27–45.

Black, D. S., Sussman, S., Johnson, C. A., & Milam, J. (2012). Trait mindfulness helps shield decision-making from translating into health-risk behavior. *Journal of Adolescent Health, 51*(6), 588–592.

Blass, E. M., Anderson, D. R., Kirkorian, H. L., Pempek, T. A., Price, I., & Koleini, M. F. (2006). On the road to obesity: Television viewing increases intake of high-density foods. *Physiology & Behavior, 88*(4–5), 597–604.

Brewer, J. A., Ruf, A., Beccia, A. L., Essien, G. I., Finn, L. M., Lutterveld, R. V., & Mason, A. E. (2018). Can mindfulness address maladaptive eating behaviors? Why traditional diet plans fail and how new mechanistic insights may lead to novel interventions. *Frontiers in Psychology, 9*, 1418.

Brown, K. W., & Ryan, R. M. (2003). The benefits of being present: Mindfulness and its role in psychological well-being. *Journal of Personality and Social Psychology, 84*(4), 822–848.

Caballero, B. (2007). The global epidemic of obesity: An overview. *Epidemiologic Reviews, 29*(1), 1–5.

Carmel, J., & Musante, G. (1980). Structured eating: A predictor of weight loss at follow-up. *Ecology of Food and Nutrition, 9*(2), 87–91.

Chatzisarantis, N. L., & Hagger, M. S. (2007). Mindfulness and the intention-behavior relationship within the theory of planned behavior. *Personality and Social Psychology Bulletin, 33*(5), 663–676.

Cheung, L., & Hanh, T. N. (2010). *Savor: Mindful eating, mindful life* (p. 304). HarperOne.

Cohen, D., & Farley, T. A. (2008). Peer reviewed: Eating as an automatic behavior. *Preventing Chronic Disease, 5*(1). http://www.cdc.gov/pcd/issues/2008/jan/07_0046.htm

Czepczor-Bernat, K., Brytek-Matera, A., Gramaglia, C., & Zeppegno, P. (2019). The moderating effects of mindful eating on the relationship between emotional functioning and eating styles in overweight and obese women. *Eating and Weight Disorders-Studies on Anorexia, Bulimia and Obesity, 25*, 1–9.

Deci, E. L., Koestner, R., & Ryan, R. M. (1999). A meta-analytic review of experiments examining the effects of extrinsic rewards on intrinsic motivation. *Psychological Bulletin, 125*, 627–668.

Egan, H., Keyte, R., Nash, E. F., Barrett, J., Regan, A., & Mantzios, M. (2020). Mindfulness moderates the relationship between emotional eating and body mass index in a sample of people with cystic fibrosis. *Eating and Weight Disorders-Studies on Anorexia, Bulimia and Obesity, 26*, 1–7.

Framson, C., Kristal, A. R., Schenk, J. M., Littman, A. J., Zeliadt, S., & Benitez, D. (2009). Development and validation of the mindful eating questionnaire. *Journal of the American Dietetic Association, 109*(8), 1439–1444.
Freitas, A. L., Gollwitzer, P., & Trope, Y. (2004). The influence of abstract and concrete mindsets on anticipating and guiding others' self-regulatory efforts. *Journal of Experimental Social Psychology, 40*(6), 739–752.
French, S. A., Epstein, L. H., Jeffery, R. W., Blundell, J. E., & Wardle, J. (2012). Eating behavior dimensions. Associations with energy intake and body weight. A review. *Appetite, 59*(2), 541–549.
Grossman, P. (2011). Defining mindfulness by how poorly I think I pay attention during everyday awareness and other intractable problems for psychology's (re) invention of mindfulness: Comment on Brown et al. (2011). *Psychological Assessment, 23*(4), 1034–1040.
Grossman, P. (2019). On the porosity of subject and object in 'mindfulness' scientific study: Challenges to 'scientific' construction, operationalization and measurement of mindfulness. *Current Opinion in Psychology, 28*, 102–107.
Grossman, P., & Van Dam, N. T. (2011). Mindfulness, by any other name...: Trials and tribulations of sati in western psychology and science. *Contemporary Buddhism, 12*(1), 219–239.
Hayes, S. C., Strosahl, K. D., & Wilson, K. G. (2011). *Acceptance and commitment therapy: The process and practice of mindful change*. Guilford Press.
Higgs, S. (2015). Manipulations of attention during eating and their effects on later snack intake. *Appetite, 92*, 287–294.
Homan, K. J., & Sirois, F. M. (2017). Self-compassion and physical health: Exploring the roles of perceived stress and health-promoting behaviors. *Health Psychology Open, 4*(2), 2055102917729542.
Hong, P. Y., Lishner, D. A., Han, K. H., & Huss, E. A. (2011). The positive impact of mindful eating on expectations of food liking. *Mindfulness, 2*(2), 103–113.
Hossain, P., Kawar, B., & El Nahas, M. (2007). Obesity and diabetes in the developing world—a growing challenge. *New England Journal of Medicine, 356*(3), 213–215.
Hulbert-Williams, L., Nicholls, W., Joy, J., & Hulbert-Williams, N. (2014). Initial validation of the mindful eating scale. *Mindfulness, 5*(6), 719–729.
Hussain, M., Egan, H., Keyte, R., & Mantzios, M. (2021a). Exploring the role of self-kindness in making healthier eating choices: A preliminary study. *International Journal of Behavioral Medicine, 28*(5), 664–669.
Hussain, M., Egan, H., Keyte, R., & Mantzios, M. (2021b). Mindful construal reflections: Reducing unhealthier eating choices. *Mindfulness, 12*(7), 1757–1767.
Hussain, M., Egan, H., Keyte, R., & Mantzios, M. (2021c). Exploring the effects of mindfulness and self-distancing on chocolate intake after a negative state affect. *Journal of Cognitive Enhancement, 5*(1), 15–24.

Hussein, M., Egan, H., & Mantzios, M. (2017). Mindful construal diaries: A less anxious, more mindful, and more self-compassionate method of eating. *Sage Open, 7*(2), 2158244017704685.

Jenkins, K. T., & Tapper, K. (2014). Resisting chocolate temptation using a brief mindfulness strategy. *British Journal of Health Psychology, 19*(3), 509–522.

Kabat-Zinn, J. (2003). Mindfulness-based interventions in context: Past, present, and future. *Clinical Psychology: Science and Practice, 10*(2), 144–156.

Keesman, M., Aarts, H., Häfner, M., & Papies, E. K. (2017). Mindfulness reduces reactivity to food cues: Underlying mechanisms and applications in daily life. *Current Addiction Reports, 4*(2), 151–157.

Keyte, R., Egan, H., & Mantzios, M. (2020). How does mindful eating without non-judgement, mindfulness and self-compassion relate to motivations to eat palatable foods in a student population? *Nutrition and Health, 26*(1), 27–34.

Kristeller, J. L. (2015). Mindfulness, eating disorders, and food intake regulation. In *Handbook of mindfulness and self-regulation* (pp. 199–215). Springer.

Kristeller, J. L., & Jordan, K. D. (2018). Mindful eating: Connecting with the wise self, the spiritual self. *Frontiers in Psychology, 9*, 1271.

Lally, P., Wardle, J., & Gardner, B. (2011). Experiences of habit formation: A qualitative study. *Psychology, Health & Medicine, 16*, 484–489.

Malinowski, P. (2013). Neural mechanisms of attentional control in mindfulness meditation. *Frontiers in Neuroscience, 7*, 8.

Mantzios, M. (2021). (Re) defining mindful eating into mindful eating behavior to advance scientific enquiry. *Nutrition and Health, 27*(4), 367–371.

Mantzios, M., Egan, H., & Asif, T. (2019). A randomised experiment evaluating the mindful raisin practice as a method of reducing chocolate consumption during and after a mindless activity. *Journal of Cognitive Enhancement, 4*(3), 250–257.

Mantzios, M., Egan, H., Bahia, H., Hussain, M., & Keyte, R. (2018). How does grazing relate to body mass index, self-compassion, mindfulness and mindful eating in a student population? *Health Psychology Open, 5*(1), 1–11.

Mantzios, M., Egan, H., Hussain, M., Keyte, R., & Bahia, H. (2018). Mindfulness, self-compassion, and mindful eating in relation to fat and sugar consumption: An exploratory investigation. *Eating and Weight Disorders-Studies on Anorexia, Bulimia and Obesity, 23*(6), 833–840.

Mantzios, M., & Giannou, K. (2014). Group vs. single mindfulness meditation: exploring avoidance, impulsivity, and weight management in two separate mindfulness meditation settings. *Applied Psychology: Health and Well-Being, 6*(2), 173–191.

Mantzios, M., & Giannou, K. (2019). A real-world application of short mindfulness-based practices: A review and reflection of the literature and a practical proposition for an effortless mindful lifestyle. *American Journal of Lifestyle Medicine, 13*(6), 520–525.

Mantzios, M., Skillett, K., & Egan, H. (2020). Examining the effects of two mindful eating exercises on chocolate consumption. *European Journal of Health Psychology, 26*, 120–128.

Mantzios, M., & Wilson, J. C. (2014). Making concrete construals mindful: A novel approach for developing mindfulness and self-compassion to assist weight loss. *Psychology & Health, 29*(4), 422–441.

Mantzios, M., & Wilson, J. C. (2015). Mindfulness, eating behaviors, and obesity: A review and reflection on current findings. *Current Obesity Reports, 4*(1), 141–146.

Marchiori, D., & Papies, E. K. (2014). A brief mindfulness intervention reduces unhealthy eating when hungry, but not the portion size effect. *Appetite, 75*, 40–45.

Mason, A. E., Jhaveri, K., Cohn, M., & Brewer, J. A. (2018). Testing a mobile mindful eating intervention targeting craving-related eating: Feasibility and proof of concept. *Journal of Behavioral Medicine, 41*(2), 160–173.

McConahy, K. L., Smiciklas-Wright, H., Mitchell, D. C., & Picciano, M. F. (2004). Portion size of common foods predicts energy intake among preschool-aged children. *Journal of the American Dietetic Association, 104*(6), 975–979.

Monroe, J. T. (2015). Mindful eating: Principles and practice. *American Journal of Lifestyle Medicine, 9*(3), 217–220.

Neff, K. D. (2009). The role of self-compassion in development: A healthier way to relate to oneself. *Human development, 52*(4), 211–214.

Nelson, J. B. (2017). Mindful eating: The art of presence while you eat. *Diabetes Spectrum, 30*(3), 171–174.

Ortega, F. B., Lavie, C. J., & Blair, S. N. (2016). Obesity and cardiovascular disease. *Circulation Research, 118*(11), 1752–1770.

Ouellette, J. A., & Wood, W. (1998). Habit and intention in everyday life: The multiple processes by which past behavior predicts future behavior. *Psychological Bulletin, 124*, 54–74.

Painter, J., & Wansink, B. (2002). How visibility and convenience influence candy consumption. *Appetite, 38*(3), 237–238.

Papies, E. K., Pronk, T. M., Keesman, M., & Barsalou, L. W. (2015). The benefits of simply observing: Mindful attention modulates the link between motivation and behavior. *Journal of Personality and Social Psychology, 108*(1), 148.

Public Health England. (2020). *Adult obesity: Patterns and trends*. HM Government. https://www.gov.uk/government/publications/adult-obesity-patterns-and-trends

Raes, F., & Williams, J. M. G. (2010). The relationship between mindfulness and uncontrollability of ruminative thinking. *Mindfulness, 1*(4), 199–203.

Robinson, E., Kersbergen, I., & Higgs, S. (2014). Eating 'attentively' reduces later energy consumption in overweight and obese females. *British Journal of Nutrition, 112*(4), 657–661.

Román, N., & Urbán, R. (2019). Mindful awareness or self-regulation in eating: An investigation into the underlying dimensions of mindful eating. *Mindfulness, 10*(10), 2110–2120.

Sirois, F. M. (2015). A self-regulation resource model of self-compassion and health behavior intentions in emerging adults. *Preventive Medicine Reports, 2*, 218–222.

Sirois, F. M., & Hirsch, J. K. (2019). Self-compassion and adherence in five medical samples: The role of stress. *Mindfulness, 10*(1), 46–54.

Spamon, J. L. (1989). Structured eating experiences in the inpatient treatment of anorexia nervosa. In: Hornyak, L.M. and Baker, E.K. (eds). *Experiential Therapies for Eating Disorders*. New York: Guilford Press, 207–233.

Tapper, K. (2017). Can mindfulness influence weight management related eating behaviors? If so, how? *Clinical Psychology Review, 53*, 122–134.

Tapper, K., & Seguias, L. (2020). The effects of mindful eating on food consumption over a half-day period. *Appetite, 145*, 104495.

Tapper, K., Shaw, C., Ilsley, J., Hill, A. J., Bond, F. W., & Moore, L. (2009). Exploratory randomised controlled trial of a mindfulness-based weight loss intervention for women. *Appetite, 52*(2), 396–404.

Tapper, K., & Turner, A. (2018). The effect of a mindfulness-based decentering strategy on chocolate craving. *Appetite, 130*, 157–162.

Taylor, M. B., Daiss, S., & Krietsch, K. (2015). Associations among self-compassion, mindful eating, eating disorder symptomatology, and body mass index in college students. *Translational Issues in Psychological Science, 1*(3), 229.

Teasdale, J. D., Segal, Z., & Williams, J. M. G. (1995). How does cognitive therapy prevent depressive relapse and why should attentional control (mindfulness) training help? *Behavior Research and Therapy, 33*(1), 25–39.

Teasdale, J. D., Segal, Z. V., Williams, J. M. G., Ridgeway, V. A., Soulsby, J. M., & Lau, M. A. (2000). Prevention of relapse/recurrence in major depression by mindfulness-based cognitive therapy. *Journal of Consulting and Clinical Psychology, 68*(4), 615–623.

Thompson, B. (2009). Mindfulness-based stress reduction for people with chronic conditions. *British Journal of Occupational Therapy, 72*(9), 405–410.

Trope, Y., & Liberman, N. (2010). Construal-level theory of psychological distance. *Psychological Review, 117*(2), 440–463.

Van Dam, N. T., Van Vugt, M. K., Vago, D. R., Schmalzl, L., Saron, C. D., Olendzki, A., Meissner, T., Lazar, S. W., Kerr, C. E., Gorchov, J., Fox, K. C., Field, B. A., Britton, W. B., Brefczynski-Lewis, J. A., & Meyer, D. E. (2018). Mind the hype: A critical evaluation and prescriptive agenda for research on mindfulness and meditation. *Perspectives on Psychological Science, 13*(1), 36–61.

Wansink, B., & Kim, J. (2005). Bad popcorn in big buckets: Portion size can influence intake as much as taste. *Journal of Nutrition Education and Behavior, 37*(5), 242–245.

Winkens, L. H., van Strien, T., Barrada, J. R., Brouwer, I. A., Penninx, B. W., & Visser, M. (2018). The mindful eating behavior scale: Development and psychometric properties in a sample of Dutch adults aged 55 years and older. *Journal of the Academy of Nutrition and Dietetics, 118*(7), 1277–1290.

Wood, S. M., Schembre, S. M., He, Q., Engelmann, J. M., Ames, S. L., & Bechara, A. (2016). Emotional eating and routine restraint scores are associated with activity in brain regions involved in urge and self-control. *Physiology & Behavior, 165*, 405–412.
Wood, W., & Neal, D. T. (2009). The habitual consumer. *Journal of Consumer Psychology, 19*, 579–592.
World Health Organization. (1998). *Obesity: Preventing and managing the global epidemic: Report of a WHO consultation on obesity, Geneva, 3–5 June 1997* (No. WHO/NUT/NCD/98.1). World Health Organization. https://apps.who.int/iris/bitstream/handle/10665/63854/WHO_NUT_NCD_98.1_%28p1-158%29.pdf?sequence=1

16

Mindfulness and Cancer

Maya Schroevers, Marije van der Lee, and Melanie Schellekens

Introduction

A diagnosis of cancer often has a great impact on those confronted with the illness and their families. The disease may affect not only people's health and physical functioning but also their psychosocial well-being and quality of life. Most people with cancer face intensive treatment, and most have severe side effects. People are also confronted with uncertainties about the future and their prognosis and need to manage the emotional impact of being diagnosed with a life-threatening illness. Moreover, people may have to make changes in their lifestyle regarding their diet and pattern of physical exercise, find a balance between keeping busy and engaging in daily activities and taking rest, and communicate their boundaries and needs with the people around them. At a more existential level, a diagnosis of cancer may affect core assumptions and beliefs that people have about themselves and the world, such as beliefs

M. Schroevers (✉)
Department of Health Sciences, Health Psychology, University of Groningen (RUG)/University Medical Center Groningen (UMCG), Groningen, Netherlands
e-mail: m.j.schroevers@umcg.nl

M. van der Lee
Department of Social and Behavioral Sciences, Medical and Clinical Psychology, Tilburg University, Tilburg, Netherlands

M. Schellekens
Helen Dowling Institute, Bilthoven, Netherlands

F. M. Sirois (ed.), *The Palgrave Handbook of Positive Psychology and Health*,
https://doi.org/10.1007/978-3-031-89095-6_16

that we are invulnerable and that life is predictable, controllable, fair, and meaningful. These physical and psychosocial challenges may vary over the course of illness and treatment as well as between individuals. A large group of people confronted with cancer are, over time, able to cope with the many consequences that cancer and its treatment may have on their life and functioning. Some experience a sense of strength, resilience, and trust in their abilities to manage the situation and sometimes even find meaning in the experience of living with cancer (Casellas-Grau et al., 2017; Lau et al., 2021). A significant group feels overwhelmed and finds it difficult to maintain emotional balance, experiencing feelings of depression and anxiety. Others may also try to ignore the impact and continue their normal life as much as possible.

In the last decades, there has been a growing interest in the human capacity for adaptation and interventions that aim to cultivate a sense of well-being and resilience. One type of interventions that focuses on resilience and living a meaningful life amid life challenges is mindfulness-based interventions. These interventions focus on cultivating present-moment awareness and acceptance. Such interventions may be especially valuable for people who face suffering in their lives, such as in the context of cancer. In this chapter, we will provide an overview of what cancer and its treatment entail and the physical and psychosocial implications of a cancer diagnosis. Then, we describe how mindfulness may play a role in adaptation to cancer. Also, the aims and content of mindfulness-based programs are pictured, possible benefits of mindfulness-based interventions for people with cancer, and empirical evidence for the efficacy of mindfulness-based interventions. This will be illustrated by case illustrations of persons diagnosed with cancer who have practiced mindfulness-based exercises to help them in their recovery. We conclude by summarizing the value and benefits of mindfulness for those people living with cancer and for cancer care.

Cancer and Its Treatment

What Is Cancer?

Cancer refers to a group of diseases characterized by the development of abnormal cells that divide uncontrollably, can infiltrate and destroy normal body tissue, and spread throughout the body (metastasis). The different types of cancer differ in their behavior, including how aggressive they are in infiltrating surrounding tissue and organs. Cancer is caused by changes (mutations) in the DNA within cells. Such gene mutations frequently occur during normal cell growth. There is a mechanism that detects when a mistake occurs and can repair the mutation. When this mechanism fails, a cell can become cancerous.

Risk Factors for Developing Cancer

Several factors may increase the risk of developing cancer, including:

- older age
- unhealthy lifestyle, including (others) smoking, alcohol consumption, unhealthy diet, lack of physical inactivity, being obese
- excessive sun exposure or use of tanning bed
- unsafe sex
- medication (e.g., immune suppressants, hormonal therapy) or presence of other chronic medical conditions or viral infections (e.g., hepatitis B-virus, human papillomavirus [HPV])
- exposure to environmental factors (e.g., harmful chemicals like asbestos and radioactive radiation)
- family history of cancer

While some factors such as aging and family history cannot be changed, lifestyle factors can. Therefore, changing lifestyle plays an important role in reducing the risks for certain cancers. Researchers in the UK found that behavior and environmental factors explained more than 40% of cancer incidence, with the highest risk factor being smoking, and to a lesser but still significant extent, a lack of fruit and vegetables, work-related exposure, obesity, and alcohol consumption (Parkin et al., 2011). It should be mentioned, however, that the role of many risk factors is complex, with some people with several risk factors never developing cancer, while others with no known risk factor do.

Research also examined the role of psychosocial factors as risk factors for developing cancer and cancer progression and survival. Existing evidence is not conclusive (McGee et al., 1994; Oerlemans et al., 2007). Overall, studies suggest a very limited role of these factors in developing cancer, with some evidence for the role of psychosocial factors in cancer progression, such as a lack of social integration and support and a pessimistic nature (Garssen & Goodkin, 1999; Nakaya, 2014; van Tuijl et al., 2023). Cancer progression will mostly depend on the type and location of the tumor, cancer stage, cancer treatment, side effects, and one's overall health status.

Cancer Incidence, Prevalence, and Survival Rates

Approximately 40% of men and women will be diagnosed with cancer at some point during their lifetimes (prevalence), with numbers of new cases increasing. This increase is, amongst others, due to the aging population, with 90% of those diagnosed with cancer being 50 years or older. In 2020, there were an estimated 18 million people diagnosed with cancer and 10 million deaths associated with cancer worldwide (Sung et al., 2021); this is expected to rise to 28 million by 2040. The most common types of cancer include breast cancer, lung cancer, colorectal cancer, prostate cancer, and stomach cancer. These numbers mean that most of us will be confronted with cancer at some point in life, either because one gets diagnosed him or herself or a close family member or friend.

While cancer is still one of the leading causes of death worldwide, the overall cancer death rate has declined in the past decades. As a result of improvements in early cancer screening and cancer treatment, survival rates have improved for many types of cancer. Overall, 64% of people with cancer are alive five years after diagnosis (which was 36% in the 1960s). This rate differs greatly for the different types of cancer. For instance, the likelihood of a person diagnosed with lung cancer to be alive after five years is only 19%, while the chance that a woman diagnosed with breast cancer is still alive after five years is 88%.

Different Trajectories of Cancer and Possible Treatment

Different trajectories can be distinguished when confronted with cancer:

1. When diagnosed timely, treatment with curative intent is often possible, with an acute treatment phase followed by a recovery phase and a follow-up period with often yearly checkups for about five years, depending on cancer type.
2. Sometimes, the cancer is of a chronic nature; think of chronic leukemia, Kahler's disease, or types of Hodgkin that will not be treated right away, but only when it will get worse, a so-called wait-and-see treatment policy.
3. Sometimes, no curative treatment is available because of the cancer type and/or stage; this is often referred to as the palliative phase. The last part of the palliative phase is the terminal phase, when symptoms progress and death is imminent. In the palliative phase, tumor-directed treatment is often possible for improvement of the length of life, and symptom-directed treatment for improvement of quality of life.

All transitions from one trajectory to another are moments that patients need to adapt, and when their resources are overloaded, psychological distress can arise. The acute phase starts with the first suspects, followed by undergoing examinations and tests for cancer. This phase is often characterized by feelings of shock, uncertainty, numbness, disbelief, and acute stress. Most people do not feel overall ill because of the cancer, but notice a lump or troublesome cough, for instance, or hear the result from participating in a cancer screening program. With the realization that something might be wrong, the question comes whether to go to the doctor or not, thinking that symptoms may not be that serious and will disappear with time.

When seeking care, most people first go to their general practitioner. This may lead to an uncertain and stressful period of examinations. Cancer may be detected by physical exams, laboratory tests (such as blood tests), imaging (such as X-ray, CT, MRI, and PET scans), and/or biopsy (during which the doctor collects a sample of cells for testing). A crucial element of diagnosis is determining the cancer stage. Cancer stage indicates how cancer cells have spread in the body, and this stage is a crucial factor in determining the prognosis and treatment. The TNM classification is used to describe the cancer stage, with T (Tumor) referring to the size and spread of the primary tumor, N (Nodes) for spread in the lymph nodes, and M (Metastasis) for spread at distance in other places of the body. Cancer stage can vary from I to IV, with higher numerals indicating more advanced cancer.

After the diagnosis of cancer has been confirmed, treatment may start (see Table 16.1 for an overview of common cancer treatments). Treatment may include surgery, radiotherapy, chemotherapy, hormone therapy, immunotherapy, and targeted therapy. Often, different cancer treatments are combined (simultaneously or sequentially). For instance, surgery is followed by a period of radiotherapy, and then hormonal therapy, or the other way around, with adjuvant hormonal therapy and chemotherapy given before surgery, or treatment starts with chemotherapy and then surgery and further chemotherapy. As a result, many people with cancer face a treatment that may last six to twelve months or even longer. The choice of treatment will depend, amongst others, on the type and stage of the cancer as well as the patient's age, general health condition, and his or her values and preferences. When possible, the aim of cancer treatment is to cure (to fully remove cancer from the body). In this phase, people are often focused on surviving and managing treatment and its side effects. In this acute phase of cancer and its treatment, about 25% of patients experience depressive symptoms, although this percentage varies strongly among the different studies (due to factors such as the type of

Table 16.1 Common cancer treatments

Surgery	For most people with cancer, surgery is the primary cancer treatment. Surgery can lead to changes in appearance (e.g., amputation of a breast) and loss of functioning of a body part (e.g., loss of voice due to surgery of head- and neck tumors or limitations in using an arm after a breast amputation)
Radiotherapy (X-rays or radioactive radiation)	Most often radiotherapy is applied from the outside of the body (external radiation), sometimes from inside the body (internal radiation). One session of radiotherapy lasts a few minutes. The number of radiations can vary from 1 to more than 30 radiations. Radiation often causes redness of the skin, hair loss, fatigue, nausea, and vomiting
Chemotherapy (using cytostatic medication)	Chemotherapy is used to kill the cancer cells or reduce cell division. These medications are often given by intravenous drip, during day treatment or during hospitalization for several days. This is followed by a period of rest. Chemotherapy exists of several periods of treatment and rest. Sometimes medications are given via injection or tablets. Chemotherapy can have many side-effects, including nausea and vomiting, fatigue, hair loss, changes in taste, weight loss, and oppression of the production of blood cells in the bone marrow, which may cause a lack of red blood cells (anemia) and white blood cells (reduced immune functioning). These effects often diminish after treatment has finished. In the long term, chemotherapy may also damage the nervous system (neuropathy) or organs (such as heart, lungs, and reproductive organs causing reduced fertility, early menopause, or sexual problems) and fatigue is a common problem
Hormonal therapy	These medications can be part of adjuvant therapy (to reduce the risk of the cancer coming back) or palliative therapy (when metastases are present). Hormonal therapy can cause menopause symptoms
Immunotherapy	This treatment uses so-called immune checkpoint inhibitors to stimulate the immune cells to attack the cancer cells Common side-effects include skin rash, inflammations of the intestines or liver, and disturbances of hormonal balance
Targeted therapy	Targeted therapy refers to the use of oral medications aiming to stop the signals by means of which cancer cells can grow. Side-effects may include fatigue, skin rash, and diarrhea

definition and assessment of symptoms, as well as sample being studied) (Caruso et al., 2017; Hartung et al., 2017).

When treatment has finished, people are faced with the long-term consequences of cancer. They have to integrate the cancer experienced in their life. This may include questions such as: "How will my health be, will the cancer come back?", "Can I take care of my family again, do tasks at home, keep working?", and "How do I want to live my life, what is important to me?". The period can be very stressful, with less contact with the medical staff, fewer medical exams, and the uncertainty about the course of illness. Psychological problems, including symptoms of depression, often reduce after medical treatment has finished (Caruso et al., 2017), and in the long term, most patients who received curative cancer treatment report the same level of depressive symptoms as people in the general population (Brandenbarg et al., 2019). Some patients maintain feelings of anxiety, especially fear of cancer recurrence (Almeida et al., 2019). Also, people may have to deal with long-term limitations and consequences, such as chronic fatigue.

When a full cure is not possible (anymore), palliative treatment may be offered to slow down cancer progression, help to relieve symptoms, such as pain and shortness of breath, and conserve a sense of quality of life as good as possible. This phase can last several weeks but also several months or years. In this period, there will often be a continued physical deterioration, and people need to deal with a short life expectancy and find peace with how they have lived their life and how they want to die.

Due to the advancements in existing treatment options and the introduction of new anti-cancer therapies (e.g., immunotherapy, targeted therapy), many patients with advanced cancer who recently would not have survived more than months are now living for years under treatment. These patients must cope with living long-term with what could be a terminal illness. Potential challenges include ongoing uncertainty about their future, physical issues related to disease burden, side effects or late effects of treatment, and changing roles in their family, social, and work life.

Consequences of Cancer and Its Treatment

Quality of life refers to perceptions people have about their physical, psychological, social, and spiritual functioning. As said earlier, a diagnosis of cancer often may have a wide range of consequences for people's physical (such as fatigue, pain, insomnia), psychological well-being (e.g., symptoms of depression, anxiety, and uncertainty) and social well-being (e.g., disruptions in daily and social activities) and bring up existential issues. As such, cancer and its treatment may make it difficult to be present in what is happening, and people's minds may be fully occupied with the cancer experience, being stressed, and worrying about what is going on and could happen. The practice of mindfulness may be a way to deal differently with cancer and reduce stress and worries by helping people to feel more present and in the moment, to relate differently to suffering, and to cultivate a sense of trust, hope, and resilience. In the next sections, first, the wide range of possible consequences of cancer will be described, followed in more detail by how mindfulness can help cancer patients.

Physical Consequences

When cancer is suspected, many cancer patients do not have specific symptoms. This changes when treatment starts, with most cancer treatments associated with severe side effects (see Table 16.1 about cancer treatment). Side effects may vary per treatment, from person to person, and over time. Fatigue is one of the most prevalent and burdensome physical problems, which may maintain after finishing treatment. Approximately one in four cancer patients suffers from severe fatigue, when treatment has ended (Abrahams et al., 2016), especially for people diagnosed with a higher stage of cancer and more intensive cancer treatment. People confronted with severe physical consequences or having difficulties managing the physical impact of cancer and its treatment may benefit from mindfulness-based interventions.

Psychological Consequences

Besides a deteriorating health, people facing cancer may experience severe distress. Such distress can express itself by feelings of uncertainty, vulnerability, irritability, anger, anxiety, helplessness, guilt, and sadness (Krebber et al., 2014; Linden et al., 2012). Especially, symptoms of depression and anxiety are common. While a majority of people seems to be able to manage the impact of cancer, a significant group of 25% of people suffers from depressive or anxiety symptoms in the year following cancer diagnosis (Hartung et al., 2017; Kuhnt et al., 2016). In the long term, most cancer survivors seem to be able to adjust to the cancer experience and report similar levels of depressive and anxiety symptoms as similar-aged healthy persons from the general population (Brandenbarg et al., 2019). It must be mentioned here that it can be difficult to recognize symptoms of anxiety and depression in cancer patients, as symptoms may overlap with those of cancer and its treatment. The network approach may be helpful to overcome this problem, proposing to turn attention toward individual symptoms and their interconnectedness, making the distinction between mental and physical symptoms obsolete (Van der Lee & Schellekens, 2020). Second, it should be noted that the number of 25% refers to a group average, with great individual variation in the report of symptoms.

Having a bad or uncertain prognosis has been related to an increased risk for depressive symptoms. In addition, psychosocial factors (including personality, history of psychological problems, coping, social sharing, and support) have been found to play a crucial role in explaining variations in depressive symptoms among people with cancer. People vulnerable to experience psychological problems may be interested in receiving psychological care, such as a mindfulness-based intervention.

Social Consequences

Cancer affects not only the person confronted with the illness but also the well-being of others close to them, such as a partner, children, other family members, and friends, and the relationships with these persons. This impact can be positive as well as negative. Regarding the negative impact, it has for instance been found that distress and depressive symptoms are also very common in partners of people with cancer (Rottmann et al., 2016). Regarding the impact on social relationships and social support, many people with cancer experience their relationships as very supportive and even an improvement in the relationship quality, whereas others experience poor marital satisfaction or a worsening of the relationship with their partner and a lack of support or being misunderstood by people in their surroundings (Ruiz-Marin et al., 2021). Cancer may also strongly affect the daily activities of the persons with cancer and role functioning at home or work or in social activities. This can cause feelings of dependence, frustration, guilt, loneliness, and sadness. Poor physical functioning, including fatigue and psychological problems, puts people with cancer at risk for problems in their social functioning (Schilstra et al., 2021).

Existential Consequences

In an existential way, a diagnosis of cancer may confront people with their vulnerability and mortality and challenge their core beliefs and fundamental assumptions about security, controllability, and priorities, which may lead to existential distress (Vehling & Philipp, 2018). Questions that may arise are: "Why (not) me?", "Who am I?", "What is important to me, what is the meaning of (my) life?", and "How do I want to live my life?". One-third to half of cancer survivors experience existential fears and concerns, and a quarter experiences demoralization and loss of meaning.

Besides such a negative existential impact, a substantial proportion of people with cancer report post-traumatic growth in the sense that they perceive positive aspects of the cancer experience. This may include a greater appreciation of life in general, a greater appreciation of small things in life, a greater appreciation of themselves or their relationships, and a greater awareness of their values, goals in life, and priorities (Casellas-Grau et al., 2017).

Summary

Cancer may pose a significant threat and numerous challenges for a person, not only to one's physical health and integrity but also at a psychosocial and existential level. Although many people seem to be able to adapt to the illness and its treatment over time on their own, with support from family and friends, many face a very difficult time in their lives, struggling with the physical burden, the fears and losses, and having intrusive memories and thoughts about an uncertain future. How can mindfulness help people with cancer? In the following section, we describe what mindfulness is, which interventions exist that aim to cultivate mindfulness, and evidence from research on the benefits of practicing mindfulness.

Mindfulness and Mindfulness-Based Interventions

What Is Mindfulness?

Mindfulness has its roots in Eastern religions and traditions of Buddhism and Hinduism, and it has entered Western culture as a secular practice by people including Jon Kabat-Zinn, Thich Nhat Hanh, Sharon Salzberg, Richard Davidson, Jack Kornfield, and Joseph Goldstein. Mindfulness refers to being fully present in the here and now. Mindfulness is described as an intentional, moment-by-moment awareness of our thoughts, feelings, bodily sensations, and the surrounding environment. This awareness is accompanied by an attitude involving openness, curiosity, and acceptance (Kabat-Zinn, 1990, 2003; Bishop et al., 2004). This means that people pay attention to experiences without judging them as being good or bad, right, or wrong.

When people are mindful, they are aware of their experiences in the present moment, rather than caught up in reliving the past or running forward to the future, as they might do most of the time. For instance, when being diagnosed with cancer, people may get lost in thoughts about how this could have happened, why did this happen to them, and the things that they should have done differently. Or they worry about all the things that could happen and could go wrong. In a state of mindfulness, thoughts, feelings, and sensations, whether pleasant or unpleasant, are observed as events in the mind, without identifying with them or denying them. Also, automatic habitual patterns of reactivity can be observed, without directly having to act upon them. This has also been referred to as non-reactivity or decentering: stepping outside of one's immediate experiences, not focusing on the content but viewing experiences as events, and taking a more objective, non-judging stance. When being mindful, the stream of thoughts about the past and future can be observed and acknowledged as thoughts, created by the mind.

By means of mindfulness, one can create a space between what is happening and how to respond. Such a way of responding relates to the quote of Victor Frankl: "Between stimulus and response there is a space. In that space is our power to choose our response. In our response lies our growth and our freedom." For example, during a mindfulness exercise, a person can observe the following: "I notice that I am tired, my mood feels heavy, I feel some tension in my belly. I notice that I judge the way I feel and that I judge myself, that I haven't taken good care of myself." By this mindful observation, recognizing and acknowledging what is going on, a person can then make a mindful choice about what to do (or not do) next, for instance, knowing how he or she feels and just continue with activities, or to do something that is soothing or restoring. For people with cancer, mindfulness can be viewed as a way to learn to better manage the challenges of having cancer. Mindfulness can also be viewed as a way of living: more present, more aware of what is happening, and more open to what life brings. This has been associated with a greater sense of appreciation, gratefulness, and feelings of connectedness.

Most of the time, people are not mindful; they act on automatic pilot and habitually. These habits are fueled by two strong motives: wanting pleasant experiences and not wanting unpleasant experiences. While often not being aware, people wish things to be different, better, more, or less. This causes a feeling of dissatisfaction and an impulse to act, for instance, to solve problems and seek things that they like. This is called the *doing-mode* (Segal et al., 2002, 2013). This doing-mode can be extremely helpful. But what if things cannot be changed or controlled? An important downside of living most of our lives on the automatic pilot and in a doing-mode, with our mind caught up in the past or future, is that we miss out the present: the pleasant things (like a friendly smile, a beautiful evening sky, or the taste of a cup of coffee in the morning) as well as signals from the body, that for instance indicate tension or fatigue and a need for rest. Being in a doing-mode, most of the time, takes a great amount of time and energy and may create endless streams of wanting, planning, worrying, and problem-solving. With mindfulness, people can recognize this doing-mode and when needed, step out of it and take a pause, into a *being-mode*. In this being-mode, people are mindfully aware of the current moment experiences.

To obtain an indication of a person's level of mindfulness, several questionnaires have been developed. The most-used questionnaire is the Five Factor Mindfulness Questionnaire (FFMQ) (Baer et al., 2006). With 39 questions, the questionnaire assesses five mindfulness facets: (1) being sensory aware; (2) labeling and describing experiences in words; (3) mindful acting; (4) holding a nonjudgmental attitude; and (5) non-reacting. While mindfulness questionnaires are widely used in scientific research and clinical practice, the validity of these questionnaires is still under debate.

Mindfulness-Based Interventions (MBSR, MBCT)

Kabat-Zinn played a crucial role in introducing mindfulness in the West by means of the secularized program he developed: Mindfulness-Based Stress Reduction (MBSR), an eight-week group program aiming to reduce stress (Kabat-Zinn, 1990). Kabat-Zinn launched this program at the University of Massachusetts Medical School in 1979. By combining Eastern practices of mindfulness with Western psychology and science, Kabat-Zinn stimulated the widespread interest in mindfulness.

MBSR consists of eight weekly group sessions that last two to three hours, with an additional practice day in silence. In addition, participants are asked to do daily practices at home for 30–60 minutes. As MBSR focuses on experiential learning (i.e., learning through direct experience), every session starts with doing a mindful exercise of 30–45 minutes, followed by a group discussion, and sharing of experiences in the practice just done (so-called "enquiry"). This is followed by a review of the experiences of doing the exercises at home, in people's own daily lives. Then, another exercise is done, and sometimes psychoeducation is provided on stress signals and our stress system, the doing- and being-modes, and automatic versus reflective responding.

The main practices are the body scan, sitting and walking meditations, and yoga exercises. During the body scan, people are invited to bring their attention to all parts of their body, starting with the toes and ending with the crown of the head, and to do this in a particular way: intentional and with an open, accepting, and curious attitude. The purpose of practicing the body scan is to improve attention regulation, to increase bodily awareness, and to develop a different relation with and perspective on our body: less judgmental, more kind and accepting. Especially when having had cancer and treatment, people may feel betrayed by their body, sad, angry, anxious, or disconnected. How doing these exercises can help a person with cancer is described in the example of Peter in the box below.

Peter is a 47-year-old, single man with no children, who was diagnosed with colon cancer two years ago. He was treated with surgery followed by three months of chemotherapy as the cancer had also spread to the lymph nodes. Treatment has been successful so far, but he still often feels very weak and tired; this fatigue hinders him in carrying out his daily activities. Also, because the surgeon had to remove a large part of his colon ("colectomy"), a stoma had to be placed. Now, a part of his bowel is brought out through an opening in the abdomen into a bag, which Peter has to regularly empty and change. The doctor told him that someday the stoma may be removed, but so far, this has not been possible. Peter hates the stoma and struggles with it almost every day. Afraid of odors or not having a bathroom nearby, he feels very limited in his activities outside the house. Because of the fatigue, he is still working fewer hours than he used to do, and he needs all his free time to recover and rest. He has stopped playing tennis every week and meeting with his best friend every Saturday. He feels his life has become very limited. Especially when he is tired, he feels gloomy and that his life has lost its meaning. He then also blames himself for getting colon cancer, as he knows obesity is a risk factor for colon cancer. He has been ignoring his weight and delaying to go on diet and more regular exercise. Sometimes, he has problems sleeping and then starts ruminating about the cancer coming back, even when the doctor said during the last visit that his results were good.

When doing the body scan at home in the first week of the program, Peter notices how tired he feels. Most of the practice times, he falls asleep. It frustrates him to fall asleep while practicing, as he expects from himself to do the exercise while being alert and awake. He wonders whether he is doing it all wrong. After several days, he stops practicing, as he feels this doesn't help him. The second group meeting starts with doing a body scan. During the sharing afterwards, Peter brings in that the body scan makes him feel very tired and fall asleep and that this frustrates him. Rather than seeking solutions, the teacher explores with Peter his experiences during the body scan he just did. He said that his body felt tired and that he didn't like to feel this. That it also brought up questions in his head, like "Why am I tired now, it is only morning, I haven't even worked yet, how can I go to work tomorrow if I feel so tired again? Perhaps they will stop my contract, what if I lose my work?" The teacher asks Peter, when doing the body scan in the coming way, to recognize when these kinds of thoughts come up, to acknowledge the thoughts, and to bring back his attention to the exercise and his body. Also, the teacher asks Peter to notice how he feels when he is awake again after having fallen asleep, notice possible thoughts and feelings about having fallen asleep and then gently bring his attention back to his body and the exercise. After the second week, Peter starts noticing that the fatigue is not always the same and does not always feel the same in his body, and that sometimes he is less frustrated than other times. Slowly, he is able to accept how his body feels, and he gets less caught up in all the thinking about it.

In other sessions, yoga exercises including gentle stretching postures are done, aiming to increase bodily awareness while doing the different postures, being aware of the possibilities and boundaries of the body and automatic responses to this (which can vary from relaxing and enjoying the movements and feeling alive to being careful and anxious, frustrated, or sad). The aim of sitting practice is to develop a greater awareness and sensitivity to internal and external experiences and our automatic judgments and responses. Doing these exercises can help to recognize and step out of automatic reacting and mind wandering, come back to the present moment, and learn how to turn gently toward difficult sensations, thoughts or feelings and hold them in awareness. This can create a sense of space and inner knowing of how to respond.

The breath plays an important role in sitting meditation and, in fact, in all exercises including the body scan and yoga. The breath can be used as an anchor, to bring the mind back to the present moment, and one can connect with the breath at any time and place and notice how the movements feel in the body. The breath often indicates how the body and mind are doing (e.g., relaxed, tense, anxious). In addition, finding ways to relax the breath can stimulate the parasympathetic nervous system and thereby give rest to body and mind.

The mindfulness-based cognitive therapy (MBCT) program is based on MBSR. This eight-week group program was introduced in 2002 by Zindel Segal, Mark Williams, and John Teasdale, with a research background and clinical expertise in cognitive behavioral therapy (CBT) (Segal et al., 2002, 2013). MBCT combines the MBSR program with psychoeducation and exercises from CBT. Though originally developed to treat recurrent depression, MBCT has proven to be acceptable and effective in the treatment of a wide range of populations and a variety of somatic and mental concerns. In this respect, it can be considered a transdiagnostic treatment for mental health. MBCT may help people to learn how to recognize changes in their mood, thoughts, and body and to separate themselves somewhat from a low mood and ruminative thinking. This may help them to deal with stressful life events and situations that are emotionally overwhelming.

Mindfulness-based interventions are foremost known as a group training. Early in the 2010s, Maya Schroevers and Joke Fleer were looking for a way to support people in managing the psychological effects of suffering from a chronic illness. They adapted the eight-week MBCT protocol into an individual eight-week MBCT intervention, which proved to be effective in several studies (Schroevers & Fleer, 2019). There are several benefits to such an individual approach. First, not every person wants to or can participate in a group training, and not everybody seems to profit to the same extent from such a group setting. Second, participants indicate that an individual training allows them to receive personal and full attention of the trainer. Trainers indicate that they have the possibility to tailor the program to individual needs, such as personal life situations and physical or mental challenges, as well as institutional settings not enabling group courses.

Another way to offer mindfulness-based interventions is by using eHealth. Due to fatigue and other barriers, it can be difficult for cancer patients to travel to a location at set times for the mindfulness-based intervention. An internet-based program could offer a valid alternative for these patients. It is easily accessible and saves travel time and costs, and patients can participate in their own environment at their own time (Toivonen et al., 2017). Specific internet-based mindfulness programs for cancer patients have been developed (Bruggeman-Everts et al., 2017).

Examples of Mindfulness-Based Programs Specifically for Cancer Patients

Two well-known mindfulness-based programs that have been developed specifically for people with cancer are mindfulness-based cancer recovery (MBCR) developed by Linda Carlson and Michael Speca from the University of Calgary in Canada (Carlson & Speca, 2011) and MBCT-Ca by Trish Bartley from Bangor University in the UK (Bartley, 2011) The programs will be described below.

Mindfulness-Based Cancer Recovery (MBCR)

The MBCR was developed in 1995 by Linda Carlson and Michael Speca. In their book, they describe the influence of stress on the prognosis and quality of life of people with cancer, and the possible benefits mindfulness may have when managing the physical consequences of cancer, side effects of treatment, and how to handle emotions (Carlson & Speca, 2011). MBCR is strongly based on MBSR. As Carlson and Speca were interested in conducting research on the value of MBCR, they wrote a structured manual for the program to standardize the content. Findings of their research are described later in this chapter.

MBCT-Ca

Trish Bartley was diagnosed with breast cancer. In her book, she openly describes her process of dealing with cancer and treatment and the role of mindfulness herein. The program she developed is strongly based on MBCT, including eight group sessions and an all-day program of 4.5 hours (Bartley, 2011). The program and themes of the weekly sessions including the exercises closely follow the original MBCT program (including the automatic pilot, dealing with barriers, the breath and the body in movement, mindfulness responding versus attachment/aversion, being with the difficult, thoughts are not facts, and taking care of oneself).

This program focuses on the so-called three-circle model. The first circle depicts the suffering that may accompany the experience with cancer and its treatment (the primary source of suffering), including four reactions: trauma (related to experiences of intense fear, intrusive memories, disbelief), rumination (often also involving self-blame), avoidance (e.g., denial of the seriousness), and distress (e.g., low mood, tension, agitation). These reactions can be viewed as secondary ways of suffering added to the cancer experience. As becomes visible from the outer ring, referring to a cognitive model of cancer distress, our mind adds extra layers of suffering by selective attention to body sensations and negative interpretations and rumination (e.g., "Perhaps the cancer is back."), thereby adding to anxiety and fueling related symptoms of tension in the body. This model is explicitly described in the group meeting, in the middle part of the program. By practicing mindfulness, people can start to recognize this chain of experiences and step out of it.

As with most mindfulness-based interventions, it has generally been recommended to participate in MBCT-Ca after the most turbulent time is over, that is, after having finished medical treatment. Cancer treatment can be demanding, and then, it may be simply too much to do a mindfulness program at the same time. MBCT-Ca program not only involves weekly sessions of 2 to 3 hours and daily homework of 30–60 minutes but also, at a mental level, can be strenuous, with exercises possibly triggering difficult issues in our lives and how we deal with life and ourselves. Mindfulness can best be developed when the living situation is somewhat stable. As the program can be intensive, it is especially important to talk with people who want to participate about their personal expectations and motivation and their intentions to attend the weekly group sessions and do home practices.

The second circle is called the circle of practice and describes what people can develop by doing the MBCT-Ca program. At the center is mindful awareness, surrounded by four aspects of mindfulness practice: intention (i.e., connecting to a deeply felt wish to do what is best for well-being), coming back (referring to recognizing and stepping out of mind wandering and stepping into the present moment), turning toward the difficult (i.e., containing what is difficult, rather than denying or pushing away), and kindness (toward oneself, and experiences in the here and now). These practices can be applied to the four dimensions of our experiences: our thinking, feeling, bodily sensations, and actions (or behaviors).

The third circle is called the circle of presence and is related to how people, after having done an MBCT-Ca program, may integrate mindfulness into their everyday lives. The inner ring is called "Being", referring to being in the present, in a direct way experiencing and knowing what is here and now, with an attitude characterized by openness and kindness. Such mindful awareness has been associated with four qualities which are described in the middle ring: appreciating the richness of experience, the ground of clarity (referring to grounding oneself, by feeling the contact of the feet on the floor, or holding a so-called "mountain standing posture"), a sense of confidence, and connecting to common humanity (i.e., feeling interconnected with others, part of a larger whole, knowing that others may be suffering as well, and wishing well-being for all). This latter contrasts with the feeling of being alone and isolated in dealing with the cancer experience that many people with cancer experience, even when feeling greatly supported by close others. With practice deepening, the body, mind, and heart can be present and integrated (the outer circle).

Empirical Evidence for Mindfulness-Based Interventions in People with Cancer

Whereas in the period from 1980 to 2000, the popularity of MBSR grew in the absence of rigorous scientific evidence, since then, research on the benefits of mindfulness has exponentially risen. The increased amount of evidence suggesting a range of positive effects of mindfulness-based interventions has further stimulated the interest and application of these types of interventions in Western countries. Specifically, in people with cancer, several studies have examined the benefits of mindfulness-based interventions, and several systematic reviews and meta-analyses have been published to summarize the existing evidence (Cillessen et al., 2019; Piet et al., 2012; Zhang et al., 2015). Overall, mindfulness-based interventions were found to be effective in reducing psychological distress (e.g., depression, anxiety, fear of cancer recurrence), although for some outcomes, effects appeared to be small. This suggests a need for optimization. Recently, several randomized controlled trials explored the effectiveness of online mindfulness-based intervention among cancer patients, showing significant effects on mood, distress, fatigue, fear of cancer recurrence, and rumination. One trial compared an individual online MBCT with face-to-face group MBCT (Compen et al., 2018), showing that online MBCT proved more effective in the long term to reduce distress than the group sessions.

The evidence for possible benefits of mindfulness-based interventions on cognitive functioning is unclear, with a recent systematic review in breast cancer survivors (Cifu et al., 2018), including six studies, concluding that there is too much heterogeneity in the cognitive skills being studied (e.g., executive functioning, memory) and the measures used to assess cognitive functioning to be able to draw conclusions. Of the six included studies, two found no effects, two found only short-term improvement, and another two found sustained improvement up until the 6-month follow-up.

Conclusions and Future Implications/Suggestions

A diagnosis of cancer may greatly impact the well-being of those confronted with this illness, as well as of their families. Mindfulness-based interventions may help people with cancer and their families to deal with the physical and psychosocial suffering that cancer generates in many people. These interventions focus on cultivating present-moment awareness with acceptance. Two well-known and widely used interventions are MBSR and MBCT. These programs have been adapted to the context of cancer and the specific issues people with cancer may face. Research suggests that mindfulness-based interventions are effective in reducing symptoms of distress, depression, and anxiety and improving quality of life.

Future studies are needed with a stronger and clearly described methodology. First, little is known about the long-term benefits, as most studies focused on short-term intervention effects (assessed directly after the end of the intervention). Second, most studies compare a mindfulness-based intervention to a passive control condition (e.g., waitlist standard care). This may inflate effects. More research is needed that includes an active control group or other well-known effective intervention such as CBT. Such research may point out whether mindfulness-based interventions are more effective than other types of interventions. Third, little is known about factors that moderate the effectiveness of mindfulness-based interventions, showing which types of people with cancer are more or less likely to benefit from these interventions. Cillessen et al. (2019) found that a wide range of factors did not significantly predict the effect size of the intervention. This included person-related factors like age and gender, cancer-related factors like type of cancer, stage, and time since diagnosis, and intervention-related factors like type of mindfulness intervention and contact hours, with some evidence of larger effect sizes in studies including younger persons. This suggests that a large group of people with cancer may benefit from mindfulness-based interventions. Fourth, in many trials, the mindfulness-based program (i.e., MBSR or MBCT) was adjusted, with poor descriptions of the adaptations. Lastly, more insight is needed into the underlying working mechanisms. For example, is it truly an increase in being mindful that is related to improvements in psychological functioning? To what extent does the intervention lead to reductions in rumination or an increase in kindness and compassion that may explain the benefits for well-being? More knowledge about the types of persons that are most likely to be interested in participating in a mindfulness-based intervention and to benefit from it, is needed to optimize the implementation of these interventions in health care.

References

Abrahams, H. J. G., Gielissen, M. F. M., Schmits, I. C., Verhagen, C. A. H. H. V. M., Rovers, M. M., & Knoop, H. (2016). Risk factors, prevalence, and course of severe fatigue after breast cancer treatment: A meta-analysis involving 12 327 breast cancer survivors. *Annals of Oncology, 27*, 965–974.

Almeida, S. N., Elliott, R., Silva, E. R., & Sales, C. (2019). Fear of cancer recurrence: A qualitative systematic review and meta-synthesis of patients' experiences. *Clinical Psychology Review, 68*, 13–24.

Baer, R. A., Smith, G. T., Hopkins, J., Krietemeyer, J., & Toney, L. (2006). Using self-report assessment methods to explore facets of mindfulness. *Assessment, 13*(1), 27–45.

Bartley, T. (2011). *Mindfulness-based cognitive therapy for cancer: Gently turning towards. Mindfulness-based cognitive therapy for cancer: Gently turning towards.* John Wiley & Sons.

Bishop, S. R., Lau, M., Shapiro, S., Carlson, L., Anderson, N. D., Carmody, J., Segal, Z. V., Abbey, S., Speca, M., Velting, D., & Devins, G. (2004). Mindfulness: A proposed operational definition. *Clinical Psychology: Science and Practice, 11*(3), 230–241.

Brandenbarg, D., Maass, S. W. M. C., Geerse, O. P., Stegmann, M. E., Handberg, C., Schroevers, M. J., & Duijts, S. F. A. (2019). A systematic review on the prevalence of symptoms of depression, anxiety and distress in long-term cancer survivors: Implications for primary care. *European Journal of Cancer Care, 28*(3), 1–14.

Bruggeman-Everts, F. Z., Wolvers, M., van de Schoot, R., Vollenbroek-Hutten, M., & Van der Lee, M. L. (2017). Effectiveness of two web-based interventions for chronic cancer-related fatigue compared to an active control condition: Results of the "fitter na Kanker" randomized controlled trial. *Journal of Medical Internet Research, 19*(10), e336.

Carlson, L. E., & Speca, M. (2011). *Mindfulness-based cancer recovery: A step-by-step MBSR approach to help you cope with Treatment & Reclaim Your Life*. New Harbinger Publications.

Caruso, R., Nanni, M. G., Riba, M., Sabato, S., Mitchell, A. J., Croce, E., & Grassi, L. (2017). Depressive spectrum disorders in cancer: Prevalence, risk factors and screening for depression: A critical review. *Acta oncologica (Stockholm, Sweden), 56*(2), 146–155.

Casellas-Grau, A., Ochoa, C., & Ruini, C. (2017). Psychological and clinical correlates of posttraumatic growth in cancer: A systematic and critical review. *Psycho-Oncology, 26*(12), 2007–2018.

Cifu, G., Power, M. C., Shomstein, S., & Arem, H. (2018). Mindfulness-based interventions and cognitive function among breast cancer survivors: A systematic review. *BMC Cancer, 18*(1), 1163.

Cillessen, L., Johannsen, M., Speckens, A., & Zachariae, R. (2019). Mindfulness-based interventions for psychological and physical health outcomes in cancer patients and survivors: A systematic review and meta-analysis of randomized controlled trials. *Psycho-Oncology, 28*(12), 2257–2222.

Compen, F., Bisseling, E., Schellekens, M., Donders, R., Carlson, L., van der Lee, M., & Speckens, A. (2018). Face-to-face and internet-based mindfulness-based cognitive therapy compared with treatment as usual in reducing psychological distress in patients with cancer: A multicenter randomized controlled trial. *Journal of Clinical Oncology, 36*(23), 2413–2421.

Garssen, B., & Goodkin, K. (1999). On the role of immunological factors as mediators between psychosocial factors and cancer progression. *Psychiatry Research, 85*(1), 51–61.

Hartung, T. J., Brähler, E., Faller, H., Härter, M., Hinz, A., Johansen, C., Keller, M., Koch, U., Schulz, H., Weis, J., & Mehnert, A. (2017). The risk of being depressed is significantly higher in cancer patients than in the general population: Prevalence and severity of depressive symptoms across major cancer types. *European Journal of Cancer, 72*, 46–53.

Kabat-Zinn, J. (2003). Mindfulness-based interventions in context: Past, present, and future. *Clinical Psychology: Science and Practice, 10*(2), 144–156.

Kabat-Zinn, J. (1990). *Full Catastrophe Living: Using the Wisdom of Your Body and Mind to Face Stress, Pain, and Illness*. Dell Publishing.

Krebber, A. M., Buffart, L. M., Kleijn, G., Riepma, I. C., de Bree, R., Leemans, C. R., Becker, A., Brug, J., van Straten, A., Cuijpers, P., & Verdonck-de Leeuw, I. M. (2014). Prevalence of depression in cancer patients: A meta-analysis of diagnostic interviews and self-report instruments. *Psycho-Oncology, 23*(2), 121–130.

Kuhnt, S., Brähler, E., Faller, H., Härter, M., Keller, M., Schulz, H., Wegscheider, K., Weis, J., Boehncke, A., Hund, B., Reuter, K., Richard, M., Sehner, S., Wittchen, H. U., Koch, U., & Mehnert, A. (2016). Twelve-month and lifetime prevalence of mental disorders in cancer patients. *Psychotherapy and Psychosomatics, 85*(5), 289–296.

Lau, J., Khoo, A. M., Ho, A. H., & Tan, K. K. (2021). Psychological resilience among palliative patients with advanced cancer: A systematic review of definitions and associated factors. *Psycho-Oncology, 30*(7), 1029–1040.

Linden, W., Vodermaier, A., Mackenzie, R., & Greig, D. (2012). Anxiety and depression after cancer diagnosis: Prevalence rates by cancer type, gender, and age. *Journal of Affective Disorders, 141*(2–3), 343–351.

McGee, R., Williams, S., & Elwood, M. (1994). Depression and the development of cancer: A meta-analysis. *Social Science & Medicine, 38*(1), 187–192.

Nakaya, N. (2014). Effect of psychosocial factors on cancer risk and survival. *Journal of Epidemiology, 24*(1), 1–6.

Oerlemans, M. E., van den Akker, M., Schuurman, A. G., Kellen, E., & Buntinx, F. (2007). A meta-analysis on depression and subsequent cancer risk. *Clinical Practice and Epidemiology in Mental Health, 3*, 29.

Parkin, D. M., Boyd, L., & Walker, L. C. (2011). 16. The fraction of cancer attributable to lifestyle and environmental factors in the UK in 2010. *British Journal of Cancer, 105*(Suppl 2), S77–S81.

Piet, J., Würtzen, H., & Zachariae, R. (2012). The effect of mindfulness-based therapy on symptoms of anxiety and depression in adult cancer patients and survivors: A systematic review and meta-analysis. *Journal of Consulting and Clinical Psychology, 80*(6), 1007–1020.

Rottmann, N., Hansen, D. G., Hagedoorn, M., Larsen, P. V., Nicolaisen, A., Bidstrup, P. E., Würtzen, H., Flyger, H., Kroman, N., & Johansen, C. (2016). Depressive symptom trajectories in women affected by breast cancer and their male partners: A nationwide prospective cohort study. *Journal of Cancer Survivorship: Research and Practice, 10*(5), 915–926.

Ruiz-Marin, C. M., Molina-Barea, R., Slim, M., & Calandre, E. P. (2021). Marital adjustment in patients with cancer: Association with psychological distress, quality of life, and sleep problems. *International Journal of Environmental Research and Public Health, 18*(13), 7089.

Schilstra, C. E., Fardell, J. E., Burns, M. A., Ellis, S. J., Anazodo, A. C., Trahair, T. N., & Sansom-Daly, U. M. (2021). Determinants of social functioning among adolescents and young adults with cancer: A systematic review. *Psycho-Oncology, 30*(10), 1626–1642.

Schroevers, M. J., & Fleer, J. (2019). Why are researchers not interested in studying individual mindfulness-based interventions? *Mindfulness, 10*(11), 2476–2478.

Segal, Z. V., Williams, J. M. G., & Teasdale, J. D. (2002). *Mindfulness-based cognitive therapy for depression: A new approach to preventing relapse.* Guilford Press.

Segal, Z. V., Williams, J. M. G., & Teasdale, J. D. (2013). *Mindfulness-based cognitive therapy for depression* (2nd ed.). The Guilford Press.

Sung, H., Ferlay, J., Siegel, R. L., Laversanne, M., Soerjomataram, I., Jemal, A., & Bray, F. (2021). Global cancer statistics 2020: GLOBOCAN estimates of incidence and mortality worldwide for 36 cancers in 185 countries. *CA: a Cancer Journal for Clinicians, 71*(3), 209–249.

Toivonen, K. I., Zernicke, K., & Carlson, L. E. (2017). Web-based mindfulness interventions for people with physical health conditions: Systematic review. *Journal of Medical Internet Research, 19*(8), e303.

Van der Lee, M., & Schellekens, M. P. J. (2020). Capturing the complexity of mental disorders in the medically ill: The network approach on behavioral medicine. *Translational Behavioral Medicine, 10*, 812–816.

van Tuijl, L. A., Basten, M., Pan, K. Y., Vermeulen, R., Portengen, L., de Graeff, A., Dekker, J., Geerlings, M. I., Hoogendoorn, A., Lamers, F., Voogd, A. C., Abell, J., Awadalla, P., Beekman, A. T. F., Bjerkeset, O., Boyd, A., Cui, Y., Frank, P., Galenkamp, H., Garssen, B., et al. (2023). Depression, anxiety, and the risk of cancer: An individual participant data meta-analysis. *Cancer.* https://doi.org/10.1002/cncr.34853

Vehling, S., & Philipp, R. (2018). Existential distress and meaning-focused interventions in cancer survivorship. *Current Opinion in Supportive and Palliative Care, 12*(1), 46–51.

Zhang, M. F., Wen, Y. S., Liu, W. Y., Peng, L. F., Wu, X. D., & Liu, Q. W. (2015). Effectiveness of mindfulness-based therapy for reducing anxiety and depression in patients with cancer: A meta-analysis. *Medicine, 94*(45), e0897.

17

Mindfulness and Adjustment to Skin Conditions

Olivia Hughes and Andrew R. Thompson

Introduction: What Are Skin Conditions?

The skin is the visible envelope around our body that can reveal information about our age, ethnicity, health, and mood (Thompson, 2012a). Furthermore, it acts as a platform by which many positive psychological processes are played out. For example, the skin is integral to the functioning of human intimacy, from early child-parent bonding to later adult sexual sensation.

There are over two thousand known skin diseases, ranging from common conditions such as eczema and acne to rarer conditions such as the depigmenting condition, vitiligo, and the blistering condition epidermolysis bullosa. The physiological and psychological impact of different skin diseases is wide ranging, and some conditions that affect the skin are systemic and involve other physiological systems, whilst others are associated with life-limiting physical (e.g., epidermal necrolysis) and/or developmental and neurological impacts (e.g., epidermolysis bullosa).

O. Hughes
School of Psychology, Cardiff University, Cardiff, Wales

A. R. Thompson (✉)
School of Psychology, Cardiff University, Cardiff, Wales

South Wales Clinical Psychology Training, Cardiff & Vale University Health Board & Cardiff University, Cardiff, Wales
e-mail: thompsona18@cardiff.ac.uk

F. M. Sirois (ed.), *The Palgrave Handbook of Positive Psychology and Health*,
https://doi.org/10.1007/978-3-031-89095-6_17

Some skin conditions can be congenital (present since birth, e.g., nemus flammeus—'port wine stain'), while other conditions are primarily of a psychological aetiology (e.g., delusions of parasitosis: see Ahmed et al., 2022) and do not fit neatly into an 'acquired' disease model. Further, if we consider other issues that can affect the skin (e.g., scarring caused by injury or medical intervention), it can be appreciated that the simple disease model does not adequately capture the range of presentations encountered. Consequently, the term 'skin condition', as opposed to 'disease', will be used throughout this chapter, in recognition of the full range of congenital, disease, injurious, iatrogenic, and psychological 'conditions' that can affect the skin and hair (Thompson, 2009, 2011, 2012b).

What Is Psychodermatology?

The importance of the skin and hair to our psychosocial development, functioning, and well-being should need no introduction, yet the skin and hair have attracted comparatively little attention from social science or psychological researchers. That said, over recent years, there has been renewed interest in 'psychodermatology', and within this specific field, some researchers have begun to investigate positive psychological variables and phenomenological accounts of positive experiences of adjustment.

In medical practice, the field of dermatology is the area of medicine that addresses conditions affecting the skin and hair. Within psychodermatology, there is a focus on the psychological aspects of skin conditions, which have historically been conceptualised into three overlapping groups: i) primarily psychological, such as delusions of parasitosis, ii) psycho-physiologic, where stress may play a significant role, such as in psoriasis and eczema, and iii) secondary psychological, where the adjustment to the skin condition is a known concern, such as in acne, vitiligo, and psoriasis (Koblenzer, 1983, 1992; Thompson, 2009). This chapter will focus mainly on the second two areas of skin-related concerns identified by Koblenzer (1983), where the primary presenting issue has a known physiological basis within the skin and requires an adjustment.

The complex nature of psychodermatological presentations is well recognised, and there exist several interprofessional organisations, such as the European Association for Dermatology and Psychiatry (European Association for Dermatology and Psychiatry [ESDaP], 2022) and the Association for Psychoneurocutaneous Medicine of North America (Association for Psychoneurocutaneous Medicine of North America [APMNA], n.d) to support the work of researchers and clinicians practicing in this area. APMNA describes itself as an association for dermatologists, psychiatrists, psychologists, and allied health professionals that is dedicated to promoting the awareness of skin and mind interaction and the role of psychoneuroimmunology in skin conditions (APMNA, n.d).

One of the issues with much of the existing psychodermatology literature is that the emphasis has largely been placed on investigating negative individual difference variables. This is problematic, as the focus on adverse quality of life could unintentionally contribute to further marginalisation (Thompson, 2011). Whilst it is essential to acknowledge the potential difficulties, the bigger picture is that most people do adapt well and live positive and happy lives with a skin condition. Providing people with this information can be empowering, although this must be done in a paced and validating way that avoids the risk of dismissing any concern or feeling of distress that may exist.

Sharpe and Curran (2006) describe adjustment to illness as "the process to maintain a positive view of the self and the world in the face of a health problem" (p. 1161), and in this chapter, we will discuss the issues faced by people with skin conditions with more emphasis placed on taking a positive psychological stance. This will include coverage of research focusing on people living well with their skin condition, and studies that have purposively investigated how innate levels of positive variables, such as mindfulness and self-compassion in particular, might promote positive adjustment.

Despite taking a positive stance, the chapter begins by briefly describing the role of stress in relation to skin conditions before detailing the psychosocial issues associated with skin conditions. However, the chapter then pays particular attention to the potential protective role of variables associated with mindfulness and includes coverage of the emerging research suggesting that self-compassion may also play an important protective role. The chapter will present a detailed summary of studies that have investigated the effectiveness of mindfulness-based psychological interventions for people living with skin conditions. It will also cover studies that have evaluated mindful parenting interventions for parents of children living with skin conditions. In addition, it will include coverage of the more limited research that has been conducted to investigate the potential effectiveness of self-compassion-based psychological interventions for people living with skin conditions.

The Role of Stress in Skin Conditions and Why Mindfulness and Self-Compassion Are Important

Living with a skin condition can cause negative emotions, including stress (Thompson, 2012a). For people with inflammatory/autoimmune skin conditions (e.g., psoriasis, acne, dermatitis, alopecia), experiencing stress can exacerbate the severity of the condition itself (Chen & Lyga, 2014; Hunter et al., 2013; Kimyai-Asadi & Usman, 2001; Schmidt et al., 2021). Being exposed to psychological stressors, such as illness, triggers the body's stress response through activating the hypothalamic-pituitary-adrenal (HPA) axis, the sympathetic-adrenal-medullary (SAM) axis, and the stress-inflammation pathways, producing cytokines (Black, 2002; Rohleder, 2019). Stress is likely to worsen and exacerbate inflammatory skin conditions via a number of different mechanisms. For example, it might exacerbate itching responses via the activation of the HPA axis (Kim et al., 2013; Golpanian et al., 2020) and may contribute to the creation of vicious cycles of itch-scratch behaviour (Golpanian et al., 2020; Sanders & Akiyama, 2018; Verhoeven et al., 2008).

Indeed, there are a large number of studies demonstrating that perceived stress is associated with a range of skin conditions. For example, a Norwegian cross-sectional study conducted by Balieva et al. (2022) reported a three-fold increase in perceived stress in patients with inflammatory skin conditions compared with controls, when adjusting for a variety of potentially confounding variables. However, there remains a dearth of fundamental scientific studies that identify the underlying mechanisms by which stress may influence specific disease onset and progression (Evers & van Beugen, 2021). Nevertheless, the existing evidence clearly demonstrates the need for interventions that promote stress tolerance or mitigate against the development of stress as a secondary impact of skin conditions.

To address psychological stress and distress, adapted versions of mindfulness have been increasingly incorporated into a range of clinical health psychology interventions (Kabat-Zinn, 1982). Mindfulness is a positive approach based on Buddhist principles, defined by Jon Kabat-Zinn (1994, pg. 4) as *"paying attention on purpose, in the present moment, non-judgementally"*. This positive approach has generally been added in alongside existing evidence-based psychological techniques, typically as used within cognitive-behavioural therapy (CBT). Several examples now exist of established mindfulness-based psychological interventions, including mindfulness-based stress reduction (MBSR: Kabat-Zinn, 1982) targeting feelings of stress and related anxiety, mindfulness-based cognitive therapy (MBCT: Segal et al., 2002) combining mindfulness practices with CBT, and more recently mindful parenting (MP: Bögels & Restifo, 2015), incorporating mindfulness practices with various parenting-focussed psychological interventions, such as developing awareness of attachment issues and underlying parental schemas. The MP approach was described by Jon Kabat-Zinn (1997, in Bögels et al., 2010) as: *"paying attention to your child and your parenting in a particular way: intentionally, here and now, and non-judgementally"*. Bringing mindful awareness into daily interactions between parents and children is *"not a project to create 'better' or 'optimal' children (whatever that might mean), or to be 'better' or 'optimal' parents, but to embrace in moment-to-moment awareness"* (Kabat-Zinn & Kabat-Zinn, 2021, pg.1). In doing this, MP could enhance parenting by improving attention and parental awareness of shared needs (Bögels et al., 2014).

Fostering self-compassion is an integral part of the mindfulness approach and has been the focus of attention in its own right by a number of researchers and therapists (e.g., Gilbert, 2009, 2010; Neff, 2003). Neff (2003) describes self-compassion as an "*emotionally positive self-attitude*"' (p. 85) and proposed that there are three important elements to it, including self-kindness, acceptance of the commonality of human suffering, and the ability to be mindful in response to distress. Self-compassion could be useful for supporting people affected by skin conditions, as being diagnosed with a condition that affects appearance and functioning has been associated with a risk of developing heightened levels of self-criticism, fear of negative evaluations from other people, and to drive negative self-comparisons (Adkins et al., 2023). Clearly, the ability to be self-compassionate in such contexts may be particularly protective and there is some preliminary evidence to suggest that this is the case (e.g. see Table 17.1 below – Clarke et al., 2024; Hudson et al., 2020; Muftin et al., 2022).

Mindfulness-based interventions are being used therapeutically for adults and children with a range of physical illnesses (e.g., Hughes et al., 2023) and might be particularly effective for targeting health conditions affected by stress, by enabling people to become better able to manage uncomfortable emotions and cognitions associated with physical symptoms (Creswell et al., 2019). From a physiological perspective, the mechanistic stress-buffering framework suggests that mindfulness-informed interventions could facilitate the development of stress resilience pathways in the brain and lessen the detrimental effect stress has on the body (Creswell & Lindsay, 2014; Creswell et al., 2019).

As hinted at earlier, the ability to be mindful may have a protective function. There is already some evidence from cross-sectional studies to suggest that mindfulness and self-compassion are associated with lower psychological distress in people with skin conditions (Clarke et al., 2020; Meneo et al., 2022; Montgomery et al., 2016; Montgomery & Thompson, 2018). For example, Montgomery et al. (2016) reported that individuals with skin conditions who had higher levels of mindfulness experienced less psychosocial distress. More specifically, the concepts of 'present-moment awareness' and 'non-judgement of inner experience' were associated with lower levels of social anxiety within the study sample (Montgomery et al., 2016).

Further, mindfulness-based interventions might assist in the management of common symptoms associated with skin conditions, such as itch, via building resilience to manage the physical sensation of itch, or by supporting the ability to modify scratching behaviour (Gallo et al., 2017; Montgomery & Thompson, 2018). Indeed, Lüßmann et al. (2021) found that the facet of mindfulness 'acting with awareness' was associated with less 'catastrophizing' in relation to itch in atopic dermatitis (e.g., worry about itch sensation). This study suggests that mindfulness interventions might have a buffering effect on itch-scratch behaviour, via reducing itch catastrophizing, which in turn could lead to lower perceived itch intensity (Lüßmann et al., 2021).

Further, for parents of children with skin conditions, dispositional mindfulness has been found to explain significant variance in levels of parental stress, depression, anxiety, and both parent and child quality of life, regardless of type of skin condition (Heapy et al., 2021). Therefore, higher levels of dispositional mindfulness could be related to improved well-being in parents of children with skin conditions and their children, suggesting that mindfulness-based interventions could be effective for families affected by skin conditions (Heapy et al., 2021). A recent study by Hughes et al., 2024, has highlighted that specific forms of mindfulness could be feasible for reducing stress and improving quality of life in parents of children with skin conditions.

We will return to the evidence base for the use of mindfulness-based interventions and self-compassion later in the chapter. In the next section, we will provide further detail on skin conditions and what has been found in studies focusing on positive adjustment. To illustrate how a skin condition can impact a person throughout their life, we will first provide a little more information on the burden of skin conditions.

Psychosocial Aspects of Skin Conditions in Children and Families

Skin conditions are common during childhood and adolescent years. Eczema is diagnosed in over 20% of children under the age of five and is the most common reason for children under ten years of age to seek initial National Health Service (NHS) consultation (All Party Parliamentary Group on Skin: APPGS, 2020). For children between the ages of ten and eighteen years, acne is particularly prevalent and commonly associated with general practitioner consultations (APPGS, 2020). Despite these statistics, consideration and support for childhood skin conditions have been overshadowed by other health conditions that might be considered (often unfairly) as more impactful, such as childhood cancers or conditions affecting physical mobility (APPGS, 2020; Ip et al., 2021; Hughes et al., 2022).

Childhood and adolescence are important times for psychological maturation and establishment of the self, self-esteem, and social confidence (De Vere Hunt et al. 2020). Having a skin condition during this important developmental period and learning to manage fluctuations or 'flares' in severity, whilst adhering to often unpleasant treatment regimens, may unsurprisingly have a significant negative impact on a child's quality of life and psychological well-being, irrespective of gender (McPherson, 2021; Hughes et al., 2021). For many children and young people, skin conditions can have a profound influence on all aspects of daily life and psychosocial development (McPherson, 2021; Bridgeman, 1994 in Fennessy et al., 2000). The physical symptoms of skin conditions can cause physical discomfort arising from having broken skin, such as bleeding, pain, and itch. These symptoms can cause problems with sleep, lead to disruptions in concentration or attention, or even directly impact upon behaviour, and as a consequence, skin conditions can adversely affect school performance (Reid & Lewis-Jones, 1995).

When considering the psychosocial development of a child, there is substantial societal value placed on attaining a flawless appearance (Kent & Thompson, 2002). Despite active lobbying by a number of charities such as Changing Faces (Changing Faces, 2022), idealised and modified images of 'perfect' bodies continue to be widely present in all forms of media. From a young age, children are repeatedly exposed to highly overworked beauty stereotypes, which, for some, may contribute to the development of appearance-related distress or concern, and anxiety associated with a perception of not having attained these (unrealistic) appearance standards (Trekels & Eggermont, 2017). This has potential to create a lot of pressure for young people whose appearance may be affected by a skin condition, and there remains a risk of stigmatisation for children that can last into later adolescence and early adulthood (Magin et al., 2008; van Beugen et al., 2022).

Experiencing stigmatisation related to having a visible skin condition may be particularly challenging for a young child learning to understand their own emerging sense of self whilst trying to manage reactions from other people (McPherson, 2021). Feeling as if they do not 'fit in' with peers could precipitate feelings of shame or in severe cases, depression, related to having a visibly different appearance (Kent & Thompson, 2002). Negative reactions from other people might be perpetuated by long-standing and incorrect myths surrounding cleanliness and fear of contagion from having visibly broken and shedding skin (McPherson, 2021; Fennessy et al., 2000; Rønnstad et al., 2018). It could be for these reasons that the All Parliamentary Group on Skin (APPGS, 2020) reported in a small survey of paediatric patients (under 18 years), that all of the responding children reported that their skin condition had negatively impacted upon their psychological well-being, and the majority also reported lowered self-esteem and difficulties connecting in school with their peers.

When considering the impact of skin conditions on children, it is important to take a systemic stance and be aware that there is likely to be stress shared within the family unit, especially held by the child's primary carers who may be responsible for administering treatment and overseeing daily care needs (e.g., applying creams and attending appointments). The family, often including siblings, may experience a loss of normality from interruptions to their own leisure activities and daily routines and, in some cases, may have to alter working hours to maintain treatment schedules (van Scheppingen et al., 2008; Tollefson et al., 2017). Caring for a child with a skin condition may also create a financial burden from the time and cost of travelling to attend appointments, replacement of treatment-damaged clothes, or the self-funding of expensive treatments (Kemp, 2003).

The responsibilities associated with caring for a child with a chronic skin condition could negatively affect family life. For example, carers may experience a range of emotions related to their child's diagnosis, such as anger, disempowerment, or even denial of the impact of the skin condition (Papadopoulos & Walker, 2003; Hughes et al., 2022). In some cases, childhood skin conditions may trigger wider issues such as sibling resentment, marital conflict, and caregiver burnout (Papadopoulos & Walker, 2003; Yang et al., 2019; Chamlin et al., 2004; Ablett & Thompson, 2016). This said, as we know from wider field of positive psychology, the family often provides a hugely protective role in adjustment to long-term conditions. For example, Hughes (2022) has highlighted that family members can provide a strong network of support for a person living with a skin condition and could even enhance coping strategies by fostering acceptance and buffering negative health outcomes. As well as relational dynamics assisting with coping, it could be that the length of time spent caring for a child with a chronic skin condition actually promotes secure attachment and healthy relational bonding with the primary caregiver (Ablett & Thompson, 2016).

Psychosocial Aspects of Skin Conditions in Adults

The experiences of a developing child living with a skin condition can undoubtedly have lasting effects across the lifespan, and there has been some evidence to suggest that skin conditions could be associated with insecure attachment styles in adulthood (Krasuska et al., 2018a). Linthorst Homan et al. (2008) reported that young adult patients with vitiligo had no difference in quality of life than controls, however those who recalled having experienced adverse childhood reactions did have significantly lowered quality of life in early adulthood. Further, the psychological impact from many of the issues described above that affect children, such as societal appearance-based pressures, could persist into adulthood, and numerous studies demonstrate that living with a skin condition can negatively affect adult quality of life (Ali et al., 2018). Psoriasis, for example, has a comparable impact on health-related quality of life as other chronic diseases, such as cancer, arthritis, diabetes, and heart disease (Rapp et al., 1999).

It is perhaps unsurprising that skin conditions have been found to be associated with heightened levels of psychological distress in adulthood (e.g., Dalgard et al., 2015; Picardi et al., 2000). For example, Dalgard et al. (2015), in a study conducted across numerous European countries, found self-reported rates of 10.1% for depression and 17.2% for anxiety in dermatological patients, and similarly high levels of depression have been reported in single country-based studies (e.g., Clarke et al., 2020).

Further in a recent UK large population-based cohort study to determine the risk and impact of psychological comorbidity in people with new adult-onset vitiligo, Thompson et al. (2022) found that people with vitiligo have a higher incidence of depression and anxiety than matched controls, and there appeared to be a heightened risk in Black and minority ethnic populations, which might relate to the higher noticeability of this condition on darker skin or issues associated with stigmatisation. In addition, the study revealed that individuals with vitiligo and documented co-morbid psychological distress had more primary care encounters, more time off work, and higher unemployment. Clearly, skin conditions in adulthood can have a huge psychological impact, akin to other long-term conditions, and studies have also found increased reports of suicidal ideation in people living with skin conditions (e.g., Picardi et al., 2013).

Self-Compassion, Positive Adjustment, and Individual Variation

Possessing a greater 'innate ability' to be self-compassionate may be protective against developing appearance-based feelings of body shame or social embarrassment (Krasuska et al., 2018b; Clarke et al., 2022). For example, Clarke et al. (2020) found in a longitudinal survey that self-compassion buffered the effects of disgust propensity on depression in people with skin conditions.

Further, in a qualitative study, Clarke et al. (2022) found that people living with skin conditions who had high levels of self-compassion used a range of strategies to achieve this. The use of self-compassionate strategies was, in some cases, effortful and consequently supports the argument that people may be more likely to maintain such strategies when they are scaffolded or supported by the use of psychological interventions (Clarke et al., 2022).

Self-compassion can clearly promote positive adjustment to a visible skin condition, as evidenced in the account contained below. The following example is not an untypical description of adaptation. It presents the case of a young child naturalistically using self-compassion strategies to accept her visibly different skin and live well with the depigmenting condition—vitiligo (Hughes et al., 2022).

Case Study: Megan Is a Nine-Year-Old Girl with Vitiligo

Megan has had vitiligo since the age of four and is currently managing her condition with her parents teaching her body positivity instead of seeking further medical treatments, which they feel might cause her further stress. However, for the most visible patches of vitiligo on Megan's face and neck, the family is still applying tacrolimus (a calcineurin inhibitor applied via an ointment). Megan regularly listens to mindfulness audio tracks as they help her to 'relax and stay calm'. Megan has also learnt to use positive affirmations such as telling herself she is 'just like everyone else', and 'it doesn't matter what we look like' but rather 'it matters is what we feel like and if we're kind', and finally, how having vitiligo contributes to her uniqueness. Megan has integrated the patches of vitiligo into her sense of self by assigning each patch a name based on the countries they resemble. Megan uses mental imagery to picture herself like her peers and reads books to focus her attention on what is happening in the story rather than on her vitiligo. For managing her skin condition, Megan thinks it would be useful to develop a 'type of mirror like a screen or something, with a robot' that can support the development of positive affirmations such as: 'you are good the way you are' and 'you are unique'. Megan is confident in showing her skin condition to anyone who asks about it and has delivered a presentation on vitiligo to her classmates in school. She has a supportive group of friends and has not experienced any bullying or negative comments. Megan's family helps her to celebrate her difference and to be confident in talking about it. Together, they have rehearsed responses to questions about vitiligo.

Megan's case study highlights the value of being kind, and of seeing one's condition as contributing to not only personal uniqueness but also part of the experience of being human. Similar to the techniques described in Megan's case study, Thompson et al. (2002) interpretative phenomenological analysis with women living with vitiligo found that the participants had spontaneously developed a range of strategies. Some of the techniques were similar to those utilised within psychological therapy, including seeking support to overcome avoidance and importantly placing emphasis on positive attributes of the self (Thompson et al., 2002).

Indeed, other qualitative studies carried out with people identifying as having positively adjusted to their skin condition (including alopecia, burn scarring, port wine stains, and psoriasis) have found that in reaching acceptance, less value was being placed on appearance and more emphasis was placed on positive personal characteristics (Egan et al., 2011; Thompson & Broom, 2009; Clarke et al., 2022). Thompson and Broom (2009) interviewed people living with a range of visible differences and found that some individuals had actively challenged the extent to which appearance was of value to them in comparison to other aspects of their self. This finding fits with several different models that seek to understand the experience of appearance-related concern and suggest that both the perceived valence and salience of appearance are important in maintaining a positive self-concept (Thompson, 2012b). Learning how to manage emotional responses is likely to be important, as shown in a study investigating psychological flexibility in people with burn injuries, where a higher level of appearance anxiety was associated with a decreased ability to 'defuse' or stand back from negative thoughts about appearance, lower mindfulness, and less engagement in meaningful activities (Shepherd et al., 2019).

The ability to be mindful and self-compassionate may therefore facilitate the use of other more positive cognitive appraisals. For example, a person might reframe their condition as a positive event or alternatively reappraise the extent to which appearance is important to their self-esteem, and place greater emphasis on the importance of their body functionality (Adkins et al., 2022; Thompson, 2012b).

Other people may also increase positive adjustment to living with a skin condition and play a role in fostering compassion. An example of how positive adjustment might occur was highlighted by Hughes and Hunter (2022), whereby people with psoriasis were interviewed and described how being in a romantic relationship had increased self-assurance and lessened feelings of anger towards their skin condition. Similarly, interviews with people living with visible difference have described the importance of family influencing their attitudes towards their conditions (as outlined in Megan's case study, with her family celebrating difference) (Hughes et al., 2022). Having access to positively adjusted role models could be important to promote acceptance of living with a chronic skin condition, as studies have demonstrated the benefit of having an informal support network of people with shared experiences (Egan et al., 2011). However, relatively little research has actively investigated positive and protective individual or systemic factors in adjustment to skin conditions.

What has been noted is that having a noticeable visible difference is *not* an impediment to attaining a good quality of life, and age, sex, and socioeconomic background are not reliable predictors of how a person adjusts (Rumsey, 2018). There may be a complex interplay of individual factors that ultimately influence how a person copes with a visible skin condition. What is most clear is that a large number of people do appear to adapt to living with a skin condition, and ascertaining how they do so is a crucial issue for future research in order to inform interventions (Harcourt & Williamson, 2019). The individual difference factors associated with mindfulness seem to play an important role and should be targets for interventions. Since the family may play an important role in supporting positive adjustment to skin conditions, it may be necessary to involve caregivers in the development and delivery of dyadic interventions (Harcourt & Williamson, 2019).

The Evidence for Mindfulness and Compassion-Based Interventions for Skin Conditions

To promote positive adjustment to living with a skin condition, mindfulness is being increasingly investigated with targeted interventions to improve psychological well-being, and our review of the literature has identified a number of examples of interventions specifically investigating mindfulness-based interventions for people with skin conditions (see Table 17.1). There are also a small number of studies evaluating self-compassion-based interventions, and these have also been included in Table 17.1.

In a qualitative study, Maddock et al. (2020) interviewed people with psoriasis after participating in their MBCT programme, and they reported feeling more able to accept difficult thoughts relating to their skin condition, reduced worry, and improved physical symptoms. Participants described feeling more compassionate towards themselves from using the mindfulness techniques they had learned in the MBCT intervention (Maddock et al., 2020).

Table 17.1 Examples of research studies using mindfulness-based interventions for people and families affected by skin conditions

Authors (year)	N (mean age in years)	Control Group	Skin Condition	Intervention	Delivery	Outcomes measured	Summary of findings
Clarke et al. (2024)	34 (38.2)	Intervention only	Eczema, Psoriasis, Autoimmune conditions, Actinic cheilitis, Contact allergies, Chronic urticaria, Lichen planus, Nodular prurigo, Pemphigus vulgaris, Vitiligo.	Compassion-Focussed Intervention (CFI)	Online	Depression, Dermatology-specific quality of life, Self-Compassion, Acceptability and feasibility.	The intervention was started by 25 participants and completed by 13. Feedback scores indicated that the website was evaluated positively and that the sessions had positive impacts on participant. Participants appreciated the skin-specific aspects of the intervention but varied as to which of the compassion-based exercises they found helpful. The online intervention was feasible to provide and facilitate. Median depression, quality of life, and self-compassion scores improved between pre- and post-intervention, although only the change in the quality of life score reached statistical significance at p0.05.
D'Alton et al. (2019)	94 (49.89)	Systemic medication psoriasis therapy alone	Psoriasis	Mindfulness-based cognitive therapy (MBCT), Mindfulness-based self-compassion therapy (MBSCT), or Self-help MBSCT (MBSCT-SH).	In-person	Anxiety and depression, Worry, Mindfulness, Compassion, Quality of life, Dermatology-specific quality of life, Psoriasis severity, Biological markers (blood)	There were no statistically significant differences reported to psychological well-being, psoriasis symptoms, or quality of life for treatment as usual (at post-treatment, 6-month or 12-month follow-up). However, participants did report favourably on the interventions.

(*continued*)

Table 17.1 (continued)

Authors (year)	N (mean age in years)	Control Group	Skin Condition	Intervention	Delivery	Outcomes measured	Summary of findings
Fordham et al. (2015)	29 (41.17)	Usual psoriasis therapy alone	Psoriasis	Mindfulness-based cognitive therapy (MBCT)	In-person	Psoriasis severity, Stress, Distress, Dermatology-specific quality of life.	There were statistically lower psoriasis severity ($p=0.05$) and quality of life impairment scores ($p=0.02$) reported by participants in the mindfulness group. There were no significant differences between groups for levels of perceived stress and distress. There was a significant improvement to psoriasis severity and quality of life for participants who received mindfulness as an adjunct to their usual psoriasis therapy.
Gojani et al. (2017)	24	Waitlist	Psoriasis	Mindfulness-based cognitive therapy (MBCT), and Schema-based therapy	In-person	General health (corporal signs, anxiety, social function, depression), Maladaptive schemas.	The mindfulness and schema-based therapy groups showed significant differences when compared to the control group. There were significant differences between the schema-based therapy groups when compared to the control group. There were also significant improvements reported for psychopathologic symptoms between the mindfulness group and the control group.
Harfensteller (2022)	9 (48.10)	Intervention only	Atopic dermatitis	Mindfulness-based training for chronic skin conditions (MBTSC) with psychoeducation on eczema/itch	In-person	Disease severity, Stress, Mindfulness, Anxiety, Depression.	There were improvements in disease severity, itch perception, and stress with small to medium effect sizes. There was a statistically significant increase in depression (post-treatment). There were mixed qualitative findings for the impact of MBTSC on symptoms. However, 100% of participants completed the intervention.

Heapy et al. (2022)	7 adults (and 7 children)	Intervention only	Psoriasis, Eczema	Mindful Parenting (MP)	In-person	Idiographic measures of parenting stress, Mindfulness, Stress, Depression, Anxiety, Dermatology-specific family quality of life, Dermatology-specific child quality of life, Qualitative exit interviews.	All parents showed improvements in idiographic measures of parenting stress from baseline to follow-up ($p=<0.001$). Improvements in parenting stress were larger at follow-up. Six out of seven parents showed improvement in at least one of the standardised measures of wellbeing from pre-intervention to post-intervention, or follow-up.
Heapy et al. (2023)	5	Intervention only	Alopecia	Mindfulness-Based cognitive therapy (MBCT)	In-person	Idiographic measures of social anxiety, Mindfulness practice, Mindfulness, Social anxiety, Depression, General anxiety, Dermatology-specific quality of life.	One participant was excluded from data analysis. Four participants showed improvements in idiographic measures of social anxiety from baseline to follow-up. Two participants showed significant improvements in standardised measures of wellbeing from baseline to follow-up, and also reported practicing mindfulness exercises most frequently at home.
Hudson et al. (2020)	176 (33.81)	Waitlist	Eczema, Psoriasis, Acne, Alopecia, 'Other.'	Compassion-based self help	Online	Stress, Anxiety and depression, Dermatology-specific quality of life, Self-compassion,	There were significant moderate improvements found for levels of stress, anxiety, depression, self-compassion and quality of life, when compared to controls. Although these results remained significant, the effect sizes decreased from moderate to small following intention-to-treat (ITT) analyses.

(*continued*)

Table 17.1 (continued)

Authors (year)	N (mean age in years)	Control Group	Skin Condition	Intervention	Delivery	Outcomes measured	Summary of findings
Hughes et al. (2024)	10 adults (and 8 children)	Intervention only	Eczema, Ectodermal Dysplasia, Ichthyosis, Alopecia.	Mindfulness-based intervention (MBI)	Online	Idiographic measures of parenting stress, Mindfulness, Dermatology-specific family quality of life, Parent Stress, Depression, Anxiety, Dermatology-specific child quality of life, Qualitative exit interviews.	Tau-U analysis showed three parents had significant improvements in positive idiographic targets, and five parents had significant improvements in negative targets. Reliable change assessment of standardised measures showed: One parent demonstrated improvement in mindful parenting, three parents demonstrated improvement in parenting stress, seven parents demonstrated improvement in anxiety, three parents demonstrated improvements in depression, six parents demonstrated improvement in QoL, and four children demonstrated improvement in QoL. Two parents demonstrated increased anxiety. Qualitative analysis suggested favourable outcomes for psychological well-being, but also shed light on the challenges associated with mindfulness, such as home practice.
Kabat-Zinn (1998)	37 (43)	Phototherapy (UVB) and photochemotherapy (PUVA) treatment without audiotapes	Psoriasis	Phototherapy (UVB) and photochemotherapy (PUVA) with mindfulness meditation-based stress reduction audiotapes	In-person	Skin severity, Psychological status.	Participants in the tape group reached the halfway point ($p=0.13$) and clearing point ($p=0.033$) significantly faster than participants in the no-tape group. Findings suggested mindfulness delivered via audiotape alongside UVB and PUVA could increase levels of skin clearance in psoriasis.

Kishimoto et al. (2023)	107 (36.3)	Wait list	Atopic dermatitis	Mindfulness and self-compassion training	Online	Dermatology-specific quality of life, Eczema severity, Itch and scratching, Self-Compassion, Mindfulness, Psychological symptoms, Treatment adherence.	Participants who took part in the mindfulness and self-compassion training group reported greater improvements in quality of life scores at 13 weeks (P < .001). Further, there were greater improvements found in all secondary outcomes for the intervention group when compared to the wait list.
Maddock et al. (2019)	101 (43.51, intervention, 44.56 control)	Usual psoriasis therapy alone	Psoriasis	Mindfulness-based cognitive therapy (MBCT)	In-person	Anxiety and depression, Psychological well-being, Psoriasis severity, Mindfulness, Acceptance, Decentering, Non-attachment, Aversion, Self-Compassion, Rumination, Worry.	Significant differences were found for each variable in the MBCT group over time, but not in the treatment as usual group.
Muftin et al. (2022)	130	Compassion-based self help	Psoriasis	Compassion-based self-help, Mindfulness-based self-help	Online	Shame, Critical and reassuring self-evaluative responses, Dermatology-specific quality of life, Acceptability.	There were small statistically significant decreases in shame (Cohen's d= 0.20) and increases in quality of life (Cohen's d= 0.40) for both the compassion-based self-help group and the mindfulness-based self-help group.

(continued)

Table 17.1 (continued)

Authors (year)	N (mean age in years)	Control Group	Skin Condition	Intervention	Delivery	Outcomes measured	Summary of findings
Offenbächer et al. (2021)	10 (53.10)	Intervention only	Atopic dermatitis	Mindfulness-based Stress Reduction (MBSR)	In-person	Atopic dermatitis severity, Frequency of symptoms, Dermatology-specific quality of life, Anxiety and depression, Stress, Mindfulness, Subjective impression regarding psychological change,	There were significant improvements found in mindfulness measures, including the constructs of presence and acceptance. There were also reports of reduced stress.
Russell et al. (2019)	69 (53.4)	Usual care	Melanoma	Mindfulness-based intervention (MBI)	Online	Fear of recurrence, Rumination, Worry, Mindfulness, Stress.	There were significant decreases in fear of recurrence in the MBI group compared to the control group ($p=0.008$). However, there were no differences between the MBI group and the control group for any of the outcome measures.
Sherman et al. (2019)	50 (27.13)	Unstructured writing	Acne, Eczema, Psoriasis, Birthmark, 'Other.'	Self-compassion writing	Online	Self-compassion, Affect, Body image disturbance, Skin severity.	There were significant improvements to self-compassion and negative affect after the self-compassion writing exercise, when compared to the control group. However, there were no significant differences between groups for positive affect at follow-up.

Although this outcome for rumination is promising, much of the existing evidence for the use of mindfulness with skin conditions has focussed on psoriasis, which raises issues of generalisability to other skin conditions. There is some evidence for the effectiveness of MBSR for adults with moderate to severe alopecia areata for improving quality of life, which was partly maintained at 6-month follow-up (Gallo et al., 2017; Heapy et al., 2023).

Recently, a randomised controlled trial (RCT) conducted by Kishimoto et al. (2023) investigated an online-based mindfulness and self-compassion training intervention for 107 adults with moderate to severe atopic dermatitis and found that dermatology-specific quality of life, disease severity, and all secondary outcomes improved (e.g., itch, eczema severity, mindfulness, self-compassion) when compared to controls. These findings were maintained over time, with a large effect size, and suggest that mindfulness combined with usual dermatological care could reduce symptoms of atopic dermatitis (Kishimoto et al., 2023). However, the biological mechanisms between the mind and the skin are complex and still not fully understood (Kishimoto et al., 2023).

MP has also been subject to preliminary investigation as a therapeutic approach for parents of children with inflammatory skin disease. In a small single-case experimental design, Heapy et al. (2022) evaluated whether MP could reduce parenting stress and improve bespoke positive outcomes, as identified by the participants. Heapy et al.'s intervention followed the MP protocol (Bögels & Restifo, 2015) that is based on MBSR and MBCT. This consists of an 8-week intensive programme made up of formal mindful practices and homework exercises. The programme involves yoga, meditations, mindful walking, breathing exercises, and also self-compassion exercises. The study reported promising results, with reductions in stress from baseline to follow-up, although caution is needed in drawing any firm conclusions from a small, uncontrolled single-case series (Heapy et al., 2022).

As with any intervention development, experts by experience must be consulted and involved from the start so as to ensure that new mindfulness- and/or compassion-focussed interventions are appropriately tailored. Recently, Hughes et al. (2022) interviewed parent and child dyads to determine the relevance of offering mindfulness-based interventions and found that whilst families appeared to be receptive to the idea of engaging in mindfulness, there were misconceptions regarding the nature of mindfulness that must be further considered when designing interventions (Hughes et al., 2022). Whilst MP interventions may show promise, care is needed in developing interventions that are going to be feasible for busy parents to undertake alongside balancing other caring responsibilities.

Concluding Comments and Directions for Future Research

Based on current evidence and theory, it can be speculated that there could potentially be a therapeutic relationship between several facets of mindfulness (acceptance, and acting with awareness), the related concept of self-compassion, and improved psychological functioning in chronic skin conditions, including lower levels of anxiety and depression. However, whilst mindfulness interventions offer promise in reducing distress associated with skin conditions, the existing studies investigating the effectiveness and feasibility of mindfulness for dermatological conditions have methodological issues such as small sample sizes and further larger-scale trials of both self-help and more intense forms of positive-based psychological interventions are needed. In addition, further research is required to fully understand the underlying mechanisms by which mindfulness might improve outcomes for people living with skin conditions. It is crucial to disentangle not only the relationship between positive psychological variables and distress but also to look at the mechanisms underlying exactly how these variables might impact upon stress and biomarkers associated with inflammatory processes. For example, future studies might use experimental designs to investigate psychoneuroimmunological pathways to explain the specific mechanisms underlying the relationship between stress and potentially protective positive psychological variables.

The chapter also draws attention to the need for further research into the naturalistic coping strategies and protective factors that are specifically relevant to people living with skin conditions. In addition to experimental and biomarker research, there remains a need to conduct qualitative studies. Such studies can play a role in demonstrating how some of the answers to treating distress already exist in the natural responses that humans have developed for achieving well-being and happiness.

Acknowledgement The authors would like to thank Dr Helen Penny, Consultant Clinical Psychologist, Aneurin Bevan University Health Board, for providing additional clinical psychology review of the areas to cover in this chapter

References

Ablett, K., & Thompson, A. R. (2016). Parental, child, and adolescent experience of chronic skin conditions: A meta-ethnography and review of the qualitative literature. *Body Image, 19*, 175–185. https://doi.org/10.1016/j.bodyim.2016.10.001

Adkins, K., Overton, P., & Thompson, A. (2022). A brief online writing intervention improves positive body image in adults living with dermatological conditions. *Frontiers in Medicine*. https://doi.org/10.3389/fmed.2022.1064012

Adkins, K., Overton, P. G., Moses, J., & Thompson, A. (2023). Investigating the role of upward comparisons and self-compassion on stigma in people with Acne: Cross-sectional Study. *JMIR Dermatology, 6*, e45368. https://doi.org/10.2196/45368

Ahmed, A., Affleck, A., Angus, J., Assalman, I., Baron, S., Bewley, A., Goulding, J. M. R., Jerrom, R., Lepping, P., Mortimer, H., Shah, R., Taylor, R., Thompson, A. R., Mohd Mustapa, M. F., & Manounah, L. (2022). British Association of Dermatologists guidelines for the management of delusional infestation. *British Journal of Dermatology*. https://doi.org/10.1111/bjd.21668

Ali, F. M., Johns, N., Salek, S., & Finlay, A. Y. (2018). Correlating the dermatology life quality index with psychiatric measures: A systematic review. *Clinics in Dermatology, 36*, 691–697. https://doi.org/10.1016/j.clindermatol.2018.08.014

All Party Parliamentary Group on Skin. (2020). *Mental health and skin disease*. http://www.appgs.co.uk/wp-content/uploads/2020/09/Mental_Health_and_Skin_Disease2020.pdf

Association for Psychoneurocutaneous Medicine of North America (APMNA n.d.). Welcome to the APMNA. Retrieved April 6, 2025, from https://psychodermatology.us/

Balieva, F., Schut, C., Kupfer, J., Lien, L., Misery, L., Sampogna, F., von Euler, L., & Dalgard, F. J. (2022). Perceived stress in patients with inflammatory and non-inflammatory skin conditions. An observational controlled study among 255 Norwegian dermatological outpatients. *Skin Health & Disease*, e162. https://doi.org/10.1002/ski2.162

Black, P. H. (2002). Stress and the inflammatory response: A review of neurogenic inflammation. *Brain, Behavior, and Immunity, 16*(6), 622–653. https://doi.org/10.1016/s0889-1591(02)00021-1

Bögels, S. M., Hellemans, J., van Deursen, S., Römer, M., & van der Meulen, R. (2014). Mindful parenting in mental health care: Effects on parental and child psychopathology, parental stress, parenting, coparenting, and marital functioning. *Mindfulness, 5*(5), 536–551. https://doi.org/10.1007/s12671-013-0209-7

Bögels, S. M., Lehtonen, A., & Restifo, K. (2010). Mindful parenting in mental health care. *Mindfulness, 1*(2), 107–120. https://doi.org/10.1007/s12671-010-0014-5

Bögels, S. M., & Restifo, K. (2015). *Mindful parenting: A guide for mental health practitioners*. Springer.

Chamlin, S. L., Frieden, I. J., Williams, M. L., & Chren, M. M. (2004). Effects of atopic dermatitis on young American children and their families. *Pediatrics, 114*(3), 607–611. https://doi.org/10.1542/peds.2004-0374

Changing Faces. (2022, December 30). *Ending appearance based discrimination*. https://www.changingfaces.org.uk/about-visible-difference/ending-appearance-related-discrimination/

Chen, Y., & Lyga, J. (2014). Brain-skin connection: Stress, inflammation and skin aging. *Inflammation & Allergy, 13*(3), 177–190. https://doi.org/10.2174/1871528113666140522104422

Clarke, E., Thompson, A. R., & Norman, P. (2020). Depression in people with skin conditions: The effects of disgust and self-compassion. *British Journal of Health Psychology, 25*(3), 540–557. https://doi.org/10.1111/bjhp.12421

Clarke, E., Thompson, A. R., & Norman, P. (2022). How does self-compassion help people adjust to chronic skin conditions? A template analysis study. *Frontiers in Medicine, 9*, 974816. https://doi.org/10.3389/fmed.2022.974816

Clarke, E., Norman, P., & Thompson, A. R. (2024). Online compassion-based self-help for depression in people with skin conditions: A feasibility study. *Pilot and Feasibility Studies, 10*, 63. https://doi.org/10.1186/s40814-024-01486-4

Creswell, J. D., & Lindsay, E. K. (2014). How does mindfulness training affect health? A mindfulness stress buffering account. *Current Directions in Psychological Science, 23*(6), 401–407. https://doi.org/10.1177/0963721414547415

Creswell, J. D., Lindsay, E. K., Villalba, D. K., & Chin, B. (2019). Mindfulness training and physical health: Mechanisms and outcomes. *Psychosomatic Medicine, 81*(3), 224–232. https://doi.org/10.1097/PSY.0000000000000675

D'Alton, P., Kinsella, L., Walsh, O., Sweeney, C., Timoney, I., Lynch, M., O'Connor, M., & Kirby, B. (2019). Mindfulness-based interventions for psoriasis: A randomized controlled trial. *Mindfulness, 10*(2), 288–300. https://doi.org/10.1007/s12671-018-0973-5

Dalgard, F. J., Gieler, U., Tomas-Aragones, L., Lien, L., Poot, F., Jemec, G. B. E., Misery, L., Szabo, C., Linder, D., Sampogna, F., Evers, A. W. M., Halvorsen, J. A., Balieva, F., Szepietowski, J., Romanov, D., Marron, S. E., Altunay, I. K., Finlay, A. Y., Salek, S. S., & Kupfer, J. (2015). The psychological burden of skin diseases: A cross-sectional multicenter study among dermatological out-patients in 13 European countries. *The Journal of Investigative Dermatology, 135*(4), 984–991. https://doi.org/10.1038/jid.2014.530

De Vere Hunt, I. J., Howard, E., & McPherson, T. (2020). The impact of chronic skin disease in adolescence and the need for specialist adolescent services. *Clinical and Experimental Dermatology, 45*(1), 5–9. https://doi-org.abc.cardiff.ac.uk/10.1111/ced.14021

Egan, K., Harcourt, D., Rumsey, N., & The Appearance Research Collaboration. (2011). Appearance Research Collaboration. A qualitative study of the experiences of people who identify themselves as having adjusted positively to a visible difference. *Journal of Health Psychology, 16*(5), 739–749. https://doi.org/10.1177/1359105310390246

European Association for Dermatology and Psychiatry. (2022, December 30). *ESDaP—European Association for Dermatology and Psychiatry.* https://www.psychodermatology.net/

Evers, A. W. M., & van Beugen, S. (2021). How stress affects the skin: From designs to mechanisms. *British Journal of Dermatology, 185*(1), 12–13. https://doi.org/10.1111/bjd.20397

Fennessy, M., Coupland, S., Popay, J., & Naysmith, K. (2000). The epidemiology and experience of atopic eczema during childhood: A discussion paper on the implications of current knowledge for health care, public health policy and research. *Journal of Epidemiology & Community Health, 54*(8), 581–589. https://doi.org/10.1136/jech.54.8.581

Fordham, B., Griffiths, C. E. M., & Bundy, C. (2015). A pilot study examining mindfulness-based cognitive therapy in psoriasis. *Psychology, Health & Medicine, 20*(1), 121–127. https://doi.org/10.1080/13548506.2014.902483

Gallo, R., Chiorri, C., Gasparini, G., Signori, A., Burroni, A., & Parodi, A. (2017). Can mindfulness-based interventions improve the quality of life of patients with moderate/severe alopecia areata? A prospective pilot study. *Journal of the American Academy of Dermatology, 76*(4), 757–759. https://doi.org/10.1016/j.jaad.2016.10.012

Gilbert, P. (2009). *The compassionate mind.* Constable.

Gilbert, P. (2010). *Compassion Focused Therapy: The CBT distinctive features series.*

Gojani, P. J., Masjedi, M., Khaleghipour, S., & Behzadi, E. (2017). Effects of the schema therapy and mindfulness on the maladaptive schemas hold by the psoriasis patients with the psychopathology symptoms. *Advanced Biomedical Research, 6*(4), 1–8. https://doi.org/10.4103/2277-9175.190988

Golpanian, R. S., Kim, H. S., & Yosipovitch, G. (2020). Effects of stress on itch. *Clinical Therapeutics, 42*(5), 745–756. https://doi.org/10.1016/j.clinthera.2020.01.025

Harcourt, D., & Williamson, H. (2019). Positive body image in people living with visible differences. In T. L. Tylka & N. Piran (Eds.), *Handbook of positive body image and embodiment* (pp. 255–262). Oxford University Press.

Harfensteller, J. (2022). An open trial on the feasibility and efficacy of a mindfulness-based intervention with psychoeducational elements on Atopic Eczema and Chronic Itch. *Psych, 4,* 160–172. https://doi.org/10.3390/psych4020014

Heapy, C., Norman, P., Cockayne, S., & Thompson, A. (2023). The effectiveness of mindfulness-based cognitive therapy for social anxiety in people with alopecia areata: A single group case-series design. *Behavioural and Cognitive Psychotherapy, 51*(5), 381–395. https://doi.org/10.1017/S1352465823000292

Heapy, C., Norman, P., Emerson, L., Murphy, R., Bögels, S., & Thompson, A. (2022). Mindful parenting intervention for parents of children with skin conditions: A single group experimental cases series. *Behavioural and Cognitive Psychotherapy,* 1–19. https://doi.org/10.1017/S1352465822000170

Heapy, C., Norman, P., Emerson, L. M., Murphy, R., Bögels, S., & Thompson, A. (2021). Is parental mindfulness associated with quality of life and itch intensity in children with Psoriasis and Eczema and well-being in parents? *Mindfulness, 12,* 2707–2717. https://doi.org/10.1007/s12671-021-01733-2

Hudson, M. P., Thompson, A. R., & Emerson, L. M. (2020). Compassion-focused self-help for psychological distress associated with skin conditions: A randomized feasibility trial. *Psychology & Health, 35*(9), 1095–1114. https://doi.org/10.1080/08870446.2019.1707829

Hughes, O. (2022). The need for psychological support in routine dermatological care across the UK. *British Journal of Dermatology*. https://doi.org/10.1111/bjd.21720

Hughes, O., & Hunter, R. (2022). Understanding the experiences of anger in the onset and progression of Psoriasis: A thematic analysis. *Skin Health and Disease*. https://doi.org/10.1002/ski2.111

Hughes, O., Hutchings, P. B., & Phelps, C. (2021). Stigma, social appearance anxiety and coping in men and women living with skin conditions: A mixed methods analysis. *Skin Health and Disease, e73*. https://doi.org/10.1002/ski2.73

Hughes, O., Shelton, K. H., Penny, H., & Thompson, A. R. (2022). Parent and child experience of skin conditions: Relevance for the provision of mindfulness-based interventions. *British Journal of Dermatology*. https://doi.org/10.1093/bjd/ljac129

Hughes, O., Shelton, K. H., Penny, H. & Thompson, A. R. (2023). Living with physical health conditions: A systematic review of mindfulness-based interventions for children, adolescents, and their parents. *Journal of Pediatric Psychology*. Advance online publication. https://doi.org/10.1093/jpepsy/jsad003

Hughes, O., Shelton, K. H., Penny, H., & Thompson, A. R. (2024). 'Living in the Present' mindfulness for parents of children with skin conditions: A single group case series. *Behavioural and Cognitive Psychotherapy, 52*(6), 561–580. https://doi.org/10.1017/S1352465824000341

Hunter, H. J., Griffiths, C. E., & Kleyn, C. E. (2013). Does psychosocial stress play a role in the exacerbation of psoriasis? *British Journal of Dermatology, 169*(5), 965–974. https://doi.org/10.1111/bjd.12478

Ip, A., Muller, I., Geraghty, A. W. A., Platt, D., Little, P., & Santer, M. (2021). Views and experiences of people with acne vulgaris and healthcare professionals about treatments: Systematic review and thematic synthesis of qualitative research. *BMJ Open, 11*(2), e041794. https://doi.org/10.1136/bmjopen-2020-041794

Kabat-Zinn, J. (1982). An outpatient program in behavioral medicine for chronic pain patients based on the practice of mindfulness meditation: Theoretical considerations and preliminary results. *General Hospital Psychiatry, 4*(1), 33–47.

Kabat-Zinn, J. (1994). *Wherever you go, there you are: Mindfulness meditation in everyday life*. Hyperion.

Kabat-Zinn, J., & Kabat-Zinn, M. (2021). Mindful parenting: Perspectives on the heart of the matter. *Mindfulness, 12*, 266–268. https://doi.org/10.1007/s12671-020-01564-7

Kabat-Zinn, J., Wheeler, E., Light, T., Skillings, A., Scharf, M. J., Cropley, T. G., Hosmer, D., & Bernhard, J. D. (1998). Influence of a mindfulness meditation-based stress reduction intervention on rates of skin clearing in patients with moderate to severe psoriasis undergoing phototherapy (UVB) and photochemotherapy (PUVA). *Psychosomatic Medicine, 60*(5), 625–632. https://doi.org/10.1097/00006842-199809000-00020

Kemp, A. S. (2003). Cost of illness of atopic dermatitis in children. *Pharmacoeconomics, 21*(2), 105–113. https://doi.org/10.2165/00019053-200321020-00003

Kent, G., & Thompson, A. R. (2002). Models of disfigurement: Implications for treatment. In P. Gilbert & J. Miles (Eds.), *Understanding body shame* (pp. 106–116). Hove, UK: Brunner-Routledge.

Kim, J. E., Cho, B. K., Cho, D. H., & Park, H. J. (2013). Expression of hypothalamic-pituitary-adrenal axis in common skin diseases: Evidence of its association with stress-related disease activity. *Acta dermato-venereologica, 93*(4), 387–393. https://doi.org/10.2340/00015555-1557

Kimyai-Asadi, A., & Usman, A. (2001). The role of psychological stress in skin disease. *Journal of Cutaneous Medicine and Surgery, 5*(2), 140–145.

Kishimoto, S., Watanabe, N., Yamamoto, Y., Imai, T., Aida, R., Germer, C., Tamagawa-Mineoka, R., Shimizu, R., Hickman, S., Nakayama, Y., Etoh, T., Sahker, E., Carnie, M. B., & Furukawa, T. A. (2023). Efficacy of integrated online mindfulness and self-compassion training for adults with Atopic Dermatitis: A randomized clinical trial. *JAMA Dermatology*, e230975. Advance online publication. https://doi.org/10.1001/jamadermatol.2023.0975

Koblenzer, C. S. (1983). Psychosomatic concepts in dermatology. A dermatologist-psychoanalyst's viewpoint. *Archives of Dermatology, 119*(6), 501–512.

Koblenzer, C. S. (1992). Cutaneous manifestations of psychiatric disease that commonly present to the Dermatologist—Diagnosis and treatment. *The International Journal of Psychiatry in Medicine, 22*(1), 47–63. https://doi.org/10.2190/JMLB-UUTJ-40PN-KQ3L

Krasuska, M., Lavda, A. C., Thompson, A. R., & Millings, A. (2018a). The role of adult attachment orientation and coping in psychological adjustment to living with skin conditions. *The British Journal of Dermatology, 178*(6), 1396–1403. https://doi.org/10.1111/bjd.16268

Krasuska, M., Millings, A., Lavda, A. C., & Thompson, A. R. (2018b). Compassion-focused self-help for skin conditions in individuals with insecure attachment: A pilot evaluation of acceptability and potential effectiveness. *The British Journal of Dermatology, 178*(2). https://doi.org/10.1111/bjd.15934

Linthorst Homan, M. W., De Korte, J., Grootenhuis, M. A., Bos, J. D., Sprangers, M. A. G., & Van Der Veen, J. P. W. (2008). Impact of childhood vitiligo on adult life. *British Journal of Dermatology, 159*(4), 915–920. https://doi.org/10.1111/j.1365-2133.2008.08788.x

Lüßmann, K., Montgomery, K., Thompson, A., Gieler, U., Zick, C., Kupfer, J., & Schut, C. (2021). Mindfulness as predictor of itch catastrophizing in patients with atopic dermatitis: Results of a cross-sectional questionnaire study. *Frontiers in Medicine, 8*. https://doi.org/10.3389/fmed.2021.627611

Maddock, A., Hevey, D., D'Alton, P., & Kirby, B. (2019). A randomized trial of mindfulness-based cognitive therapy with psoriasis patients. *Mindfulness, 10*(12), 2606–2619. https://doi.org/10.1007/s12671-019-01242-3

Maddock, A., Hevey, D., D'Alton, P., & Kirby, B. (2020). Mindfulness-based cognitive therapy as a clinical intervention with psoriasis patients through the lens of the clinically modified Buddhist psychological model: A qualitative study. *Mental*

Health, Religion & Culture, 1–20. https://doi.org/10.1080/13674676.2020.1823950

Magin, P., Adams, J., Heading, G., Pond, D., & Smith, W. (2008). Experiences of appearance-related teasing and bullying in skin diseases and their psychological sequelae: Results of a qualitative study. *Scandinavian Journal of Caring Sciences, 22*, 430–436. https://doi.org/10.1111/j.1471-6712.2007.00547.x

McPherson, T. (2021). *Skin conditions in young people: A practical guide on how to be comfortable in your own skin*. Oxford University Press.

Meneo, D., Martoni, M., Giannandrea, A., Tengattini, V., & Baglioni, C. (2022). Mindfulness and self-compassion in dermatological conditions: A systematic narrative review. *Psychology & Health*. https://doi.org/10.1080/08870446.2022.2070619

Montgomery, K., Norman, P., Messenger, A. G., & Thompson, A. R. (2016). The importance of mindfulness in psychosocial distress and quality of life in dermatology patients. *British Journal of Dermatology, 175*(5), 930–936. https://doi.org/10.1111/bjd.14719

Montgomery, K., & Thompson, A. R. (2018). The potential role of mindfulness in psychosocial support for dermatology patients. *Clinics in Dermatology, 36*(6), 743–747. https://doi.org/10.1016/j.clindermatol.2018.08.010

Muftin, Z., Gilbert, P., & Thompson, A. R. (2022). A randomised controlled feasibility trial of online compassion-focused self-help for Psoriasis. *British Journal of Dermatology, 186*, 955–962. https://doi.org/10.1111/bjd.21020

Neff, K. D. (2003). Self-compassion: An alternative conceptualization of a healthy attitude toward oneself. *Self Identity, 2*, 85–101. https://doi.org/10.1080/15298860309032

Offenbächer, M., Seitlinger, M., Münch, D., Schnopp, C., Darsow, U., Harfensteller, J., Schmid-Grendelmeier, P., Ring, J., & Kohls, N. (2021). A Pilot Study of a mindfulness-based stress reduction programme in patients suffering from Atopic Dermatitis. *Psych, 3*, 663–672. https://doi.org/10.3390/psych3040042

Papadopoulos, L., & Walker, C. (2003). *Understanding skin problems; Acne, Eczema, Psoriasis and related conditions*. Wiley.

Picardi, A., Abeni, D., Melchi, C., Puddu, P., & Pasquini, P. (2000). Psychiatric morbidity in dermatological outpatients: An issue to be recognized. *British Journal of Dermatology, 143*, 983–991. https://doi.org/10.1046/j.1365-2133.2000.03831.x

Picardi, A., Lega, I., & Tarolla, E. (2013). Suicide risk in skin disorders. *Clinics in Dermatology, 31*(1), 47–56. https://doi.org/10.1016/j.clindermatol.2011.11.006

Rapp, S. R., Feldman, S. R., Exum, M. L., Fleischer, A. B., & Reboussin, D. M. (1999). Psoriasis causes as much disability as other major medical diseases. *Journal of the American Academy of Dermatology, 41*, 401–407. https://doi.org/10.1016/S0190-9622(99)70112-X

Reid, P., & Lewis-Jones, M. S. (1995). Sleep difficulties and their management in preschoolers with atopic eczema. *Clinical and Experimental Dermatology, 20*(1), 38–41. https://doi.org/10.1111/j.1365-2230.1995.tb01280.x

Rohleder, N. (2019). Stress and inflammation—The need to address the gap in the transition between acute and chronic stress effects. *Psychoneuroendocrinology, 105*, 164–171. https://doi.org/10.1016/j.psyneuen.2019.02.021

Rønnstad, A. T. M., Halling-Overgaard, A. S., Hamann, C. R., Skov, L., Egeberg, A., & Thyssen, J. P. (2018). Association of atopic dermatitis with depression, anxiety, and suicidal ideation in children and adults: A systematic review and meta-analysis. *Journal of the American Academy of Dermatology, 79*(3), 448–456. https://doi.org/10.1016/j.jaad.2018.03.017

Rumsey, N. (2018). Psychosocial adjustment to skin conditions resulting in visible difference (disfigurement): What do we know? Why don't we know more? How shall we move forward? *International Journal of Women's Dermatology, 4*, 2–7. https://doi.org/10.1016/j.ijwd.2017.09.005

Russell, L., Ugalde, A., Orellana, L., Milne, D., Krishnasamy, M., Chambers, R., Austin, D. W., & Livingston, P. M. (2019). A pilot randomised controlled trial of an online mindfulness-based program for people diagnosed with melanoma. *Supportive Care in Cancer, 27*(7), 2735–2746. https://doi.org/10.1007/s00520-018-4574-6

Sanders, K. M., & Akiyama, T. (2018). The vicious cycle of itch and anxiety. *Neuroscience and Biobehavioral Reviews, 87*, 17–26. https://doi.org/10.1016/j.neubiorev.2018.01.009

Schmidt, S. A. J., Sorensen, H. T., Langan, S. M., & Vestergaard, M. (2021). Perceived psychological stress and risk of herpes zoster: A nationwide population-based cohort study. *British Journal of Dermatology, 185*(1), 130–138. https://doi.org/10.1111/bjd.19832

Segal, Z. V., Williams, J. M., & Teasdale, J. (2002). *Mindfulness-based cognitive therapy for depression: A new approach to preventing relapse*. Guilford Press.

Sharpe, L., & Curran, L. (2006). Understanding the process of adjustment to illness. *Social Science & Medicine, 62*, 153–166. https://doi.org/10.1016/j.socscimed.2005.07.010

Shepherd, L., Reynolds, D. P., Turner, A., O'Boyle, C. P., & Thompson, A. R. (2019). The role of psychological flexibility in appearance anxiety in people who have experienced a visible burn injury. *Burns, 45*, 942–949. https://doi.org/10.1016/j.burns.2018.11.015

Sherman, K. A., Roper, T., & Kilby, J. (2019). Enhancing self-compassion in individuals with visible skin conditions: Randomised pilot of the 'My Body Changed' self-compassion writing intervention. *Health Psychology and Behavioural Medicine, 7*(1), 62–77. https://doi.org/10.1080/21642850.2019.1587298

Thompson, A. R. (2009). Psychosocial impact of skin conditions. *Dermatological Nursing, 8*, 43–48.

Thompson, A. R. (2011). Adaptation in long-term conditions: The role of stigma particularly in conditions that affect appearance. In S. Randall & H. Ford (Eds.), *The textbook of long-term conditions* (pp. 121–137). Wiley.

Thompson, A. R. (2012a). Skin conditions. In T. Cash (Ed.), *The encyclopaedia of body image and human appearance* (Vol. 2, pp. 738–744).

Thompson, A. R. (2012b). Researching appearance: Models, theories, and frameworks. In Self-help for management of distress associated with skin conditions. In A. Bewley, R. E. Taylor, J. S. Reichenberg, & M. Magid (Eds.), *Practical psychodermatology* (pp. 60–66). Wiley.

Thompson, A. R., & Broom, L. (2009). Positively managing intrusive reactions to disfigurement: An interpretative phenomenological analysis of naturalistic coping. *Diversity in Health & Care, 6*, 171–180.

Thompson, A. R., Eleftheriadou, V., & Nesnas, J. (2022). The mental health associations of vitiligo: A population-based cohort study in the UK. *BJPsych Open, 8*(6), E190. https://doi.org/10.1192/bjo.2022.591

Thompson, A. R., Kent, G., & Smith, J. A. (2002). Living with vitiligo: Dealing with difference. *British Journal of Health Psychology, 7*, 213–225. https://doi.org/10.1348/135910702169457

Tollefson, M. M., Finnie, D. M., Schoch, J. J., & Eton, D. T. (2017). Impact of childhood psoriasis on parents of affected children. *Journal of the American Academy of Dermatology, 76*(2), 286–289.e5. https://doi.org/10.1016/j.jaad.2016.09.014

Trekels, J., & Eggermont, S. (2017). Linking magazine exposure to social appearance anxiety: The role of appearance norms in early adolescence. *Journal of Research on Adolescence, 27*(4), 736–751. https://doi.org/10.1111/jora.12311

van Beugen, S., Schut, C., Kupfer, J., Bewley, S., Finlay, A., Gieler, U., Thompson, A. R., Gracia-Cazana, T., Balieva, F., Ferreira, B., Jemec, G., Lien, L., Misery, L., Marron, S., Stander, S., Zeidler, C., Szaba, C., Szepietowski, J., Reich, A, …, Dalgard, F. (2022, In review). Perceived stigmatisation among dermatological outpatients compared to controls: An observational multicenter study in 17 European countries. *Acta Dermato-Venereologica.*

van Scheppingen, C., Lettinga, A. T., Duipmans, J. C., Maathuis, K. G., & Jonkman, M. F. (2008). The main problems of parents of a child with epidermolysis bullosa. *Qualitative Health Research, 18*(4), 545–556. https://doi.org/10.1177/1049732308315110

Verhoeven, E. W., de Klerk, S., Kraaimaat, F. W., van de Kerkhof, P. C., de Jong, E. M., & Evers, A. W. (2008). Biopsychosocial mechanisms of chronic itch in patients with skin diseases: A review. *Acta Dermato-Venereologica, 88*(3), 211–218. https://doi.org/10.2340/00015555-0452

Yang, E. J., Beck, K. M., Sekhon, S., Bhutani, T., & Koo, J. (2019). The impact of pediatric atopic dermatitis on families: A review. *Pediatric Dermatology, 36*(1), 66–71. https://doi.org/10.1111/pde.13727

18

The Beneficial Effects of Yoga on Stress: A Positive Psychology Perspective

Crystal L. Park and C. Sophie Skoggard

Classical yoga was originally designed to create mind-body harmony and aid in the ultimate goal of "enlightenment" (Birdee et al., 2008). In recent decades, yoga has evolved considerably, and much greater emphasis is typically placed on its physical aspects. Hatha yoga, the modality most often practiced in the United States, involves the practice of yoga postures together with breathing techniques and concentration/meditation (Gard et al., 2014). Based on a national survey (the NHIS, conducted every 5 years), in 2012, over 31 million Americans reported that they had ever practiced yoga and 21 million had practiced within the past year. These numbers represented a substantial increase from the previous NHIS in 2007, and the number of practitioners is expected to continue increasing (Cramer et al., 2016). The reasons people are drawn to yoga practice are many. In one national survey, desire to exercise and relieve stress were the most common reasons beginners reported for seeking out yoga, followed by getting more flexible, getting into shape, and relieving depression and anxiety (Park et al., 2016a).

Although yoga has been shown to exert favorable influences on myriad aspects of health and well-being, stress is perhaps the most well-documented aspect of health shown to be improved by yoga. Yet, we know little about *how* yoga brings about these reductions in stress. Positive psychology—an area of psychology that emphasizes human strengths and flourishing—may provide

C. L. Park (✉) • C. S. Skoggard
Department of Psychological Sciences, University of Connecticut, Storrs, CT, USA
e-mail: crystal.park@uconn.edu

F. M. Sirois (ed.), *The Palgrave Handbook of Positive Psychology and Health*,
https://doi.org/10.1007/978-3-031-89095-6_18

insights into important yet often overlooked pathways between yoga practice and stress. Little research to date has taken a positive psychology perspective on yoga, yet its mutual focus on promoting optimal and holistic health makes this linkage an obvious approach (Ivtzan & Papantoniou, 2014). In this chapter, we take a positive psychology perspective to illuminate relevant potential pathways through which yoga influences stress. First, we review the role of stress in health and the influences of yoga on stress and then describe the potential utility of a positive psychology approach to understanding the mechanisms through which yoga may affect stress. We then review the evidence linking yoga with nine specific positive-psychology-related constructs that may account for its salutary effects on stress. We conclude with potential intervention implications and directions for future research.

Yoga Improves Many Health Conditions, Including Stress

Applied as a mind-body intervention, yoga has been demonstrated to improve the health and well-being of people with many different health concerns. Although the quality and depth of evidence supporting yoga for treating different conditions varies, and yoga is sometimes used as an adjunctive treatment, systematic reviews have concluded that yoga is effective and safe for treating aspects of depression (Cramer et al., 2013), chronic low back pain (Skelly et al., 2018; Wieland et al., 2017), chronic neck pain (Cramer et al., 2017), osteoarthritis (Kan et al., 2016), diabetes (Thind et al., 2017), heart failure (Metin et al., 2018), hypertension (Tyagi et al., 2014), and cancer-treatment side effects (Lin et al., 2018). Other studies suggest that yoga is a promising therapy for many other conditions, including anxiety (Cramer et al., 2018b), PTSD (Cramer et al., 2018a; Cushing & Braun, 2018), insomnia (Zhou et al., 2017), multiple sclerosis (Miller & Soundy, 2017), and irritable bowel syndrome (Ewais et al., 2019; Schumann et al., 2016). However, reviews typically conclude with the notion that results to date are promising, but that more high-quality evidence is needed.

Stress underlies many of these above-listed health problems. Stress—feeling overwhelmed and unable to meet the demands being placed on oneself—is purported to impact the course of disease and illness at a systemic level (Cohen et al., 2015; Muscatell & Eisenberger, 2012). Indeed, many of the health conditions for which yoga has been shown effective are directly related to stress (e.g., PTSD, hypertension), and even those health conditions that are not overtly related to stress have close linkages. For example, the experience of pain is highly influenced by the amount of physiological stress an individual is experiencing (Woda et al., 2016). In addition, stress is widely considered to constitute a major health problem in itself (Goyal et al., 2014).

Yoga is effective in alleviating stress. In fact, stress is one of the most commonly studied outcomes in yoga research (Domingues, 2018), and systematic reviews of yoga interventions to alleviate stress have generally demonstrated favorable effects (Chong et al., 2011; Pascoe & Bauer, 2015; Pascoe et al., 2017; Sharma, 2014). Stress is most commonly measured by self-report (Sharma, 2014), and many yoga interventions have demonstrated reductions in perceived stress. Randomized controlled trials (RCTs) of yoga conducted with many groups, including healthy stressed individuals, employees, students, pregnant women, people in treatment for cancer, and people with hypertension, arthritis, headaches, and asthma, have demonstrated reductions in perceived stress (see Pascoe & Bauer, 2015, for a review).

However, the magnitude of yoga intervention effect sizes on stress has varied, and not all studies have demonstrated significant stress-reducing effects. The range of effect sizes noted (and occasional lack of statistically significant effects) may be due in part to the very different types of yoga tested in each study as well as methodological shortcomings (e.g., including a sample not particularly high in stress). Still, it appears that yoga's broad effects on stress are observable across multiple domains. In addition to generally demonstrating positive effects on self-reported stress, many yoga interventions have also yielded positive results in reducing biomarkers of stress, including endocrine and cardiovascular markers, across many different populations (see Pascoe et al., 2017, for a review). A few studies have even demonstrated improvements in physiological reactivity to stress. For example, one study found a yoga intervention improved acute stress responses (specifically, the production of the stress hormone cortisol) in the face of a laboratory challenge (Hopkins et al., 2016).

Mechanisms Through Which Yoga Reduces Stress

Despite this considerable body of research on yoga and stress, we actually know little about *how* yoga reduces stress. Until recently, yoga research primarily focused on testing its efficacy for improving a variety of health problems and conditions. As efficacy has been increasingly demonstrated, the need to understand *how* yoga produces salutary effects is emerging as a central concern of yoga research. To date, very few studies have focused on identifying the mechanisms through which yoga reduces stress. In our recent review (Riley & Park, 2015), we identified just a handful of studies that tested such mechanisms. Although the methodology of those studies was generally of low quality, this review found some evidence for both physiological and psychological pathways of yoga's influence on stress.

Moreover, multiple theoretical perspectives have been advanced regarding mechanisms that might underlie yoga's effects on stress, including both physiological and psychological mediators of its effects (Gard et al., 2014; Kinser et al., 2012; Streeter et al., 2012). Although these linkages remain to be fully tested (i.e., yoga to a mediator to a stress outcome), likely mediators can be identified by examining evidence indicating that yoga has been associated with the potential stress-reducing variable (i.e., mediator) and that the potential mediator, in turn, has reliably been linked to lower levels of stress (see the NIH Science of Behavior Change [Nielsen et al., 2018]). In this chapter, we examine an array of potential mediators that either have been demonstrated to relate to lower levels of stress or that plausibly could be related to lower levels of stress (e.g., Kiecolt-Glaser et al., 2020).

A Positive Psychology Approach to Yoga's Mechanisms of Effect

For this review, we have adopted a positive psychology approach. Positive psychology is a subfield of psychology that encompasses the scientific study of the conditions and processes contributing to flourishing or optimal functioning (Gable & Haidt, 2005). The mutual focus on promoting optimal holistic health taken by both yoga and positive psychology makes this approach a promising one for identifying key pathways of yoga's salutary influence on stress. Based on the positive psychology and yoga literatures, which are quite separate, we summarized literature on nine mechanisms (see Fig. 18.1). As we discuss below, there are other potential positive-psychology-related mediators of the yoga-reduced stress relationship, but to date, there is little research to review.

Physical Health/Fitness

Increased physical fitness—being as physically healthy or fit as one can be—promotes stress resilience. While physical health/fitness is not often talked about as an aspect of positive psychology (Seligman & Fowler, 2011), it is, in

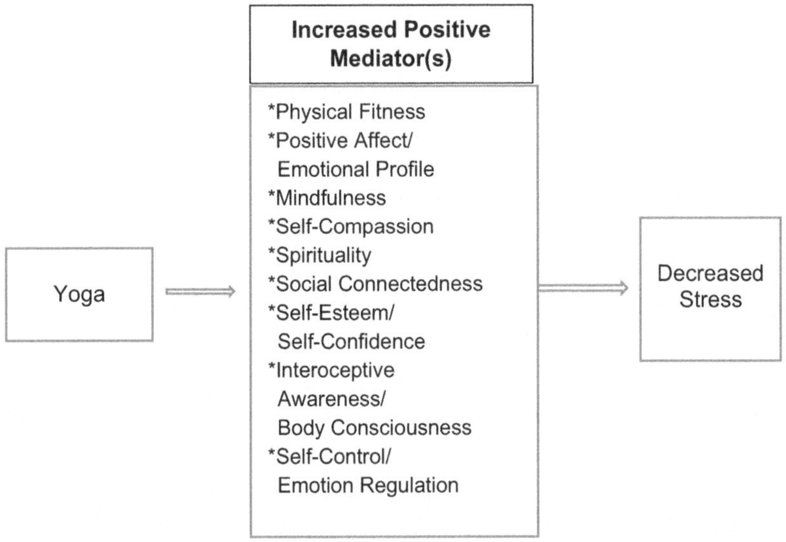

Fig. 18.1 Potential mediators of yoga's effects drawn from positive psychology

fact, often conceptualized as an aspect of flourishing (Vanderweele et al., 2019) and therefore highly relevant to positive psychology. Thus, a positive psychology-related way that yoga may promote lower stress is through its function as whole-body physical exercise that improves physical health and fitness. The literature is replete with examples of yoga's promotion of better health and fitness. One study of an 8-week twice-weekly Iyengar yoga intervention for older adults found that, post-intervention, yoga practitioners experienced an increase in muscle strength, active range of motion, physical well-being, and perceived benefits regarding body awareness, balance and walking, posture, body shape and ability to undertake daily activities, which also correlated with an increase in emotional well-being and self-care (Vogler et al., 2011). In an 8-week Hatha yoga intervention consisting of at least two classes per week, the yoga group saw significant improvement in muscle strength, endurance, flexibility and cardiorespiratory endurance (Tran et al., 2001). Even among college athletes, yoga was found to increase flexibility, balance and aerobic fitness (Polsgrove et al., 2016). One 8-week intervention using Bikram yoga (a type of hot yoga) reported improvement in flexibility, balance, and cardiorespiratory endurance that corresponded with a decrease in perceived stress (Hewett et al., 2011).

Beyond improving strength and fitness levels, yoga affects specific health functions such as improved quality of sleep, aerobic respiration, lung function, heart rate, and blood pressure. In a 7-week Tibetan yoga intervention for patients with lymphoma, participants receiving the yoga intervention improved in their subjective sleep quality, faster sleep latency, and longer sleep duration, and reduced their use of sleep medications (Cohen et al., 2004). Longer sleep duration and better-quality sleep are not only essential for physical health (allowing for muscle repair and memory consolidation) but also impact memory, judgment, and mood, with sleep deprivation increasing emotional sensitivity to stress (Worley, 2018). Another yoga intervention that emphasized pranayama—breathing exercises that are generally included in yoga classes—found that the added attention to pranayama not only increased overall respiratory functions but improved inspiratory muscle strength (Yamamoto-Morimoto et al., 2019). Improved breathing capacity, and specifically the use of pranayama, has been identified as a key mediator to reducing stress (Tellhed et al., 2019). In an intensive 3-month, 6-days-per-week yoga intervention for coronary artery disease patients, the experimental group (yoga intervention and dietary modifications plus conventional medication) demonstrated significant improvements in lung functions and diffusion capacity as well as improved heart rate, systolic, and diastolic blood pressure versus control group (who only received conventional medicine) (Yadav et al., 2015).

These studies demonstrate that yoga has beneficial physiological effects upon the body that increase the physical health and fitness of individuals, reduce cortisol levels, and may thereby boost emotional resilience and protect against stress. Considering that physical fitness has been demonstrated to improve resilience to stress (e.g., Crowley et al., 2020; Mücke et al., 2018; Sharon-David & Tenebaum, 2017), physical health and fitness are a theoretically convincing mediator between yoga and stress, although we were unable to find any studies that directly tested this mediation.

Positive Affect/Emotional Profile

Research has linked yoga with more general favorable emotion profiles (i.e., higher positive and lower negative emotion). In turn, experiencing high positive affect/low negative affect is associated with lower stress levels (Blevins et al., 2017; Fiori et al., 2015). In multiple clinical trials, yoga practice has been associated with more positive affect and more favorable emotional profiles, promoting positive emotions like happiness and contentment and reducing negative emotions like depression and anxiety, in many different populations, including women with chronic stress (Harkess et al., 2016a) and breast cancer (Bower et al., 2012; Danhauer et al., 2009), college students

(Park et al., 2017), and hospital employees (Riley et al., 2017). One randomized, double-blinded study of engineers in India examining the effect of 10 weeks of daily mindful yoga found that relative to the control group (primarily physical activity), those in the yoga condition increased in positive affect (Dwivedi et al., 2015). In another study, boys between the ages of 12 and 15 assigned to 1 month of yoga practice improved substantially on positive-negative affect compared to those in a no-treatment control, who did not change in affect (Kale & Kumari, 2017). In a trial of women experiencing moderate to severe chronic stress levels, those in the yoga group experienced increases in positive affect and decreases in negative affect relative to those in a waitlist control condition (Harkess et al., 2016b). However, female university students in a 10-week yoga intervention showed no increase in positive affect but a decrease in negative affect (Csala et al., 2020). Hatha yoga has been shown to increase mood scores in experienced yoga practitioners after just a single session (Luu & Hall, 2016). In a study of chronic low back pain patients, levels of positive states of mind did not change relative to control groups nor did they mediate effects of the intervention on back pain (Sherman et al., 2013).

Inducing more positive or less negative affect is often a key mechanism by which physical activity reduces stress (Rosenbaum et al., 2015), and studies have demonstrated that improved emotional profiles are associated with reduced stress in physical activity stress reduction interventions (e.g., Asmundson et al., 2013), Thus, improving participants' emotional profiles appears a promising mechanism of yoga's salutary effects on stress reduction, although we were unable to find any studies that explicitly tested the yoga-positive affect-stress pathway, so this linkage remains to be tested.

Mindfulness

Mindfulness—having present-moment awareness with acceptance and without judgment—is often suggested as a mechanism of yoga's effects (e.g., Gaiswinkler & Unterrainer, 2016). A large observational literature links higher levels of mindfulness to lower levels of stress as measured by self-report (Chamberlain et al., 2016; Finkelstein-Fox et al., 2022; Jarrett et al., 2017) and biomarkers (Laurent et al., 2016, 2017). Further, RCTs of yoga have demonstrated increased mindfulness in samples ranging from women with PTSD (Mitchell et al., 2014) and cancer (Moadel et al., 2007) to cardiac patients (Toise et al., 2014) and healthy populations (Bowden et al., 2012; Shelov et al., 2009). Thus, the linkage between yoga practice and stress appears plausibly mediated by increased mindfulness, but research has yet to demonstrate this full mediational path.

Although mindfulness is commonly linked with yoga (e.g., Kinser et al., 2012), surprisingly few studies have actually examined increased mindfulness as a mediator of yoga's effects or even documented increases in mindfulness as a result of practicing yoga. Several observational studies have shown that length of yoga practice (e.g., Brisbon & Lowery, 2011) or intensity of integration of yoga into daily life (Gaiswinkler & Unterrainer, 2016) is associated with higher levels of mindfulness. One single-arm study showed increases in mindfulness across an 8-week Bikram intervention (Hewett et al., 2011), but an 8-week yoga intervention with a healthy population found increases in mindfulness for both the intervention and control (no treatment) groups, while another study of women showed no changes in mindfulness in a 10-week intervention (Csala et al., 2020). One small study of participants in a 4-month residential yoga program found that increases in mindfulness mediated effects on perceived stress and quality of life (Gard et al., 2012). Another small study of a 12-week yoga intervention for women with PTSD found that mindfulness increased slightly in both the intervention and assessment-only arms, but it did *not* mediate the noted improvements in post-traumatic stress symptoms in the yoga group (Mitchell et al., 2014). One clinical trial of stressed community residents found that practicing Kripalu yoga was associated with increased mindfulness across the 12-week intervention, and these increases in mindfulness mediated the reductions in both perceived stress and stress reactivity (Park et al., 2021).

Self-Compassion

Researchers have suggested that self-compassion—taking a loving and kind approach toward oneself, especially when encountering difficulties or suffering (Neff, 2003)—may be yet another mediator through which yoga lowers stress (Braun et al., 2016). Yoga interventions have shown increases in self-compassion from pre- to post-intervention in samples of college students (Kramer & Cuccolo, 2019), nursing students (Mathad et al., 2017), and health care providers (Riley et al., 2017). Two additional intervention studies tested self-compassion as a mediator of yoga's effects on stress. One, a study of young adults in a 4-month residential yoga intervention program showed that self-compassion increased over time and mediated yoga's effects on stress (Gard et al., 2012). The other, a study of stressed community adults found that self-compassion did not increase over time on average, but increases in self-compassion did mediate pre-post reductions in stress (Park et al., 2021).

Spirituality

Spirituality—the extent to which one feels connected to others or a higher power—may mediate some of yoga's effects on stress. Most forms of yoga originated as methods for developing contemplative states of consciousness and spirituality (Büssing et al., 2012). Yet few studies have focused on yoga's effects on spirituality. Studies of motivations for yoga practice have found that although yoga practitioners report having begun yoga for physical health benefits, they report continuing their practices for spiritual reasons (Park et al., 2016; Penman et al., 2012). Survey studies of yoga practitioners have found that longer time practicing (Ivtzan & Papantoniou, 2014) and higher levels of integrating yoga into their lives (Gaiswinkler & Unterrainer, 2016) were associated with higher levels of spirituality and meaning in life.

Few clinical trials of yoga have assessed spirituality, but those that have consistently shown favorable effects. For example, one randomized controlled trial of breast cancer patients found that while their spiritual well-being was stable from baseline through a 3-month intervention, the waitlist control group showed significant declines in spiritual well-being, potentially demonstrating a protective effect of the yoga (Moadel et al., 2007), while another study of breast cancer patients found that, relative to a waitlist control, spiritual well-being increased for those in a restorative yoga intervention (Danhauer et al., 2009). Compared to a waitlist control, university employees in a 6-week yoga intervention group experienced increased levels of meaning in life (Hartfiel et al., 2011). Similarly, in a 10-week yoga intervention, female college students showed increases in spirituality relative to a control group (Csala et al., 2020), and a 12-week clinical trial of stressed community residents found that practicing Kripalu yoga was associated with increased spirituality (Park et al., 2021). Importantly, the latter study tested mediation and demonstrated that increases in spirituality mediated the observed reductions in both perceived stress and stress reactivity (Park et al., 2021).

Social Connectedness

Social connectedness—broadly defined as objective and subjective social support—has also been posited as a mechanism by which yoga may lead to lower stress (e.g., Meister & Juckel, 2018), yet social connection is rarely measured in studies of yoga. In several studies, yoga practitioners qualitatively reported experiencing yoga as leading to more positive relations with others as a result of their practice (Kishida et al., 2018; Ross et al., 2013). One small pilot study found some evidence for increased social connection as a result of a yoga intervention in a sample of counselors (Thompson et al., 2018). However, a large clinical trial of yoga for breast cancer patients found that those in the yoga group did not increase in social support, even compared to waitlist control (Kiecolt-Glaser et al., 2014). In another trial for breast cancer patients, social well-being was stable from baseline through a 3-month intervention, while the waitlist control showed significant declines in social well-being (Moadel et al., 2007). Thus, whether social connection or support is a mediator of yoga's stress reduction effects remains unestablished.

Self-Esteem/Self-Confidence

Increases in self-esteem/self-confidence—the extent to which one holds oneself in regard and feels capable of positive actions—is a widely suggested mediator of yoga's salutary effects, including its reduction of stress. In one 6-week yoga intervention targeting university employees, the yoga group improved in self-confidence when dealing with stressful situations as compared to a waitlist control (Hartfiel et al., 2011). One 12-week yoga program found that self-efficacy had a greater mediating effect than physical or affect-related mediators on relieving low back pain (often considered a somaticized expression of stress or depression; Sherman et al., 2013). Self-esteem mediated the effects of yoga on menopausal symptoms and quality of life in breast cancer survivors in one trial (Koch et al., 2017). Another intervention found that over the course of a 12-week yoga intervention, elderly women in a hospice in India experienced increased self-esteem along with decreased depression and anxiety (Ramanathan et al., 2017). In one intervention consisting of twice-weekly Ashtanga yoga classes over a 9-week period, participants experienced quick and significant improvement in self-esteem and anxiety (Jarry et al., 2017). This body of research suggests that yoga may reduce stress through improving self-esteem or self-confidence and thus alleviate stress, although no studies have yet directly tested these linkages.

Interoceptive Awareness/Body Consciousness

Some theorists have posited that yoga practice may foster increased body consciousness or interoceptive awareness (i.e., consciousness of internal body states) (e.g., Gard et al., 2014; Neukirch et al., 2019). One study found that women yoga practitioners had healthier body awareness than did comparison samples of aerobic exercise practitioners or those practicing neither yoga nor aerobic exercise (Daubenmier, 2005). A single-arm trial of a yoga intervention found that higher amounts of yoga practice produced greater improvements in body consciousness (Impett et al., 2006), but female university students in a 10-week yoga intervention did not increase in body awareness (Csala et al., 2020). A study of first-year college students showed improvements in emotion regulation in a yoga intervention relative to cognitive behavioral stress management and a waitlist control (Park et al., 2017). One clinical trial of stressed community residents found that practicing Kripalu yoga was associated with increased interoceptive awareness across the 12-week intervention, and these increases in interoceptive awareness mediated reductions in both perceived stress and stress reactivity (Park et al., 2021).

Self-Control/Emotion Regulation

Self-control refers to the ability to deliberately override or change one's initial emotional and behavioral responses, particularly in circumstances in which they are misaligned with one's goals (Tangney et al., 2004). Self-control and emotion regulation capacities are related to lower levels of stress (e.g., Park et al., 2016b). Many elements of yoga can help develop self-control and emotion regulation abilities (Menezes et al., 2015), including meditative movement, body and emotion awareness, reappraisal, distress tolerance, attention allocation, and acceptance (Gard et al., 2014). Through these elements, practitioners strengthen their capacity for emotional stability and equanimity and are able to cultivate emotions that are helpful and manage emotions that are harmful (Gross, 2013). The more participants practice yoga, the greater their tendency for adaptive emotion regulation both on and off the yoga mat (Daly et al., 2015; Park et al., 2018). Yoga combines these different aspects, rendering it a highly potent intervention for improving self-control and emotion regulation capacities.

Yet little research has examined yoga's potential to increase self-control. Several pilot studies of adolescents provide some support for the notion that yoga can increase self-control (Khalsa et al., 2012; Ramadoss & Bose, 2010).

A study of first-year college students showed improvements in emotion regulation in a yoga intervention relative to cognitive behavioral stress management and a waitlist control (Park et al., 2017). One clinical trial of stressed community residents found that practicing Kripalu yoga was associated with increased self-control across the 12-week intervention, but increases in self-control did not mediate the reductions in perceived stress or stress reactivity (Park et al., 2021).

Conclusions and Future Research Directions

We used a positive psychology framework to identify constructs that may mediate the salutary effects of yoga practice on stress. Specifically, we identified nine constructs drawn from positive psychology that may mediate this linkage: physical fitness, positive affect, mindfulness, self-compassion, spirituality, social connection, self-esteem/self-confidence, interoceptive awareness/body consciousness, and self-control. Overall, our review demonstrated that each of these constructs has at least some empirical support as increasing with yoga practice, based on results from observational and interventional studies. However, the evidence remains quite preliminary: for many of these constructs, just a handful of studies exist, and many of these studies rely on fairly weak methods. Further, only a few studies have explicitly tested whether these positive psychological constructs mediate the effects of yoga practice on stress (e.g., Park et al., 2021).

Thus, the current support for these constructs as mediators is best characterized as "promising" and deserving of further investigation and elaboration. Research on yoga is becoming increasingly sophisticated; as this field continues to mature, the need for rigorous research testing these potential mediators becomes increasingly urgent. Identifying the most potent mediators of its effects will expand our understanding of yoga, adding to its scientific credibility in the Western health care arena. Increasing credibility should, in turn, increase access to yoga as it becomes established as conventional health promotion (Khalsa et al., 2016). Understanding mediators will also assist interventionists in optimizing yoga therapies and perhaps in tailoring yoga practices for individuals with particular needs.

Our review indicated that many additional potential mediators drawn from positive psychology deserve consideration. For example, many core positive psychology constructs were included in just a few studies (e.g., gratitude; Ivtzan & Papantoniou, 2014) or none at all (e.g., patience, humility). Yoga researchers should carefully consider theoretical models of yoga's effects from a positive psychology perspective and select potential mediators that yoga might influence and that are either known to be associated with stress reduction or plausibly may be. Then, studies of yoga's effect on stress must be conducted that explicitly assess and test these mediational pathways (Nielsen et al., 2018); this mediational work can be readily incorporated into clinical trials. Along with the increasing rigor of yoga research, this focus on strong psychological theories will enrich our understanding of positive psychological principles and how they may play out in mind-body applications.

References

Asmundson, G. J., Fetzner, M. G., DeBoer, L. B., Powers, M. B., Otto, M. W., & Smits, J. A. (2013). Let's get physical: A contemporary review of the anxiolytic effects of exercise for anxiety and its disorders. *Depression and Anxiety, 30*(4), 362–373.

Birdee, G. S., Legedza, A. T., Saper, R. B., Bertisch, S. M., Eisenberg, D. M., & Phillips, R. S. (2008). Characteristics of yoga users: Results of a national survey. *Journal of General Internal Medicine, 23*, 1653–1658.

Blevins, C. L., Sagui, S. J., & Bennett, J. M. (2017). Inflammation and positive affect: Examining the stress-buffering hypothesis with data from the National Longitudinal Study of Adolescent to Adult Health. *Brain, Behavior, and Immunity, 61*, 21–26.

Bowden, D., Gaudry, C., An, S. C., & Gruzelier, J. (2012). A comparative randomised controlled trial of the effects of brain wave vibration training, Iyengar yoga, and mindfulness on mood, well-being, and salivary cortisol. *Evidence-Based Complementary and Alternative Medicine*, Article ID 234713.

Bower, J. E., Garet, D., Sternlieb, B., Ganz, P. A., Irwin, M. R., Olmstead, R., & Greendale, G. (2012). Yoga for persistent fatigue in breast cancer survivors: A randomized controlled trial. *Cancer, 118*(15), 3766–3775.

Braun, T. D., Park, C. L., & Gorin, A. (2016). Self-compassion, body image, and disordered eating: A review of the literature. *Body Image, 17*, 117–131.

Brisbon, N. M., & Lowery, G. A. (2011). Mindfulness and levels of stress: A comparison of beginner and advanced hatha yoga practitioners. *Journal of Religion and Health, 50*(4), 931–941.

Büssing, A., Hedtstück, A., Khalsa, S.B., Ostermann, T., Heusser, P. (2012). Development of specific aspects of spirituality during a 6-month intensive yoga practice. *Evidence-Based Complementary and Alternative Medicine*, Article 981523.

Chamberlain, D., Williams, A., Stanley, D., Mellor, P., Cross, W., & Siegloff, L. (2016). Dispositional mindfulness and employment status as predictors of resilience in third year nursing students: A quantitative study. *Nursing Open, 3*(4), 212–221.

Chong, C., Tsunaka, M., Tsang, H., Chan, E., & Cheung, W. (2011). Effects of yoga on stress management in healthy adults: A systematic review. *Alternative Therapies in Health and Medicine, 17*(1), 32–38.

Cohen, B., Edmondson, D., & Kronish, I. (2015). State of the art review: Depression, stress, anxiety, and cardiovascular disease. *American Journal of Hypertension, 28*(11), 1295–1302.

Cohen, L., Warneke, C., Fouladi, R. T., Rodriguez, M. A., & Chaoul-Reich, A. (2004). Psychological adjustment and sleep quality in a randomized trial of the effects of a Tibetan yoga intervention in patients with lymphoma. *Cancer, 100*, 2253–2260.

Cramer, H., Anheyer, D., Saha, F. J., & Dobos, G. (2018a). Yoga for posttraumatic stress disorder: A systematic review and meta-analysis. *BMC Psychiatry, 18*(1), 72.

Cramer, H., Klose, P., Brinkhaus, B., Michalsen, A., & Dobos, G. (2017). Effects of yoga on chronic neck pain: A systematic review and meta-analysis. *Clinical Rehabilitation, 31*(11), 1457–1465.

Cramer, H., Lauche, R., Anheyer, D., Pilkington, K., de Manincor, M., Dobos, G., & Ward, L. (2018b). Yoga for anxiety: A systematic review and meta-analysis of randomized controlled trials. *Depression and Anxiety, 35*(9), 830–843.

Cramer, H., Lauche, R., Langhorst, J., & Dobos, G. (2013). Yoga for depression: A systematic review and meta-analysis. *Depression and Anxiety, 30*(11), 1068–1083.

Cramer, H., Ward, L., Steel, A., Lauche, R., Dobos, G., & Zhang, Y. (2016). Prevalence, patterns, and predictors of yoga use: Results of a US nationally representative survey. *American Journal of Preventive Medicine, 50*(2), 230–235.

Crowley, S. K., Rebellon, J., Huber, C., Leonard, A. J., Henderson, D., & Magal, M. (2020). Cardiorespiratory fitness, sleep, and physiological responses to stress in women. *European Journal of Sport Science, 20*, 1368–1377.

Csala, B., Ferentzi, E., Tihanyi, B. T., Drew, R., & Köteles, F. (2020). Verbal cuing is not the path to enlightenment. Psychological effects of a 10-session hatha yoga practice. *Frontiers in Psychology, 11*, 1375.

Cushing, R. E., & Braun, K. L. (2018). Mind–body therapy for military veterans with post-traumatic stress disorder: A systematic review. *The Journal of Alternative and Complementary Medicine, 24*(2), 106–114.

Daly, L. A., Haden, S. C., Hagins, M., Papouchis, N., & Ramirez, P. M. (2015). Yoga and emotion regulation in high school students: A randomized controlled trial. *Evidence-Based Complementary and Alternative Medicine*, Article 794928.

Danhauer, S. C., Mihalko, S. L., Russell, G. B., Campbell, C. R., Felder, L., Daley, K., & Levine, E. A. (2009). Restorative yoga for women with breast cancer: Findings from a randomized pilot study. *Psycho-Oncology, 18*(4), 360–368.

Daubenmier, J. (2005). The relationship of yoga, body awareness, and body responsiveness to self-objectification and disordered eating. *Psychology of Women Quarterly, 29*, 207–219.

Domingues, R. B. (2018). Modern postural yoga as a mental health promoting tool: A systematic review. *Complementary Therapies in Clinical Practice, 31*, 248–255.

Dwivedi, U., Kumari, S., Akhilesh, K. B., & Nagendra, H. R. (2015). Well-being at workplace through mindfulness: Influence of yoga practice on positive affect and aggression. *Ayu, 36*(4), 375.

Ewais, T., Begun, J., Kenny, M., Rickett, K., Hay, K., Ajilchi, B., & Kisely, S. (2019). A systematic review and meta-analysis of mindfulness based interventions and yoga in inflammatory bowel disease. *Journal of Psychosomatic Research, 116*, 44–53.

Finkelstein-Fox, L., Park, C. L., & Huedo-Medina, T. B. (2022). Appraisal and coping link sexual victimization history to emotional experience: A multilevel daily diary study. *Journal of Interpersonal Violence, 37*(9–10), NP6159–NP6185.

Fiori, M., Bollmann, G., & Rossier, J. (2015). Exploring the path through which career adaptability increases job satisfaction and lowers job stress: The role of affect. *Journal of Vocational Behavior, 91*, 113–121.

Gable, S. L., & Haidt, J. (2005). What (and why) is positive psychology? *Review of General Psychology, 9*(2), 103–110.

Gaiswinkler, L., & Unterrainer, H. F. (2016). The relationship between yoga involvement, mindfulness and psychological well-being. *Complementary Therapies in Medicine, 26*. https://doi.org/10.1016/j.ctim.2016.03.011

Gard, T., Brach, N., Hölzel, B. K., Noggle, J. J., Conboy, L. A., & Lazar, S. W. (2012). Effects of a yoga-based intervention for young adults on quality of life and perceived stress: The potential mediating roles of mindfulness and self-compassion. *Journal of Positive Psychology, 7*(3), 165–175.

Gard, T., Noggle, J. J., Park, C. L., Vago, D. R., & Wilson, A. (2014). Potential self-regulatory mechanisms of yoga for psychological health. *Frontiers in Human Neuroscience, 8*. https://doi.org/10.3389/fnhum.2014.00770

Goyal, M., Singh, S., Sibinga, E., Gould, N., Rowland-Seymour, A., Sharma, R., et al. (2014). Meditation programs for psychological stress and well-being: A systematic review and meta-analysis. *Deutsche Zeitschrift Für Akupunktur, 57*(3), 26–27.

Gross, J. J. (2013). Emotion regulation: Taking stock and moving forward. *Emotion, 13*(3), 359–365.

Harkess, K. N., Delfabbro, P., & Cohen-Woods, S. (2016a). The longitudinal mental health benefits of a yoga intervention in women experiencing chronic stress: A clinical trial. *Cogent Psychology, 3*(1), 1256037.

Harkess, K. N., Ryan, J., Delfabbro, P. H., & Cohen-Woods, S. (2016b). Preliminary indications of the effect of a brief yoga intervention on markers of inflammation and DNA methylation in chronically stressed women. *Translational Psychiatry, 6*(11), e965–e965.

Hartfiel, N., Havenhand, J., Khalsa, S. B., Clarke, G., & Krayer, A. (2011). The effectiveness of yoga for the improvement of well-being and resilience to stress in the workplace. *Scandinavian Journal of Work, Environment & Health, 37*, 70–76.

Hewett, Z. L., Ransdell, L. B., Gao, Y., & Petlichkoff, L. M. (2011). An examination of the effectiveness of an 8-week Bikram yoga program on mindfulness, perceived stress, and physical fitness. *Journal of Exercise Science and Fitness, 9*(2), 87–92.

Hopkins, L. B., Medina, J. L., Baird, S. O., Rosenfield, D., Powers, M. B., & Smits, J. A. (2016). Heated hatha yoga to target cortisol reactivity to stress and affective eating in women at risk for obesity-related illnesses: A randomized controlled trial. *Journal of Consulting and Clinical Psychology, 84*(6), 558–564.

Impett, E. A., Daubenmier, J. J., & Hirschman, A. L. (2006). Minding the body: Yoga, embodiment, and well-being. *Sexuality Research and Social Policy, 3*, 39–48.

Ivtzan, I., & Papantoniou, A. (2014). Yoga meets positive psychology: Examining the integration of Hedonic (gratitude) and Eudaimonic (meaning) wellbeing in relation to the extent of yoga practice. *Journal of Bodywork and Movement Therapies, 18*(2), 183–189.

Jarrett, N. L., Pickett, S. M., Amsbaugh, H., & Afzal, B. (2017). Mindfulness and forgiveness buffer distress: Associations with interpersonal transgression blameworthiness. *Counseling and Values, 62*(2), 198–215.

Jarry, J. L., Chang, F. M., & La Civita, L. (2017). Ashtanga yoga for psychological well-being: Initial effectiveness study. *Mindfulness, 8*, 1269–1279.

Kale, D., & Kumari, S. (2017). Effect of 1-month yoga practice on positive-negative affect and attitude toward violence in schoolchildren: A randomized control study. *International Journal of Educational and Psychological Researches, 3*(3), 180–186.

Kan, L., Zhang, J., Yang, Y., & Wang, P. (2016). The effects of yoga on pain, mobility, and quality of life in patients with knee osteoarthritis: A systematic review. *Evidence-Based Complementary and Alternative Medicin*e, Article 6016532.

Khalsa, S. B. S., Cohen, L., McCall, T., & Telles, S. (2016). *Principles and practice of yoga in health care*. Handspring Publishing Limited.

Khalsa, S. B. S., Hickey-Schultz, L., Cohen, D., Steiner, N., & Cope, S. (2012). Evaluation of the mental health benefits of yoga in a secondary school: A preliminary randomized controlled trial. *The Journal of Behavioral Health Services & Research, 39*(1), 80–90.

Kiecolt-Glaser, J. K., Bennett, J. M., Andridge, R., Peng, J., Shapiro, C. L., Malarkey, W. B., et al. (2014). Yoga's impact on inflammation, mood, and fatigue in breast cancer survivors: A randomized controlled trial. *Journal of Clinical Oncology, 32*(10), 1040–1049.

Kiecolt-Glaser, J. K., Renna, M. E., Shrout, M. R., & Madison, A. A. (2020). Stress reactivity: What pushes us higher, faster, and longer—And why it matters. *Current Directions in Psychological Science, 29*, 492–498.

Kinser, P. A., Goehler, L. E., & Taylor, A. G. (2012). How might yoga help depression? A neurobiological perspective. *Explore, 8*(2), 118–126.

Kishida, M., Mama, S. K., Larkey, L. K., & Elavasky, S. (2018). "Yoga resets my inner peace barometer": A qualitative study illuminating the pathways of how yoga impacts one's relationship to oneself and to others. *Complementary Therapies in Medicine, 40*, 215–221.

Koch, A. K., Rabsilber, S., Lauche, R., Kümmel, S., Dobos, G., Langhorst, J., & Cramer, H. (2017). The effects of yoga and self-esteem on menopausal symptoms and quality of life in breast cancer survivors. *Maturitas, 105*, 95–99.

Kramer, R., & Cuccolo, K. (2019). Yoga practice in a college sample: Associated changes in eating disorder, body image, and related factors over time. *Eating Disorders, 28*, 494–512.

Laurent, H. K., Duncan, L. G., Lightcap, A., & Khan, F. (2017). Mindful parenting predicts mothers' and infants' hypothalamic-pituitary-adrenal activity during a dyadic stressor. *Developmental Psychology, 53*(3), 417–424.

Laurent, H. K., Hertz, R., Nelson, B., & Laurent, S. M. (2016). Mindfulness during romantic conflict moderates the impact of negative partner behaviors on cortisol responses. *Hormones and Behavior, 79*, 45–51.

Lin, P. J., Peppone, L. J., Janelsins, M. C., Mohile, S. G., Kamen, C. S., Kleckner, I. R., …, & Mustian, K. M. (2018). Yoga for the management of cancer treatment-related toxicities. *Current Oncology Reports, 20*(1), Article 5.

Luu, K., & Hall, P. A. (2016). Hatha yoga and executive function: A systematic review. *Journal of Alternative and Complementary Medicine, 22*, 125–133.

Mathad, M. D., Pradhan, B., & Sasidharan, R. K. (2017). Effect of yoga on psychological functioning of nursing students: A randomized wait list control trial. *Journal of Clinical and Diagnostic Research, 11*(5), KC01–KC05.

Meister, K., & Juckel, G. (2018). A systematic review of mechanisms of change in body-oriented yoga in major depressive disorders. *Pharmacopsychiatry, 51*(03), 73–81.

Menezes, C. B., Dalpiaz, N. R., Rossi, N. T., & De Oliveira, A. A. (2015). Yoga and the interplay between attentional load and emotion interference. *Psychological Reports, 117*(1), 271–289.

Metin, Z. G., Ejem, D., Dionne-Odom, J. N., Turkman, Y., Salvador, C., Pamboukian, S., & Bakitas, M. (2018). Mind-body interventions for individuals with heart failure: A systematic review of randomized trials. *Journal of Cardiac Failure, 24*(3), 186–201.

Miller, P., & Soundy, A. (2017). The pharmacological and non-pharmacological interventions for the management of fatigue related multiple sclerosis. *Journal of the Neurological Sciences, 381*, 41–54.

Mitchell, K. S., Dick, A. M., DiMartino, D. M., Smith, B. N., Niles, B., Koenen, K. C., & Street, A. (2014). A pilot study of a randomized controlled trial of yoga as an intervention for PTSD symptoms in women. *Journal of Traumatic Stress, 27*(2), 121–128.

Moadel, A. B., Shah, C., Wylie-Rosett, J., Harris, M. S., Patel, S. R., Hall, C. B., & Sparano, J. A. (2007). Randomized controlled trial of yoga among a multiethnic sample of breast cancer patients: Effects on quality of life. *Journal of Clinical Oncology, 25*(28), 4387–4395.

Mücke, M., Ludyga, S., Colledge, F., & Gerber, M. (2018). Influence of regular physical activity and fitness on stress reactivity as measured with the Trier Social Stress Test protocol: A systematic review. *Sports Medicine, 48*(11), 2607–2622.

Muscatell, K. A., & Eisenberger, N. I. (2012). A social neuroscience perspective on stress and health. *Social and Personality Psychology Compass, 6*(12), 890–904.

Neff, K. D. (2003). The development and validation of a scale to measure self-compassion. *Self and Identity, 2*, 223–250.

Neukirch, N., Reid, S., & Shires, A. (2019). Yoga for PTSD and the role of interoceptive awareness: A preliminary mixed-methods case series study. *European Journal of Trauma & Dissociation, 3*(1), 7–15.

Nielsen, L., Riddle, M., King, J. W., Aklin, W. M., Chen, W., Clark, D., et al. (2018). The NIH Science of Behavior Change Program: Transforming the science through a focus on mechanisms of change. *Behaviour Research and Therapy, 101*, 3–11.

Park, C. L., Finkelstein-Fox, L., Sacco, S., Braun, T., & Lazar, S. (2021). How does yoga reduce stress? A clinical trial testing psychological mechanisms. *Stress and Health, 37*, 116–126.

Park, C. L., Lee, S. Y., Finkelstein-Fox, L., & Sanderson, K. (2018). Yoga to promote physical, mental and spiritual well-being: Self-regulation on and off the mat. In T. G. Plante (Ed.), *Healing with spiritual practices: Proven techniques for disorders from addictions and anxiety to cancer and chronic pain* (pp. 72–85). Praeger/ABC-CLIO.

Park, C. L., Riley, K. E., Bedesin, E., & Stewart, V. M. (2016a). Why practice yoga? Practitioners' motivations for adopting and maintaining yoga practice. *Journal of Health Psychology, 21*(6), 887–896.

Park, C. L., Riley, K. E., Braun, T. D., Jung, J. Y., Suh, H. G., Pescatello, L. S., & Antoni, M. H. (2017). Yoga and cognitive-behavioral interventions to reduce stress in incoming college students: A pilot study. *Journal of Applied Biobehavioral Research, 22*(4), e12068.

Park, C. L., Wright, B. E. W., Pais, J., & Ray, D. M. (2016b). Reciprocal relations between daily stressful events and ego depletion: A smartphone-based experience sampling study. *Journal of Social and Clinical Psychology, 35*, 738–753.

Pascoe, M. C., & Bauer, I. E. (2015). A systematic review of randomised control trials on the effects of yoga on stress measures and mood. *Journal of Psychiatric Research, 68*, 270–282.

Pascoe, M. C., Thompson, D. R., & Ski, C. F. (2017). Yoga, mindfulness-based stress reduction and stress-related physiological measures: A meta-analysis. *Psychoneuroendocrinology, 86*, 152–168.

Penman, S., Cohen, M., Stevens, P., & Jackson, S. (2012). Yoga in Australia: Results of a national survey. *International Journal of Yoga, 5*(2), 92–101.

Polsgrove, M. J., Eggleston, B. M., & Lockyer, R. J. (2016). Impact of 10-weeks of yoga practice on flexibility and balance of college athletes. *International Journal of Yoga Therapy, 9*(1), 27–34.

Ramadoss, R., & Bose, B. (2010). Transformative life skills: Pilot study of a yoga model for reduced stress and improving self-control in vulnerable youth. *International Journal of Yoga Therapy, 20*(1), 73–78.

Ramanathan, M., Bhavanani, A. B., & Trakroo, M. (2017). Effect of a 12-week yoga therapy program on mental health status in elderly women inmates of a hospice. *International Journal of Yoga Therapy, 10*(1), 24–28.

Riley, K. E., & Park, C. L. (2015). How does yoga reduce stress? A systematic review of mechanisms of change and guide to future inquiry. *Health Psychology Review, 9*(3), 379–396.

Riley, K. E., Park, C. L., Wilson, A., Sabo, A. N., Antoni, M. H., Braun, T. D., et al. (2017). Improving physical and mental health in frontline mental health care providers: Yoga-based stress management versus cognitive behavioral stress management. *Journal of Workplace Behavioral Health, 32*(1), 26–48.

Rosenbaum, S., Vancampfort, D., Steel, Z., Newby, J., Ward, P. B., & Stubbs, B. (2015). Physical activity in the treatment of post-traumatic stress disorder: A systematic review and meta-analysis. *Psychiatry Research, 230*(2), 130–136.

Ross, A., Friedmann, E., Bevans, M., & Thomas, S. (2013). National survey of yoga practitioners: Mental and physical health benefits. *Complementary Therapies in Medicine, 21*(4), 313–323.

Schumann, D., Anheyer, D., Lauche, R., Dobos, G., Langhorst, J., & Cramer, H. (2016). Effect of yoga in the therapy of irritable bowel syndrome: A systematic review. *Clinical Gastroenterology and Hepatology, 14*(12), 1720–1731.

Seligman, M. E., & Fowler, R. D. (2011). Comprehensive Soldier Fitness and the future of psychology. *American Psychologist, 66*(1), 82–86.

Sharma, M. (2014). Yoga as an alternative and complementary approach for stress management: A systematic review. *Journal of Evidence-Based Complementary & Alternative Medicine, 19*(1), 59–67.

Sharon-David, H., & Tenebaum, G. (2017). The effectiveness of exercise interventions on coping with stress: Research synthesis. *Studies in Sport Humanities, 22*, 19–29.

Shelov, D. V., Suchday, S., & Friedberg, J. P. (2009). A pilot study measuring the impact of yoga on the trait of mindfulness. *Behavioural and Cognitive Psychotherapy, 37*(5), 595–598.

Sherman, K. J., Wellman, R. D., Cook, A. J., Cherkin, D. C., & Ceballos, R. M. (2013). Mediators of yoga and stretching for chronic low back pain. *Evidence-based Complementary and Alternative Medicine*, Article 130818.

Skelly, A. C., Chou, R., Dettori, J. R., Turner, J. A., Friedly, J. L., Rundell, S. D., Fu, R., Brodt, E. D., Wasson, N., Winter, C., & Ferguson, A. (2018). *Noninvasive nonpharmacological treatment for chronic pain: A systematic review.* Agency for Healthcare Research and Quality.

Streeter, C. C., Gerbarg, P. L., Saper, R. B., Ciraulo, D. A., & Brown, R. P. (2012). Effects of yoga on the autonomic nervous system, gamma-aminobutyric-acid, and allostasis in epilepsy, depression, and post-traumatic stress disorder. *Medical Hypotheses, 78*(5), 571–579.

Tangney, J. P., Baumeister, R. F., & Boone, A. L. (2004). High self-control predicts good adjustment, less pathology, better grades, and interpersonal success. *Journal of Personality, 72*(2), 271–324.

Tellhed, U., Daukantaitė, D., Maddux, R. E., Svensson, T., & Melander, O. (2019). Yogic breathing and mindfulness as stress coping mediate positive health outcomes of yoga. *Mindfulness, 10*, 2703–2715.

Thind, H., Lantini, R., Balletto, B. L., Donahue, M. L., Salmoirago-Blotcher, E., Bock, B. C., & Scott-Sheldon, L. A. (2017). The effects of yoga among adults with type 2 diabetes: A systematic review and meta-analysis. *Preventive Medicine, 105*, 116–126.

Thompson, I. A., Wolf, C. P., Mott, E., Baggs, A. S., Thompson, E. S., Callueng, C., & Puig, A. (2018). Luna yoga: A wellness program for female counselors and counselors-in-training to foster self-awareness and connection. *Journal of Creativity in Mental Health, 13*(2), 169–184.

Toise, S. C., Sears, S. F., Schoenfeld, M. H., Blitzer, M. L., Marieb, M. A., Drury, J. H., et al. (2014). Psychosocial and cardiac outcomes of yoga for ICD patients: A randomized clinical control trial. *Pacing and Clinical Electrophysiology, 37*(1), 48–62.

Tran, M. D., Holly, R. G., Lashbrook, J., & Amsterdam, E. A. (2001). Effects of hatha yoga practice on the health-related aspects of physical fitness. *Preventive Cardiology, 4*(4), 165–170.

VanderWeele, T. J., McNeely, E., & Koh, H. K. (2019). Reimagining health—Flourishing. *JAMA, 321*(17), 1667–1668.

Vogler, J., O'Hara, L., Gregg, J., & Burnell, F. (2011). The impact of a short-term Iyengar yoga program on the health and well-being of physically inactive older adults. *International Journal of Yoga Therapy, 21*, 61–72.

Wieland, L. S., Skoetz, N., Pilkington, K., Vempati, R., D'Adamo, C. R., & Berman, B. M. (2017). Yoga treatment for chronic non-specific low back pain. *Cochrane Database of Systematic Reviews, 1*.

Woda, A., Picard, P., & Dutheil, F. (2016). Dysfunctional stress responses in chronic pain. *Psychoneuroendocrinology, 71*, 127–135.

Worley, S. L. (2018). The extraordinary importance of sleep. *Pharmacy and Therapeutics, 43*(12), 758–763.

Yadav, A., Singh, S., Singh, K. P., & Pai, P. (2015). Effect of yoga regimen on lung functions including diffusion capacity in coronary artery disease patients: A randomized controlled study. *International Journal of Yoga Therapy, 8*(1), 62–67.

Yamamoto-Morimoto, K., Horibe, S., Takao, R., & Anami, K. (2019). Positive effects of yoga on physical and respiratory functions in healthy inactive middle-aged people. *International Journal of Yoga Therapy, 12*(1), 62–67.

Zhou, E. S., Gardiner, P., & Bertisch, S. M. (2017). Integrative medicine for insomnia. *Medical. Clinics, 101*(5), 865–879.

19

Self-Compassion and Health Behaviours

Marios Biskas, Fuschia M. Sirois, and Thomas L. Webb

Introduction

The importance of health behaviours for lifelong health and overall well-being cannot be overstated. As key modifiable risk factors for a number of chronic and long-term health conditions and related mortality, engaging in health-promoting behaviours such as healthy eating, taking regular exercise, and getting adequate sleep, as well as reducing health-risk behaviours such as excessive alcohol consumption and smoking, are crucial for ensuring lasting health (World Health Organisation, 2021). Yet, despite common knowledge of the dangers of not adopting health-promoting behaviours and of reducing

M. Biskas (✉)
Department of Psychology, Durham University, Durham, UK

Department of Psychology, Bradford University, Bradford, UK
e-mail: m.biskas@bradford.ac.uk

F. M. Sirois
Department of Psychology, Durham University, Durham, UK

T. L. Webb
Department of Psychology, The University of Sheffield, Sheffield, UK

F. M. Sirois (ed.), *The Palgrave Handbook of Positive Psychology and Health*,
https://doi.org/10.1007/978-3-031-89095-6_19

health-risk behaviours, many people struggle to make the sustainable changes to their health behaviours that can foster long-term health.

There are a number of barriers to successful health behaviour change, including low motivation (Hardcastle et al., 2015), not considering current progress (Harkin et al., 2016; Webb et al., 2013) or future consequences of behaviour (Baird et al., 2021), as well as unwanted social influences (Sheeran et al., 2005) and habits (Gardner, 2015). However, one often overlooked factor is the way that people respond to the inevitable lapses and setbacks that can occur on the path towards engaging in healthier behaviours. For example, when people break their diets or miss a scheduled exercise session, they can get caught in a self-perpetuating cycle of self-criticism, guilt, and shame that can trigger avoidance or abandonment of their health goals (e.g., Dickson & Shulman, 2016; Duarte et al., 2017).

One way to address this issue is to help people to replace their default self-critical and negative emotional response with one that is kind and accepting, understanding of the imperfection of being human, and takes a balanced emotional perspective. Our review of the evidence suggests that this self-compassionate stance can provide the motivation, self-regulation resources, and coping skills necessary to navigate the often bumpy challenges of adopting a healthier set of behaviours. After discussing how self-compassion can be conceptualised and outlining processes and pathways that provide insights into the question of *why* self-compassion may help people make and maintain changes in their health behaviour, we review evidence on the potential barriers that some people face when trying to respond with kindness, connectedness, and mindfulness to their health behaviour lapses. We then propose a new framework for understanding when and why people have difficulties being self-compassionate as well as discuss the implications of this for interventions targeting health behaviour change.

Self-Regulation and the Challenges of Health Behaviour Change

Despite the obvious benefits of certain patterns of behaviour, such as being physically active, eating a healthy diet, and abstaining from ingesting harmful substances like tobacco and alcohol, people often behave in ways that potentially damage their health (e.g., Lippke et al., 2012; Owen et al., 2010). Some of these actions are intentional (e.g., indulgence as part of a celebration), but many are unintentional (e.g., people are more sedentary than they would like). Thus, it is clear that intentions do not always translate into action (Sheeran & Webb, 2016; Webb & Sheeran, 2006). One key challenge is that the (health) benefits of behaviours such as physical activity and a healthy diet only accrue in the long term, and engaging in these behaviours may be unappealing in the moment (e.g., they have short-term costs, such as requiring effort). In contrast, behaviours that can damage health in the long term (e.g., consumption of fried food) are often rewarding in the short term (e.g., fried food tastes good). In this sense, striving to reach health goals is the quintessential self-regulation task.

Self-regulation is "the general process by which people adopt and manage various goals and standards for their thoughts, feelings, and behaviour, and then ensure that these goals and standards are met" (p. 353; Fujita, 2011). The focus of this chapter is primarily on the volitional aspect of self-regulation—that is, the process of translating intentions, once decided upon, into action. This is because we are interested in understanding how people respond to setbacks, lapses, and failures, which are usually defined with respect to a goal. For example, if someone intends to cook at home during the week but orders a takeaway on Thursday, then this would be deemed a lapse with respect to the goal. However, if someone did not have the goal to cook at home, then ordering a takeaway would not be considered a lapse (assuming that doing so was not inconsistent with other goals, such as to save money or avoid fried food). In short, because lapses are only construed as such if they reflect responses and behaviours that are inconsistent with achieving a desired outcome, how people respond to such lapses reflects a volitional process.

What Is Self-Compassion?

Current theory and research provide different conceptualisations of self-compassion. For example, Gilbert (2019) describes self-compassion in the context of compassion more generally. For Gilbert, compassion is viewed as flowing from self to others, others to self, and self to self, with the latter flow of compassion reflecting self-compassion. The definition that is more prevalent in research examining the associations between self-compassion and health-related outcomes is that of Neff (2003). According to this definition, self-compassion involves taking a kind, non-judgmental, and accepting stance towards oneself in the face of perceived failures or difficulties. In particular, self-compassion involves six key components organised along three bipolar dimensions. First, self-kindness versus self-judgement, which refers to responding to difficulties and personal weaknesses with understanding and acceptance, instead of self-criticism and self-blame. Second, common humanity versus isolation, which refers to the recognition that all people experience difficulties and make mistakes, instead of viewing difficulties and shortcomings as unique, and thus feeling isolated. Third, mindfulness versus over-identification, which refers to being aware of one's current emotional state and suffering without becoming over-identified with the negative feelings that derive from experiencing a difficult situation. Together these three bipolar dimensions of self-compassion are posited to operate synergistically to provide an alternative response to challenges that can help reduce negative emotions and enhance well-being (Neff, 2003).

Particularly relevant for our discussion of the implications of self-compassion for health behaviour is that self-compassion can be viewed as falling along a continuum from an enduring tendency to a momentary way of responding to difficulties and challenges. The dispositional or "trait" form of self-compassion, as it is often referred to, reflects a relatively stable capacity to respond to difficulties and personal shortcomings in the characteristic accepting, connected, and mindful ways. This generalised tendency can become the default response to facing setbacks and lapses across a variety of settings. In contrast, the momentary or "state" form of self-compassion refers to responding with self-compassion to a specific difficulty or challenging situation.

Before discussing how self-compassion may facilitate health behaviour, it is worth clarifying some common misconceptions, which often distort people's understanding of the nature of self-compassion (Neff, 2015). For example, self-compassion is often considered as being synonymous with self-pity. Although self-pity and self-compassion both reflect ways of responding to personal suffering, they are distinct in the sense that self-pity involves exaggerating personal suffering and the associated negative feelings as well as forgetting that others face similar, or perhaps worse, difficulties (Stöber, 2003). In contrast, self-compassion involves accepting a difficulty as it is and viewing it as part of life that others may experience too (Neff, 2003). People may view self-compassion as taking an overly self-centred stance, and so it is also sometimes confused with narcissism, despite research showing no link between narcissism and self-compassion (Neff, 2011; Neff & Vonk, 2009). While narcissism emphasises on maintaining a positive and inflated self-view (Morf & Rhodewalt, 2001), self-compassion involves accepting and embracing a personal inadequacy or weakness.

Perhaps one of the most common misconceptions is between self-compassion and complacency. That is, people often believe that being kind towards themselves when facing a difficulty, instead of being self-critical, will undermine their motivation to push themselves to do better and successfully pursue their goals (Bayir & Lomas, 2016; Kelly et al., 2021). However, people with higher levels of self-compassion may view a challenge in pursuing a health goal less negatively, because they realise that everyone encounters such lapses (common humanity) and, thus, do not become overly self-critical (self-kindness) or embroiled in self-directed negative feelings (mindfulness). Indeed, evidence supports this proposition (e.g., Breines & Chen, 2012; Chwyl et al., 2021; Hope et al., 2014; Miyagawa et al., 2018; Moffitt et al., 2018; Neely et al., 2009; Zhang & Chen, 2016, 2017). For example, Miyagawa et al. (2018) found that people high in trait levels of self-compassion are more likely to disengage from unattained goals and re-engage in alternative meaningful goals. In a more stringent test, Breines and Chen (2012) conducted a series of experiments and found that self-compassion fostered motivation to improve oneself following identification of a personal weakness, increased studying time following failure on an academic test, and raised a desire to make amends after reflecting on a moral transgression.

Current Evidence on Self-Compassion and Health Behaviours

The growing interest in the implications of self-compassion for health has led to a number of studies investigating whether, how, and why self-compassion is linked to various health behaviours. Research and theory tend to differentiate health behaviours based on whether they refer to health-promoting behaviours, that is, behaviours that maintain or promote health (e.g., healthy eating, regular exercise, adherence to medical regimens), or health-risk behaviours, that is behaviours that increase the risk of negative health outcomes (e.g., smoking, excessive alcohol use, substance use; Lippke et al., 2012; Vickers et al., 1990). Evidence indicates that self-compassion is associated with the two classes of health behaviours in different ways.

With respect to health-promoting behaviours, research has shown that self-compassion fosters various health-promoting behaviours. For example, a meta-analysis of 15 student and community samples demonstrated that trait levels of self-compassion were positively linked to healthy eating and sleeping habits, regular exercise, and stress management (Sirois et al., 2015). Another meta-analysis of 25 studies showed that both dispositional and induced self-compassion predicted greater engagement in physical activity (Wong et al., 2021), with additional evidence indicating that self-compassionate people are more likely to exercise for intrinsic, rather than extrinsic, reasons (Magnus et al., 2010; Mosewich et al., 2011). People who are self-compassionate also tend to be more proactive about their health, seek medical advice sooner, and exert greater effort to follow the recommendations of their doctors when they identify a health problem (Terry et al., 2013).

Self-compassion is also linked to engaging in fewer health-risk behaviours. For example, a systematic review of 28 studies showed that dispositional and induced self-compassion predicted greater satisfaction with body image, lower body mass index, and less eating disorder symptomatology (e.g., weight and eating concerns, restrictive eating, binge eating; Braun et al., 2016). Additionally, evidence from a study of smokers who were trying to quit showed that a 3-week self-compassion intervention, in which participants were asked to engage in self-compassionate imagery and self-talk at every urge to smoke, reduced daily consumption of cigarettes (Kelly et al., 2010). Studies examining other health-risk behaviours have found similar findings, with higher levels of self-compassion linked to fewer alcohol-related problems and fewer sexual risk behaviours (Dawson Rose et al., 2014; Phelps et al., 2018; Wisener & Khoury, 2019, 2020).

There is also evidence that self-compassion is associated with a broad array of disease management behaviours, which are central for managing symptoms and minimising the risk of disease progression or complications. For example, Sirois and Hirsch (2019) found that higher levels of self-compassion were related to better adherence to physician recommendations across five different samples of people with cancer, chronic fatigue syndrome, and fibromyalgia. The benefits of self-compassion for adherence have also been tested longitudinally. Specifically, Dowd and Jung (2017) investigated the link between self-compassion and dietary adherence for people with coeliac disease over time. Lifelong adherence to a strict gluten-free diet is the only available and effective treatment for people with celiac disease. They assessed trait levels of self-compassion at baseline and dietary adherence 1 month later, finding that self-compassion predicted stricter adherence to a gluten-free diet.

In addition to this correlational research, evidence to date suggests a promising role for self-compassion as a tool for supporting health behaviour change. For example, two recent systematic reviews assessed the effectiveness of interventions designed to cultivate a self-compassionate mindset on eating-related outcomes. These reviews demonstrated that self-compassion interventions had a positive impact on body image, eating pathology, nutrition behaviours, and weight loss for normal-weight or overweight people (Brenton-Peters et al., 2021; Rahimi-Ardabili et al., 2018). Relatedly, an intervention study found that participants who attended a 1-week mindfulness and self-compassion programme exhibited higher levels of perceived health as well as lower stress and improved immune system functioning, as assessed by physiological measures (Bellosta-Batalla et al., 2018).

In a similar vein, a systematic review of seven studies examined the effectiveness of self-compassion interventions versus traditional interventions on health behaviours (Biber & Ellis, 2019). In all seven studies, self-compassion interventions had a positive impact on health behaviours such as physical activity, eating disorder symptomatology, smoking cessation, and self-care behaviours across samples of students, community adults, and people with eating disorders. Importantly, the results from three of these studies further showed that self-compassion interventions were as—or more—effective than other well-established behavioural interventions. For example, one study compared the effects of a 3-week self-compassion intervention to behavioural intervention on eating disorder pathology (Kelly & Carter, 2015). Both interventions led to fewer binge days, but those who received the self-compassion intervention exhibited less general eating disorder pathology as well as weight and eating concerns compared to those who received the behavioural intervention. Another study compared the effects of a 3-week self-compassion intervention to self-monitoring intervention on smoking cessation (Kelly et al., 2010). Self-monitoring has been found to be effective in smoking cessation programmes (Edmunds et al., 1991), yet participants who received the self-compassion intervention reported reducing their daily consumption of cigarettes more rapidly than those who received the self-monitoring intervention. Overall, this evidence suggests that self-compassion interventions can be at least as effective as other well-established interventions targeting health behaviours.

Taken together, it is clear that responding with self-compassion supports patterns of behaviour that benefit people's health. Current research indicates that those who respond with self-compassion are more likely to engage in health-promoting behaviours, less likely to engage in health-risk behaviours, and better able to manage their health problems. The obvious question, then, is why? Why does responding with self-compassion help people to behave in ways that benefit their health? This is an important question to be addressed for both theoretical and practical reasons. For example, self-compassion interventions may also affect intermediate health-related outcomes, such as efficacy beliefs and psychological distress, in addition to health behaviours. In the next section, we explore the idea that self-compassion helps people to regulate their emotions—particularly, in response to difficulties when striving for a goal—and therefore enables people to stay on track.

Emotion Regulation and Health Behaviours

Striving for health goals requires continued efforts on a long-term basis, with the consequence that people inevitably encounter lapses (e.g., overindulging in food when intending to lose weight). As such, people often end up abandoning their health goals, mainly because of their emotional responses to these lapses (Sirois & Giguère, 2018). That is, people typically respond with self-criticism and self-blame to these lapses, which can increase shame, guilt, and overall distress (e.g., Powers et al., 2007, 2012). These negative feelings can, in turn, impair self-regulation because the person's focus shifts to how to alleviate or diminish these negative feelings in order to feel good in the present—something that is potentially at the expense of making progress towards their longer-term health goals (Sirois & Pychyl, 2013; Tice et al., 2001; Wagner & Heatherton, 2015).

In line with these propositions, accumulating evidence highlights the important role of affect in health behaviours. For example, negative affect is associated with engaging in harmful cardiovascular-related health behaviours, such as unhealthy diet, smoking, and low physical activity (Kiecolt-Glaser et al., 2002). Furthermore, daily diary studies found that people are more likely to engage in binge drinking on days when they experience stressful events and feel distressed (Armeli et al., 2000; Carney et al., 2000; Grzywacz & Almeida, 2008). Studies on substance use have also shown that experiencing negative life events may predict relapses in smoking and drinking alcohol (Sinha, 2007; Shiffman & Waters, 2004; Witkiewitz & Villarroel, 2009). Additionally, longitudinal research has demonstrated links between positive affect and engaging in physical activity, as well as medication adherence in patients with coronary patients over a 5-year period (Sin et al., 2015).

Together, this evidence highlights the value of the capacity to regulate emotions for supporting health-promoting behaviours and discouraging health-risk behaviours. According to the process model of emotion regulation (Gross, 1998, 2014), emotion regulation refers to how people influence the specific emotions that they have, when they have them, and how they experience and/or express them. Adaptive emotion regulation strategies, such as changing the meaning of a situation to modify its emotional impact (i.e., cognitive reappraisal), involve down-regulating negative emotions and up-regulating positive emotions. In the context of health, emotion regulation strategies that diminish negative emotional responses to lapses in pursuing a health behaviour and promote overall positive feelings have the potential to help people to overcome these lapses and successfully pursue their health goals.

Self-Compassion and Emotion Regulation

Some theorists have posited that self-compassion can promote adaptive emotion regulation (Finlay-Jones et al., 2015; Sirois et al., 2015; Sirois & Hirsch, 2019), whilst others have conceptualised self-compassion as an emotion regulation strategy that is similar to cognitive reappraisal (Diedrich et al., 2014). However, as Finlay-Jones et al. (2015) have argued, self-compassion focuses on the implications of the situation for the self rather than exclusively on emotions, with the latter being a hallmark of emotion regulation. Thus, although self-compassion may promote adaptive emotion regulation, it is not synonymous with this process—responding to health lapses with self-kindness, accepting them as a normal part of engaging in health behaviours, and taking a balanced view of the lapses in the context of making progress can reduce negative emotions and increase positive feelings, but it is the process of relating to oneself in a kinder, more connected, and mindful manner that leads to healthier emotion regulation.

A large body of research supports the view that self-compassion promotes adaptive emotional responses. For example, systematic reviews of studies assessing the link between self-compassion and well-being have found that self-compassion predicts lower levels of negative emotions such as anger, anxiety, and negative affect, as well as higher levels of positive emotions such as optimism, happiness, and positive affect (Barnard & Curry, 2011; Zessin et al., 2015). Relatedly, self-compassion has been associated with lower levels of negative affect in the face of everyday difficult events and reduces negative emotional responses to distressing situations involving embarrassment and personal failure (Leary et al., 2007; see also Diedrich et al., 2014; Odou & Brinker, 2015). The aforementioned findings are consistent with those of studies that used physiological measures to assess whether self-compassion supports adaptive emotion regulation. In particular, trait levels of self-compassion have been associated with higher vagally mediated heart rate variability (vmHRV), which is an index of healthy heart function and adaptive emotion regulation (Appelhans & Luecken, 2006), and brief training in self-compassion has been found to result in smaller decreases in vmHRV following an exposure to a psychological stressor (Arch et al., 2014; Svendsen et al., 2016).

Self-compassion also appears to support adaptive emotion regulation in the health domain. For example, two meta-analyses of studies examining the relations between self-compassion and health-related outcomes found that self-compassion promotes health-promoting behaviours and health management behaviours, partly because it is associated with lower levels of negative affect and perceived stress as well as higher levels of positive affect (Sirois et al., 2015; Sirois & Hirsch, 2019). Relatedly, Friis et al. (2017) examined how instructions to respond with self-compassion or self-criticism affected mood following a manipulated failure to engage in a health behaviour (in this case, teeth flossing). They found that participants who responded to the failure with self-compassion showed lower levels of negative affect and greater positive affect. In contrast, those who responded to the failure with self-criticism reported greater negative affect and lower levels of positive affect.

Self-Compassion as a Self-Regulation Resource

Given that self-compassion can support adaptive emotion regulation, some researchers have proposed that self-compassion may serve as a self-regulation resource that facilitates engaging in health-promoting behaviours (Sirois, 2015a; Sirois et al., 2015). Specifically, the link between self-compassion and health behaviours has been viewed through the lens of the Temporal-Affective Self-Regulation Resource Model (TASRR; Sirois, 2015a, b; Sirois & Hirsch, 2015). According to the TASRR, qualities and traits that are associated with higher levels of positive affect and future-oriented thinking, and lower levels of negative affect, will promote the self-regulation of health behaviours. In other words, health behaviours are supported when there is a healthy affective balance.

Research to date provides some support for the idea that self-compassion serves as a resource for self-regulation. For example, in a study of undergraduate students, the link between self-compassion and stronger intentions to engage in health behaviours was explained in part by lower levels of negative affect, even after accounting for current levels of health behaviours and body mass index (Sirois, 2015a). Similarly, a study of mothers with young children found that higher levels of self-compassion were associated with lower levels of guilt regarding taking the time to engage in health-promoting behaviours (Miller & Strachan, 2020). Importantly, lower levels of guilt accounted for the mothers' more frequent practice of health behaviours.

There is also research testing the links between self-compassion and affective balance in relation to health behaviours. In the meta-analysis of 15 samples presented previously (Sirois et al., 2015), additional analyses were conducted with eight data sets that included a measure of positive and negative affect. In each of the eight samples, higher positive affect and lower negative affect partly explained the association between self-compassion and more frequent health-promoting behaviours. When considered in the context of theory and evidence on the role of emotions in health behaviours, these cross-sectional findings provide preliminary support for a self-regulation resource explanation of how self-compassion can support health behaviours. Examining these associations over time would provide further and more rigorous support. For example, it is possible that self-compassion and health behaviours are reciprocally and dynamically related with self-compassion, potentially increasing in response to increased practice of health behaviours, which could be viewed as a way of expressing kindness to oneself.

Barriers to Responding with Self-Compassion

The theory and evidence presented thus far shows a promising role for self-compassion in supporting people in their efforts to change and maintain health behaviours. By providing an alternative, more adaptive response to inevitable lapses encountered when striving for health goals, self-compassion can help people to manage the negative emotions that can derail self-regulation of health behaviours and provide a resource for maintaining changes. Yet, despite this promise, an emerging body of research suggests that responding with self-compassion may be challenging for some individuals. For example, prior work suggests that some people are not aware of the concept of self-compassion (Campion et al., 2017; Kelly et al., 2021). Others may be familiar with the concept but believe that responding with self-compassion will lower their personal standards, undermine their personal growth and development, and thus mean that they fail to accomplish their goals (Kelly et al., 2021). Furthermore, some people may associate self-compassionate responding with negative attributes (e.g., weakness, selfishness, or self-indulgence), poor performance, and/or as going against their cultural norms or family expectations (Bayir & Lomas, 2016; Campion & Glover, 2017; Gilbert et al., 2011; Kelly et al., 2021; Robinson et al., 2016; Simpson et al., 2021). Even if people like the idea of being self-compassionate, they may nonetheless find it challenging because they lack confidence in their ability to be self-compassionate (Campion & Glover, 2017; Kelly et al., 2021; Pauley & McPherson, 2010). Finally, some people tend, or even prefer, to respond with self-criticism when they experience difficulties (Bayir & Lomas, 2016; Kelly et al., 2021; Tobin & Dunkley, 2021), despite its detrimental effects on goal pursuit (e.g., Powers et al., 2007, 2012).

To better understand the difficulties that many people encounter when responding with self-compassion, we suggest that responding with self-compassion can be viewed as a behaviour, much like phoning a friend or going for a walk. Doing so provides an opportunity to apply classic health behaviour change theories and models to better understand when and why someone may or may not respond to lapses with self-compassion. In particular, we propose that taking action control perspective (Webb et al., 2012) may provide valuable insights for dealing with difficulties in responding with self-compassion. This view suggests that responding with self-compassion involves distinct tasks, including (i) seeing a need to change, (ii) deciding how to change, and (iii) enacting change. A similar perspective has been applied to understand the challenges that people experience in regulating their emotions (Sirois & Giguère, 2018; Webb et al., 2012). Accordingly, we propose that people may not respond with self-compassion to lapses in goal pursuit because they: (i) do not see the need to change how they respond to lapses, (ii) are unwilling to respond to lapses with self-compassion, and/or (iii) are prepared to believe that self-compassion may be effective and are willing to respond in this way, but struggle to actually be self-compassionate in the critical moment.

Following this approach, we posited that social cognition models, such as the Theory of Planned Behaviour (Ajzen, 1991) and the Prototype Willingness Model (Gibbons et al., 1998, 2009), could explain why some people struggle to respond with self-compassion. Social cognition models propose that behaviour is often a function of people's beliefs—or thoughts and feelings—about that behaviour. For example, the Theory of Planned Behaviour suggests that positive attitudes (e.g., responding with self-compassion would be worthwhile), norms (e.g., those important to me would want me to respond with self-compassion), and control beliefs (e.g., I feel capable of responding with self-compassion) lead people to intend to engage in the respective behaviour (e.g., I intend to respond with self-compassion). The strength of these intentions then predicts the likelihood of behaviour (i.e., whether people will respond with self-compassion), assuming that they have the opportunity to do so in the relevant context (i.e., they have actual control over the behaviour). However, if attitudinal, normative, or control beliefs are more negative, then the person is less likely to intend to engage in the behaviour and, subsequently, to do so. Social cognition models therefore have the potential to help understand why some people are not willing to respond with self-compassion.

To test this proposition, we recently conducted a large-scale prospective study consisting of two-time points (Biskas et al., 2022). At time 1, we assessed participants' attitudes towards self-compassion as well as their normative and control beliefs about self-compassion. Next, we instructed participants to write about a lapse that they experienced in pursuing a personal goal and subsequently indicate their willingness to respond with self-compassion to the lapse before prompting them to respond so. Afterwards, we assessed whether they actually responded self-compassionately and then their willingness to respond self-compassionately in future lapses in pursuing their goal. At time 2, 2 weeks later, we assessed whether they responded with self-compassion to lapses that they faced during the follow-up period. The results demonstrated that participants who had more positive attitudes towards self-compassion as well as normative and control beliefs about self-compassion were more willing to respond with self-compassion to both a recalled and future lapse and, in turn, more likely to actually respond self-compassionately to these lapses. Taken together, these findings provide evidence that social cognition models, such as the Theory of Planned Behaviour, can predict whether people respond with self-compassion to lapses and difficulties.

One key challenge for social cognition models is that, while behaviour may sometimes be driven by intentions (e.g., someone decides to try to respond with self-compassion), intentions do not always translate into action (Sheeran & Webb, 2016; Webb & Sheeran, 2006); for example, someone finds themselves defaulting back to a self-critical way of thinking. Therefore, our action control perspective on self-compassion is also clear that, while people may believe that self-compassion could be effective and intend to respond in this way, they may still struggle to actually be self-compassionate in the critical moment. In other words, they have a problem with enactment. Therefore, in the study presented previously (Biskas et al., 2022), we also measured the extent to which participants experienced difficulties enacting self-compassion (e.g., "My critical inner voice gets in the way of seeing experiencing difficulties as part of being human") and found that enactment difficulties independently predicted whether or not participants responded with self-compassion to lapses in goal pursuit.

In the same study, we also found evidence that certain individuals are more likely to hold negative beliefs about self-compassion and, therefore, have difficulty being self-compassionate. Perfectionistic concerns are a broad dimension of perfectionism that is characterised by unrealistically high expectations, chronic and harsh self-scrutiny, and an excessive preoccupation with the expectations, criticism, and evaluations that they perceive others have of them (Sirois & Molnar, 2016). Research has demonstrated that those high in perfectionistic concerns tend to also score lower on measures of dispositional self-compassion (e.g., Stoeber et al., 2020; Tobin & Dunkley, 2021). In line with this research, our study (Biskas et al., 2022) indicated that those high in perfectionistic concerns were less likely to respond self-compassionately to a goal lapse (low enactment), and that negative beliefs about self-compassion explained in part this difficulty (Biskas et al., 2022). Relevant to our discussion of self-compassion and health behaviour lapses, when we conducted additional analyses examining only lapses to health goals, the same pattern of results emerged (Sirois et al., 2022). These findings highlight that responding with self-compassion to health goal lapses may be particularly difficult for individuals who hold negative beliefs about self-compassion, and that certain personality traits characterised by self-criticism may provide useful indicators of who is more likely to hold such beliefs.

Implications of Self-Compassion for Health Behaviour Change: Some Caveats

Understanding the barriers to being self-compassionate can both support and inform interventions designed to increase self-compassion for the purpose of health behaviour change. For example, the demonstrated effectiveness of self-compassion interventions for health behaviour change (e.g., Biber & Ellis, 2019) could be further enhanced by addressing the barriers to being self-compassionate prior to or as an adjunct to the delivery of such interventions. Specifically, the barriers can serve as targets for interventions (e.g., an intervention might try to make it easier for people who appreciate the potential value of self-compassion to enact the intended response). Moreover, understanding who is likely to encounter particular barriers (e.g., people high in perfectionistic concerns may have negative attitudes towards self-compassion) can help to target interventions towards those most likely to benefit. In the absence of taking into consideration the barriers to being self-compassionate, the effectiveness of self-compassion interventions may be underestimated, as not everyone will respond favourably to self-compassion training, prompts, or other instructions aimed at enhancing people's capacity to be self-compassionate in the face of health goal failures and lapses. This can have important implications for clinical applications, feasibility trials, and research on the role of self-compassion in health contexts more generally.

In summary, some people who could benefit from receiving a self-compassion intervention (including those who potentially have the most to gain, as they typically respond in a highly critical fashion) may struggle to respond to the intervention. The current chapter proposes an action control perspective (Sirois & Giguère, 2018; Webb et al., 2012) which suggests that this struggle may occur because people (i) do not recognise the need to respond with self-compassion, (ii) hold negative beliefs about being self-compassionate, which mean that they are unwilling to respond in this way, and/or (iii) experience difficulties enacting self-compassion when facing a difficult time. Developing strategies to address these barriers and incorporating them in existing or new self-compassion interventions could lead to significant improvements in the delivery and effectiveness of interventions aimed at increasing self-compassion and thus help more people to harvest the benefits of self-compassion for improving health behaviours.

Conclusions

The way that people respond to lapses and setbacks that they inevitably face in pursuing a health goal plays a crucial role in their efforts to make and maintain changes in their health behaviours. The evidence reviewed in this chapter indicated that responding with self-compassion, instead of self-criticism, facilitates positive changes in health behaviours by promoting adaptive emotional responses to lapses. Despite emerging evidence demonstrating the benefits of self-compassion interventions for health behaviours, responding with self-compassion can be challenging for some people. We therefore introduced a theoretical framework for understanding the potential barriers to being self-compassionate and how they might be addressed. Considering and addressing these barriers is particularly important for future self-compassion interventions in order to optimise their effectiveness in cultivating a self-compassionate mindset and thus promoting healthy behaviours.

References

Ajzen, I. (1991). The theory of planned behavior. *Organizational Behavior and Human Decision Processes, 50*(2), 179–211. https://doi.org/10.1016/0749-5978(91)90020-T

Appelhans, B. M., & Luecken, L. J. (2006). Heart rate variability as an index of regulated emotional responding. *Review of General Psychology, 10*(3), 229–240. https://doi.org/10.1037/1089-2680.10.3.229

Arch, J. J., Brown, K. W., Dean, D. J., Landy, L. N., Brown, K. D., & Laudenslager, M. L. (2014). Self-compassion training modulates alpha-amylase, heart rate variability, and subjective responses to social evaluative threat in women. *Psychoneuroendocrinology, 42,* 49–58. https://doi.org/10.1016/j.psyneuen.2013.12.018

Armeli, S., Tennen, H., Affleck, G., & Kranzler, H. R. (2000). Does affect mediate the association between daily events and alcohol use? *Journal of Studies on Alcohol, 61*(6), 862–871. https://doi.org/10.15288/jsa.2000.61.862

Baird, H. M., Webb, T. L., Sirois, F. M., & Gibson-Miller, J. (2021). Understanding the effects of time perspective: A meta-analysis testing a self-regulatory framework. *Psychological Bulletin, 147*(3), 233–267. https://doi.org/10.1037/bul0000313

Barnard, L. K., & Curry, J. F. (2011). Self-compassion: Conceptualizations, correlates, & interventions. *Review of General Psychology, 15*(4), 289–303. https://doi.org/10.1037/a0025754

Bayir, A., & Lomas, T. (2016). Difficulties generating self-compassion: An interpretative phenomenological analysis. *The Journal of Happiness & Well-Being, 4*(1), 15–33.

Bellosta-Batalla, M., Ruiz-Robledillo, N., Sariñana-González, P., Capella-Solano, T., Vitoria-Estruch, S., Hidalgo-Moreno, G., et al. (2018). Increased salivary IgA response as an indicator of immunocompetence after a mindfulness and self-compassion-based intervention. *Mindfulness, 9*(3), 905–913. https://doi.org/10.1007/s12671-017-0830-y

Biber, D. D., & Ellis, R. (2019). The effect of self-compassion on the self-regulation of health behaviors: A systematic review. *Journal of Health Psychology, 24*(14), 2060–2071. https://doi.org/10.1177/1359105317713361

Biskas, M., Sirois, F. M., & Webb, T. L. (2022). Using social cognition models to understand why people, such as perfectionists, struggle to respond with self-compassion. *British Journal of Social Psychology, 61*(4), 1160–1182. https://doi.org/10.1111/bjso.12531

Braun, T. D., Park, C. L., & Gorin, A. (2016). Self-compassion, body image, and disordered eating: A review of the literature. *Body Image, 17*, 117–131. https://doi.org/10.1016/j.bodyim.2016.03.003

Breines, J. G., & Chen, S. (2012). Self-compassion increases self-improvement motivation. *Personality and Social Psychology Bulletin, 38*(9), 1133–1143. https://doi.org/10.1177/0146167212445599

Brenton-Peters, J., Consedine, N. S., Boggiss, A., Wallace-Boyd, K., Roy, R., & Serlachius, A. (2021). Self-compassion in weight management: A systematic review. *Journal of Psychosomatic Research, 150*, 110617. https://doi.org/10.1016/j.jpsychores.2021.110617

Campion, M., & Glover, L. (2017). A qualitative exploration of responses to self-compassion in a non-clinical sample. *Health & Social Care in the Community, 25*(3), 1100–1108. https://doi.org/10.1111/hsc.12408

Carney, M. A., Armeli, S., Tennen, H., Affleck, G., & O'Neil, T. P. (2000). Positive and negative daily events, perceived stress, and alcohol use: A diary study. *Journal of Consulting and Clinical Psychology, 68*(5), 788–798. https://doi.org/10.1037/0022-006X.68.5.788

Chwyl, C., Chen, P., & Zaki, J. (2021). Beliefs About Self-Compassion: Implications for Coping and Self-Improvement. *Personality and Social Psychology Bulletin, 47*(9), 1327–1342. https://doi.org/10.1177/0146167220965303

Dawson Rose, C., Webel, A., Sullivan, K. M., Cuca, Y. P., Wantland, D., Johnson, M. O., et al. (2014). Self-compassion and risk behavior among people living with HIV/AIDS. *Research in Nursing & Health, 37*(2), 98–106. https://doi.org/10.1002/nur.21587

Dickson, D. J., & Shulman, S. (2016). Directions of effects between self-criticism and parental support on adaptive goal pursuit among emerging adults. *Personality and Individual Differences, 101*, 327–332. https://doi.org/10.1016/j.paid.2016.06.018

Diedrich, A., Grant, M., Hofmann, S. G., Hiller, W., & Berking, M. (2014). Self-compassion as an emotion regulation strategy in major depressive disorder. *Behaviour Research and Therapy, 58*, 43–51. https://doi.org/10.1016/j.brat.2014.05.006

Dowd, A. J., & Jung, M. E. (2017). Self-compassion directly and indirectly predicts dietary adherence and quality of life among adults with celiac disease. *Appetite, 113*, 293–300. https://doi.org/10.1016/j.appet.2017.02.023

Duarte, C., Matos, M., Stubbs, R. J., Gale, C., Morris, L., Gouveia, J. P., & Gilbert, P. (2017). The impact of shame, self-criticism and social rank on eating behaviours in overweight and obese women participating in a Weight Management Programme. *PloS one, 12*(1), e0167571. https://doi.org/10.1371/journal.pone.0167571

Edmunds, M., Conner, H., Jones, C., Gorayeb, R., & Waranch, H. R. (1991). Evaluation of a multicomponent group smoking cessation program. *Preventive Medicine, 20*(3), 404–413. https://doi.org/10.1016/0091-7435(91)90038-6

Finlay-Jones, A. L., Rees, C. S., & Kane, R. T. (2015). Self-Compassion, Emotion Regulation and Stress among Australian Psychologists: Testing an Emotion Regulation Model of Self-Compassion Using Structural Equation Modeling. *PloS one, 10*(7), e0133481. https://doi.org/10.1371/journal.pone.0133481

Friis, A. M., Johnson, M. H., & Consedine, N. S. (2017). Paradoxical effects of self-compassion on mood and teeth flossing behavior in an experimental setting. *Mindfulness, 8*(1), 150–158. https://doi.org/10.1007/s12671-016-0585-x

Fujita, K. (2011). On conceptualizing self-control as more than the effortful inhibition of impulses. *Personality and Social Psychology Review, 15*(4), 352–366. https://doi.org/10.1177/1088868311411165

Gardner, B. (2015). A review and analysis of the use of 'habit' in understanding, predicting and influencing health-related behaviour. *Health Psychology Review, 9*(3), 277–295. https://doi.org/10.1080/17437199.2013.876238

Gibbons, F. X., Gerrard, M., Blanton, H., & Russell, D. W. (1998). Reasoned action and social reaction: Willingness and intention as independent predictors of health risk. *Journal of Personality and Social Psychology, 74*(5), 1164–1180. https://doi.org/10.1037/0022-3514.74.5.1164

Gibbons, F. X., Houlihan, A. E., & Gerrard, M. (2009). Reason and reaction: The utility of a dual-focus, dual-processing perspective on promotion and prevention of adolescent health risk behaviour. *British Journal of Health Psychology, 14*(2), 231–248. https://doi.org/10.1348/135910708X376640

Gilbert, P. (2019). Explorations into the nature and function of compassion. *Current Opinion in Psychology, 28*, 108–114. https://doi.org/10.1016/j.copsyc.2018.12.002

Gilbert, P., McEwan, K., Matos, M., & Rivis, A. (2011). Fears of compassion: Development of three self-report measures. *Psychology and Psychotherapy: Theory, Research and Practice, 84*(3), 239–255. https://doi.org/10.1348/147608310X526511

Gross, J. J. (1998). The Emerging Field of Emotion Regulation: An Integrative Review. *Review of General Psychology, 2*(3), 271–299. https://doi.org/10.1037/1089-2680.2.3.271

Gross, J. J. (2014). Emotion regulation: Conceptual and empirical foundations. In J. J. Gross (Ed.), *Handbook of emotion regulation* (pp. 3–20). The Guilford Press.

Grzywacz, J. G., & Almeida, D. M. (2008). Stress and binge drinking: A daily process examination of stressor pile-up and socioeconomic status in affect regulation. *International Journal of Stress Management, 15*(4), 364–380. https://doi.org/10.1037/a0013368

Hardcastle, S. J., Hancox, J., Hattar, A., Maxwell-Smith, C., Thøgersen-Ntoumani, C., & Hagger, M. S. (2015). Motivating the unmotivated: How can health behavior be changed in those unwilling to change? *Frontiers in Psychology, 6*, 835. https://doi.org/10.3389/fpsyg.2015.00835

Harkin, B., Webb, T. L., Chang, B. P., Prestwich, A., Conner, M., Kellar, I., et al. (2016). Does monitoring goal progress promote goal attainment? A meta-analysis of the experimental evidence. *Psychological Bulletin, 142*(2), 198–229. https://doi.org/10.1037/bul0000025

Hope, N., Koestner, R., & Milyavskaya, M. (2014). The role of self-compassion in goal pursuit and well-being among University Freshmen. *Self & Identity, 13*(5), 579–593. https://doi.org/10.1080/15298868.2014.889032

Kelly, A., Katan, A., Sosa Hernandez, L., Nightingale, B., & Geller, J. (2021). Why would I want to be more self-compassionate? A qualitative study of the pros and cons to cultivating self-compassion in individuals with anorexia nervosa. *British Journal of Clinical Psychology, 60*(1), 99–115. https://doi.org/10.1111/bjc.12275

Kelly, A. C., & Carter, J. C. (2015). Self-compassion training for binge eating disorder: A pilot randomized controlled trial. *Psychology and Psychotherapy: Theory, Research and Practice, 88*(3), 285–303. https://doi.org/10.1111/papt.12044

Kelly, A. C., Zuroff, D. C., Foa, C. L., & Gilbert, P. (2010). Who benefits from training in self-compassionate self-regulation? A study of smoking reduction. *Journal of Social and Clinical Psychology, 29*(7), 727–755. https://doi.org/10.1521/jscp.2010.29.7.727

Kiecolt-Glaser, J. K., McGuire, L., Robles, T. F., & Glaser, R. (2002). Psychoneuroimmunology: Psychological influences on immune function and health. *Journal of Consulting and Clinical Psychology, 70*(3), 537–547. https://doi.org/10.1037/0022-006X.70.3.537

Leary, M. R., Tate, E. B., Adams, C. E., Batts Allen, A., & Hancock, J. (2007). Self-compassion and reactions to unpleasant self-relevant events: The implications of treating oneself kindly. *Journal of Personality and Social Psychology, 92*(5), 887–904. https://doi.org/10.1037/0022-3514.92.5.887

Lippke, S., Nigg, C. R., & Maddock, J. E. (2012). Health-promoting and health-risk behaviors: Theory-driven analyses of multiple health behavior change in three international samples. *International Journal of Behavioral Medicine, 19*(1), 1–13. https://doi.org/10.1007/s12529-010-9135-4

Magnus, C. M., Kowalski, K. C., & McHugh, T. L. F. (2010). The role of self-compassion in women's self-determined motives to exercise and exercise-related outcomes. *Self and Identity, 9*(4), 363–382. https://doi.org/10.1080/15298860903135073

Miller, C. L., & Strachan, S. M. (2020). Understanding the role of mother guilt and self-compassion in health behaviors in mothers with young children. *Women & Health, 60*(7), 763–775. https://doi.org/10.1080/03630242.2020.1713966

Miyagawa, Y., Taniguchi, J., & Niiya, Y. (2018). Can self-compassion help people regulate unattained goals and emotional reactions toward setbacks? *Personality and Individual Differences, 134*, 239–244. https://doi.org/10.1016/j.paid.2018.06.029

Moffitt, R. L., Neumann, D. L., & Williamson, S. P. (2018). Comparing the efficacy of a brief self-esteem and self-compassion intervention for state body dissatisfaction and self-improvement motivation. *Body Image, 27*, 67–76. https://doi.org/10.1016/j.bodyim.2018.08.008

Morf, C. C., & Rhodewalt, F. (2001). Unraveling the paradoxes of narcissism: A dynamic self-regulatory processing model. *Psychological Inquiry, 12*(4), 177–196. https://doi.org/10.1207/S15327965PLI1204_1

Mosewich, A. D., Kowalski, K. C., Sabiston, C. M., Sedgwick, W. A., & Tracy, J. L. (2011). Self-compassion: A potential resource for young women athletes. *Journal of Sport and Exercise Psychology, 33*(1), 103–123. https://doi.org/10.1123/jsep.33.1.103

Neely, M. E., Schallert, D. L., Mohammed, S. S., Roberts, R. M., & Chen, Y. J. (2009). Self-kindness when facing stress: The role of self-compassion, goal regulation, and support in college students' well-being. *Motivation and Emotion, 33*(1), 88–97. https://doi.org/10.1007/s11031-008-9119-8

Neff, K. D. (2003). Self-compassion: An alternative conceptualization of a healthy attitude toward oneself. *Self and Identity, 2*(2), 85–101. https://doi.org/10.1080/15298860309032

Neff, K. D. (2011). Self-compassion, self-esteem, and well-being. *Social and Personality Psychology Compass, 5*(1), 1–12. https://doi.org/10.1111/j.1751-9004.2010.00330.x

Neff, K. D. (2015). The five myths of self-compassion. *Psychotherapy Networker, 39*(5), 30–35.

Neff, K. D., & Vonk, R. (2009). Self-compassion versus global self-esteem: Two different ways of relating to oneself. *Journal of Personality, 77*(1), 23–50. https://doi.org/10.1111/j.1467-6494.2008.00537.x

Odou, N., & Brinker, J. (2015). Self-compassion, a better alternative to rumination than distraction as a response to negative mood. *The Journal of Positive Psychology, 10*(5), 447–457. https://doi.org/10.1080/17439760.2014.967800

Owen, N., Sparling, P. B., Healy, G. N., Dunstan, D. W., & Matthews, C. E. (2010). Sedentary behavior: Emerging evidence for a new health risk. *Mayo Clinic Proceedings, 85*(12), 1138–1141.·https://doi.org/10.4065/mcp.2010.0444

Pauley, G., & McPherson, S. (2010). The experience and meaning of compassion and self-compassion for individuals with depression or anxiety. *Psychology and Psychotherapy: Theory, Research and Practice, 83*(2), 129–143. https://doi.org/10.1348/147608309X471000

Phelps, C. L., Paniagua, S. M., Willcockson, I. U., & Potter, J. S. (2018). The relationship between self-compassion and the risk for substance use disorder. *Drug and Alcohol Dependence, 183*, 78–81. https://doi.org/10.1016/j.drugalcdep.2017.10.026

Powers, T. A., Koestner, R., & Zuroff, D. C. (2007). Self–criticism, goal motivation, and goal progress. *Journal of Social and Clinical Psychology, 26*(7), 826–840. https://doi.org/10.1521/jscp.2007.26.7.826

Powers, T. A., Milyavskaya, M., & Koestner, R. (2012). Mediating the effects of self-criticism and self-oriented perfectionism on goal pursuit. *Personality and Individual Differences, 52*(7), 765–770. https://doi.org/10.1016/j.paid.2011.12.031

Rahimi-Ardabili, H., Reynolds, R., Vartanian, L. R., McLeod, L. V. D., & Zwar, N. (2018). A systematic review of the efficacy of interventions that aim to increase self-compassion on nutrition habits, eating behaviours, body weight and body image. *Mindfulness, 9*(2), 388–400. https://doi.org/10.1007/s12671-017-0804-0

Robinson, K. J., Mayer, S., Allen, A. B., Terry, M., Chilton, A., & Leary, M. R. (2016). Resisting self-compassion: Why are some people opposed to being kind to themselves? *Self and Identity, 15*(5), 505–524. https://doi.org/10.1080/15298868.2016.1160952

Sheeran, P., Aarts, H., Custers, R., Rivis, A., Webb, T. L., & Cooke, R. (2005). The goal-dependent automaticity of drinking habits. *British Journal of Social Psychology, 44*, 47–64. https://doi.org/10.1348/014466604X23446

Sheeran, P., & Webb, T. L. (2016). The intention-behavior gap. *Social and Personality Psychology Compass, 10*(9), 503–518. https://doi.org/10.1111/spc3.12265

Shiffman, S., & Waters, A. J. (2004). Negative affect and smoking lapses: A prospective analysis. *Journal of Consulting and Clinical Psychology, 72*(2), 192–201. https://doi.org/10.1037/0022-006X.72.2.192

Simpson, K. M., Semenchuk, B. N., & Strachan, S. M. (2021). Put MY mask on first: Mothers' reactions to prioritizing health behaviours as a function of self-compassion and fear of self-compassion. *Journal of Health Psychology, 27*(5), 1259–1266. https://doi.org/10.1177/1359105321995979

Sin, N. L., Moskowitz, J. T., & Whooley, M. A. (2015). Positive affect and health behaviors across 5 years in patients with coronary heart disease: The Heart and Soul Study. *Psychosomatic Medicine, 77*(9), 1058–1066. https://doi.org/10.1097/PSY.0000000000000238

Sinha, R. (2007). The role of stress in addiction relapse. *Current Psychiatry Reports, 9*(5), 388–395. https://doi.org/10.1007/s11920-007-0050-6

Sirois, F. M. (2015a). A self-regulation resource model of self-compassion and health behavior intentions in emerging adults. *Preventive Medicine Reports, 2*, 218–222. https://doi.org/10.1016/j.pmedr.2015.03.006

Sirois, F. M. (2015b). Perfectionism and health behaviors: a self-regulation resource perspective. In F. M. Sirois & D. S. Molnar (Eds.), *Perfectionism, health and well-being* (pp. 45–68). Cham: Springer.

Sirois, F. M., Biskas, M., & Webb, T. L. (2022, August). *Why do people struggle to be self-compassionate to health goal lapses? A social cognitive perspective.* Paper presented at the 36th Conference of the European Health Psychology Society, Bratislava, Slovakia.

Sirois, F. M., & Giguère, B. (2018). Giving in when feeling less good: Procrastination, action control, and social temptations. *British Journal of Social Psychology, 57*(2), 404–427. https://doi.org/10.1111/bjso.12243

Sirois, F. M., & Hirsch, J. K. (2015). Big five traits, affect balance and health behaviors: a self-regulation resource perspective. Personality and Individual Differences, 87, 59–64. https://doi.org/10.1016/j.paid.2015.07.031

Sirois, F. M., & Hirsch, J. K. (2019). Self-compassion and adherence in five medical samples: The role of stress. *Mindfulness, 10*(1), 46–54. https://doi.org/10.1007/s12671-018-0945-9

Sirois, F. M., Kitner, R., & Hirsch, J. K. (2015). Self-compassion, affect, and health-promoting behaviors. *Health Psychology, 34*(6), 661–669. https://doi.org/10.1037/hea0000158

Sirois, F. M., & Molnar, D. S. (2016). Conceptualizations of perfectionism, health, and well-being: An introductory overview. In F. M. Sirois & D. S. Molnar (Eds.), *Perfectionism, health and well-being* (pp. 45–68). Springer.

Sirois, F. M., & Pychyl, T. (2013). Procrastination and the priority of short-term mood regulation: Consequences for future self. *Social and Personality Psychology Compass, 7*(2), 115–127. https://doi.org/10.1111/spc3.12011

Stöber, J. (2003). Self-pity: Exploring the links to personality, control beliefs, and anger. *Journal of Personality, 71*(2), 183–220. https://doi.org/10.1111/1467-6494.7102004

Stoeber, J., Lalova, A. V., & Lumley, E. J. (2020). Perfectionism, (self-) compassion, and subjective well-being: A mediation model. *Personality and Individual Differences, 154*. https://doi.org/10.1016/j.paid.2019.109708

Svendsen, J. L., Osnes, B., Binder, P. E., Dundas, I., Visted, E., Nordby, H., et al. (2016). Trait self-compassion reflects emotional flexibility through an association with high vagally mediated heart rate variability. *Mindfulness, 7*(5), 1103–1113. https://doi.org/10.1007/s12671-016-0549-1

Terry, M. L., Leary, M. R., Mehta, S., & Henderson, K. (2013). Self-compassionate reactions to health threats. *Personality and Social Psychology Bulletin, 39*(7), 911–926. https://doi.org/10.1177/0146167213488213

Tice, D. M., Bratslavsky, E., & Baumeister, R. F. (2001). Emotional distress regulation takes precedence over impulse control: If you feel bad, do it! *Journal of Personality and Social Psychology, 80*(1), 53–67. https://doi.org/10.1037/0022-3514.80.1.53

Tobin, R., & Dunkley, D. M. (2021). Self-critical perfectionism and lower mindfulness and self-compassion predict anxious and depressive symptoms over two years. *Behaviour Research and Therapy, 136*, 103780. https://doi.org/10.1016/j.brat.2020.103780

Vickers, R. R., Conway, T. L., & Hervig, L. K. (1990). Demonstration of replicable dimensions of health behaviors. *Preventive Medicine, 19*, 377–401. https://doi.org/10.1016/0091-7435(90)90037-K

Wagner, D. D., & Heatherton, T. F. (2015). Self-regulation and its failure: The seven deadly threats to self-regulation. In M. Mikulincer, P. R. Shaver, E. Borgida, & J. A. Bargh (Eds.), *APA handbook of personality and social psychology, Vol. 1. Attitudes and social cognition* (pp. 805–842). American Psychological Association. https://doi.org/10.1037/14341-026

Webb, T. L., Chang, B. P., & Benn, Y. (2013). 'The ostrich problem': Motivated avoidance or rejection of information about goal progress. *Social and Personality Psychology Compass, 7*(11), 794–807. https://doi.org/10.1111/spc3.12071

Webb, T. L., Schweiger Gallo, I., Miles, E., Gollwitzer, P. M., & Sheeran, P. (2012). Effective regulation of affect: An action control perspective on emotion regulation. *European Review of Social Psychology, 23*(1), 143–186. https://doi.org/10.1080/10463283.2012.718134

Webb, T. L., & Sheeran, P. (2006). Does changing behavioral intentions engender behavior change? A meta-analysis of the experimental evidence. *Psychological Bulletin, 132*(2), 249–268. https://doi.org/10.1037/0033-2909.132.2.249

Wisener, M., & Khoury, B. (2019). Associations between specific mindfulness facets, self-compassion, internally motivated drinking, and alcohol-related problems. *Mindfulness, 10*(1), 2073–2081. https://doi.org/10.1007/s12671-019-01172-0

Wisener, M., & Khoury, B. (2020). Is self-compassion negatively associated with alcohol and marijuana-related problems via coping motives? *Addictive Behaviors, 111*, 106554. https://doi.org/10.1016/j.addbeh.2020.106554

Witkiewitz, K., & Villarroel, N. A. (2009). Dynamic association between negative affect and alcohol lapses following alcohol treatment. *Journal of Consulting and Clinical Psychology, 77*(4), 633–644. https://doi.org/10.1037/a0015647

Wong, M. Y. C., Chung, P.-K., & Leung, K.-M. (2021). The relationship between physical activity and self-compassion: A systematic review and meta-analysis. *Mindfulness, 12*(3), 547–563. https://doi.org/10.1007/s12671-020-01513-4

World Health Organisation. (2021). Noncommunicable diseases. Retrieved July 27, 2022, from https://www.who.int/news-room/fact-sheets/detail/noncommunicable-diseases

Zessin, U., Dickhäuser, O., & Garbade, S. (2015). The relationship between self-compassion and well-being: A meta-analysis. *Applied Psychology: Health and Well-Being, 7*(3), 340–364. https://doi.org/10.1111/aphw.12051

Zhang, J. W., & Chen, S. (2016). Self-compassion promotes personal improvement from regret experiences via acceptance. *Personality and Social Psychology Bulletin, 42*(2), 244–258. https://doi.org/10.1177/0146167215623271

Zhang, J. W., & Chen, S. (2017). Self-compassion promotes positive adjustment for people who attribute responsibility of a romantic breakup to themselves. *Self and Identity, 16*(6), 732–759. https://doi.org/10.1080/15298868.2017.1305985

20

Self-Compassion, Body Compassion, and Body Image

Nicholas A. Troop and Emily S. Beadle

The reactions people make towards their emotional responses when they experience stress, difficulty, or failure are important in psychological adjustment. *Self-compassion* is one such response. Self-compassion is a kind of self-to-self relating that regulates negative emotions. A considerable literature has emerged in recent years and meta-analysis has shown there is a large effect size in the link between self-compassion and mental well-being (MacBeth & Gumley, 2012).

Negative subjective evaluations of one's physical body are common in both men and women and can lead to overeating, binge eating, restrictive eating, eating disorders, and psychological distress (Stice, 1994; APPG, 2012). Recently, therefore, studies have explored a role for self-compassion in eating- and body-related pathology. The present chapter explores self-compassion as an affect regulatory process in relation to eating pathology as well as other health consequences of body image issues.

N. A. Troop (✉)
School of Psychology, University of Plymouth, Plymouth, UK
e-mail: Nicholas.troop@plymouth.ac.uk

E. S. Beadle
Department of Psychology, Sports and Geography, University of Hertfordshire, Hatfield, UK
e-mail: e.beadle@herts.ac.uk

F. M. Sirois (ed.), *The Palgrave Handbook of Positive Psychology and Health*,
https://doi.org/10.1007/978-3-031-89095-6_20

To contextualise what follows in this chapter, we will first briefly describe Gilbert's (2005, 2010) model of affect regulation. This model includes a threat-focused component that triggers safety seeking behaviour, and two positive affect components, an affiliation-focused system and a drive- or incentive-focused system. The affiliation-focused system is associated with feeling safe and content and tones down the threat system by self-soothing (self-compassion). The incentive-focused system is associated with seeking reward, resources, and achievements. Where the soothing system cannot regulate threat-based emotions such as shame, people may rely on the drive/incentive system and focus on achieving social status or rank (Steindl et al., 2017). There is already considerable evidence for the links between shame and self-perceived low social rank in eating disorders and eating pathology (Troop et al., 2003; Goss & Allan, 2009). Exploring the role of self-compassion in relation to eating pathology is therefore warranted.

Definition of Self-Compassion

Gilbert (2014, p. 19) defines *compassion* as "a sensitivity to suffering in self and others, with a commitment to try to alleviate and prevent it". In describing four components of compassion, Jazaieri et al. (2013) also emphasise these elements:

1. Cognitive—an awareness of suffering
2. Affective—sympathy with or being moved by suffering
3. Intention—desire to see relief of suffering
4. Motivation—responsiveness to relieve suffering

Both of these definitions therefore incorporate what Gilbert (2009, 2017) terms the *psychologies of compassion*—the motivated sensitivity to suffering and the motivated action to alleviate and prevent suffering.

Retaining these motivational elements, Neff (2003a, 2003b) therefore defines *self-compassion* as being open to and touched by one's own suffering and a desire to alleviate this and to heal with kindness. Neff suggests there are three bipolar components to self-compassion: *self-kindness* (rather than critical self-judgement), common humanity (where failure and pain are accepted as part of the human experience rather than feelings of isolation), and mindful awareness (negative emotional states are faced rather than over-identified, e.g. exaggerated).

Self-Compassion, Eating Pathology, and Body Image

In an early study on self-compassion in eating behaviour, Adams and Leary (2007) examined the effect of a simple self-compassion induction in restrained and unrestrained eaters. Restrained eaters are those who set limits or rules on their eating whereas unrestrained eaters are more likely to base decisions about eating on hunger and preference (Herman & Mack, 1975). However, individuals with high levels of dietary restraint (restrained eaters) are prone to overeat under various conditions relative to individuals who are low in dietary restraint (unrestrained eaters) (see Ruderman, 1986, for a review). For example, early studies showed that giving individuals a milkshake preload led to overeating (disinhibition) in a subsequent bogus taste test in restrained but not unrestrained eaters (e.g. Herman & Mack, 1975). It was proposed that this disinhibition effect was due to the preload taking restrained eaters past their self-imposed diet boundary (Herman & Polivy, 1984). Since their diet had already been blown, it was argued, restrained eaters give up on their resolve to diet and eat until they reached satiety (the so-called *what-the-hell* effect).

Participants in Adams and Leary's (2007) study were told that the study was testing the effects of television viewing upon mood and taste perception and were given doughnuts to eat. While the control group received no additional information, participants in the self-compassion group were given the following rationale that tapped into self-kindness, common humanity, and mindful awareness:

> You may wonder why doughnuts were picked to be used in this study. They were chosen because they are typical of the high-calorie, high-fat unhealthy foods that people often tend to eat while watching TV. We thought it would be more like the "real world" to have people eat a dessert or junk food. Several people so far have said they feel bad about eating doughnuts in this study, so I hope you won't be hard on yourself. Everyone eats unhealthily sometimes, and everyone in this study eats this stuff, so I don't think there's any reason to really feel bad about it. The little amount of food doesn't really matter anyway.

Restrained eaters given the self-compassion induction compensated for eating a pre-load in a subsequent taste test (compared with those not given a pre-load) and also reported lower negative affect. Restrained eaters not given a self-compassion induction did not show these effects.

Many naturalistic studies have subsequently explored self-compassion in eating pathology and body image, examining direct associations or testing moderator or mediator effects. In terms of direct associations, higher levels of self-compassion correlate with lower body dissatisfaction and eating concerns in female college students (Wasylkiw et al., 2012) and lower body consciousness, body surveillance, and body shame in young women athletes (Mosewich et al., 2011). The negative subscales of self-compassion (self-judgement, isolation, and over-identification) are also related to higher levels of grazing behaviour (such as eating when not hungry) (Mantzios, Egan, Bahia et al., 2018). Curiously, the same authors also found that higher levels of isolation and over-identification were related to lower levels of fat and sugar consumption (Mantzios, Egan, Hussain et al., 2018).

In terms of moderator effects, Holtham and Dyck (2014) found that self-compassion moderated the effect of risk factors (self-esteem, perfectionism, and experiential avoidance) on disordered eating. Similarly, Daye et al. (2014) found that self-compassion moderated the effect of retrospective recall of restrictive/critical comments (e.g. "that you were eating too much") on body shame and body surveillance. In particular, high levels of self-compassion reduced the impact of high levels of critical comments on body surveillance while low levels of self-compassion increased the impact of high levels of critical comments on body shame. Common to several sociocultural theories (e.g. Stice, 1994; Fredrickson & Roberts, 1997; Thompson et al., 1999) is the role of external pressures to be thin. Self-compassion moderated the effect on media pressures to be thin on internalisation of the thin ideal as well as moderating the effects of media and family pressures to be thin on disordered eating (Tylka et al., 2015). Furthermore, the effect of body mass index on eating pathology and body image flexibility (ability to tolerate negative body-related thoughts and feelings) was also moderated by self-compassion (Kelly et al., 2014a).

Self-compassion also moderates the effect of depression on eating pathology. In one study there was a stronger association in women low in self-compassion than in those high in self-compassion (Geller et al., 2015). Other studies looking at gender differences found that self-compassion moderated the effect of body shame on depression in women but not men (Sick et al., 2020), while self-compassion moderated the effect of overvaluation of weight and shape on eating pathology, distress, and psychosocial impairment in both men and women (Linardon et al., 2020). Finally, self-compassion moderated the effect on body appreciation of the tendency to compare one's body to others, and the belief that one's self-worth is contingent on one's appearance (Homan & Tylka, 2015). Interestingly, however, self-compassion also had a mediating effect on the tendency to compare the body with others; specifically, the mindfulness component partially mediated the effect on body satisfaction (Dijkstra & Bartelds, 2011).

Other studies have found mediating effects. For example, one study found that self-compassion partially mediated the relation between body preoccupation and depressive symptoms (Wasylkiw et al., 2012, study 2). The link between shame and drive for thinness was also mediated by self-compassion in both women with an eating disorder and women in the general population (Ferreira et al., 2013). Relatedly, other authors have found self-criticism (indicative of a lack of self-compassion) mediates the effect of shame on disordered eating, body dissatisfaction, and binge eating disorder (Dunkley et al., 2010; Gois et al., 2018; Duarte & Pinto-Gouveia, 2017).

As a consequence of this literature, Braun et al. (2016) conclude that self-compassion may influence eating disorder outcomes by decreasing the outcomes directly, preventing the occurrence of risk factors, interrupting the effects of risk factors, and disrupting the mediation train through which these risk factors operate. Most of the studies leading to this summary, however, and including those above, were cross-sectional. This limits the confidence in conclusions around the aetiological role of self-compassion. In addition, studies used general measures of self-compassion which ask about self-compassion in relation to negative mood. It's not clear whether self-compassion directly related to negative feelings around body image would make a useful contribution to understanding the aetiology of eating disorder (or other) outcomes. The next section therefore discusses the notion of *body compassion*.

Body Compassion

Definition

Although the studies described above have demonstrated the importance of self-compassion in relation to body-related outcomes, the term *body compassion* has recently emerged. Strictly speaking, the correct term should be *body self-compassion* since *body compassion* could be taken to mean compassion for other people's bodies. Indeed, some authors have referred to *body self-compassion* (e.g. Berry et al., 2010) although, more recently, researchers have come to refer simply to *body compassion*. While arguably ambiguous, this is essentially consistent with the use of the terms *body esteem* and *body image* rather than the technically more correct *body self-esteem* and *body self-image*.

Since the term *body compassion* is already becoming more widely used, and since there is precedent for similar terms neglecting reference to the "self", we also adopt the term *body compassion* in this chapter.

Murn (2013) defined body compassion as reflecting self-kindness, common humanity, and mindfulness to one's own body, in contrast to being critical, isolating, and over-identifying with negative feelings and emotions. Altman et al. (2017, p. 3) similarly refer to "the regarding of one's own body, in appearance, competence and health, with mindfulness, kindness and awareness of common humanity". However, these do not explicitly reflect the motivational elements described by Gilbert (2010, 2017) and Neff (2003a, 2003b) in their definitions of *compassion* and *self-compassion*, respectively. Therefore, we (Beadle et al., 2021) define body compassion more comprehensively:

> Body compassion is compassion directed to one's own body, incorporating elements of kindness, common humanity and mindful awareness, as well as elements of sensitivity to body-related distress, pain and suffering, and the motivation and ability to combat this

Qualitative Studies

The term body compassion and body self-compassion particularly emerged in qualitative research. In young women exercisers, for example, Berry et al. (2010) identified four themes that were consistent with, rather than mirrored, Neff's (2003a, 2003b) three components. Specifically, women described an *appreciation of their bodies being unique*, not just in terms of appearance (i.e. different body types) but also in terms of their body's capabilities, creating feelings of empowerment. They also described *taking ownership of their bodies* in terms of developing an understanding of their bodies and taking responsibility for their physical and psychological well-being. Women reported using *less social comparison*, often unintentionally, and discussed *the importance of others*. While other people were not essential for their experience of self-compassion, the presence of supportive others and positive role models was a facilitator or catalyst to developing body self-compassion.

Woekel and Ebbeck (2013) investigated body self-compassion in postpartum women. Since they explored this in relation to Neff' (2003a, 2003b) definition of self-compassion, unsurprisingly the themes identified broadly conformed to this structure. However, these were expressed in interesting ways. For example, self-kindness included themes around being *non-judgmental* in relation to bodily changes as well as having a *self-focused moment*, a "mental nap". Common humanity included a consideration of other mothers as well as women struggling with their weight more generally and included both personal as well as virtual (social media) connections. Mindful awareness reflected a balanced emotional perspective, acknowledging anxieties but also finding humour, as well as a recognition these feelings were transitory. The flip-side was also expressed, of course, self-criticism about appearance, over-identification (e.g. "getting worked up"), and unfavourable comparisons (feelings of inadequacy at others' successes). A final theme also emerged, one of caring motivation. This reflected an acknowledgement that, while they do not always take the time to care for themselves, it was something they would strive towards achieving.

In men with spinal cord injury, Smith (2013) identified body self-compassion as a theme that motivated men's leisure time physical activity. Specifically, and consistent with Berry et al.'s (2010) study on women exercisers, body self-compassion involved taking ownership of, and appreciating the uniqueness of their bodies, rather than criticism of their perceived imperfections and limitations. It also helped them develop a sense of "a productive body", so they could feel socially connected and develop a stronger satisfaction with life.

In her unpublished MSc thesis, Stokes (2013) was concerned with the connection to nature by naturists and its impact on well-being. She also addressed, in part, the link between naturism and body image. Interestingly, people did not take up naturism because they already had a positive body image but, rather, developed a positive body image as a result of becoming naturists. In her small qualitative interview study, Stokes (2013) found that the improvement in body image and self-acceptance appeared to be achieved through acceptance by others and a sense of inclusion, a similar process to that described in Berry et al.'s (2010) study on women exercisers. Participants described compassionate processes such as lack of judgment from others, common humanity, and a mindful awareness of their negative feelings towards their own bodies as important in developing a positive body image.

Measuring Body Compassion

There are currently two measures of body compassion, the Body Compassion Scale (BCS: Altman et al., 2017) and the Body Compassion Questionnaire (BCQ: Beadle et al., 2021).

The Body Compassion Scale (BCS)

Altman et al. (2017) developed the Body Compassion Scale (BCS) following Neff's (2003a, 2003b) definition of self-compassion combined with Cash's (2002) definition of body image including evaluative, cognitive, and behavioural components of appearance, competence, fitness and health, or illness. Items for the BCS were developed by the authors. It has 23 items and high scores indicate a greater level of body compassion. Factor analysis identified a three-factor solution (see Table 20.1). The 3-factor structure has also been replicated in a sample of Italian women (Policardo et al., 2022), a mixed (mostly male) sample of Chinese adolescents (Wong et al., 2022), and a mixed (mostly female) sample of Portuguese adults (Ferresra et al., 2018). Although a single-factor solution was not a good fit to the data in Altman et al.'s (2017) study, the BCS is nevertheless often used by summing the subscales to give a total BCS score. In fact, Wong et al. (2022) carried out a second-order confirmatory factor analysis on the subscale scores in their sample of Chinese adolescents and supported this approach. Descriptions and sample items are given in Table 20.1.

The BCS cements itself with mindfulness and acceptance-based (MAB) approaches. This is stated from the outset in developing the measure but is also reflected in the *defusion* and *acceptance* subscales of the measure. Indeed, the measure is also validated against measures of mindfulness and acceptance (as well as self-compassion). Although related (Germer & Barnhofer, 2017; Germer & Neff, 2013; Neff & Germer, 2013), mindfulness focuses on the experience while compassion focuses on the experiencer, with compassion

Table 20.1 Subscales, descriptions, and example items for the Body Compassion Scale (Altman et al., 2017)

Subscale	Description	Example item
Defusion	Focuses largely on feelings of being cut off from others (although it also includes items relating to self-criticism and feelings of inadequacy	"When I feel frustrated with my body's inability to do something, I tend to feel separate and cut off from other people"
Common humanity	Focuses on the sense that the experience of inadequacy, frustration, or failing is something that everyone feels	"When I am frustrated with some aspect of my appearance, I try to remind myself most people feel this way at some time"
Acceptance	Reflects feelings of acceptance and tolerance in the body's appearance and flaws	"I am accepting of my looks just the way they are"

being more emotionally activating than mindfulness and compassion training being uniquely able to help with shame (Germer & Barnhofer, 2017; Gilbert & Procter, 2006).

Body Compassion Questionnaire (BCQ)

In developing the BCQ, we (Beadle et al., 2021) were informed by definitions of compassion and self-compassion, including motivational elements (Gilbert, 2009, 2010, 2014, 2017; Jazaieri et al., 2013; Neff, 2003a, 2003b). The items were generated from the transcriptions written by participants in an expressive writing study (Ouwens et al., 2025). This is described in more detail below but, briefly, participants were asked to write for 15 minutes per day on three consecutive days, once about body image from a perspective of self-kindness, once from a perspective of common humanity, and once from a perspective of mindful awareness of emotional states. We tried to retain the original wording of participants' sentences but removed references to evaluation and (as much as possible) specific elements of one's body (e.g. explicit references to appearance or function) in order to make items as widely applicable as possible.

Exploratory and confirmatory factor analyses identified a bi-factor model in which the BCQ could be computed to give an overall BCQ score (higher scores indicating more body compassion) or three subscales. Descriptions and sample items are given in Table 20.2.

Table 20.2 Subscales, descriptions, and example items for the Body Compassion Questionnaire (Beadle et al., 2021)

Subscale	Description	Example item
Body kindness	Incorporates self-kindness, non-judgement, acceptance, and sensitivity and distress tolerance	"I accept my body the way it is and am comfortable in my own skin"
Common humanity	Incorporates accepting that one's feelings and concerns about one's body are normal, common, and a part of the greater human experience	"I am sure everyone has insecurities about their bodies"
Motivated action	Incorporates attention, reasoning, feelings, behaviour, imagery, and sensory skills to help develop body compassion, and also mindful awareness, keeping painful thoughts and feelings in balanced awareness	"I am working on making myself feel better about the way I look"

In validation studies, both the BCS and BCQ correlated positively with measures self-compassion and positive mood and negatively with measures of eating pathology and negative mood. Beadle et al. (2021) also showed that the BCS and BCQ total scores correlated with each other. Subscales of the BCS and BCQ also generally correlated with each other although the *motivated action* subscale of the BCQ is not reflected in the BCS.

Correlates and Outcomes of Body Compassion

A number of studies have begun using either the BCS or the BCQ. Denu et al. (2019) explored body compassion (using the BCS) among endometrial cancer survivors. Body compassion was unrelated to pain and quality of life variables. However, obese patients reported lower body compassion than non-obese patients. Using the BCQ, we also found a negative correlation between body compassion and body mass index (Beadle et al., 2021) but only in women, not men. In other words, women with larger BMI report lower levels of body compassion than women with lower BMI. Body compassion (using the BCS) correlated directly and negatively with body image shame in men and women referred for cosmetic surgery (Khanjani et al., 2020), while it also moderated the effect of general (external) shame on body image shame as well as on eating pathology (i.e. there was a stronger effect in those with lower body compassion) in women in the general population (Oliveira et al., 2018)

Beadle et al. (2021) found that body compassion (using the BCQ) was negatively related to measures of eating pathology and body image avoidance. However, in another study, de Carvalho Barreto et al. (2018) also included a measure of self-compassionate attributes (the sensitivity and motivation to deal with suffering with a compassionate attitude) and self-compassionate actions (the commitment and skills to alleviate suffering). Self-compassionate attributes had an impact on body compassion (BCS) that was partially mediated by self-compassionate actions (i.e. attributes had both a direct and an indirect effect). Body compassion fully mediated the association with eating pathology.

In a prospective study, Beadle (2020) found that body shame predicted levels of physical activity at 1-month follow-up and this effect was mediated by motivation (internal motivation predicted higher physical activity and external motivation predicted lower physical activity). Motivation itself was predicted by body compassion (this study used an early version of the measure that went on to become the BCQ) which was mediated by body shame. In contrast to these direct effects, an online study looking at the effect of

Instagram images of fitness versus weight-inclusivity on exercise motives did not find a moderating effect of body compassion (Wood & Pila, 2022).

Beadle et al. (2025a) examined the impact of body compassion (using the BCQ) on mood in a study of 451 participants where 59 self-identified as disabled (disabilities included mental health, visual, learning, pain, hearing, and mobility). Body compassion moderated the effect of self-identified disability on mood. In those with low levels of body compassion, participants with a disability reported lower mood than those without. In those with moderate levels of body compassion, there was no significant difference in mood between participants with and without a disability. Interestingly, in those with high levels of body compassion, participants with a disability reported a more positive mood than those without.

Evidence for another role for body compassion, this time in relation to eating pathology, concerns its impact on life events. Life events and difficulties play an important role in the aetiology of psychological disorders generally (Tennant, 2002), including eating disorders (Schmidt et al., 1997; Welch et al., 1997; Rojo et al., 2006) and disordered eating in non-clinical samples (Kupeli et al., 2017). A recent study also showed that body compassion (using the BCS) moderated the effect of both the number and the negative appraisal of life events on severity of binge eating (Barata-Santos et al., 2019).

However, stress research that considers only the *number* of negative life events, or a general *negative appraisal* of these events, is somewhat limited. The precise *meaning* of an event may also be important. Our research shows that events that involve a loss of self-perceived social rank may be particularly important in eating pathology. In social rank theory (Gilbert, 2006), when low social rank is imposed, involuntary and inescapable, this can lead to a submissive stance and passivity as a means of avoiding conflict (Allan & Gilbert, 1997). Patients with eating disorders report a lower self-perceived social rank (Connan et al., 2007; Troop et al., 2003). Self-perceived low social rank also predicts an increase in symptoms over 6 months in women with a history of eating disorders (Troop et al., 2014). We have also found that life events only predicted eating pathology if women perceived these events to have had a detrimental effect on their social rank (e.g. shame, loss of reputation) (Troop, 2016). Furthermore, this was only true in women who already perceived themselves to have low social rank. Further studies are already underway to determine whether this effect is mediated by body compassion as would be expected on the basis of the self-regulatory model described above. However, interestingly, in a prospective study with a non-clinical sample of over 1000 women, increases in stress were associated with weight loss, whereas increases in stress itself was predicted by baseline levels of self-perceived low social rank and high levels of self-criticism (the inverse of self-kindness) (Kupeli, 2014; Kupeli et al., 2017).

Although we have focused on body compassion in this section, this does not necessarily deny the importance of self-compassion more generally. In a series of studies on coping with life events in the aetiology of eating disorders (Troop & Treasure 1997a, 1997b; Troop et al., 1998), women spontaneously reported responses that reflect self-compassion in relation to life events that did not reflect body image issues (Troop, 1996). For example, in two women describing the end of a relationship, in response to a general question about becoming upset or distressed, one woman who did not develop an eating disorder replied that, "of course [she] was upset, [her] boyfriend had just dumped [her]". Another woman who developed anorexia nervosa after a similar experience replied, "yeah, I just felt so stupid letting it get to me". Although self-compassion was not being asked about systematically (these studies predated the growth in interest in self-compassion), they reflect spontaneous expressions of common humanity and critical self-judgement, respectively. They therefore allude to the significance of self-compassion in the aetiology of eating disorders that is not directly body related but related to the stressful events that may have provoked the onset of an eating disorder.

The degree to which both self-compassion and body compassion may be involved in the link between social rank and stress in relation to eating- and body-related pathology needs to be further unpacked. The implications may relate to the roles of self-compassion versus body compassion more generally.

Changing Self-Compassion and Body Compassion

In eating disorder patients treated with the gold standard cognitive behaviour therapy, early improvement in self-compassion predicted response to treatment (Kelly et al., 2012). In addition, increases in self-compassion over the 12 weeks of treatment lead to reductions in shame in eating disorder patients (Kelly et al., 2014b).

More directly, there is evidence for the effectiveness of interventions designed to address self-compassion. For example, Albertson et al. (2014) recruited women who wanted to feel better about their bodies. Compared with a waiting list control, participants who had three weeks of self-compassion meditation showed improvements in body dissatisfaction and body shame that were maintained at 3 months.

Compassion-focused therapy (CFT) explicitly addresses difficulties in affect regulation, shame, self-directed hostility, and self-criticism as described in Gilbert's (2005, 2010) model above. Originally developed for depression, it has been modified specifically for eating disorders (CFT-E: Goss & Allan, 2010). With CFT added to group Cognitive Behavioural Therapy, Gale et al. (2012) found a clinically significant decrease in eating disorder symptoms and psychological distress. Used as an adjunct to treatment as usual, CFT also leads to greater improvements in self-compassion, shame, and eating pathology (Kelly et al., 2017). Combinations of CFT with other treatments such as acceptance and commitment therapy (ACT), mindfulness, and guided imagery lead to a range of improvements in eating pathology and other aspects of well-being and quality of life (Gilbert & Choden, 2013; Goss, 2011; Palmeira et al., 2017).

In a pilot study, five individuals with obesity participated in 12 sessions of group CFT for body weight shame (Carter et al., 2020). Although the sample size was too small to determine clinically reliable change, there was improvement in body shame and external shame. Qualitative analysis identified a number of themes relating to the development of self-compassion in group CFT. These included: feelings of safeness to explore feelings of shame (knowing that they won't be judged); common humanity (knowing that they were not alone with the struggle); developing compassionate wisdom to move from self-criticism to self-compassion in making healthy choices; compassion directed to oneself from others feels uncomfortable but becomes easier over time; and becoming mindfully aware of switching from self-criticism to self-compassion.

Kelly and Carter (2015) also compared brief 3-week self-help interventions for binge eating disorder (BED). One group had planning and self-monitoring plus self-compassion to counteract urges to binge; a second group had planning and self-monitoring plus behavioural strategies to counteract urges to binge; a third group acted as a waiting list control. The two intervention groups were equal to each and better than the control in reducing the number of binge days. However, the first (self-compassion) group was better than both the second (behavioural strategies) and third (control) groups in reducing eating pathology.

Successfully adapting a compassion-based therapy into a self-help intervention opens up the possibility to deliver other light-touch compassion-based approaches when psychotherapy is either not needed or not routinely provided. The next section explores one such approach.

Expressive Writing

Pennebaker and Beall (1986) developed a paradigm in which participants write about trauma for 15–20 minutes a day for 3–4 consecutive days. Over 300 studies have shown that writing about stress and trauma leads to significant improvements in a range of outcomes including health centre visits, immune function, exam grades, and return to work following redundancy (Frattaroli, 2006; Smyth, 1998), with benefits lasting several months.

A number of studies have used expressive writing in relation to eating pathology in both clinical and non-clinical samples. Participants write either about emotionally upsetting topics, positive topics, or about body image directly, and generally show an improvement (e.g. East et al., 2010; Kupeli et al., 2018), though not always (e.g. O'Connor et al., 2010; Frayne & Wade, 2006). However, this approach largely adopts the "insight theory" approach in which improvement is proposed to be due to actively processing and reappraising an event (Tausczik & Pennebaker, 2010).

In contrast, an affect regulatory approach involves participants first describing stress/trauma and then writing to incorporate self-compassion in relation to this. Experimental and real-world settings show that self-compassionate writing increases the benefit of expressive writing (e.g. Leary et al., 2007; Imrie & Troop, 2012). Self-compassionate letter writing is already an element of compassion-focused interventions. Even as a standalone activity, writing a letter about one's body from a self-compassionate perspective leads to increased mood and body satisfaction (Stern & Engeln, 2018; Seekis et al., 2017).

We carried out two expressive writing studies to stimulate body compassion directly (Ouwens et al., 2025). In the first study we randomised female students to write about body image alone or to write about body image from a self-compassionate perspective for 15 minutes. State levels of body image improved from pre- to post-experiment. In a second study, we gave female students a notepad to take home and asked them to write for 15 minutes per day for three consecutive days either about body image alone or about body image from a self-compassionate perspective. Specifically, for those writing compassionately, on day one the instructions tapped into self-kindness, on day two the instructions tapped into common humanity, and on day three the instructions tapped into mindful awareness. We then followed participants up three months later with the intervention being carried out in November and the follow-up in January/February. We have previously found female students often gain weight during this time (Roberts et al., 2007) and so felt this would be an optimum time to evaluate this intervention. In this study, participants in the control group gained weight and reported a worsening of their mood. Participants in the body compassion group, however, maintained their weight and mood. There were no other effects (e.g. on self-compassion, eating behaviour, or eating pathology).

Furthermore, on the basis that body image has a significant effect on physical activity (Beadle, 2020), we carried out our body compassion expressive writing approach, again in female students, but this time to examine its effects on physical activity (Beadle et al., 2025b). All participants were given NHS guidelines on recommended levels of physical activity and were asked to increase physical activity to these levels. All participants also wrote for 15 minutes on a single occasion about body image, half writing about body image alone and half writing compassionately. Half of the participants in each group were also given an implementation intention instruction, being asked to write down when, where, and how they would implement their goals to increase their physical activity levels (Gollwitzer, 1999). Implementation intentions had no effect on physical activity. However, participants who wrote about body image from a self-compassionate perspective increased their physical activity levels at the 1-month follow-up relative to participants writing about body image alone.

Other researchers using body compassionate expressive writing have adopted a slightly different approach. Przezdziecki et al. (2016) describe the development and acceptability (to breast cancer survivors and physicians) of a web-based expressive writing intervention called *My Changed Body* (MyCB). This is a one-off 30-minute writing task which participants can complete at their own pace. In MyCB, individuals write about a negative body image experience followed by a series of prompts that address self-kindness, common humanity, and mindful awareness.

In breast cancer survivors, MyCB led to improvements in body image distress and self-compassion over 1-month follow-up and improvement in body appreciation over 3 months (Sherman et al., 2018). In another study in breast cancer survivors, the effect of MyCB on self-compassion and anxiety were enhanced with the inclusion of self-compassionate meditation (Mifsud et al., 2021). MyCB also led to an improvement in self-compassion over 1 month in patients with head and neck cancer but there was no effect on body image distress (Melissant et al., 2021). In adults with a visible skin condition (e.g. eczema, psoriasis, acne) and who had experienced at least one negative event related to their skin condition (entailing feelings of failure, humiliation, or rejection), MyCB also led to an increase in self-compassion and a decrease in negative mood post-writing (Sherman et al., 2019).

Since the ultimate goal is to determine whether such an intervention can be recommended to the general public, we are cautious about the notion that participants should write about the negative experience first, before being self-compassionate. There is a possible risk that asking vulnerable people to describe something that provokes anxiety and distress may cause them to discontinue the activity without reaching the self-compassionate task. Because it is not possible to rule out vulnerable people participating in such an intervention delivered to the general public, we have preferred to ask participants to consider a self-compassionate perspective from the start of their writing. One could also argue that this more closely reflects the experience of people who already have high levels of body compassion since they bring this cognitive resource to bear from the outset which then limits the degree to which they become distressed in the first place. On the other hand, the MyCB approach may be closer to the principal of self-compassion in which the distress is experienced which then leads to implementing the compassionate resource. Of course, how closely a compassionate writing task in non-compassionate individuals mirrors the process of *being* compassionate in compassionate individuals is an empirical issue and one that has not yet been addressed.

Exposure to Body Images

Two other recent but equivocal studies are worth noting. Ogden and colleagues examined the effect of exposure to images of diverse body shapes/sizes versus slim bodies. Using photographic images, there was an increase in body compassion in the diverse body shape condition relative to the thin-ideal condition (Ogden et al., 2020). However, there was no such interaction in a similar study that used video images (Stewart & Ogden, 2021).

These studies used an early version of the measure that went on to become the BCQ and which, in correspondence with the authors, we had re-worded to pick up state changes on body compassion in an experimental setting rather than the trait version described above. In addition to our ongoing work on developing a state version of the BCQ, its use in experimental studies such as Ogden and colleagues' use of body-diversity will also be useful in identifying processes for improving body compassion. Whether this is in conjunction with, or separate from, expressive writing approaches is for future research to address.

Future Directions

There are many questions still to address. These can be broadly grouped into those relating to (1) understanding where body compassion fits in the aetiology of relevant outcomes, (2) understanding how body compassion develops, and relatedly (3) how to improve body compassion in those who lack it.

Much of the research described here is cross-sectional. While these studies may be useful in determining the range of body-relevant circumstances where body compassion may play a role, we need to be moving towards an understanding of precisely how body compassion develops and how it impacts on outcomes. A related issue is the sheer diversity of outcomes that are measured against self-compassion without elaborating explicitly on a plausible aetiological chain. It is difficult to get a sense of an emerging model because researchers use different predictors and different outcomes (e.g. body shame itself is sometimes an outcome and sometimes a predictor).

Bringing these two points together it is possible to think of body compassion in the same way as social support, as a resource that is perceived to be available should the need arise, as well as a process that is enacted at the time of a crisis. As such, body compassion may mitigate against a body-related challenge (e.g. weight change, weight-related teasing, pressure to adopt a thin-ideal) in the development of body shame. It may further mitigate against the experience of body shame at the time body shame is provoked, for example, by a self-compassionate intervention or the presence of compassionate others. This is far from a formal model but may at least guide subsequent research.

In terms of the development of body compassion, two of the qualitative studies described above (Berry et al., 2010; Stokes, 2013) suggest that body compassion can develop spontaneously without the need for a formal intervention, partly as a result of the presence of compassionate others. In fact, this brings us back to Gilbert's (2006) model, which suggests that we develop the ability to self-soothe by internalising being soothed by caregivers to whom we are securely attached. But it tells us that this development of a self-compassionate perspective may occur even in adulthood.

However, Jeziorek-Wozny (2019) recruited women who were overweight and had attempted weight loss a number of times in the past. In describing struggles with self-compassion, a number of themes were identified: (1) participants reported prioritising other responsibilities (other needs, other people, and feeling guilty about prioritising self-compassion); (2) participants reported that learning a new way of life was difficult because of habits as well as past trauma; (3) there were also difficulties due to maintaining high standards which involved negative judgments from both self and others. Difficulties in developing body compassion therefore also needs to be explored and strategies developed to overcome these. Indeed, CFT and the use of letter and other expressive writing procedures often use the strategy of suggesting that people (especially those who struggle with self-compassion) may find it helpful to write from the perspective of a compassionate other. These factors suggest there may be something fruitful in tapping into developing body compassion with the involvement of compassionate others. How this can be achieved and what this might look like in a formal intervention is something that needs to be considered very carefully.

Another question that has not received much attention is the relationship between self-compassion and body compassion more broadly. Do we develop self-compassion which then generalises to all domains of our lives wherever we may experience negative feelings? Or do we develop self-compassion separately in multiple domains which then sum to an overall level of self-compassion? This would seem an inefficient way to develop affect regulatory skills. Nevertheless, we could explore whether it is possible for individuals to have self-compassion in relation to negative feelings in one domain (such as achievements, work, or study) but lack it in another (such as relationships or body image) and what the implications of this are for general versus domain-specific interventions.

Body compassion's importance relative to body image is also open to future research. For example, where we find that body compassion underpins body image (e.g. body shame) but that it is body shame that predicts health behaviours such as physical activity (Beadle, 2020), one could argue that we need only develop interventions to improve body image and forget about body compassion altogether. However, liking one's body and being kind to one's body are entirely different. If bodies change, such as in the case of illness, disability and injury, aging, and childbirth, then body image must change too. However, body compassion could remain a stable trait regardless of bodily changes and may even be the process that supports the development of a positive change in body image following such bodily changes. Clearly this is an empirical question for future research to address.

Conclusions

Much of the work on self-compassion in relation to body image, both in terms of naturalistic studies and interventions, has focused on the kind of body-image that is related to eating pathology (disordered eating as well as eating disorders) and/or is appearance-based. Interestingly, and pleasingly, the introduction of the concept of body compassion seems to have shifted its attention to a wider concept of body image to accommodate function as well as appearance. There seems also to be a tendency to consider conditions where body image may be affected and for which the outcomes could be well-being more generally rather than, say, issues to do with weight and shape in which the outcomes are predominantly about eating pathology. There is room for both, of course. The literature on self-compassion and body image may simply reflect the fact that compassion-based interventions were developed in clinical psychology, initially to improve outcomes for depressed patients who did not respond to cognitive-behaviour therapy, but now adopted for eating disorders. The application of body compassion to other physical or body-related conditions that are not psychopathology but about adaptation to health conditions and the adoption of healthy behaviours opens up whole new opportunities for research. The development of measures of body compassion (as opposed to self-compassion) and the development of light touch interventions should also prove useful in supporting this research.

References

Adams, C. E., & Leary, M. R. (2007). Promoting self–compassionate attitudes toward eating among restrictive and guilty eaters. *Journal of Social and Clinical Psychology, 26*(10), 1120–1144. https://doi.org/10.1521/jscp.2007.26.10.1120

Albertson, E. R., Neff, K. D., & Dill-Shackleford, K. E. (2014). Self-compassion and body dissatisfaction in women: A randomized controlled trial of a brief meditation intervention. *Mindfulness*. https://doi.org/10.1007/s12671-014-0277-3

All Party Parliamentary Group on Body Image. (2012). *Reflections on body image.*

Allan, S., & Gilbert, P. (1997). Submissive behaviour and psychopathology. *British Journal of Clinical Psychology, 36*, 467–488. https://doi.org/10.1111/j.2044-8260.1997.tb01255.x

Altman, J. K., Linfield, K., Salmon, P. G., & Beacham, A. O. (2017). The body compassion scale: Development and initial validation. *Journal of Health Psychology*, 1–11. https://doi.org/10.1177/1359105317718924

Barata-Santos, M., Marta-Simoes, J., & Ferreira, C. (2019). Body compassion safeguards against the impact of major life events on binge eating. *Appetite, 134*, 34–39.

Beadle, E. S. (2020). *Body shame, body compassion and physical activity.* Unpublished PhD Thesis. University of Hertfordshire. https://doi.org/10.18745/th.22613

Beadle, E. S., Cain, A., Akhtar, S., Lennox, J., McGuire, L., & Troop, N. A. (2021). Development and validation of the body compassion questionnaire. *Health Psychology and Behavioral Medicine*. https://doi.org/10.1080/21642850.2021.1993229

Beadle, E. S., Cain, A., & Troop, N. A. (2025a). *Body compassion, mood and disability*. In preparation.

Beadle, E. S., Cain, A., & Troop, N. A. (2025b). *Body compassionate expressive writing and physical activity*. In preparation.

Berry, K. A., Kowalski, K. C., Ferguson, L. J., & McHugh, T. L. F. (2010). An empirical phenomenology of young adult women exercisers' body self-compassion. *Qualitative Research in Sport and Exercise, 2*(3), 293–312. https://doi.org/10.1080/19398441.2010.517035

Braun, T. D., Park, C. L., & Gorin, A. (2016). Self-compassion, body image, and disordered eating: A review of the literature. *Body Image*. https://doi.org/10.1016/j.bodyim.2016.03.003

Carter, A., Gilbert, P., & Kirby, J. N. (2020). Compassion-focused therapy for body weight shame: A mixed methods pilot trial. *Clinical Psychology and Psychotherapy*, 1–16. https://doi.org/10.1002/cpp.2488

Cash, T. F. (2002). Body image assessments: MBSRQ. Available at: http://www.body-images.com/assessments/mbsrq.html

Connan, F., Troop, N. A., Landau, S., Campbell, I. C., & Treasure, J. L. (2007). Poor social comparison and the tendency to submissive behavior in anorexia nervosa. *International Journal of Eating Disorders, 40*, 733–793. https://doi.org/10.1002/eat.20427

Daye, C. A., Webb, J. B., & Jafari, N. (2014). Exploring self-compassion as a refuge against recalling the body-related shaming of caregiver eating messages on dimensions of objectified body consciousness in college women. *Body Image, 11*, 547–556.

de Carvalho Barreto, M., Ferreira, C., Marta-Simoes, J., & Mendes, A. L. (2018). Exploring the paths between self-compassionate attributes and actions, body compassion and disordered eating. *Eating and Weight Disorders - Studies on Anorexia, Bulimia and Obesity*. https://doi.org/10.1007/s40519-018-0581-3

Denu, S. L., Dacey, C. M., Beacham, A. O., & Zucchero, R. (2019). Acceptance and body compassion improve quality of life in endometrial cancer patients. https://doi.org/10.31234/osf.io/kw2sm

Dijkstra, P., & Bartelds, D. P. H. (2011). Examining a model of dispositional mindfulness, body comparison, and body satisfaction. *Body Image, 8*, 419–422.

Duarte, C., Pinto-Gouveia, J., & Stubbs, R. J. (2017). Compassionate attention and regulation of eating behaviour: A pilot study of a brief low-intensity intervention for binge eating. *Clinical Psychology and Psychotherapy, 24*, O1437–O1447. https://doi.org/10.1002/cpp.2094

Dunkley, D. M., Masheb, R. M., & Grilo, C. M. (2010). Childhood maltreatment, depressive symptoms, and body dissatisfaction in patients with binge eating disorder: The mediating role of self-criticism. *International Journal of Eating Disorders, 43*(3), 274–281. https://doi.org/10.1002/eat.20796

East, P., Startup, H., Roberts, C., & Schmidt, U. (2010). Expressive writing and eating disorder features: A preliminary trial in a student sample of the impact of three writing tasks on eating disorder symptoms and associated cognitive, affective and interpersonal factors. *European Eating Disorders Review, 18*, 180–196.

Ferreira, C., Marta-Simões, J., & Oliveira, S. (2018). The body compassion scale: A confirmatory factor analysis with a sample of Portuguese adults. *European Psychiatry, S*, 48.

Ferreira, C., Pinto-Gouveia, J., & Duarte, C. (2013). Self-compassion in the face of shame and body image dissatisfaction: Implications for eating disorders. *Eating Behaviors, 14*(2), 207–210.

Frattaroli, J. (2006). Experimental disclosure and its moderators: A meta-analysis. *Psychological Bulletin, 132*(6), 823–865. https://doi.org/10.1037/0033-2909.132.6.823

Frayne, A., & Wade, T. D. (2006). A comparison of written emotional expression and planning with respect to bulimic symptoms and associated psychopathology. *European Eating Disorders Review, 14*, 329–340.

Fredrickson, B. L., & Roberts, T. (1997). Objectification theory: Toward understanding women's lived experiences and mental health risks. *Psychology of Women Quarterly, 21*(1997), 173–206. https://doi.org/10.1111/j.1471-6402.1997.tb00108.x

Gale, C., Gilbert, P., Read, N., & Goss, K. (2012). An evaluation of the impact of introducing compassion focused therapy to a standard treatment programme for people with eating disorders. *Clinical Psychology and Psychotherapy, 21*, 1–12. https://doi.org/10.1002/cpp.1806

Geller, J., Srikameswaran, S., & Zelichowska, J. (2015). Resilience to shape and weight concerns and disordered eating: The role of self-compassion. *Advances in Eating Disorders: Theory, Research and Practice, 3*, 4–12. https://doi.org/10.1080/21662630.2014.945604

Germer, C. K., & Barnhofer, T. (2017). Mindfulness and compassion: Similarities and differences. In *Compassion: Concepts, research and applications* (pp. 69–86). Routledge. https://doi.org/10.4324/9781315564296

Germer, C. K., & Neff, K. D. (2013). The mindful self-compassion training program. In T. Singer & M. Bolz (Eds.), *Compassion: Bridging theory and practice: A multimedia book* (pp. 365–396). Max-Planck Institute.

Gilbert, P. (2005). Compassion and cruelty: A biopsychosocial approach. In P. Gilbert (Ed.), *Compassion: Conceptualisations, Research and Use in Psychotherapy* (pp. 3–74). Routledge.

Gilbert, P. (2006). Evolution and depression: Issues and implications. *Psychological Medicine, 36*, 287–297. https://doi.org/10.1017/S0033291705006112

Gilbert, P. (2009). Introducing compassion-focused therapy. *Advances in Psychiatric Treatment, 15*(3), 199–208. https://doi.org/10.1192/apt.bp.107.005264

Gilbert, P. (2010). An introduction to compassion focused therapy in cognitive behavior therapy. *International Journal of Cognitive Therapy, 3*(2), 97–112. https://doi.org/10.1521/ijct.2010.3.2.97

Gilbert, P. (2014). The origins and nature of compassion focused therapy. *British Journal of Clinical Psychology, 53*(1), 6–41. https://doi.org/10.1111/bjc.12043

Gilbert, P. (2017). Compassion: definitions and controversies. In P. Gilbert (Ed.), *Compassion: Concepts, research and applications* (pp. 3–15). Routledge.

Gilbert, P., & Choden. (2013). *Mindful compassion*. Robinson.
Gilbert, P., & Procter, S. (2006). Compassionate mind training for people with high shame and self-criticism: Overview and pilot study of a group therapy approach. *Clinical Psychology and Psychotherapy*. https://doi.org/10.1002/cpp.507
Gois, A. C., Ferreira, C., & Mendes, A. (2018). Steps toward understanding the impact of early emotional experiences on disordered eating: The role of self-criticism, shame, and body image shame. *Appetite, 125*, 10–17. https://doi.org/10.1016/j.appet.2018.01.025
Gollwitzer, P. (1999). Implementation intentions: Strong effects of simple plans. *American Psychologist, 54*, 493–503.
Goss, K. (2011). *The compassionate-mind guide to ending overeating*. New Harbinger Publications.
Goss, K., & Allan, S. (2009). Shame, pride and eating disorders. *Clinical Psychology and Psychotherapy, 16*, 303–316.
Goss, K., & Allan, S. (2010). Compassion focused therapy for eating disorders. *International Journal of Cognitive Therapy, 3*(2), 141–158. https://doi.org/10.1521/ijct.2010.3.2.141
Herman, C. P., & Mack, D. (1975). Restrained and unrestrained eating. *Journal of Personality, 43*, 646–660.
Herman, C. P., & Polivy, J. (1984). A boundary model for the regulation of eating. In A. J. Stunkard & E. Stellar (Eds.), *Eating and its disorders* (pp. 141–156). Raven Press.
Holtham, T., & Dyck, M. (2014). The positive impact of self-compassion on disordered eating and associated risk factors. *Journal of Eating Disorders, 2*, 4.
Homan, K. J., & Tylka, T. L. (2015). Self-compassion moderates body comparison and appearance self-worth's inverse relationships with body appreciation. *Body Image, 15*, 1–7. https://doi.org/10.1016/j.bodyim.2015.04.007
Imrie, S., & Troop, N. A. (2012). A pilot study on the effects and feasibility of compassion-focused expressive writing in Day Hospice patients. *Palliative and Supportive Care, 10*(2), 115–122. https://doi.org/10.1017/S1478951512000181
Jazaieri, H., Jinpa, G. T., McGonigal, K., Rosenberg, E. L., Finkelstein, J., Simon-Thomas, E., Cullen, M., Doty, J. R., Gross, J. J., & Goldin, P. R. (2013). Enhancing compassion: A randomized controlled trial of a compassion cultivation training program. *Journal of Happiness Studies, 14*, 1113–1126. https://doi.org/10.1007/s10902-012-9373-z
Jeziorek-Wozny, A. (2019). *The lived experience of barriers to self-compassion in women experiencing weight difficulties*. Unpublished Doctoral (DClinPsy) thesis. Royal Holloway, University of London.
Kelly, A. C., & Carter, J. C. (2015). Self-compassion training for binge eating disorder: A pilot randomized controlled trial. *Psychology and Psychotherapy: Theory, Research and Practice, 88*(3), 285–303. https://doi.org/10.1111/papt.12044

Kelly, A. C., Vimalakanthan, K., & Miller, K. E. (2014a). Self-compassion moderates the relationship between body mass index and both eating disorder pathology and body image flexibility. *Body Image, 11*, 446–453.

Kelly, A. C., Carter, J. C., & Borairi, S. (2014b). Are improvements in shame and self-compassion early in eating disorders treatment associated with better patient outcomes? *International Journal of Eating Disorders, 47*(1), 54–64. https://doi.org/10.1002/eat.22196

Kelly, A. C., Carter, J. C., Zuroff, D. C., & Borairi, S. (2012). Self-compassion and fear of self-compassion interact to predict response to eating disorders treatment: A preliminary investigation. *Psychotherapy Research*. https://doi.org/10.1080/10503307.2012.717310

Kelly, A. C., Wisniewski, L., Martin-Wagar, C., & Hoffman, E. (2017). Group-based compassion-focused therapy as an adjunct to outpatient treatment for eating disorders: A pilot randomized controlled trial. *Clinical Psychology and Psychotherapy, 24*, 475–487.

Khanjani, S., Gharraee, B., Ramezani Farani, A., & Foroughi, A. (2020). Psychometric properties of Persian version of body image shame scale: A study in cosmetic surgery clinics. *Iranian Journal of Psychiatry and Behavioral Science*, 14(2), e99492. https://doi.org/10.5812/ijpbs.99492

Kupeli, N. (2014). *Stress, affect systems and eating pathology in problematic weight regulation*. Unpublished PhD thesis. University of Hertfordshire.

Kupeli, N., Norton, S., Chilcot, J., Campbell, I. C., Schmidt, U. H., & Troop, N. A. (2017). Affect systems, changes in body mass index, disordered eating and stress: An 18-month longitudinal study in women. *Health Psychology and Behavioral Medicine., 5*(1), 214–228. https://doi.org/10.1080/21642850.2017.1316667

Kupeli, N., Schmidt, U. H., Campbell, I. C., Chilcot, J., Roberts, C., & Troop, N. A. (2018). The impact of an emotionally expressive writing intervention on eating pathology in female students. *Health Psychology and Behavioral Medicine, 6*, 162–179.

Leary, M. R., Tate, E. B., Adams, C. E., Allen, A. B., & Hancock, J. (2007). Self-compassion and reactions to unpleasant self-relevant events: The implications of treating oneself kindly. *Journal of Personality and Social Psychology, 92*(5), 887–904. https://doi.org/10.1037/0022-3514.92.5.887

Linardon, J., Susanto, L., Tepper, H., & Fuller-Tyszkiewicz, M. (2020). Self-compassion as a moderator of the relationships between shape and weight overvaluation and eating disorder psychopathology, psychosocial impairment, and psychological distress. *Body Image, 33*, 183–189.

MacBeth, A., & Gumley, A. (2012). Exploring compassion: A meta-analysis of the association between self-compassion and psychopathology. *Clinical Psychology Review, 32*, 545–552.

Mantzios, M., Egan, H., Bahia, H., Hussain, M., & Keyte, R. (2018). How does grazing relate to body mass index, self-compassion, mindfulness and mindful eating in a student population? *Health Psychology Open*. https://doi.org/10.1177/2055102918762701

Mantzios, M., Egan, H., Hussain, M., Keyte, R., & Bahia, H. (2018). Mindfulness, self-compassion, and mindful eating in relation to fat and sugar consumption: An exploratory investigation. *Eating and Weight Disorders - Studies on Anorexia, Bulimia and Obesity, 23*, 833–840.

Melissant, H. C., Jansen, F., Eerenstein, S. E. J., Cuijpers, P., Lissenberg-Witte, B. I., Sherman, K. A., Laan, E. T. M., Leemans, C. R., & Verdonck-de Leeuw, I. M. (2021). A structured expressive writing activity targeting body image-related distress among head and neck cancer survivors: who do we reach and what are the effects? *Support Care Cancer, 29*, 5763–5776. https://doi.org/10.1007/s00520-021-06114-y

Mifsud, A., Pehlivan, M. J., Fam, P., O'Grady, M., van Steensel, A., Elder, E., Gilchrist, J., & Sherman, K. A. (2021). Feasibility and pilot study of a brief self-compassion intervention addressing body image distress in breast cancer survivors. *Health Psychology and Behavioral Medicine, 9*, 498–526. https://doi.org/10.1080/21642850.2021.1929236

Mosewich, A. D., Kowalski, K. C., Sabiston, C. M., Sedgwick, W. A., & Tracy, J. L. (2011). Self-compassion: A potential resource for young women athletes. *Journal of Sport and Exercise Psychology, 33*(1), 103–123. https://doi.org/10.1123/jsep.33.1.103

Murn, L. T. (2013). *Increasing self-compassion and positive body esteem: An expressive writing intervention*. Unpublished PhD thesis: Oklahoma State University.

Neff, K. D. (2003a). Self-compassion: An alternative conceptualization of a healthy attitude toward oneself. *Self and Identity, 2*(2), 85–101. https://doi.org/10.1080/15298860309032

Neff, K. D. (2003b). The development and validation of a scale to measure self-compassion. *Self and Identity, 2*(3), 223–250. https://doi.org/10.1080/15298860390209035

Neff, K. D., & Germer, C. K. (2013). A pilot study and randomized controlled trial of the mindful self-compassion program. *Journal of Clinical Psychology, 69*(1), 28–44. https://doi.org/10.1002/jclp.21923

O'Connor, D. B., Hurling, R., Hendrickx, H., Osborne, G., Hall, J., Walklet, E., Whaley, A., & Wood, H. (2010). Effects of written emotional disclosure on implicit self-esteem and body-image. *British Journal of Health Psychology, 16*, 488–501.

Ogden, J., Gosling, C., Hazelwood, M., & Atkins, E. (2020). Exposure to body diversity images as a buffer against the thin-ideal: An experimental study. *Psychology Health and Medicine, 25*, 1165–1178. https://doi.org/10.1080/13548506.2020.1734219

Oliveira, S., Trindade, I. A., & Ferresra, C. (2018). The buffer effect of body compassion on the association between shame and body and eating difficulties. *Appetite, 125*, 118–123.

Ouwens, M., Kupeli, N., Beadle, E., & Troop, N. A. (2025). *Body compassion through expressive writing*. Submitted.

Palmeira, L., Pinto-Gouveia, J., & Cunha, M. (2017). Exploring the efficacy of an acceptance, mindfulness and compassionate-based group intervention for women struggling with their weight (kg-Free): A randomised control trial. *Appetite, 112*, 107–116. https://doi.org/10.1016/j.appet.2017.01.027

Pennebaker, J. W., & Beall, S. K. (1986). Confronting a traumatic event: Toward an understanding of inhibition and disease. *Journal of Abnormal Psychology, 95*(3), 274–281. https://doi.org/10.1037/0021-843X.95.3.274

Policardo, G. R., Nerini, A., Di Gesto, C., & Matera, C. (2022). Body compassion scale: A validation study in the Italian context. *European Journal of Health Psychology, 29*, 88–98. https://doi.org/10.1027/2512-8442/a000088

Przezdziecki, A., Alcorso, J., & Sherman, K. A. (2016). My changed body: Background, development and acceptability of a self-compassion based writing activity for female survivors of breast cancer. *Patient Education and Counseling, 99*(5), 870–874. https://doi.org/10.1016/j.pec.2015.12.011

Roberts, C. R., Troop, N. A., Connan, F., Treasure, J. L., & Campbell, I. (2007). The effects of stress on body weight: Biological and psychological predictors of BMI. *Obesity, 15*, 3045–3055.

Rojo, L., Conesa, L., Bermudez, O., & Livianos, L. (2006). Influence of stress in the onset of eating disorders: Data from a two-stage epidemiologic controlled study. *Psychosomatic Medicine, 68*, 628–635. https://doi.org/10.1097/01.psy.0000227749.58726.41

Ruderman, A. J. (1986). Dietary restraint: A theoretical and empirical review. *Psychological Bulletin, 99*, 247–262.

Schmidt, U. H., Tiller, J. M., Andrews, B., Blanchard, M., & Treasure, J. L. (1997). Is there a specific trauma precipitating onset of anorexia nervosa? *Psychological Medicine, 27*, 523–530.

Seekis, V., Bradley, G. L., & Duffy, A. (2017). The effectiveness of self-compassion and self-esteem writing tasks in reducing body image concerns. *Body Image, 23*, 206–213. https://doi.org/10.1016/j.bodyim.2017.09.003

Sherman, K. A., Przezdziecki, A., Alcorso, J., Kilby, C. J., Elder, E., Boyages, J., Koelmeyer, L., & Mackie, H. (2018). Reducing body image–related distress in women with breast cancer using a structured online writing exercise: Results from the My Changed Body randomized controlled trial. *Journal of Clinical Oncology, 36*(19), 1930–1940. https://doi.org/10.1200/jco.2017.76.3318

Sherman, K. A., Roper, T., & Kilby, C. J. (2019). Enhancing self-compassion in individuals with visible skin conditions: randomised pilot of the 'My Changed Body' self-compassion writing intervention. *Health Psychology and Behavioral Medicine, 7*(1), 62–77. https://doi.org/10.1080/21642850.2019.1587298

Sick, K., Pila, E., Nesbitt, A., & Sabiston, C. (2020). Does self-compassion buffer the detrimental effect of body shame on depressive symptoms? *Body Image, 34*, 175–183.

Smith, B. (2013). Disability, sport and men's narratives of health: A qualitative study. *Health Psychology, 32*(1), 110–119. https://doi.org/10.1037/a0029187

Smyth, J. M. (1998). Written emotional expression: Effect sizes, outcome types, and moderating variables. *Journal of Consulting and Clinical Psychology, 66*(1), 174–184. https://doi.org/10.1037/0022-006X.66.1.174

Steindl, S. R., Buchanan, K., Goss, K., & Allan, S. (2017). Compassion focused therapy for eating disorders: A qualitative review and recommendations for further applications. *Clinical Psychologist, 21*(2), 62–73. https://doi.org/10.1111/cp.12126

Stern, N. G., & Engeln, R. (2018). Self-compassionate writing exercises increase college women's body satisfaction. *Psychology of Women Quarterly, 42*(3), 326–341. https://doi.org/10.1177/0361684318773356

Stewart, S. J., & Ogden, J. (2021). The impact of body diversity vs thin-idealistic media messaging on health outcomes: An experimental study. *Psychology, Health & Medicine, 26*, 631–643. https://doi.org/10.1080/13548506.2020.1859565

Stice, E. (1994). Review of the evidence for a sociocultural model of bulimia nervosa and an exploration of the mechanisms of action. *Clinical Psychology Review, 14*, 633–661.

Stokes, E. (2013). *The relationship between connectedness to nature, happiness, self-concept and self-esteem in naturist and non-naturist samples: A mixed method approach*. Unpublished MSc Thesis. Keele University.

Tausczik, Y. R., & Pennebaker, J. W. (2010). The psychological meaning of words: LIWC and computerised text analysis methods. *Journal of Language and Social Psychology, 29*, 24–53.

Tennant, C. (2002). Life events, stress and depression: A review of recent findings. *Australian and New Zealand Journal of Psychiatry, 36*, 173–182. https://doi.org/10.1046/j.1440-1614.2002.01007.x

Thompson, J. K., Heinberg, L. J., Altabe, M., & Tantleff-Dunn, S. (1999). *Exacting beauty: Theory, assessment, and treatment of body image disturbance*. American Psychological Association.

Troop, N. A. (1996). *Coping and crisis support in eating disorders*. Unpublished PhD Thesis. IoP.

Troop, N. A. (2016). Social rank, rank-related life events and eating pathology. *European Eating Disorders Review, 24*, 75–77.

Troop, N. A., Allan, S., Treasure, J. L., & Katzman, M. (2003). Social comparison and submissive behaviour in eating disorder patients. *British Journal of Clinical Psychology, 76*, 237–249. https://doi.org/10.1348/147608303322362479

Troop, N. A., Andrews, L., Hiskey, S., & Treasure, J. L. (2014). Social rank and symptom change in eating disorders: A 6-month longitudinal study. *Clinical Psychology & Psychotherapy, 21*, 115–122. https://doi.org/10.1002/cpp.1830

Troop, N. A., Holbrey, A., & Treasure, J. L. (1998). Stress, coping and crisis support in eating disorders. *International Journal of Eating Disorders, 24*, 157–166.

Troop, N. A., & Treasure, J. L. (1997a). Psychosocial factors in the onset of eating disorders: Responses to life events and difficulties. *British Journal of Medical Psychology, 70*, 373–385.

Troop, N. A., & Treasure, J. L. (1997b). Setting the scene for eating disorders II: Childhood helplessness and mastery. *Psychological Medicine, 27*, 531–538.

Tylka, T.L., Russell, H.L., & Neal, A.A. (2015). Self-compassion as a moderator of thinness-related pressures' associations with thin-ideal internalization and disordered eating. *Eating Behaviors, 17*, 23–26.

Wasylkiw, L., MacKinnon, A. L., & MacLellan, A. M. (2012). Exploring the link between self-compassion and body image in university women. *Body Image, 9*, 236–245. https://doi.org/10.1016/j.bodyim.2012.01.007

Welch, S. L., Doll, H. A., & Fairburn, C. G. (1997). Life events and the onset of bulimia nervosa: A controlled study. *Psychological Medicine, 27*, 515–522. https://doi.org/10.1017/S0033291796004370

Woekel, E., & Ebbeck, V. (2013). Transitional bodies: A qualitative investigation of postpartum body self-compassion. *Qualitative Research in Sport, Exercise and Health, 5*(2), 245–266. https://doi.org/10.1080/2159676X.2013.766813

Wong, M., Chung, P. K., & Leung, K. M. (2022). Psychometric properties of Chinese translated body compassion scale (BCS) among Hong Kong adolescents. *Journal of Exercise Science & Fitness, 20*, 54–61. https://doi.org/10.1016/j.jesf.2021.10.001

Wood, M., & Pila, E. (2022). Investigating the effects of fit-normative and weight-inclusive Instagram images on women's exercise motivations. *Body Image, 41*, 460–471. https://doi.org/10.1016/j.bodyim.2022.04.003

21

The Role of Self-Compassion for Adjustment to Inflammatory Bowel Disease

Rebecca Yeates and Georgina Rowse

Life with a chronic illness is challenging for individuals across both physical and psychological aspects of daily life. The symptoms themselves often encompass pain, limit daily functioning, and treatments and medication are often associated with side-effects. Potential limitations on diet and restrictions on time place individuals under significant strain due to their prolonged and uncertain trajectories. Many chronic health conditions are relapsing and remitting, with uncertain trajectories, presenting their own stressors and posing difficulties in coping. There is also a psychological impact of chronic ill health, managing compromise and self-management, with implications for individuals' wellbeing, quality of life and potential life-course (education, employment, relationships and family plans).

This chapter sets out to specifically look at living with the chronic illness inflammatory bowel disease, a chronic condition, encompassing Crohn's disease and ulcerative colitis, and how self-compassion may have a role in self-management and positive outcomes, both for physical disease outcomes and

---

R. Yeates (✉)
Leeds Clinical Psychology Training Programme, School of Medicine, The University of Leeds, Leeds, UK
e-mail: r.a.yeates@leeds.ac.uk

G. Rowse
Clinical and Applied Psychology, University of Sheffield Cathedral Court, Sheffield, UK
e-mail: g.rowse@sheffield.ac.uk

F. M. Sirois (ed.), *The Palgrave Handbook of Positive Psychology and Health*,
https://doi.org/10.1007/978-3-031-89095-6_21

their associated psychological impact. The limited, but growing, evidence base for self-compassion, the act of taking a kind, balanced and non-judgemental stance towards oneself (Neff, 2016), as a resource for successful living with IBD will be outlined, along with considerations of the potential future clinical implications and next avenues for research in this field. Specifically, it will outline the theoretical rationale for this clinical approach, its existing evidence and what is required to advance the field.

Inflammatory Bowel Disease

Inflammatory bowel disease (IBD) is a broad term used to refer to a group of chronic and relapsing-remitting conditions that affect the digestive system, the two most prevalent conditions being Crohn's disease and ulcerative colitis (Goodhand et al., 2011). The conditions have previously been considered as having unknown aetiology and no cure (NICE; Mayberry et al., 2013). However, more recently the cause of IBD is proposed to result from an over-active immune response in the gut (El Menyiy et al., 2022). IBD affects the digestive tract and when active (in a 'flare'), erodes the lining of the colon causing ulcers, inflammation of areas of the digestive tract, and can result in lesions and strictures of the bowel wall. Ulcerative colitis affects the large intestine whereas Crohn's disease can affect any part of the digestive system (McCombie et al., 2013). A number of associated symptoms are also common, including inflammation of the mouth, skin, joints and liver, and weight loss and fatigue. Whilst IBD is rarely fatal, the impact of the disease can be profound and cause considerable physical, psychological and social impacts for individuals. IBD treatments can generate additional physical complications for individuals: corticosteroid treatment can result in weight gain and acne and surgery may lead to ileostomies (Greenley et al., 2010; Mackner & Crandall, 2007).

Around 1 in 100 people have a diagnosis of IBD, with the average age of diagnosis in adolescence. A recent European study identified around 37% of those with Crohn's Disease alone need to have surgery on diseased areas of bowel within 10 years of diagnosis (Odes et al., 2006) although a range of between 29% and 61% has been identified across studies (Bernstein et al., 2012), with a small number resulting in a stoma, which brings with it challenges and further psychological impact. The symptoms of IBD can be distressing for individuals to manage, with nearly a quarter experiencing incontinence at some point during a disease flare up (24%; Gu et al., 2018), and with individuals reporting the stigma surrounding the condition resulting in feelings of shame.

IBD affects individuals across the lifespan; however, a large proportion of IBD patients are young people (Ghione et al., 2018). Twenty-five percent of individuals with IBD are diagnosed by the age of 16 years (IBD Standards Group, 2009). Research has found that IBD poses some specific developmental challenges for young people: delays to physical growth and puberty; reduced autonomy; and lower self-worth (Loonen et al., 2002; Pfefferkorn et al., 2009; Nicholas et al., 2007). These challenges occur for young people at a crucial time in their psychological development when they are establishing their independence, identity and forming relationships (Arnett, 2000; Goodhand et al., 2011). The impacts on adults with IBD are also not insubstantial, impacting on relationships, parenting and employment (Trindade et al., 2017).

Treatment for IBD

There is no cure for IBD, though several treatments and interventions are available. These are largely focused on achieving relief from, and stability of, physical symptoms and maintenance and extension of periods of remission. Treatment management varies according to individual disease factors, such as the severity, location of the inflammation and the individuals' age. First line interventions are usually pharmaceutical to induce remission, often administered via regular infusion or injection, surgery to remove or repair affected sections of the digestive tract and tube feeding (Kapasi et al., 2020; Martins et al., 2019). Surgical interventions, when strictures result in obstructions in the bowel, are frequent, occurring in between 29% and 61% of those diagnosed with IBD (Bernstein et al., 2012). However, diet and lifestyle changes are increasingly being utilised in combination with pharmaceutical options; however, sometimes these are restrictive in nature (e.g., eliminating a food group) which whilst helpful for disease control may contribute to an overall reliance upon avoidant coping, and have been associated with disordered eating patterns and their associated impact on mental health (Ilzarbe et al., 2017).

The treatment and interventions themselves also have a number of side-effects, such as headache, nausea, fatigue and rashes (Pithadia & Jain, 2011). Pharmacological interventions for both disease activity and distress (e.g., antidepressants) are associated with improvements in wellbeing and quality of life (Calvet et al., 2006). However, there is evidence to suggest up to 45% of IBD patients do not adhere to their prescribed medications (Gracie et al., 2018).

Medication non-adherence is multi-factorial but psychological factors such as holding negative beliefs about medications and experiencing or anticipating unpleasant side effects are believed to reduce adherence (Lehane & McCarthy, 2007). Additionally, there are further burdens on the patients in the receipt of these treatments, infusions are delivered in hospital out-patient settings, with a frequency of between 4 and 12 weeks, and a duration of up to 4 hours per visit. These can have an ongoing impact on daily life for the individual, potentially impacting education and employment, as discussed below.

Psychological Impact of IBD

Living with a chronic illness like IBD is a profoundly stressful experience for individuals due to uncertain trajectories and prognoses of the illnesses (Keeton et al., 2015). Stress is a state of disharmony or threat to living organisms' homeostasis generated by stressors (Chrousos & Gold, 1992). Stress activates bodily hormones such as cortisol and the brain's 'threat system' which has a powerful impact on the way individuals interact with the environment and themselves (Gilbert, 2005). When the threat system is activated, physiological, emotional, cognitive and behavioural responses are triggered which aim to 'fight' the threat or escape it. Whilst the fight-flight response has long had important evolutionary utility in instances where there is a threat to life, many 'new brain' threats such as stressors posed by chronic health conditions quickly reoccur and do not pose immediate threat to life (Gilbert, 2009). Prolonged activation of the threat system can lead the system to become the dominant emotional regulation system over alternative active and restorative responses, manifesting in clinical symptoms such as low mood or anxiety.

Unsurprisingly, IBD has been shown to have psychosocial consequences. Qualitative studies find that individuals with IBD face illness stigma and consequently either choose not to disclose their illness and isolate themselves to prevent its discovery, or face anguish deciding how much and when to disclose, fearing shaming responses (Guo et al., 2020). Many subsequently view the body as flawed or damaged and hold fears over what their future may hold (Fourie et al., 2018). The impact on education and employment can be complex, for example, one study conducted identified individuals with IBD losing 4.8 working days per year more than their healthy counterparts (Gunnarsson et al., 2013), but also IBD having an impact, in that they would choose employment that is manageable within the restrictions of the disease (van Gennep et al., 2021). Rates of sickness leave from work are high in adults with IBD and children and young people have been found to exhibit lower educational functioning with greater absences from educational settings (Bassi et al., 2004; Diederen et al., 2018). Concerns about the duration of a flare, being able to control it and access to toilets have often been found to underpin these education and employment difficulties (van Erp et al., 2017; Barnes et al., 2020). Social interactions and relationships are also impacted in myriad ways (Devlen et al., 2014).

A recent systematic review estimated that 1 in 3 adults with IBD experience clinically significant anxiety and 1 in 4 experience depression (Barberio et al., 2021). Young people with IBD are also estimated to have a 4.6 times greater odds of having clinically significant symptoms of anxiety or depression than healthy peers (Mackner & Crandall, 2007; Raymer et al., 1984). Individuals with IBD have also been found to higher rates of psychological distress and reduced quality of life when compared to healthy individuals without IBD (Graff et al., 2009; Knowles et al., 2018; Mikocka-Walus et al., 2016). This is unsurprising given the prolonged stressors they face: such as obtaining a diagnosis, ongoing symptoms, extended physical treatments, recovery and risk of relapse (Casati et al., 2000; Drossman et al., 1989; Kemp et al., 2012; Larsson et al., 2008). In addition to anxiety and depression, the pain that is associated with eating and drinking can also be associated with disordered eating, with the majority of those living with IBD limiting their diet in some way, in an attempt to manage their symptoms, the more extreme of these experiencing eating disorders (Ilzarbe et al., 2017).

A number of factors have been identified as elevating the risk of psychological distress. Illness activity, nonadherence to treatment, unemployment and lower socioeconomic status have all been associated with increased risk in adults (Nahon et al., 2012). A systematic review identified that increased illness activity, being diagnosed younger, having lower socioeconomic status, being prescribed corticosteroids and parental stress were all risk factors for young people (Brooks et al., 2016; Hoogkamer et al., 2018). These findings highlight that across the lifespan, the severity of the illness, treatment status and an individual's living conditions and/or access to resources play key roles in an individual's ability to live well.

The relationship between disease activity and distress is not believed to be unidirectional. Poor psychological wellbeing has also been associated with shorter time-to-'flare', more severe disease and greater hospitalisations, creating a 'vicious cycle' which can prolong both distress and disease duration (Graff et al., 2009; Dubinsky et al., 2021). The 'brain-gut axis' which proposes a physiological link between the central nervous system and the gut is understood to underpin this relationship within Irritable Bowel Syndrome (IBS) but has been less applied to IBD (Gracie et al., 2018). However, with increasing awareness of the link between inflammation and mood (Alinaghi et al., 2020), the relationship between IBD and mental health has garnered more recent interest, and the bi-directional impacts identified with improvements in mental wellbeing having positive associations with disease outcomes and vice versa emphasise the need for a focus on psychological factors.

Bi-directional Relationship Between Disease Activity and Distress in IBD

Recent longitudinal survey research has supported a bi-directional link between distress and disease activity in which active disease and distress both precede one another; however, the results were based on self-reported disease indices (Gracie et al., 2018). Nevertheless, the clear adverse links between psychological distress and symptom severity, and the associated costs of relapse to individuals and the National Health Service (NHS), is causing attention to be increasingly paid to how psychological wellbeing may be linked to IBD (Bassi et al., 2004; Ghosh & Premchand, 2015).

One possible link between IBD and distress may be how the disease is viewed by the individual. The Common Sense Model (CSM) of self-regulation in health and illness proposes that in response to an illness, an individual develops ideas about the nature of their illness which informs the way they assess the threats presented by it and in turn how they cope with them (Leventhal et al., 2016). Appraisals of stressors and mechanisms for coping can therefore reduce or amplify the impact of stressors like chronic health conditions and are therefore important determinants of quality of life (Skinner et al., 2003; Compas et al., 2012; Goodhand & Rampton, 2008). One study has found that when individuals perceived more serious consequences to IBD, had a greater perception of control over it and had a weaker understanding of the illness, they decreased their physical activity more which in turn was associated with poorer mental and physical wellbeing (van Erp et al., 2017). These findings suggest that fear-based appraisals may lead to greater use of avoidant coping styles which when relied upon are widely associated with poorer mental health. Both adults and young people diagnosed with IBD make greater use of avoidant coping styles (e.g., minimising, social withdrawal) when compared to healthy controls (Jones et al., 2006). Higher IBD illness activity has also been linked with greater use of avoidant strategies and in turn poorer psychological adjustment (Voth & Sirois, 2009). This suggests that individuals with IBD may retreat both physically and psychologically at times of stress in an attempt to generate feelings of greater control over the illness in the short term but this may ultimately limit their connections to others and meaningful activity and lead to deteriorations in their quality of life. Interventions which raise awareness of the connections between fear, shame, avoidant coping and its maintenance of distress are likely to be helpful to individuals with IBD.

In summary, research into the psychological needs of individuals with IBD is developing and key themes are emerging from both the qualitative and quantitative literature. Both stress and distress are high amongst individuals living with the condition, particularly when the disease is active. Common fears are the unpredictability of the condition, subsequent levels of control over both day-to-day life and long-term goals and appraisals of the body (Brooks et al., 2015). These stressors are exacerbated by the stigma surrounding the condition and subsequent fears about how others will respond to the discovery of the condition. Active approaches to practical and emotional challenges, like problem solving and meditation (Gerbarg et al., 2015), are associated with improved emotional wellbeing whilst avoidant coping is associated with poorer wellbeing outcomes (Voth & Sirois, 2009). Positive psychology approaches such as compassion, mindfulness and acceptance are garnering increasing interest as interventions for chronic health conditions. These approaches encourage individuals to turn towards and connect with their psychological pain, acknowledge underlying stressors in a balanced way and take a flexible approach to coping.

The Benefits of Self-Compassion for Living with IBD

Self-compassion as conceptualised by Kristen Neff comprises of three distinct but inter-related qualities: 'mindfulness', 'self-kindness' and 'common humanity' as well as reduced counter-states of 'over-identification', 'self-judgement' and 'isolation' (Neff, 2023). The concept originates from Buddhist psychology and in essence involves turning towards difficulties, such as a perceived shortcoming or uncontrollable circumstance, and treating oneself with warmth and compassion, in contrast to criticism or blame, and recognising oneself to not be alone in experiencing psychological pain (Neff, 2023).

Self-compassion holds a number of theoretical benefits for individuals with IBD. The relapsing and remitting nature of IBD presents a number of challenges, many of which are unforeseen, sudden and disrupt an individual's ability to live their life in the way they want. Individuals diagnosed with IBD frequently describe feeling their thoughts to be dominated by concerns over when and how the disease will become active again in both the short and long term (Keeton et al., 2015). Periods of remission are so varied in IBD, and the uncertainty of not knowing when the next flare may occur can be agonising for many. Day-to-day life is also affected by fears of losing control of the bowel and the potential for perceived humiliation, this leads many individuals to avoid meaningful work and leisure activities (Fourie et al., 2018; van der Zaag-Loonen et al., 2004; Trindade et al., 2017). Experiential avoidance, the act of trying to escape or control unwanted internal experiences, is considered an underpinning maintenance process in a number of mental health difficulties since efforts to control the unwanted experiences only provide temporary relief and typically create unintended consequences which impact psychological wellbeing (Hayes-Skelton & Eustis, 2020). IBD has been frequently associated with greater experiential avoidance, and associated coping strategies like minimisation and social withdrawal (e.g., Trindade et al., 2018).

Experiential avoidance can manifest in different ways. For example, one qualitative study with young people with IBD found that many attempted to be stoic, and hide emotions, which may be in part a desire to avoid the emotional experience itself but also avoid revealing it to others in an effort to fit in (Brooks et al., 2015). A meta-synthesis of qualitative studies investigating the experience of living with IBD found a prevalent theme across the data to be the experience of being entangled in an internal war with the disease, fighting to feel and be known as 'normal' (Kemp et al., 2012). This inner fight reflects an understandable attempt to control and avoid the disease and its associated psychological pain but this is likely to be all-consuming, leading to over-identification with this pain and leave individuals with little psychological space to disentangle themselves from it and acknowledge it in a balanced mindful way.

One component of self-compassion, mindfulness, aims to enable individuals to both acknowledge and experience their distress as opposed to attempting to escape it (Baer, 2010). It can also help individuals to step back from their fears about the past and future, which is likely to take them away from their present moment experiences, and instead help them connect with what they can be doing to live optimally in the here-and-now. That may be fully enjoying what life in remission can offer them, increased freedoms and opportunities without fears of whether this will be interrupted by an unexpected flare dominating, or connecting with what they can be doing to take care of themselves in relapse. In order to be able to adopt a self-compassionate stance, the suffering must first be identified in a balanced way. Avoiding, exaggerating or minimising pain is psychologically effortful and keeps the individual close to their suffering. In contrast, when individuals are able to identify their painful thoughts and feelings they are typically able to create a helpful distance from them. This space is hypothesised to prevent over-identification and fusion with the distress which serve to prolong the distressed state as the individual remains consumed and entangled with their suffering (Chishima et al., 2018.).

Self-kindness, as opposed to self-judgement, is the ability to unconditionally treat oneself with warmth and kindness in response to challenges or setbacks that arise from within (e.g., negative thoughts) or externally (e.g., losing out on a work promotion) (Neff, 2023). Individuals with IBD are typically living with chronic pain, fatigue, intrusive and prolonged physical treatments, altered bodies and restrictions to work, and leisure activities. These experiences often understandably leave individuals feeling different to their peers which for some cultivates feelings of inferiority and shame (Muse et al., 2021). Shame is thought to arise in circumstances where people have an experience which prevents them from feeling accepted by and connected to those around them (Miller & Tangney, 1994). Negative self-evaluations may develop as a possible internal explanation for these experiences, 'it's me', and lead individuals to develop a cold, critical inner dialogue with themselves, 'I'm a failure', which compounds feelings of distress. Individuals with IBD often express they 'should' be able to do more, feel frustration with perceived lack of fulfilment of responsibilities and express self-criticism at their own perceived limitations (Brooks et al., 2015). Many qualitative studies have also identified that individuals with IBD who can adopt a critical or uncaring attitude towards themselves may not prioritise their health. They may neglect aspects of their care, such as their medication. Others may engage in stoic over-exertion in an effort to continue life as normal (Allison et al., 2013; Brooks et al., 2017). These actions risk compromising an individual's health further which may perpetuate underlying fears of the self being flawed or inadequate. Setbacks which may have resulted from these acts of neglect may then be considered as further evidence of inadequacy.

Self-kindness contrasts with self-judgment and can offer individuals an alternative perspective by enabling them to first mindfully acknowledge these feelings of unworthiness when they arise and then to recognise them as momentary thoughts or feelings and shift their response from complicit self-criticism to loving understanding and taking action to care and nurture the self (Neff, 2023). Mistakes are accepted as an inevitable part of humanity and opportunities for learning. By adopting a self-compassionate stance, individuals can view their IBD as just one part of their existence and reflect that every human is or will experience life challenges in one or more areas of their life (Sirois & Rowse, 2016). This shift in perception can prevent individuals from becoming preoccupied by negative thoughts linked to their chronic illness, such as 'my body has been ruined by my illness' and instead recognise its implications in a balanced way and ignite a motivation to alleviate associated distress using adaptive means. Additionally, this perspective is more likely to help regulate subsequent emotional states and bring about a more thoughtful and flexible approach to coping and adjustment (Terry & Leary, 2011).

Common humanity is the view that psychological suffering is a shared human experience and unavoidable. In contrast, when an individual is struggling to connect with psychological pain being a shared experience, they may believe it to be unique to them and lead them to feel isolated and disconnected from society. The symptoms of IBD can be embarrassing and taboo to discuss which is compounded by it being an invisible illness to others, leading many individuals to hide their diagnosis (Brooks et al., 2015; Saunders, 2014). The secrecy and stigma surrounding the disease often leads individuals to feel misunderstood and at a distance from others (Lynch & Spence, 2008). This sense of isolation has the capacity to magnify one's own difficulties and not see the suffering of others. This increases the likelihood of individuals internalising that challenging life events happen more frequently to them when compared to other people and there is a risk that blame for IBD events is attributed to the individual, 'I'm flawed', and not the condition itself. This can create disconnection from support networks and provide fewer opportunities to notice other people's suffering. Isolation from others is often cited as a key stressor by individuals with IBD (Nass et al., 2022).

With a more self-compassionate lens, individuals are encouraged to see IBD challenges as part of the common human experience and that all individuals make mistakes and experience challenges. Common humanity encourages individuals to remain connected to their communities and other individuals because this offers them with a knowledge of other people's suffering, even if their triggers differ. This ultimately serves to broaden an individual's perspective beyond their own experience which helps reduce the likelihood of people viewing their challenges or shortcomings as their fault or necessarily within their control. This approach would enable individuals to feel less alone in their experiences and may reduce negative self-talk. For example, a kind inner voice may tell themselves, 'at the moment my IBD is flaring, I did nothing wrong, this happens to everyone who has IBD'. This is supported by many IBD psychological intervention studies which find that individuals with IBD describe finding it helpful to discuss living with IBD in psychological group interventions, as it serves to normalise the symptoms, thereby reducing loneliness and shame (Schoultz et al., 2016).

Taken all together, these findings suggest self-compassion has an important role to play in the self-management of IBD and research is beginning to support these theoretical links. Higher levels of trait self-compassion have been found to be associated with reduced psychological distress in both adults and young people diagnosed with IBD (Prentice et al., 2021). This suggests that those who are naturally more able to adopt a self-compassionate stance have better psychological outcomes than those who are less naturally inclined in this way. Sirois et al. (2015) also found adults with chronic illness who were higher in trait self-compassion made greater use of active, acceptance and positive reframing coping and less use of avoidance and self-blame which in turn was associated with reduced stress. Self-compassion has also been associated with reduced pain interference and distress in young adults diagnosed with IBD, with self-compassion accounting for significant proportions of variance over and above disease-related factors (Wren et al., 2021). These findings need to be replicated with an adult population and over time.

However, there is some evidence that these effects are maintained over time. One study has found these effects hold over a nine-month period, and longer disease duration was associated with greater self-compassion (Trindade & Sirois, 2021). This study also examined the individual facets of self-compassion and their relationships with wellbeing markers for people with IBD. Isolation was found to be most predictive of depression symptoms and mindfulness had greatest potential to reduce low mood and anxiety symptoms. These findings concur with other IBD research which has found individuals to be immersed in fears over the future, which disconnects individuals from their present moment awareness, and that high levels of avoidant coping strategies such as social withdrawal leave individuals feeling isolated (Fourie et al., 2018; Kemp et al., 2012). These findings together suggest that self-compassion interventions have potential value for this group and Trindade and Sirois's (2021) provide preliminary evidence to begin tailoring compassion-based interventions according to the needs of the group.

Compassion-Based Approaches for IBD

Self-compassion overlaps with other 'third-wave' concepts such as mindfulness and acceptance and is often cultivated as part of broader third-wave interventions (such as a mindfulness-based cognitive therapy; MBCT; Kuyken et al., 2010). However, it can also be the sole treatment target. Specific self-compassion interventions typically focus on supporting individuals to acknowledge and notice their tendencies to be self-critical, over-identify with their suffering and view their pain in an isolating way and then practice adopting a self-compassionate mind-set and responding to new stressors from this perspective (Neff et al., 2007). The evidence base for self-compassion interventions is still relatively small, and of limited quality within the chronic illness literature (when compared with health adult sample literature) (Ferrari et al., 2019; Wilson et al., 2019), with a lack of randomisation, intention-to-treat analyses and unclear study processes. However, a meta-analysis of self-compassion interventions for adults with chronic health conditions found moderate within-subject effects for improved self-compassion and quality of life and reduced depression, anxiety and pain (Mistretta & Davis, 2021).

Third-wave and compassion-based intervention studies which include individuals with IBD as a part of their samples are small in number, but show promising early results. However, changes in self-compassion itself is rarely a collected quantitative outcome. Untailored mindfulness interventions have been found to be effective in reducing psychological distress and improving mindfulness and quality of life (QoL) in small samples of adults with IBD when compared to individuals in the control condition and improvements were also maintained at 6-month follow-up (Jedel et al., 2014; Berrill et al., 2014; Schoultz et al., 2015).

There has also been an increase in tailored IBD-mindfulness programmes. Neilson et al. (2016) conducted a small trial of an eight-week IBD-mindfulness intervention and found a reduction in depression and improvements in quality of life and mindfulness when compared to a wait-list control condition, which was maintained at follow-up. These studies found the mindfulness interventions to be acceptable in most cases, but there was unexplored drop-out in all samples, and the relationship with disease activity was not explored. Ewais et al. (2021) recently found that young people with IBD reported significantly lower depression, stress and higher active coping, positive reframing and mindfulness, when compared to active control condition, following an adapted MBCT programme. The key adaptation was the inclusion of psycho-education about the 'gut-brain axis'. This study also collected biological markers for disease activity, including faecal calprotectin, a sensitive biomarker which when present in faeces indicates gut inflammation is present, and intestinal ultrasound; however, no significant differences were found in gut inflammation between the intervention and control groups. The results were potentially impacted by attrition and low levels of disease activity at baseline. One mindfulness intervention study found a positive impact of disease activity; González-Moret et al. (2020) found that following an eight-session hybrid face-to-face and online mindfulness intervention, adults with IBD experienced significant decreases in faecal calprotectin and in C-reactive protein levels, a protein produced by the liver which when elevated indicates gut inflammation, when compared to an active control group. This suggests that mindfulness does have the potential to improve disease outcomes, but this does require further research.

Whilst mindfulness interventions are known to cultivate self-compassion in other chronic illness groups (Merkes, 2010), the majority of existing studies investigating IBD samples have not measured changes in self-compassion. Therefore, it is unknown to what extent this is occurring within IBD samples and to what degree self-compassion contributes to overall therapeutic gains. In a recent trial which compared two brief online interventions, four-session acceptance and commitment therapy (ACT) and four-session CFT, 32.4% (n = 16) had diagnoses of IBD and self-compassion outcome data was collected (Trindade et al., 2021). No reliable clinically significant changes occurred in psychological wellbeing or self-compassion across either group which suggests that brief third-wave interventions may have limited value to this group when compared to longer therapist led third-wave interventions, although more research is needed to determine optimal treatment lengths.

At the time of writing, there were two ongoing feasibility trials investigating whether longer third-wave-based interventions can reduce distress and improve self-compassion in adults and young people with IBD. The first builds upon Trindade et al.'s (2021) study and examines an 8-session tailored ACT for IBD online group (Evans et al., 2022) and the second seeks to examine whether a 16-week sequential mindfulness and self-compassion (MBCL) intervention can improve the wellbeing of young people diagnosed with IBD (Rowse et al., 2018). The results of these trials will provide important insights and advances in the field of third-wave psychological interventions for IBD.

These studies aim to suggest that self-compassion can be cultivated in adults and young people with IBD and that both third-wave and compassion-based interventions can similarly cultivate self-compassion to produce improved outcomes in IBD. In the chronic health samples to date however the effects are not as robust as in healthy adult or mental health samples. This could be due to study quality being lower (e.g., low sample sizes), factors relating to the chronic illnesses themselves or that individuals living with chronic illnesses may require different treatment considerations (Ferrari et al., 2019). More research is required into the process of therapeutic change for individuals living with chronic illnesses such as IBD and whether there are certain factors that moderate the magnitude of change achieved.

The Benefits and Challenges to Cultivating Self-Compassion

Research encouragingly suggests that self-compassion can be taught (Germer & Neff, 2013). However, individuals with IBD may require different treatment foci and adaptations to maximise its effectiveness. In a mixed-methods systematic review where qualitative data from intervention studies with chronic illness samples was analysed, self-compassion interventions were credited with helping individuals to: accept their chronic illness and their post-condition body and its limitations; regulate threat-based emotions such as anger; and feel a sense of community and companionship amongst peers in a group setting (Austin et al., 2021). However, few studies monitor or analyse adverse effects in intervention studies or follow-up individuals who drop-out, which limits understanding of whether there are conditions in which compassion-based interventions are not as accepted or effective.

Other studies have begun to consider what may be underpinning treatment drop-out or limited gains for some individuals with chronic illnesses who engage in compassion-based interventions. Some authors have hypothesised that some individuals may experience some barriers to adopting a self-compassionate stance (Mistretta & Davis, 2021). One barrier may be the 'backdraft effect', which occurs when learning and attempting a loving and kind relationship with oneself may reveal some unexpected pain (Germer & Neff, 2013). This may be because the individual realises they have been treating themselves critically for a long time and feel a sense of grief about this, particularly if the roots of the critical voice are underpinned by traumatic experiences. Other individuals may experience a fear of positive emotions like compassion, both from others and themselves (Gilbert et al., 2014). This may be rooted in a fear of the positive emotion being taken from them or that they are undeserving of the emotion. This can lead individuals to feel a sense of threat when they are invited to show themselves kindness or when others treat them with compassion. Since individuals with IBD have been found to use more avoidant coping when compared to healthy peers (McCombie et al., 2013) and avoidance is often fused with a sense of threat, it is possible that these experiences may have some influence on the therapeutic process in compassion-based therapies.

This potential sense of threat may suggest that individuals with IBD may require more time and therapist support to cultivate a self-compassionate stance and this is supported by the finding that longer compassion-based interventions of over eight weeks produce greater effects on psychological wellbeing for this group (Mistretta & Davis, 2021). One intervention which may meet the needs of individuals with chronic illnesses is an eight-week, group-based self-compassion intervention called mindfulness-based compassionate living (MBCL), developed by Van den Brink and Koster (2015). The programme was designed to act as adjunct intervention for individuals who have already completed an eight-week mindfulness intervention such as Mindfulness Based Stress Reduction (MBSR) or Mindfulness Based Cognitive Therapy (MBCT). When delivered together, across 16 weeks, the two-part programme intends to initially lay a foundation of mindfulness skills (i.e., present moment and non-judgemental awareness) before inviting individuals to undertake the more challenging task of cultivating a self-compassionate stance. The intervention requires investment from participants, involving regular practice in-between group sessions. This sequential treatment has been piloted with physically healthy adults experiencing recurrent depression and promising findings of pre-post intervention reductions in depression and increases in self-compassion were found (Schuling et al., 2016). In a follow-up qualitative study, Schuling et al. (2021) found that participants described finding mindfulness initially helped cultivate a neutral awareness of their difficulties and MBCL then provided individuals with the psychological tools they needed to approach difficult experiences and emotions with kindness. This sequential mindfulness and MBCL approach is currently being piloted with young people with IBD (Rowse et al., 2018).

Whilst the evidence base for self-compassion interventions for IBD is developing steadily, there is still considerable work to be done to understand the full benefits of self-compassion for IBD. Rigorously conducted intervention studies are needed which analyse the effects of self-compassion over time, in both relapse and remission, and whether gains can be amplified when specific adaptations are made based on our understanding of which facets of self-compassion particularly benefit living with IBD.

Future Research Directions

Further research is needed to corroborate the preliminary findings from compassion-based interventions in larger samples of adults and young people with IBD to determine whether the smaller effects observed in chronic illness samples like IBD are due to study limitations or other factors. Many of the intervention studies conducted thus far have had significant drop-out, and understanding whether this reflects aspects of the feasibility and acceptability of compassion-based interventions needs to be understood using post-intervention qualitative studies. It is possible that greater adaptations are required to standardise compassion-based interventions to scaffold individuals with IBD's engagement with these interventions, as they experience high levels of experiential avoidance. Improvements in study quality are also required; for example, the use of active control conditions, longer follow-up intervals and monitoring both physical and psychological outcomes to further understanding as to whether psychological therapies have the capacity to influence gut health. Finally, greater research is required into the mechanisms of change in interventions to improve understanding of what the 'active ingredients' are. This will enable future researchers to further tailor IBD interventions to maximise engagement and potential for therapeutic change.

Conclusion

Individuals diagnosed with IBD face distressing symptoms and uncertain long-term disease trajectories. There is considerable stigma surrounding the condition leaving many to feel shame about their bodies and experiences. Rates of depression and anxiety are high amongst young people and adults diagnosed with the disease and absence from school and employment is common. Recent research supports a bi-directional relationship between mood and disease activity which suggests that identifying psychological coping mechanisms which can buffer against distress, to complement pharmaceutical treatments, is essential to improving long-term physical and psychological outcomes for this group. Self-compassion is one promising target. Self-compassion encourages individuals to mindfully connect with their present moment experiences, consider their experiences as part of the broader human experience and treat oneself with loving kindness. Research supports the theory that a self-compassionate mindset may provide individuals diagnosed with IBD with the skillset to recognise and challenge self-critical thoughts and tendencies to withdraw when the disease flares and enable them to instead take compassionate actions which serve their health. Current research is focused on determining whether compassion-based interventions are capable of cultivating greater self-compassion within individuals with IBD, and whether this learning ultimately translates into improved long-term psychological and physical outcomes. Robust methodologies and rich analysis of treatment engagement are required to determine optimal treatment components and length.

References

Alinaghi, F., Tekin, H. G., Burisch, J., Wu, J. J., Thyssen, J. P., & Egeberg, A. (2020). Global prevalence and bidirectional association between psoriasis and inflammatory bowel disease—A systematic review and meta-analysis. *Journal of Crohn's and Colitis, 14*(3), 351–360.

Allison, M., Lindsay, J., Gould, D., & Kelly, D. (2013). Surgery in young adults with inflammatory bowel disease: A narrative account. *International Journal of Nursing Studies, 50*(11), 1566–1575.

Arnett, J. J. (2000). Emerging adulthood: A theory of development from the late teens through the twenties. *American Psychologist, 55*(5), 469.

Austin, J., Drossaert, C. H. C., Schroevers, M. J., Sanderman, R., Kirby, J. N., & Bohlmeijer, E. T. (2021). Compassion-based interventions for people with long-term physical conditions: A mixed methods systematic review. *Psychology & Health, 36*(1), 16–42.

Baer, R. A. (2010). Self-compassion as a mechanism of change in mindfulness-and acceptance-based treatments. *Assessing mindfulness and acceptance processes in clients: Illuminating the theory and practice of change, 2*(1), 135–153.

Barberio, B., Zamani, M., Black, C. J., Savarino, E. V., & Ford, A. C. (2021). Prevalence of symptoms of anxiety and depression in patients with inflammatory bowel disease: A systematic review and meta-analysis. *The Lancet Gastroenterology & Hepatology, 6*(5), 359–370.

Barnes, E. L., Lightner, A. L., & Regueiro, M. (2020). Perioperative and postoperative management of patients with Crohn's disease and ulcerative colitis. *Clinical Gastroenterology and Hepatology, 18*(6), 1356–1366.

Bassi, A., Dodd, S., Williamson, P., & Bodger, K. (2004). Cost of illness of inflammatory bowel disease in the UK: A single Centre retrospective study. *Gut, 53*(10), 1471–1478.

Bernstein, C. N., Loftus, E. V., Ng, S. C., Lakatos, P. L., & Moum, B. (2012). Hospitalisations and surgery in Crohn's disease. *Gut, 61*(4), 622–629.

Berrill, J. W., Sadlier, M., Hood, K., & Green, J. T. (2014). Mindfulness-based therapy for inflammatory bowel disease patients with functional abdominal symptoms or high perceived stress levels. *Journal of Crohn's and Colitis, 8*(9), 945–955.

Brooks, A. J., Rowse, G., Ryder, A., Narula, P., Corfe, B. M., Norman, P., & Lobo, A. J. (2015). PTU-059 "I can cope right now, because I know where I have come from"; a qualitative exploration of the lived experience of young adults with inflammatory bowel disease.

Brooks, A. J., Rowse, G., Ryder, A., Peach, E. J., Corfe, B. M., & Lobo, A. J. (2016). Systematic review: Psychological morbidity in young people with inflammatory bowel disease–risk factors and impacts. *Alimentary Pharmacology & Therapeutics, 44*(1), 3–15.

Brooks, A. J., Sebastian, S., Cross, S. S., Robinson, K., Warren, L., Wright, A., Marsh, A. M., Tsai, H., Majeed, F., McAlindon, M. E., Preston, C., & Lobo, A. J. (2017). Outcome of elective withdrawal of anti-tumour necrosis factor-α therapy in patients with Crohn's disease in established remission. *Journal of Crohn's and Colitis, 11*(12), 1456–1462.

Calvet, X., Gallardo, O., Coronas, R., Casellas, F., Montserrat, A., Torrejon, A., Vergara, M., Campo, R., & Brullet, E. (2006). Remission on thiopurinic immunomodulators normalizes quality of life and psychological status in patients with Crohn's disease. *Inflammatory Bowel Diseases, 12*(8), 692–696.

Casati, J., Toner, B. B., De Rooy, E. C., Drossman, D. A., & Maunder, R. G. (2000). Concerns of patients with inflammatory bowel disease. *Digestive Diseases and Sciences, 45*, 26–31.

Chishima, Y., Mizuno, M., Sugawara, D., & Miyagawa, Y. (2018). The influence of self-compassion on cognitive appraisals and coping with stressful events. *Mindfulness, 9*, 1907–1915.

Chrousos, G. P., & Gold, P. W. (1992). The concepts of stress and stress system disorders: Overview of physical and behavioral homeostasis. *JAMA, 267*(9), 1244–1252.

Compas, B. E., Jaser, S. S., Dunn, M. J., & Rodriguez, E. M. (2012). Coping with chronic illness in childhood and adolescence. *Annual Review of Clinical Psychology, 8*, 455–480.

Devlen, J., Beusterien, K., Yen, L., Ahmed, A., Cheifetz, A. S., & Moss, A. C. (2014). The burden of inflammatory bowel disease: A patient-reported qualitative analysis and development of a conceptual model. *Inflammatory Bowel Diseases, 20*(3), 545–552.

Diederen, K., Haverman, L., Grootenhuis, M. A., Benninga, M. A., & Kindermann, A. (2018). Parental distress and quality of life in pediatric inflammatory bowel disease: Implications for the outpatient clinic. *Journal of paediatric gastroenterology and nutrition, 66*(4), 630–636.

Drossman, D. A., Patrick, D. L., Mitchell, C. M., Zagami, E. A., & Appelbaum, M. I. (1989). Health-related quality of life in inflammatory bowel disease: Functional status and patient worries and concerns. *Digestive Diseases and Sciences, 34*, 1379–1386.

Dubinsky, M. C., Dotan, I., Rubin, D. T., Bernauer, M., Patel, D., Cheung, R., Modesto, I., Latymer, M., & Keefer, L. (2021). Burden of comorbid anxiety and depression in patients with inflammatory bowel disease: A systematic review. *Expert Review of Gastoenterology & Hepatology, 15*(9), 985–997.dub.

El Menyiy, N., El Allam, A., Aboulaghras, S., Jaouadi, I., Bakrim, S., El Omari, N., Shariati, M. A., Miftakhutdinov, A., Wilairatana, P., Mubarak, M. S., & Bouyahya, A. (2022). Inflammatory auto-immune diseases of the intestine and their management by natural bioactive compounds. *Biomedicine & Pharmacotherapy, 151*, 113158.

Evans, S., Olive, L., Dober, M., Knowles, S., Fuller-Tyszkiewicz, M., Eric, O., Gibson, P., Raven, L., Gearry, R., McCombie, A., Van Niekerk, L., Chesterman, S., & Mikocka-Walus, A. (2022). Acceptance commitment therapy (ACT) for psychological distress associated with inflammatory bowel disease (IBD): Protocol for a feasibility trial of the ACTforIBD programme. *BMJ Open, 12*(6), e060272.

Ewais, T., Begun, J., Kenny, M., Hay, K., Houldin, E., Chuang, K. H., Tefay, M., & Kisely, S. (2021). Mindfulness based cognitive therapy for youth with inflammatory bowel disease and depression-findings from a pilot randomised controlled trial. *Journal of Psychosomatic Research, 149*, 110594.

Ferrari, M., Hunt, C., Harrysunker, A., Abbott, M. J., Beath, A. P., & Einstein, D. A. (2019). Self-compassion interventions and psychosocial outcomes: A meta-analysis of RCTs. *Mindfulness, 10*, 1455–1473.

Fourie, S., Jackson, D., & Aveyard, H. (2018). Living with inflammatory bowel disease: A review of qualitative research studies. *International Journal of Nursing Studies, 87*, 149–156.

Gerbarg, P. L., Jacob, V. E., Stevens, L., Bosworth, B. P., Chabouni, F., DeFilippis, E. M., Warren, R., Trivellas, M., Patel, P. V., Webb, C. D., Harbus, M. D., & Scherl, E. J. (2015). The effect of breathing, movement, and meditation on psychological and physical symptoms and inflammatory biomarkers in inflammatory bowel disease: A randomized controlled trial. *Inflammatory Bowel Diseases, 21*(12), 2886–2896.

Germer, C. K., & Neff, K. D. (2013). Self-compassion in clinical practice. *Journal of Clinical Psychology, 69*(8), 856–867.

Ghione, S., Sarter, H., Fumery, M., Armengol-Debeir, L., Savoye, G., Ley, D., Spyckerelle, C., Pariente, B., Peyrin-Biroulet, L., Turck, D., Gower-Rousseau, C., & El Farisi, M. (2018). Dramatic increase in incidence of ulcerative colitis and Crohn's disease (1988–2011): A population-based study of French adolescents. *Official journal of the American College of Gastroenterology| ACG, 113*(2), 265–272.

Ghosh, N., & Premchand, P. (2015). A UK cost of care model for inflammatory bowel disease. *Frontline Gastroenterology, 6*(3), 169–174.

Gilbert, P. (2005). Compassion and cruelty: A biopsychosocial approach. In P. Gilbert (Ed.), *Compassion: Conceptualisations, research and use in psychotherapy* (pp. 9–74). Routledge.

Gilbert, P. (2009). *The compassionate mind.* Constable & Robinson Ltd..

Gilbert, P., McEwan, K., Catarino, F., & Baião, R. (2014). Fears of compassion in a depressed population: Implication for psychotherapy. *Journal of Depression and Anxiety.*

González-Moret, R., Cebolla, A., Cortés, X., Baños, R. M., Navarrete, J., de la Rubia, J. E., Lisón, J. F., & Soria, J. M. (2020). The effect of a mindfulness-based therapy on different biomarkers among patients with inflammatory bowel disease: A randomised controlled trial. *Scientific Reports, 10*(1), 1–7.

Goodhand, J., Hedin, C. R., Croft, N. M., & Lindsay, J. O. (2011). Adolescents with IBD: The importance of structured transition care. *Journal of Crohn's and Colitis, 5*(6), 509–519.

Goodhand, J., & Rampton, D. (2008). Psychological stress and coping in IBD. *Gut, 57*(10), 1345–1347.

Gracie, D. J., Guthrie, E. A., Hamlin, P. J., & Ford, A. C. (2018). Bi-directionality of brain–gut interactions in patients with inflammatory bowel disease. *Gastroenterology, 154*(6), 1635–1646.

Graff, L. A., Walker, J. R., & Bernstein, C. N. (2009). Depression and anxiety in inflammatory bowel disease: A review of comorbidity and management. *Inflammatory Bowel Diseases, 15*(7), 1105–1118.

Greenley, R. N., Hommel, K. A., Nebel, J., Raboin, T., Li, S. H., Simpson, P., & Mackner, L. (2010). A meta-analytic review of the psychosocial adjustment of youth with inflammatory bowel disease. *Journal of paediatric psychology, 35*(8), 857–869.

Gu, P., Kuenzig, M. E., Kaplan, G. G., Pimentel, M., & Rezaie, A. (2018). Faecal incontinence in inflammatory bowel disease: A systematic review and meta-analysis. *Inflammatory Bowel Diseases, 24*(6), 1280–1290.

Gunnarsson, C., Chen, J., Rizzo, J. A., Ladapo, J. A., Naim, A., & Lofland, J. H. (2013). The employee absenteeism costs of inflammatory bowel disease: Evidence from US national survey data. *Journal of Occupational and Environmental Medicine, 55*(4), 393–401. https://www.jstor.org/stable/48510284

Guo, L., Rohde, J., & Farraye, F. A. (2020). Stigma and disclosure in patients with inflammatory bowel disease. *Inflammatory Bowel Diseases, 26*(7), 1010–1016.

Hayes-Skelton, S. A., & Eustis, E. H. (2020). Experiential avoidance. In J. S. Abramowitz & S. M. Blakey (Eds.), *Clinical handbook of fear and anxiety: Maintenance processes and treatment mechanisms* (pp. 115–131). American Psychological Association. https://doi.org/10.1037/0000150-007

Hoogkamer, A. B., Rowse, R., Brooks, A. J., & Lobo, A. J. (2018). Systematic review: Predicting the development of psychological morbidity in inflammatory bowel disease. *UEG J, 6*(1), P0956.

IBD Standards Group. (2009). *Quality care: Service standards for the healthcare of people who have inflammatory bowel disease (IBD).* The IBD Standards Group.

Ilzarbe, L., Fàbrega, M., Quintero, R., Bastidas, A., Pintor, L., García-Campayo, J., Gomollón, F., & Ilzarbe, D. (2017). Inflammatory bowel disease and eating disorders: A systematized review of comorbidity. *Journal of Psychosomatic Research, 102*, 47–53.

Jedel, S., Hoffman, A., Merriman, P., Swanson, B., Voigt, R., Rajan, K. B., Shaikh, M., Li, H., & Keshavarzian, A. (2014). A randomized controlled trial of mindfulness-based stress reduction to prevent flare-up in patients with inactive ulcerative colitis. *Digestion, 89*(2), 142–155.

Jones, M. P., Wessinger, S., & Crowell, M. D. (2006). Coping strategies and interpersonal support in patients with irritable bowel syndrome and inflammatory bowel disease. *Clinical Gastroenterology and Hepatology, 4*(4), 474–481.

Kapasi, R., Glatter, J., Lamb, C. A., Acheson, A. G., Andrews, C., Arnott, I. D., Barrett, K. J., Bell, G., Bhatnagar, G., Bloom, S., Brookes, M. J., & Hawthorne, A. B. (2020). Consensus standards of healthcare for adults and children with inflammatory bowel disease in the UK. *Frontline Gastroenterology, 11*(3), 178–187.

Keeton, R. L., Mikocka-Walus, A., & Andrews, J. M. (2015). Concerns and worries in people living with inflammatory bowel disease (IBD): A mixed methods study. *Journal of Psychosomatic Research, 78*(6), 573–578.

Kemp, K., Griffiths, J., & Lovell, K. (2012). Understanding the health and social care needs of people living with IBD: A meta-synthesis of the evidence. *World Journal of Gastroenterology: WJG, 18*(43), 6240.

Knowles, S. R., Graff, L. A., Wilding, H., Hewitt, C., Keefer, L., & Mikocka-Walus, A. (2018). Quality of life in inflammatory bowel disease: A systematic review and meta-analyses—Part I. *Inflammatory Bowel Diseases, 24*(4), 742–751.

Kuyken, W., Watkins, E., Holden, E., White, K., Taylor, R. S., Byford, S., Evans, A., Radford, S., Teasdale, J. D., & Dalgleish, T. (2010). How does mindfulness-based cognitive therapy work? *Behaviour Research and Therapy, 48*(11), 1105–1112.

Larsson, K., Lööf, L., Rönnblom, A., & Nordin, K. (2008). Quality of life for patients with exacerbation in inflammatory bowel disease and how they cope with disease activity. *Journal of Psychosomatic Research, 64*(2), 139–148.

Lehane, E., & McCarthy, G. (2007). Intentional and unintentional medication non-adherence: A comprehensive framework for clinical research and practice? A discussion paper. *International Journal of Nursing Studies, 44*(8), 1468–1477.

Leventhal, H., Phillips, L. A., & Burns, E. (2016). The common-sense model of self-regulation (CSM): A dynamic framework for understanding illness self-management. *Journal of Behavioral Medicine, 39*, 935–946.

Loonen, H. J., Grootenhuis, M. A., Last, B. F., Koopman, H. M., & Derkx, H. H. F. (2002). Quality of life in paediatric inflammatory bowel disease measured by a generic and a disease-specific questionnaire. *Acta Paediatrica, 91*(3), 348–354.

Lynch, T., & Spence, D. (2008). A qualitative study of youth living with Crohn disease. *Gastroenterology Nursing, 31*(3), 224–230.

Mackner, L. M., & Crandall, W. V. (2007). Psychological factors affecting pediatric inflammatory bowel disease. *Current Opinion in Pediatrics, 19*(5), 548–552.

Martins, R., Carmona, C., George, B., & Epstein, J. (2019). Management of Crohn's disease: Summary of updated NICE guidance. *BMJ, 367*.

Mayberry, J. F., Lobo, A., Ford, A. C., Thomas, A., & Guideline Development Group. (2013). NICE clinical guideline (CG152): The management of Crohn's disease in adults, children and young people. *Alimentary Pharmacology & Therapeutics, 37*(2), 195–203.

McCombie, A. M., Mulder, R. T., & Gearry, R. B. (2013). How IBD patients cope with IBD: A systematic review. *Journal of Crohn's and Colitis, 7*(2), 89–106.

Merkes, M. (2010). Mindfulness-based stress reduction for people with chronic diseases. *Australian Journal of Primary Health, 16*(3), 200–210.

Mikocka-Walus, A., Knowles, S. R., Keefer, L., & Graff, L. (2016). Controversies revisited: A systematic review of the comorbidity of depression and anxiety with inflammatory bowel diseases. *Inflammatory Bowel Diseases, 22*(3), 752–762.

Miller, R. S., & Tangney, J. P. (1994). Differentiating embarrassment and shame. *Journal of Social and Clinical Psychology, 13*(3), 273–287.

Mistretta, E. G., & Davis, M. C. (2021). Meta-analysis of self-compassion interventions for pain and psychological symptoms among adults with chronic illness. *Mindfulness*, 1–18.

Muse, K., Johnson, E., & David, A. L. (2021). A feeling of otherness: A qualitative research synthesis exploring the lived experiences of stigma in individuals with inflammatory bowel disease. *International Journal of Environmental Research and Public Health, 18*(15), 8038.

Nahon, S., Lahmek, P., Durance, C., Olympie, A., Lesgourgues, B., Colombel, J. F., & Gendre, J. P. (2012). Risk factors of anxiety and depression in inflammatory bowel disease. *Inflammatory Bowel Diseases, 18*(11), 2086–2091.

Nass, B. Y. S., Dibbets, P., & Markus, C. R. (2022). Impact of the COVID-19 pandemic on inflammatory bowel disease: The role of emotional stress and social isolation. *Stress and Health, 38*(2), 222–233.

Neff, K. D. (2016). Self-compassion definition of self-compassion. *Mindfulness in positive psychology: The Science of meditation and wellbeing, 37.*

Neff, K. D. (2023). Self-compassion: Theory, method, research, and intervention. *Annual Review of Psychology, 74*, 193–218.

Neff, K. D., Kirkpatrick, K. L., & Rude, S. S. (2007). Self-compassion and adaptive psychological functioning. *Journal of Research in Personality, 41*(1), 139–154.

Neilson, K., Ftanou, M., Monshat, K., Salzberg, M., Bell, S., Kamm, M. A., Connell, W., Knowles, S. R., Sevar, K., Mancuso, S. G., & Castle, D. (2016). A controlled study of a group mindfulness intervention for individuals living with inflammatory bowel disease. *Inflammatory Bowel Diseases, 22*(3), 694–701.

Nicholas, D. B., Otley, A., Smith, C., Avolio, J., Munk, M., & Griffiths, A. M. (2007). Challenges and strategies of children and adolescents with inflammatory bowel disease: A qualitative examination. *Health and Quality of Life Outcomes, 5*(1), 1–8.

Odes, S., Vardi, H., Friger, M., Wolters, F., Russel, M. G., Riis, L., Munkholm, P., Politi, P., Tsianos, E., Clofent, J., Vermeire, S., & European Collaborative Study on Inflammatory Bowel Disease. (2006). Cost analysis and cost determinants in a European inflammatory bowel disease inception cohort with 10 years of follow-up evaluation. *Gastroenterology, 131*, 719e28.

Pfefferkorn, M., Burke, G., Griffiths, A., Markowitz, J., Rosh, J., Mack, D., Otley, A., Kugathasan, S., Evans, J., Bousvaros, A., Moyer, M. S., & Hyams, J. (2009). Growth abnormalities persist in newly diagnosed children with Crohn disease despite current treatment paradigms. *Journal of Pediatric Gastroenterology and Nutrition, 48*(2), 168–174.

Pithadia, A. B., & Jain, S. (2011). Treatment of inflammatory bowel disease (IBD). *Pharmacological Reports, 63*(3), 629–642.

Prentice, K., Rees, C., & Finlay-Jones, A. (2021). Self-compassion, wellbeing, and distress in adolescents and young adults with chronic medical conditions: The mediating role of emotion regulation difficulties. *Mindfulness, 12*, 2241–2252.

Raymer, D., Weininger, O., & Hamilton, J. R. (1984). Psychological problems in children with abdominal pain. *The Lancet, 323*(8374), 439–440.

Rowse, G., Yeates, R., Sirois, F., Lobo, A., & Brooks, A. (2018). A pilot and feasibility trial of a group mindfulness and self-compassion intervention for young people diagnosed with inflammatory bowel disease. *Clinical Trials, 159047.*

Saunders, B. (2014). Stigma, deviance and morality in young adults' accounts of inflammatory bowel disease. *Sociology of Health & Illness, 36*(7), 1020–1036.

Schoultz, M., Atherton, I., & Watson, A. (2015). Mindfulness-based cognitive therapy for inflammatory bowel disease patients: Findings from an exploratory pilot randomised controlled trial. *Trials, 16*, 1–13.

Schoultz, M., Macaden, L., & Hubbard, G. (2016). Participants' perspectives on mindfulness-based cognitive therapy for inflammatory bowel disease: A qualitative study nested within a pilot randomised controlled trial. *Pilot and Feasibility Studies, 2*, 1–13.

Schuling, R., Huijbers, M. J., van Ravesteijn, H., Donders, R., Kuyken, W., & Speckens, A. E. (2016). A parallel-group, randomized controlled trial into the effectiveness of mindfulness-based compassionate living (MBCL) compared to treatment-as-usual in recurrent depression: Trial design and protocol. *Contemporary Clinical Trials, 50*, 77–83.

Schuling, R., Huijbers, M. J., van Ravesteijn, H., Kuyken, W., & Speckens, A. E. (2021). Mindfulness-based compassionate living (MBCL): A qualitative study into the added value of compassion in recurrent depression. *Mindfulness, 12*(9), 2196–2206.

Sirois, F. M., Molnar, D. S., & Hirsch, J. K. (2015). Self-compassion, stress, and coping in the context of chronic illness. *Self and Identity, 14*(3), 334–347.

Sirois, F. M., & Rowse, G. (2016). The role of self-compassion in chronic illness care. *Journal of Clinical Outcomes Management, 23*(11), 521–527.

Skinner, E. A., Edge, K., Altman, J., & Sherwood, H. (2003). Searching for the structure of coping: A review and critique of category systems for classifying ways of coping. *Psychological Bulletin, 129*(2), 216.

Terry, M. L., & Leary, M. R. (2011). Self-compassion, self-regulation, and health. *Self and Identity, 10*(3), 352–362.

Trindade, I. A., Ferreira, C., & Pinto-Gouveia, J. (2017). Chronic illness-related shame: Development of a new scale and novel approach for IBD patients' depressive symptomatology. *Clinical Psychology & Psychotherapy, 24*(1), 255–263.

Trindade, I. A., Ferreira, C., & Pinto-Gouveia, J. (2018). The longitudinal effects of emotion regulation on physical and psychological health: A latent growth analysis exploring the role of cognitive fusion in inflammatory bowel disease. *British Journal of Health Psychology, 23*(1), 171–185.

Trindade, I. A., Pereira, J., Galhardo, A., Ferreira, N. B., Lucena-Santos, P., Carvalho, S. A., Oliveira, S., Skvarc, D., Rocha, B. S., Portela, F., & Ferreira, C. (2021). The LIFEwithIBD intervention: Study protocol for a randomized controlled trial of a face-to-face acceptance and commitment therapy and compassion-based intervention tailored to people with inflammatory bowel disease. *Frontiers in Psychiatry, 12*, 699367.

Trindade, I. A., & Sirois, F. M. (2021). The prospective effects of self-compassion on depressive symptoms, anxiety, and stress: A study in inflammatory bowel disease. *Journal of Psychosomatic Research, 146*, 110429.

Van den Brink, E., & Koster, F. (2015). *Mindfulness-based compassionate living.* Routledge.

Van der Zaag-Loonen, H. J., Grootenhuis, M. A., Last, B. F., & Derkx, H. H. F. (2004). Coping strategies and quality of life of adolescents with inflammatory bowel disease. *Quality of Life Research, 13*, 1011–1019.

van Erp, S. J., Brakenhoff, L. K. M. P., Vollmann, M., van der Heijde, D., Veenendaal, R. A., Fidder, H. H., Hommes, D. W., Kaptein, A. A., van der Meulen-de Jong, A. E., & Scharloo, M. (2017). Illness perceptions and outcomes in patients with inflammatory bowel disease: Is coping a mediator? *International Journal of Behavioral Medicine, 24*, 205–214.

van Gennep, S., Evers, S. W., Rietdijk, S. T., Gielen, M. E., de Boer, N. K., Gecse, K. B., Ponsioen, C. I., Duijvestein, M., D'Haens, G. R., de Boer, A. G., & Löwenberg, M. (2021). High disease burden drives indirect costs in employed inflammatory bowel disease patients: The WORK-IBD study. *Inflammatory Bowel Diseases, 27*(3), 352–363.

Voth, J., & Sirois, F. M. (2009). The role of self-blame and responsibility in adjustment to inflammatory bowel disease. *Rehabilitation Psychology, 54*(1), 99.

Wilson, A. C., Mackintosh, K., Power, K., & Chan, S. W. (2019). Effectiveness of self-compassion related therapies: A systematic review and meta-analysis. *Mindfulness, 10*, 979–995.

Wren, A. A., Neiman, N., Caruso, T. J., Rodriguez, S., Taylor, K., Madill, M., Rives, H., & Nguyen, L. (2021). Mindfulness-based virtual reality intervention for children and young adults with inflammatory bowel disease: A pilot feasibility and acceptability study. *Children, 8*(5), 368.

22

Facing Cancer-Related Adversity with Kindness and Understanding: The Promising Benefits of Self-Compassion for People with Cancer

Inês A. Trindade, Maria Inês Caçador, and Helena Moreira

Introduction

Cancer has been broadly described as a group of heterogeneous diseases characterized by an uncontrolled division of abnormal cells in a specific part of the body, which can invade nearby tissues or spread to other parts of the body (National Cancer Institute, 2021). The latest estimates of the worldwide cancer incidence and mortality point to 18.1 million new cases and 9.6 million deaths in 2018. The most frequently diagnosed cancer was lung cancer (11.6% of all new cases; 14.5% of all new male cases); among women, the most frequently diagnosed cancer was breast cancer (24.2% of new cases; Ferlay et al., 2019). Although the global incidence and mortality estimates are still

I. A. Trindade (✉)
Center for Research in Neuropsychology and Cognitive and Behavioral Intervention (CINEICC), Faculty of Psychology and Education Sciences, University of Coimbra, Coimbra, Portugal

EMBRACE Lab, School of Behavioural, Social and Legal Sciences, Örebro University, Örebro, Sweden

M. I. Caçador • H. Moreira
Center for Research in Neuropsychology and Cognitive and Behavioral Intervention (CINEICC), Faculty of Psychology and Education Sciences, University of Coimbra, Coimbra, Portugal

F. M. Sirois (ed.), *The Palgrave Handbook of Positive Psychology and Health*,
https://doi.org/10.1007/978-3-031-89095-6_22

considerably high, technical and scientific advances in the early detection and treatment of cancer in recent decades have resulted in a very significant decrease in mortality and, consequently, in a significant increase in the number of survivors (Firkins et al., 2020). It is estimated that the 5-year survival is approximately 70% (Miller et al., 2017).

The diagnosis of cancer is an adverse and potentially traumatic event that can affect several areas of an individual's life, including emotional and social well-being, marital and family functioning, body image, sexuality, and physical functioning (Essue et al., 2020). The patient's adjustment to cancer can vary according to the type of cancer (e.g., body image concerns are particularly common among patients with breast cancer), cancer treatment (e.g., adverse physical effects might be more intense among patients undergoing chemotherapy), and the phase of the disease (e.g., higher levels of anxiety are more common in the diagnosis and initial treatment phases). Several other factors (e.g., personality, coping strategies, social support) may also account for individual differences in the adjustment to cancer and may explain why some patients are more vulnerable to experiencing poorer adjustment results, such as poor quality of life (QoL) or high levels of negative emotions, while others are more resilient (Brandão et al., 2017b). In recent years, it has been suggested that some psychological resources, such as self-compassion, may have an important protective effect on the adjustment of people with cancer.

In this chapter, we focus on the role of self-compassion in the adjustment to cancer. First, we summarize the implications of cancer on several areas of the psychosocial adjustment of patients, including their mental health, marital relationship, sexual functioning, stigma, and body image. Next, we review the empirical evidence that supports the protective role of self-compassion in the adjustment to cancer. Finally, we review the results of studies investigating the efficacy of compassion-based interventions in this population.

The Impact of Cancer on Different Dimensions of Life

Cancer is currently considered a chronic disease with different phases (diagnosis, treatment, and survivorship) that progress over time and are characterized by different medical, emotional, and psychosocial challenges (Frost et al., 2000). Therefore, the adjustment process along the cancer trajectory depends upon the particular experiences, demands, and threats that define each particular phase (Veach et al., 2002). For example, the treatment phase is usually associated with invasive medical interventions (e.g., chemotherapy, surgery) that can cause several painful symptoms (e.g., nausea and vomiting, fatigue) and body image changes (e.g., hair loss, weight changes), which can negatively interfere with the patient's adjustment, leading to poorer QoL and higher levels of negative emotions (Krebber et al., 2014; Niedzwiedz et al., 2019; Pitman et al., 2018; Reece et al., 2013). Factors such as body image changes, which may interfere with one's sense of attractiveness (Rumsey & Harcourt, 2005), as well as cancer-related stigma (especially in lung and prostate cancer; e.g., Chambers et al., 2012; Ettridge et al., 2018) and compromised sexual functioning (Bober & Varela, 2012), are known to contribute considerably to poor mental health outcomes in cancer populations. Disruption in sexual functioning might also be due to the negative impact of cancer on other life domains, such as body image and mental health (Fobair et al., 2006; Paterson et al., 2016).

The survivorship phase presents distinct challenges and difficulties for cancer survivors (Naughton & Weaver, 2014). Concerns about pain and fatigue may continue to be relevant (Bjerkeset et al., 2020), as may concerns about changes in sexual functioning (Rajotte et al., 2017) or body image (Paterson et al., 2016). However, other issues may emerge only at the survivorship phase, such as difficulties in coping with the physical consequences of treatments (e.g., early menopause or infertility, heart failure, atherosclerosis, cognitive dysfunction, chronic pain, endocrine dysfunction, sexual dysfunction, and/or secondary cancers; Arndt et al., 2017) and fear of recurrence (Simard et al., 2013).

The challenges and difficulties that cancer survivors face can strongly impact their mental health and QoL (Arndt et al., 2017; Naughton & Weaver, 2014). A recent meta-analysis revealed that the QoL of cancer survivors continues to be significantly impacted 2 to 26 years post-diagnosis, particularly in the domains of physical and mental health (Firkins et al., 2020). A population-based study found that cancer survivors (ranging from less than 2 years to more than 20 years after diagnosis) were more than twice as likely to report incapacitating psychological problems compared with individuals without a history of cancer or other chronic diseases (Hewitt et al., 2003). However, there is also evidence that although depression, anxiety, and distress symptoms occur frequently in the first years after the diagnosis, the prevalence of these symptoms among long-term survivors is similar to that found in the general population (Brandenbarg et al., 2019).

Self-Compassion and Its Importance in Cancer

Self-compassion has emerged as a quality that may attenuate the impact of cancer on psychosocial and mental health outcomes through the promotion of adaptive emotion regulation. Self-compassion, which can be conceptualized as an enduring trait or as a changeable dynamic process that can be cultivated, allows individuals to accept their personal suffering and perceived failures and self-direct kindness while facing adversity (Neff, 2003). The most common definition of self-compassion is the one proposed by Neff (2003), which comprises three components: self-kindness (as opposed to self-judgment), mindfulness (as opposed to overidentification), and common humanity (as opposed to isolation). Self-kindness is characterized by the extension of kindness and understanding when facing difficulties instead of engaging in self-blame or self-criticism. Mindfulness comprises awareness of one's internal experiences (e.g., thoughts, emotions, memories) rather than being carried away by them. Common humanity refers to the acknowledgment that suffering is a universal, shared experience of all human beings and not a unique or individualized aspect of one's experience.

Most studies on self-compassion assess this construct at the trait level using the Self-Compassion Scale (SCS; Neff, 2003). The majority of research has measured self-compassion through the total score of the 6 facets of the SCS, although some studies divide the 6 facets into 2 factors: a positive one, referring to compassionate self-responding (which includes self-kindness, mindfulness, and common humanity), and a negative one, referring to uncompassionate self-responding (that comprises self-judgment, overidentification, and isolation). Differences in the employment of the SCS among studies are rooted in the different empirical findings on the factor structure of the SCS. Several studies have supported the use of a common overarching factor that includes the six components of the scale (e.g., Castilho et al., 2015; Kotsou & Leys, 2016; Kumlander et al., 2018; Neff et al., 2017; Petrocchi et al., 2014), while others indicate the presence of two separate overarching factors—compassionate and uncompassionate responding (e.g., Brenner et al., 2017; Coroiu et al., 2018; Costa et al., 2016; Hayes et al., 2016; Zhang et al., 2019).

The debate on the SCS scoring and the conceptualization of self-compassion is ongoing. Authors defending the use of two separate factors argue that the SCS's compassionate responding dimension refers to aspects of positive cognitive coping and healthy psychological functioning, and that the uncompassionate responding dimension is an indicator of vulnerability and psychopathology (Muris et al., 2018). For these authors, the use of the SCS total score may conceal the full extent of the effects of self-compassion as a positive protective quality against mental health problems (Muris & Otgaar, 2020). In turn, authors defending the use of the total score of the SCS argue that self-compassion encompasses both compassionate and reduced uncompassionate self-responding components, and that both components contribute to explain the link between self-compassion and mental health (Neff et al., 2017). This conceptualization sees the SCS's six components as a balanced, coherent system within individuals (Neff, 2020).

In the context of cancer, self-compassion involves self-directing kindness and empathy while experiencing challenging symptoms, emotions, or thoughts, mindfully accepting these experiences without self-blame or judgment, and perceiving the cancer diagnosis and cancer-related suffering as a result of the human condition rather than a personal injustice, weakness, or failure. In 2011, Terry and Leary highlighted the potential role of self-compassion in medical conditions and proposed that the cultivation of self-compassion in people with such conditions may increase their ability to regulate negative affect, manage health-related behavior, and deal effectively with medical problems. In their paper, Terry and Leary (2011) proposed that self-compassion may facilitate each step in Baumeister and Heatherton's (1996) process of self-regulation: people with more self-compassion may set appropriate health goals more efficiently, engage in goal-directed behavior (e.g., seeking medical treatment when needed; adhering to treatment), monitor their progress toward each goal with less defensiveness, and adjust behavior and goals when required.

Since then, empirical research on self-compassion in medical conditions has blossomed over time, especially during the past 3 years. Nevertheless, studies on self-compassion have mostly focused on non-disease populations (e.g., Ferrari et al., 2019; Raes, 2011; Shonin et al., 2015). Further research in disease contexts, including cancer, must be conducted to more clearly understand the effects of self-compassion in these populations. Furthermore, the vast majority of research on self-compassion in cancer has used cross-sectional designs, limiting inferences on causality between variables. In the next two sections, we present the currently available empirical evidence on the link between self-compassion and psychological functioning in cancer populations and the efficacy of compassion-based interventions in this setting.

Evidence in Cancer Populations

Psychological Distress

The first study to provide evidence on the link between self-compassion and outcomes in cancer was conducted in 2014 by Pinto-Gouveia et al. Trait self-compassion was found to be associated with fewer psychopathological symptoms and higher quality of life levels in a mixed sample of people with cancer. Self-compassion also explained the variance of depressive and stress symptoms and of psychological and social quality of life (Pinto-Gouveia et al., 2014). Further corroborative findings on the relationship between self-compassion and indicators of psychological well-being have been provided by a number of studies on different cancer populations, such as breast cancer survivors (Arambasic et al., 2019; Brown et al., 2020; Przezdziecki et al., 2013; Todorov et al., 2019), men with prostate cancer (Lennon et al., 2018), people with lung cancer (Siwik et al., 2021), individuals undergoing antineoplastic chemotherapy (Garcia et al., 2021), and other heterogeneous cancer samples (van der Donk et al., 2020; Zhu et al., 2020). The study by van der Donk et al. (2020), conducted with 245 people with cancer and 245 matched controls, additionally demonstrated that mindfulness and self-compassion were about equally strongly related to depressive symptoms and affect among the groups. This evidence indicates that these characteristics are basic human resources linked with psychological functioning regardless of the presence or absence of a cancer diagnosis (van der Donk et al., 2020).

The only longitudinal study conducted to date on this topic examined a heterogeneous cancer sample with 153 participants and revealed that self-compassion appeared to be more than a correlate of psychological functioning in these populations; it was also a predictor (Zhu et al., 2019). Positive self-compassion (or compassionate responding) measured at the time of diagnosis predicted lower levels of depression, anxiety, and fatigue at the end of medical treatment (Zhu et al., 2019). Interestingly, no significant predictive role of negative self-compassion (or uncompassionate responding) was found in the study, which the authors interpreted as suggesting that for people who are facing "a life-threatening disease, being kind and understanding toward themselves, recognizing that suffering is part of life, and holding an open, accepting, mindful attitude towards difficulties in life, are more powerful for our future functioning than merely not being self-critical, not getting caught up by our negative experiences, and not feeling different and isolated" (Zhu et al., 2019, p. 1923).

Also interesting were the findings of a study in a heterogeneous sample of adults who had experienced cancer that measured self-compassion using the SCS total score. In that study, self-compassion was associated with lower psychological distress and higher quality of life, but not after controlling for variables such as cognitive distress, cognitive avoidance, emotional distress, avoidance coping, and cognitive fusion (Gillanders et al., 2015). Controlling for these predictors might have resulted in a more rigorous test of self-compassion; at the same time, the way self-compassion is measured might substantially influence the results of studies.

The literature on self-compassion in cancer has also examined self-compassion as a mediator or moderator of known associations between important variables in cancer as well as the mechanisms by which self-compassion may be linked to these variables. We present these findings by topic.

Body Image

Body image disturbance is another cancer dimension in which self-compassion seems to be a protective factor, especially in women who survive breast cancer (Todorov et al., 2019). A study conducted with women who had completed active treatment for breast cancer (Przezdziecki et al., 2013) showed the mediating role of self-compassion between body image disturbance and psychological distress and proposed that self-compassion is a potentially protective characteristic for women at risk of experiencing body image disturbance. In this study, among all tested variables (which included comfort with weight and pressure from others), only self-compassion emerged as a mediator of anxiety and stress. As the authors note, this finding suggests that breast cancer survivors may have a unique body image experience that differs from that found among non-cancer populations (such as women with eating disorders; Striegel-Moore et al., 2004) and for which self-compassion may be a particular determinant (Przezdziecki et al., 2013).

Findings from a more recent study corroborated the apparent importance of self-compassion for a positive body image in women with breast cancer. Self-compassion and appearance investment both moderated the association between body image disturbance and psychological distress in women with breast cancer who had undergone nipple-sparing mastectomy with immediate breast reconstruction (Sherman et al., 2017). This suggests that these characteristics may help to minimize the negative impacts of a mastectomy.

Illness Perceptions

Self-compassion also appears to influence the known association of threatening illness perceptions with anxiety, depression, and quality of life (e.g., Gray et al., 2014). Higher self-compassion buffers the effects of threat appraisals on avoidant coping, resulting in less anxiety and depression and higher quality of life scores (Gillanders et al., 2015). Interestingly, these associations appear to be bidirectional. Another study provided evidence in the opposite direction, showing the mediational role of illness perceptions on the relationship between self-compassion and psychological distress (Zhu et al., 2020). One's perception of a cyclical timeline of cancer and of the consequences of cancer seems to be a strong mediator of the relationship between self-compassion and symptoms of depression. This suggests that people higher in self-compassion tend to perceive cancer as a condition that is less cyclical and with fewer major consequences, which may subsequently lead to better psychological outcomes (Zhu et al., 2020).

Worry and Rumination

Worry and rumination (depressive brooding) have also been tested as mediators of the link between self-compassion and anxiety and depression in breast cancer survivors. Worry and depressive brooding appear to mediate the association between two facets of self-compassion (kindness and mindfulness) and anxiety, while depressive brooding appears to mediate their effects on depression (Brown et al., 2020). Common humanity predicted fewer depression symptoms but without mediation. The researchers speculated that this might be due to self-kindness and mindfulness operating as self-guided responses to difficulties, while common humanity operates through affiliative responses rather than by reducing threat arousal (Brown et al., 2020; Kim et al., 2012).

Shame

In people with lung cancer, a population especially prone to guilt and shame due to the link between smoking and this type of cancer (Chapple et al., 2004), greater self-compassion appears to act as a mediator between less shame and fewer depressive symptoms. However, this does not seem to happen with guilt (Siwik et al., 2021). The researchers did not consider this finding to be surprising given that shame is a negative feeling about the self and guilt is a negative feeling about a behavior (Siwik et al., 2021). These findings are in line with the existing literature on the negative link between self-compassion and shame in several other populations (Luoma & Platt, 2015; Woods & Proeve, 2014).

Gender-Role Conflict

In men with prostate cancer, a study by Lennon et al. (2018) tested whether self-compassion moderated the association between gender role conflict and emotional approach coping. Gender role conflict (i.e., the negative intrapersonal conflict that occurs when men rigidly subscribe to traditional gender roles; O'Neil et al., 1986) was significantly associated with men's cancer-related distress due to a decreased ability to portray traditional masculine stereotypes (Wall & Kristjanson, 2005). Gender role conflict was linked to poor emotional approach coping, although this relationship was not moderated by self-compassion (Lennon et al., 2018). Self-compassion was nonetheless negatively linked to gender role conflict (indicating that the internalization of traditional masculine values is linked to difficulties in self-directing kindness and accepting perceived personal flaws or failures), and moderated the association between gender role conflict and distress. Self-compassion may thus help men with high gender role conflict perceive aspects of cancer that may be seen as emasculating as part of this medical condition rather than as personal weaknesses or challenges to masculinity, which in turn may lead to less cancer-related distress (Lennon et al., 2018).

Attachment Styles

Self-compassion has been found to be a mediator of the relationship between insecure attachment style and stress and the perceived negative impact of cancer in survivors of breast cancer (Arambasic et al., 2019). Participants with higher attachment anxiety (which involves worry about being abandoned or rejected by others) or higher attachment avoidance (involving discomfort with closeness, dependence, and intimacy) presented less ability to self-direct compassion during adversity, which in turn appeared to lead to greater stress and a more negative perception of the impact of cancer. These associations have also been demonstrated in non-cancer populations (Raque-Bogdan et al., 2011; Wei et al., 2011).

Self-Care and Medical Adherence

A study of women with breast cancer (Abdollahi et al., 2020) revealed self-compassion as a moderator of the known link between higher perceived stress and fewer self-care behaviors (e.g., lack of adequate rest, physical activity, and personal hygiene; Johnston et al., 2009). Self-compassion appears to attenuate this link. For the same level of perceived stress, women with higher self-compassion abilities appear to be better able to adhere to adaptive health behaviors (Abdollahi et al., 2020). Another study demonstrated that the trait self-compassion is linked to better medical adherence in five different groups of medical conditions, in which were included people with cancer and cancer survivors (Sirois & Hirsch, 2019). This link was partially due to decreased stress and highlights the importance of self-compassion in the engagement of adaptive health behaviors.

Caregivers

Caregivers of individuals with cancer may also benefit from self-compassion. The link between the caregiver burden and depression appears to be moderated by self-compassion by decreasing the effect of the caregiving burden on this outcome (Xu et al., 2020). Caregivers with higher self-compassion may be more likely to extend kindness and acceptance toward themselves and their care recipients, leading to a positive and warm attitude that seems to attenuate the impact of the caregiving burden on depressive symptomatology. The authors also postulate that a self-compassionate attitude may facilitate the development of resilience in caregivers (Xu et al., 2020).

Relationship with the Partner

The diagnosis and treatment of cancer not only affects the individual's psychological adjustment but also has a significant impact on all family members, particularly on couple relationships (Brandão et al., 2017a). Although research on the role of self-compassion on the dyadic outcomes of people with cancer remains scarce, there is preliminary evidence that self-compassion can facilitate communication between partners. For instance, Schellekens et al. (2017), in a dyadic study of people with lung cancer and their partners, found that higher levels of patients' self-compassion predicted lower levels of psychological distress and higher levels of communication about the cancer with the partner. Interestingly, the association between the patient's self-compassion and psychological distress decreased as the self-compassion levels of the partner increased. These results may suggest that when one partner exhibits less self-compassion, the other compensates by exhibiting more compassion, which contributes to reducing the psychological distress of both (Schellekens et al., 2017). Self-compassion was also found to be an important determinant of a woman's ability to form new romantic relationships after breast cancer. Shaw et al. (2018), in a study with unpartnered survivors of breast cancer, found that self-compassion was a significant predictor of greater perceived interpersonal competence in a romantic relationship.

Compassion-Based Interventions for People with Cancer

Considering the promising results from observational studies, in recent years, several compassion-based interventions, including Mindful Self-Compassion (MSC; Neff & Germer, 2013), Compassion-Focused Therapy (CFT; Gilbert, 2009), Cognitively-Based Compassion Training (CBCT; Negi, 2013), and adaptations of these interventions, have been tested in several cancer populations. These interventions were developed to promote well-being through the increase in self-compassion levels and can be applied to any population. Overall, compassion-based interventions applied to the cancer context have shown promise in enhancing well-being and reducing the distress of individuals with this condition. We will next present the available data on the interventions tested to date.

The feasibility, acceptability, and preliminary efficacy of adaptations of the MSC program, an eight-week group-based intervention aimed at cultivating self-compassion through mindfulness and self-compassion practices (Neff & Germer, 2013), were examined among adult (Brooker et al., 2020) and young adult cancer survivors (Campo et al., 2017). Brooker et al. (2020) showed that the adaptation of the MSC program was feasible and acceptable for a heterogeneous sample of cancer survivors diagnosed with nonadvanced cancer. Specifically, the retention rate was 90%, program completers attended an average of seven out of eight sessions, and the satisfaction rates regarding several aspects of the program (e.g., content, teacher, venue) were high. In addition, the program was found to improve depressive and stress symptoms, fear of recurrence, loneliness, mindfulness, and self-compassion (small to medium effects) from pre- to post-intervention.

Another intervention based on the adult MSC program (Neff & Germer, 2013) and its adaptation for teenagers (Making Friends With Yourself; Bluth et al., 2016) was specifically developed for young adult survivors (ages 18–29; Campo et al., 2017). This 8-week intervention was delivered online and was found to be feasible (84% of participants attended six out of eight sessions) and acceptable (high scores were obtained for aspects related to the intervention design, perceived usefulness, and enjoyment). Significant improvements were found in body image, anxiety, self-compassion, mindfulness, depression, social isolation, and posttraumatic growth from baseline to post-intervention (mostly with large effect sizes). In addition, a qualitative study that examined participants' experiences during this program supported its acceptability and utility and suggested that the program offers important coping skills that promote the mental health of young adult survivors (Lathren et al., 2018).

The 8-week CBCT program, a compassion training program that incorporates intellectual analysis into meditation practice (Negi, 2013), has also been adapted to survivors of cancer. A pilot feasibility study (Dodds et al., 2015) suggested that CBCT is a feasible and highly satisfactory intervention for survivors of breast cancer. Compared to a waitlist control group, participants in the CBCT group showed significant improvements in depression, avoidance of intrusive thoughts, functional impairment due to fear of recurrence, mindfulness, and vitality/fatigue. Gonzalez-Hernandez et al. (2018) also conducted a randomized clinical trial to test the efficacy of a CBCT intervention versus a treatment-as-usual control group on several indicators of the psychosocial adjustment of survivors of cancer. This program was found to be feasible (e.g., 96.4% of participants attended five or more of the 8 sessions of the program) and highly acceptable (e.g., 92.9% of participants were satisfied with the program and said that they would recommend the program to other participants). In addition, the program was found to be efficacious in reducing the stress caused by the fear of cancer recurrence and depressive and general distress symptomatology and in increasing self-compassion and mindfulness skills compared with the control group.

Recently, an integrative intervention combining elements of CFT (Gilbert, 2009), Mindfulness-Based Stress Reduction (Kabat-Zinn, 2003), and Acceptance and Commitment Therapy (Hayes et al., 1999) was adapted for women with nonmetastatic breast cancer (Mind program; Trindade et al., 2020). This 8-week program was shown to be feasible and highly acceptable: the retention rate was 100%, and most participants found the Mind program very useful and relevant, and believed that it helped them deal with cancer-related issues, difficult thoughts and emotions, and social relationships. The preliminary results of the efficacy of the program were promising, suggesting that the Mind program can result in improvements in psychological and physical health, quality of social relationships, depression symptoms, and stress (Trindade et al., 2025).

Although not explicitly compassion-based, some mindfulness interventions also comprise loving-kindness (Mettā) training, a meditation technique for cultivating unconditional kindness toward the self and all human beings (Hofmann et al., 2011) and have been developed for individuals with cancer. For instance, a 6-week Mindful Awareness Practices program (Bower et al., 2015; Boyle et al., 2017) that included loving-kindness meditation for young breast cancer survivors aged 50 or younger was found to be efficacious in improving positive affect, peace, and meaning compared to a wait-list condition. This program was also successful in reducing perceived stress, depressive symptoms, fatigue, sleep disturbance, vasomotor symptoms, proinflammatory gene expression, and inflammatory signaling (Bower et al., 2015). A subsequent study exploring the mediators of intervention effects showed that increased self-kindness mediated declines in depressive symptoms and in perceived stress (Boyle et al., 2017). Wren et al. (2019) also developed a loving-kindness meditation intervention for women with breast cancer undergoing biopsy and breast cancer surgery. The authors conducted a randomized controlled pilot study that showed that this intervention was feasible and efficacious in improving self-compassion and in maintaining pain levels and stable heart rate over time compared to treatment-as-usual and music control groups.

With the aim of reducing body image disturbance and increasing the body appreciation of survivors of breast cancer, an online self-compassion focused writing activity (My Changed Body; MyCB) was developed by Przezdziecki et al. (2016). In this 30-minute online writing activity, participants are invited to write about their body image after cancer treatment following five self-compassionate prompts (e.g., connection with others experiencing difficulties with body image; Przezdziecki et al., 2016). A randomized controlled trial provided evidence of the feasibility and acceptability of MyCB (the compliance rate was 88%) as well as its efficacy. Specifically, a significant reduction in body image disturbance and a significant improvement in body appreciation and self-compassion were found compared to an unstructured expressive writing control group. A significant reduction in psychological distress (depression and anxiety) was also found, but only among participants with lymphedema (Sherman et al., 2018).

Conclusions

The evidence suggests that self-compassion is an important characteristic to have and to foster in the face of a cancer diagnosis and during cancer survivorship. The cultivation of self-compassion in these contexts may theoretically support a healthy regulation of negative affect, effective health behavior management, and coping with symptomatology. Most empirical research on this topic is promising as it indicates that a self-compassionate attitude may protect people with cancer against psychological distress and within domains such as body image, cancer-related shame, relationship with the partner, and self-care. Evidence from the testing of compassion-based interventions in cancer corroborates these suggestions. The interventions that have been tested to date in different cancer populations (e.g., breast cancer, young adults, survivors) have resulted in improvements in outcomes such as depression, perceived stress, fear of recurrence, social isolation, body image, posttraumatic growth, sleep disturbance, fatigue, vasomotor symptoms, and inflammatory markers. However, most of these studies were preliminary and used inactive control groups as comparators and were not subjected to meta-analytical analysis. It would be of interest for future studies to conduct randomized controlled trials with active comparators such as active control conditions or even other interventions, to better understand the effects of compassion-based interventions on relevant outcomes in cancer. Self-compassion appears able to drive exciting further and much needed research in oncology settings, with current findings strongly suggesting its prominent role in affect regulation in people with cancer.

References

Abdollahi, A., Taheri, A., & Allen, K. A. (2020). Self-compassion moderates the perceived stress and self-care behaviors link in women with breast cancer. *Psycho-Oncology, 29*(5), 927–933. https://doi.org/10.1002/pon.5369

Arambasic, J., Sherman, K. A., Elder, E., & Breast Cancer Network Australia. (2019). Attachment styles, self-compassion, and psychological adjustment in long-term breast cancer survivors. *Psycho-Oncology, 28*(5), 1134–1141. https://doi.org/10.1002/pon.5068

Arndt, V., Koch-Gallenkamp, L., Jansen, L., Bertram, H., Eberle, A., Holleczek, B., Schmid-Höpfner, S., Waldmann, A., Zeissig, S. R., & Brenner, H. (2017). Quality of life in long-term and very long-term cancer survivors versus population controls in Germany. *Acta Oncologica, 56*(2), 190–197. https://doi.org/10.1080/0284186X.2016.1266089

Baumeister, R. F., & Heatherton, T. F. (1996). Self-regulation failure: An overview. *Psychological Inquiry, 7*(1), 1–15. https://doi.org/10.1207/s15327965pli0701_1

Bjerkeset, E., Röhrl, K., & Schou-Bredal, I. (2020). Symptom cluster of pain, fatigue, and psychological distress in breast cancer survivors: Prevalence and characteristics. *Breast Cancer Research and Treatment, 180*(1), 63–71. https://doi.org/10.1007/s10549-020-05522-8

Bluth, K., Gaylord, S. A., Campo, R. A., Mullarkey, M., & Hobbs, L. (2016). Making friends with yourself: A mixed methods pilot study of a mindful self-compassion program for adolescents. *Mindfulness, 7*(2), 479–492. https://doi.org/10.1007/s12671-015-0476-6

Bober, S. L., & Varela, V. S. (2012). Sexuality in adult cancer survivors: Challenges and intervention. *Journal of Clinical Oncology, 30*(30), 3712–3719. https://doi.org/10.1200/JCO.2012.41.7915

Bower, J. E., Crosswell, A. D., Stanton, A. L., Crespi, C. M., Winston, D., Arevalo, J., Ma, J., Cole, S. W., & Ganz, P. A. (2015). Mindfulness meditation for younger breast cancer survivors: A randomized controlled trial. *Cancer, 121*(8), 1231–1240. https://doi.org/10.1002/cncr.29194

Boyle, C. C., Stanton, A. L., Ganz, P. A., Crespi, C. M., & Bower, J. E. (2017). Improvements in emotion regulation following mindfulness meditation: Effects on depressive symptoms and perceived stress in younger breast cancer survivors. *Journal of Consulting and Clinical Psychology, 85*(4), 397–402. https://doi.org/10.1037/ccp0000186

Brandão, T., Pedro, J., Nunes, N., Martins, M. V., Costa, M. E., & Matos, P. M. (2017a). Marital adjustment in the context of female breast cancer: A systematic review. *Psycho-Oncology, 26*(12), 2019–2029. https://doi.org/10.1002/pon.4432

Brandão, T., Schulz, M. S., & Matos, P. M. (2017b). Psychological adjustment after breast cancer: A systematic review of longitudinal studies. *Psycho-Oncology, 26*(7), 917–926. https://doi.org/10.1002/pon.4230

Brandenbarg, D., Maass, S. W. M. C., Geerse, O. P., Stegmann, M. E., Handberg, C., Schroevers, M. J., & Duijts, S. F. A. (2019). A systematic review on the prevalence of symptoms of depression, anxiety and distress in long-term cancer survivors: Implications for primary care. *European Journal of Cancer Care, 28(3), Article e13086*. https://doi.org/10.1111/ecc.13086

Brenner, R. E., Heath, P. J., Vogel, D. L., & Crede, M. (2017). Two is more valid than one: Examining the factor structure of the self-compassion scale (SCS). *Journal of Counseling Psychology, 64*, 696–707. https://doi.org/10.1037/cou0000211

Brooker, J., Julian, J., Millar, J., Prince, H. M., Kenealy, M., Herbert, K., Graham, A., Smith, R., Kissane, D., Taylor, K., Frydenberg, M., Porter, I., Fletcher, J., Haines, I., & Burney, S. (2020). A feasibility and acceptability study of an adaptation of the mindful self-compassion program for adult cancer patients. *Palliative & Supportive Care, 18*(2), 130–140. https://doi.org/10.1017/S1478951519000737

Brown, S. L., Hughes, M., Campbell, S., & Cherry, M. G. (2020). Could worry and rumination mediate relationships between self-compassion and psychological distress in breast cancer survivors? *Clinical Psychology & Psychotherapy, 27*(1), 1–10. https://doi.org/10.1002/cpp.2399

Campo, R. A., Bluth, K., Santacroce, S. J., Knapik, S., Tan, J., Gold, S., Philips, K., Gaylord, S., & Asher, G. N. (2017). A mindful self-compassion videoconference intervention for nationally recruited posttreatment young adult cancer survivors:

Feasibility, acceptability, and psychosocial outcomes. *Supportive Care in Cancer, 25*(6), 1759–1768. https://doi.org/10.1007/s00520-017-3586-y

Castilho, P., Pinto-Gouveia, J., & Duarte, J. (2015). Evaluating the multifactor structure of the long and short versions of the self-compassion scale in a clinical sample. *Journal of Clinical Psychology, 71*, 856–870. https://doi.org/10.1002/jclp.22187

Chambers, S. K., Dunn, J., Occhipinti, S., Hughes, S., Baade, P., Sinclair, S., Aitken, J., You, P., & O'Connell, D. L. (2012). A systematic review of the impact of stigma and nihilism on lung cancer outcomes. *BMC Cancer, 12, Article 184.*

Chapple, A., Ziebland, S., & McPherson, A. (2004). Stigma, shame, and blame experienced by patients with lung cancer: Qualitative study. *BMJ, 328*, Article 1470. https://doi.org/10.1136/bmj.38111.639734.7C.

Coroiu, A., Kwakkenbos, L., Moran, C., Thombs, B., Albani, C., Bourkas, S., Zenger, M., Brahler, E., & Körner, A. (2018). Structural validation of the self-compassion scale with a German general population sample. *PLoS One, 13*, e0190771. https://doi.org/10.1371/journal.pone.0190771

Costa, J., Maroco, J., Pinto-Gouveia, J., Ferreira, C., & Castilho, P. (2016). Validation of the psychometric properties of the self-compassion scale. Testing the factorial validity and factorial invariance of the measure among borderline personality disorder, anxiety disorder, eating disorder, and general populations. *Clinical Psychology and Psychotherapy, 23*, 460–468. https://doi.org/10.1002/cpp.1974

Dodds, S. E., Pace, T. W. W., Bell, M. L., Fiero, M., Negi, L. T., Raison, C. L., & Weihs, K. L. (2015). Feasibility of cognitively-based compassion training (CBCT) for breast cancer survivors: A randomized, wait list controlled pilot study. *Supportive Care in Cancer, 23*(12), 3599–3608. https://doi.org/10.1007/s00520-015-2888-1

Essue, B. M., Iragorri, N., Fitzgerald, N., & de Oliveira, C. (2020). The psychosocial cost burden of cancer: A systematic literature review. *Psycho-Oncology, 29*(11), 1746–1760. https://doi.org/10.1002/pon.5516

Ettridge, K. A., Bowden, J. A., Chambers, S. K., Smith, D. P., Murphy, M., Evans, S. M., Roder, D., & Miller, C.L. (2018). "Prostate cancer is far more hidden…": Perceptions of stigma, social isolation and help-seeking among men with prostate cancer. *European Journal of Cancer Care, 27*(2), Article e12790. https://doi.org/10.1111/ecc.12790.

Ferlay, J., Colombet, M., Soerjomataram, I., Mathers, C., Parkin, D. M., Piñeros, M., Znaor, A., & Bray, F. (2019). Estimating the global cancer incidence and mortality in 2018: GLOBOCAN sources and methods. *International Journal of Cancer, 144*(8), 1941–1953. https://doi.org/10.1002/ijc.31937

Ferrari, M., Hunt, C., Harrysunker, A., Abbott, M. J., Beath, A. P., & Einstein, D. A. (2019). Self-compassion interventions and psychosocial outcomes: A meta-analysis of RCTs. *Mindfulness, 10*(8), 1455–1473. https://doi.org/10.1007/s12671-019-01134-6

Firkins, J., Hansen, L., Driessnack, M., & Dieckmann, N. (2020). Quality of life in "chronic" cancer survivors: A meta-analysis. *Journal of Cancer Survivorship, 14*(4), 504–517. https://doi.org/10.1007/s11764-020-00869-9

Fobair, P., Stewart, S. L., Chang, S., D'Onofrio, C., Banks, P. J., & Bloom, J. R. (2006). Body image and sexual problems in young women with breast cancer. *Psycho-Oncology, 15*(7), 579–594. https://doi.org/10.1002/pon.991

Frost, M. H., Suman, V. J., Rummans, T. A., Dose, A. M., Taylor, M., Novotny, P., Johnson, R., & Evans, R. E. (2000). Physical, psychological and social well-being of women with breast cancer: The influence of disease phase. *Psycho-Oncology, 9*(3), 221–231. https://doi.org/10.1002/1099-1611(200005/06)9:3<221::aid-pon456>3.0.co;2-t

Garcia, A. C. M., Junior, J. B. C., Sarto, K. K., Marcelo, C. A. S., Paiva, E. M. C., Nogueira, D. A., & Mills, J. (2021). Quality of life, self-compassion and mindfulness in cancer patients undergoing chemotherapy: A cross-sectional study. *European Journal of Oncology Nursing, 51*, Article 101924. https://doi.org/10.1016/j.ejon.2021.101924.

Gilbert, P. (2009). Introducing compassion-focused therapy. *Advances in Psychiatric Treatment, 15*(3), 199–208. https://doi.org/10.1192/apt.bp.107.005264

Gillanders, D. T., Sinclair, A. K., MacLean, M., & Jardine, K. (2015). Illness cognitions, cognitive fusion, avoidance and self-compassion as predictors of distress and quality of life in a heterogeneous sample of adults, after cancer. *Journal of Contextual Behavioral Science, 4*(4), 300–311. https://doi.org/10.1016/j.jcbs.2015.07.003

Gonzalez-Hernandez, E., Romero, R., Campos, D., Burychka, D., Diego-Pedro, R., Baños, R., Negi, L. T., & Cebolla, A. (2018). Cognitively-based compassion training (CBCT(®)) in breast cancer survivors: A randomized clinical trial study. *Integrative Cancer Therapies, 17*(3), 684–696. https://doi.org/10.1177/1534735418772095

Gray, N. M., Hall, S. J., Browne, S., Johnston, M., Lee, A. J., Macleod, U., Mitchell, E. D., Samuel, L., & Campbell, N. C. (2014). Predictors of anxiety and depression in people with colorectal cancer. *Supportive Care in Cancer, 22*(2), 307–314. https://doi.org/10.1007/s00520-013-1963-8

Hayes, J. A., Lockard, A. J., Janis, R. A., & Locke, B. D. (2016). Construct validity of the self-compassion scale-short form among psychotherapy clients. *Counselling Psychology Quarterly, 29*, 405–422. https://doi.org/10.1080/09515070.2016.1138397

Hayes, S. C., Strosahl, K. D., & Wilson, K. G. (1999). *Acceptance and commitment therapy: An experiential approach to behavior change*. Guilford Press.

Hewitt, M., Rowland, J. H., & Yancik, R. (2003). Cancer survivors in the United States: Age, health, and disability. *The Journals of Gerontology, Series A: Biological Sciences and Medical Sciences, 58*(1), 82–91. https://doi.org/10.1093/gerona/58.1.m82

Hofmann, S. G., Grossman, P., & Hinton, D. E. (2011). Loving-kindness and compassion meditation: Potential for psychological interventions. *Clinical Psychology Review, 31*(7), 1126–1132. https://doi.org/10.1016/j.cpr.2011.07.003

Johnston, B., McGill, M., Milligan, S., McElroy, D., Foster, C., & Kearney, N. (2009). Self care and end of life care in advanced cancer: Literature review. *European Journal of Oncology Nursing, 13*(5), 386–398. https://doi.org/10.1016/j.ejon.2009.04.003

Kabat-Zinn, J. (2003). Mindfulness-based interventions in context: Past, present, and future. *Clinical Psychology: Science and Practice, 10*(2), 144–156. https://doi.org/10.1093/clipsy.bpg016

Kim, E., Han, J. Y., Moon, T. J., Shaw, B., Shah, D. V., McTavish, F. M., & Gustafson, D. H. (2012). The process and effect of supportive message expression and reception in online breast cancer support groups. *Psycho-Oncology, 21*(5), 531–540. https://doi.org/10.1002/pon.1942

Kotsou, I., & Leys, C. (2016). Self-compassion scale (SCS): Psychometric properties of the French translation and its relations with psychological well-being, affect, and depression. *PLoS One, 11*, e0152880. https://doi.org/10.1371/journal.pone.0152880

Krebber, A. M. H., Buffart, L. M., Kleijn, G., Riepma, I. C., de Bree, R., Leemans, C. R., Becker, A., Brug, J., van Straten, A., Cuijpers, P., & Verdonck-de Leeuw, I. M. (2014). Prevalence of depression in cancer patients: A meta-analysis of diagnostic interviews and self-report instruments. *Psycho-Oncology, 23*(2), 121–130. https://doi.org/10.1002/pon.3409

Kumlander, S., Lahtinen, O., Turunen, T., & Salmivalli, C. (2018). Two is more valid than one, but is six even better? The factor structure of the self-compassion scale (SCS). *PLoS One, 13*, e0207706. https://doi.org/10.1371/journal.pone.0207706

Lathren, C., Bluth, K., Campo, R., Tan, W., & Futch, W. (2018). Young adult cancer survivors' experiences with a mindful self-compassion (MSC) video-chat intervention: A qualitative analysis. *Self and Identity, 17*(6), 646–665. https://doi.org/10.1080/15298868.2018.1451363

Lennon, J., Hevey, D., & Kinsella, L. (2018). Gender role conflict, emotional approach coping, self-compassion, and distress in prostate cancer patients: A model of direct and moderating effects. *Psycho-Oncology, 27*(8), 2009–2015. https://doi.org/10.1002/pon.4762

Luoma, J. B., & Platt, M. G. (2015). Shame, self-criticism, self-stigma, and compassion in acceptance and commitment therapy. *Current Opinion in Psychology, 2*, 97–101. https://doi.org/10.1016/j.copsyc.2014.12.016

Miller, K., Mehta, R., Abraham, J., Opneja, A., & Jain, R. K. (2017). Patterns of long-term cancer survivorship care in a National Cancer Institute-designated Comprehensive Cancer Center. *American Journal of Clinical Oncology, 40*(6), 639–643. https://doi.org/10.1097/COC.0000000000000217

Muris, P., & Otgaar, H. (2020). The process of science: A critical evaluation of more than 15 years of research on self-compassion with the self-compassion scale. *Mindfulness, 11*(6), 1469–1482. https://doi.org/10.1007/s12671-020-01363-0

Muris, P., Van den Broek, M., Otgaar, H., Oudenhoven, I., & Lennartz, J. (2018). Good and bad sides of self-compassion: A face validity check of the self-compassion scale and an investigation of its relations to coping and emotional symptoms in non-clinical adolescents. *Journal of Child and Family Studies, 27*, 2411–2421. https://doi.org/10.1007/s10826-018-1099-z

National Cancer Institute. (2021). Cancer. In *NCI dictionary of cancer terms*. https://www.cancer.gov/publications/dictionaries/cancer-terms/def/cancer

Naughton, M. J., & Weaver, K. E. (2014). Physical and mental health among cancer survivors: Considerations for long-term care and quality of life. *North Carolina Medical Journal, 75*(4), 283–286. https://doi.org/10.18043/ncm.75.4.283

Neff, K. D. (2003). Self-compassion: An alternative conceptualization of a healthy attitude toward oneself. *Self and Identity, 2*(2), 85–101. https://doi.org/10.1080/15298860309032

Neff, K. D. (2020). Commentary on Muris and Otgaar (2020): Let the empirical evidence speak on the self-compassion scale. *Mindfulness, 11*(1), 1900–1909. https://doi.org/10.1007/s12671-020-01411-9

Neff, K. D., & Germer, C. K. (2013). A pilot study and randomized controlled trial of the mindful self-compassion program. *Journal of Clinical Psychology, 69*(1), 28–44. https://doi.org/10.1002/jclp.21923

Neff, K. D., Whittaker, T., & Karl, A. (2017). Evaluating the factor structure of the self-compassion scale in four distinct populations: Is the use of a total self-compassion score justified? *Journal of Personality Assessment, 99*, 596–607. https://doi.org/10.1080/00223891.2016.1269334

Negi, L. T. (2013). *Emory compassion meditation protocol: Cognitively-based compassion training manual.* Emory University.

Niedzwiedz, C. L., Knifton, L., Robb, K. A., Katikireddi, S. V., & Smith, D. J. (2019). Depression and anxiety among people living with and beyond cancer: A growing clinical and research priority. *BMC Cancer, 19*, Article 943. https://doi.org/10.1186/s12885-019-6181-4.

O'Neil, J., Helms, B., Gable, R., David, L., & Wrightsman, L. (1986). Gender-role conflict scale: College men's fear of femininity. *Sex Roles, 14*(5–6), 335–350. https://doi.org/10.1007/BF00287583

Paterson, C. L., Lengacher, C. A., Donovan, K. A., Kip, K. E., & Tofthagen, C. S. (2016). Body image in younger breast cancer survivors: A systematic review. *Cancer Nursing, 39*(1), E39–E58. https://doi.org/10.1097/NCC.0000000000000251

Petrocchi, N., Ottaviani, C., & Couyoumdjian, A. (2014). Dimensionality of self-compassion: Translation and construct validation of the self-compassion scale in an Italian sample. *Journal of Mental Health, 23*, 72–77. https://doi.org/10.3109/09638237.2013.841869

Pinto-Gouveia, J., Duarte, C., Matos, M., & Fráguas, S. (2014). The protective role of self-compassion in relation to psychopathology symptoms and quality of life in chronic and in cancer patients. *Clinical Psychology & Psychotherapy, 21*(4), 311–323. https://doi.org/10.1002/cpp.1838

Pitman, A., Suleman, S., Hyde, N., & Hodgkiss, A. (2018). Depression and anxiety in patients with cancer. *Bmj, 361*, Article 1415. https://doi.org/10.1136/bmj.k1415.

Przezdziecki, A., Alcorso, J., & Sherman, K. A. (2016). My changed body: Background, development and acceptability of a self-compassion based writing activity for female survivors of breast cancer. *Patient Education and Counseling, 99*(5), 870–874. https://doi.org/10.1016/j.pec.2015.12.011

Przezdziecki, A., Sherman, K. A., Baillie, A., Taylor, A., Foley, E., & Stalgis-Bilinski, K. (2013). My changed body: Breast cancer, body image, distress and self-compassion. *Psycho-Oncology, 22*(8), 1872–1979. https://doi.org/10.1002/pon.3230

Raes, F. (2011). The effect of self-compassion on the development of depression symptoms in a non-clinical sample. *Mindfulness, 2*(1), 33–36. https://doi.org/10.1007/s12671-011-0040-y

Rajotte, E. J., Baker, K. S., Heron, L., & Syrjala, K. L. (2017). Sexual function in adult cancer survivors. *Journal of Clinical Oncology, 35*(5, Suppl), S123–S123. https://doi.org/10.1200/JCO.2017.35.5_suppl.123

Raque-Bogdan, T. L., Ericson, S. K., Jackson, J., Martin, H. M., & Bryan, N. A. (2011). Attachment and mental and physical health: Self-compassion and mattering as mediators. *Journal of Counseling Psychology, 58*(2), 272–278. https://doi.org/10.1037/a0023041

Reece, J. C., Chan, Y.-F., Herbert, J., Gralow, J., & Fann, J. R. (2013). Course of depression, mental health service utilization and treatment preferences in women receiving chemotherapy for breast cancer. *General Hospital Psychiatry, 35*(4), 376–381. https://doi.org/10.1016/j.genhosppsych.2013.03.017

Rumsey, N., & Harcourt, D. (2005). *The psychology of appearance*. Open University Press.

Schellekens, M. P. J., Karremans, J. C., van der Drift, M. A., Molema, J., van den Hurk, D. G. M., Prins, J. B., & Speckens, A. E. M. (2017). Are mindfulness and self-compassion related to psychological distress and communication in couples facing lung cancer? A dyadic approach. *Mindfulness, 8*(2), 325–336. https://doi.org/10.1007/s12671-016-0602-0

Shaw, L.-K., Sherman, K. A., Fitness, J., Elder, E., & Breast Cancer Network Australia. (2018). Factors associated with romantic relationship formation difficulties in women with breast cancer. *Psycho-Oncology, 27*(4), 1270–1276. https://doi.org/10.1002/pon.4666

Sherman, K. A., Przezdziecki, A., Alcorso, J., Kilby, C. J., Elder, E., Boyages, J., Koelmeyer, L., & Mackie, H. (2018). Reducing body image-related distress in women with breast cancer using a structured online writing exercise: Results from the my changed body randomized controlled trial. *Journal of Clinical Oncology, 36*(19), 1930–1940. https://doi.org/10.1200/JCO.2017.76.3318

Sherman, K. A., Woon, S., French, J., & Elder, E. (2017). Body image and psychological distress in nipple-sparing mastectomy: The roles of self-compassion and appearance investment. *Psycho-Oncology, 26*(3), 337–345. https://doi.org/10.1002/pon.4138

Shonin, E., Van Gordon, W., Compare, A., Zangeneh, M., & Griffiths, M. D. (2015). Buddhist-derived loving-kindness and compassion meditation for the treatment of psychopathology: A systematic review. *Mindfulness, 6*(5), 1161–1180. https://doi.org/10.1007/s12671-014-0368-1

Simard, S., Thewes, B., Humphris, G., Dixon, M., Hayden, C., Mireskandari, S., & Ozakinci, G. (2013). Fear of cancer recurrence in adult cancer survivors: A systematic review of quantitative studies. *Journal of Cancer Survivorship, 7*(3), 300–322. https://doi.org/10.1007/s11764-013-0272-z

Sirois, F. M., & Hirsch, J. K. (2019). Self-compassion and adherence in five medical groups: The role of stress. *Mindfulness, 10*, 46–54. https://doi.org/10.1007/s12671-018-0945-9

Siwik, C. J., Phillips, K., Zimmaro, L., Salmon, P., & Sephton, S. E. (2021). Depressive symptoms among patients with lung cancer: Elucidating the roles of shame, guilt, and self-compassion. *Journal of Health Psychology*. Advance online publication. https://doi.org/10.1177/1359105320988331.

Striegel-Moore, R., Franko, D., Thompson, D., Barton, B., Schreiber, G., & Daniels, S. (2004). Changes in weight and body image over time in women with eating disorders. *International Journal of Eating Disorders, 36*(3), 315–327. https://doi.org/10.1002/eat.20053

Terry, M. L., & Leary, M. R. (2011). Self-compassion, self-regulation, and health. *Self and Identity, 10*(3), 352–362. https://doi.org/10.1080/15298868.2011.558404

Todorov, N., Sherman, K. A., Kilby, C. J., & Breast Cancer Network Australia. (2019). Self-compassion and hope in the context of body image disturbance and distress in breast cancer survivors. *Psycho-Oncology, 28*(10), 2025–2032. https://doi.org/10.1002/pon.5187

Trindade, I. A., Ferreira, C., & Pinto-Gouveia, J. (2020). Acceptability and preliminary test of efficacy of the mind programme in women with breast cancer: An acceptance, mindfulness, and compassion-based intervention. *Journal of Contextual Behavioral Science, 15*, 162–171. https://doi.org/10.1016/j.jcbs.2019.12.005

Trindade, I. A., Soares, A., & Skvarc, D. (2025). Efficacy and cost-effectiveness of an ACT and compassion-based intervention for women with breast cancer: study protocol of two randomised controlled trials {1}. *Trials, 26*, 5. https://doi.org/10.1186/s13063-024-08626-4

van der Donk, L. J., Fleer, J., Tovote, A., Ranchor, A. V., Smink, A., Mul, V. E. M., Sanderman, R., & Schroevers, M. J. (2020). The role of mindfulness and self-compassion in depressive symptoms and affect: A comparison between cancer patients and healthy controls. *Mindfulness, 11*(4), 883–894. https://doi.org/10.1007/s12671-019-01298-1

Veach, T. A., Nicholas, D. R., & Barton, M. A. (2002). *Cancer and the family life cycle: A practitioner's guide*. Brunner-Routledge.

Wall, D., & Kristjanson, L. (2005). Men, culture and hegemonic masculinity: Understanding the experience of prostate cancer. *Nursing Inquiry, 12*(2), 87–97. https://doi.org/10.1111/j.1440-1800.2005.00258.x

Wei, M., Liao, K. Y.-H., Ku, T.-Y., & Shaffer, P. A. (2011). Attachment, self-compassion, empathy, and subjective well-being among college students and community adults. *Journal of Personality, 79*(1), 191–221. https://doi.org/10.1111/j.1467-6494.2010.00677.x

Woods, H., & Proeve, M. (2014). Relationships of mindfulness, self-compassion, and meditation experience with shame-proneness. *Journal of Cognitive Psychotherapy, 28*(1), 20–33. https://doi.org/10.1891/0889-8391.28-1.20

Wren, A. A., Shelby, R. A., Soo, M. S., Huysmans, Z., Jarosz, J. A., & Keefe, F. J. (2019). Preliminary efficacy of a lovingkindness meditation intervention for patients undergoing biopsy and breast cancer surgery: A randomized controlled pilot study. *Supportive Care in Cancer, 27*(9), 3583–3592. https://doi.org/10.1007/s00520-019-4657-z

Xu, S., Zhang, H., & Wang, J. (2020). Caregiver burden and depression among Chinese family caregivers: The role of self-compassion. *Mindfulness, 11*(7), 1647–1654. https://doi.org/10.1007/s12671-020-01378-7

Zhang, H., Dong, L., Watson-Singleton, N. N., Tarantino, N., Carr, E. R., Niles-Carnes, L. V., Patterson, B., & Kaslow, N. J. (2019). Psychometric properties of the self-compassion scale in an African American sample. *Mindfulness, 10*, 1395–1405. https://doi.org/10.1007/s12671-019-01099-6

Zhu, L., Wang, J., Liu, S., Xie, H., Hu, Y., Yao, J., Ranchor, A. V., Schroevers, M. J., & Fleer, J. (2020). Self-compassion and symptoms of depression and anxiety in Chinese cancer patients: The mediating role of illness perceptions. *Mindfulness, 11*(10), 2386–2396. https://doi.org/10.1007/s12671-020-01455-x

Zhu, L., Yao, J., Wang, J., Wu, L., Gao, Y., Xie, J., Liu, A., Ranchor, A. V., & Schroevers, M. J. (2019). The predictive role of self-compassion in cancer patients' symptoms of depression, anxiety, and fatigue: A longitudinal study. *Psycho-Oncology, 28*(9), 1918–1925. https://doi.org/10.1002/pon.5174

23

Applying Self-Compassion: Does Self-Compassion Influence Other-Focused Care in Healthcare?

Jane E. Cha and Nathan S. Consedine

Introduction

Compassion is central to healthcare. Compassion can enhance doctor–patient relationships, reduce healthcare expenses, and offer a range of benefits to physicians, patients, and healthcare systems (Fernando & Consedine, 2017; Sinclair et al., 2016). However, while many providers train for careers in healthcare *precisely because* they care for others, modern healthcare environments present numerous challenges to well-being and the provision of compassionate care (Fernando & Consedine, 2014a). The challenges in healthcare are extensive, ranging from exposure to trauma (Showalter, 2010) and complex cases (Brownie et al., 2016) to difficult colleagues and conflicts (Jones et al., 2016), poor leadership (Papadopoulos et al., 2017), long hours (Davison & Williams, 2009), and unrealistic employer expectations (Bynum IV & Sukhera, 2021); the demands of the COVID-19 pandemic likely compound such difficulties (Alrawashdeh et al., 2021). Inevitably, such factors collectively contribute to physical, psychological, and emotional difficulties among healthcare professionals (West et al., 2018), almost certainly impacting their capacity to provide compassionate care.

J. E. Cha (✉) • N. S. Consedine
Department of Psychological Medicine, Faculty of Medical and Health Sciences, The University of Auckland, Auckland, New Zealand
e-mail: j.cha@auckland.ac.nz

F. M. Sirois (ed.), *The Palgrave Handbook of Positive Psychology and Health*, https://doi.org/10.1007/978-3-031-89095-6_23

As importantly, while providing compassionate care to others is a social and professional expectation in healthcare, providing compassion for oneself has historically been missing from medical curricula. Although it seems logical to suggest that self-care is necessary to sustain the ability to work in healthcare, self-directed compassion may be stigmatized as being "selfish" or "narcissistic" in healthcare environments (Mills et al., 2015). Of course, as conceptualized by leading writers (Gilbert, 2014; Neff, 2003), self-compassion is neither selfish nor narcissistic. Rather, it is a way of relating to the self during times of failure or challenge that has the potential to both enhance the well-being of professionals (Pavlova & Consedine, 2023), as well as, more speculatively, their capacity to provide care to others (Kemper et al., 2015; Neff et al., 2007; Seppala et al., 2014).

Indeed, one of the common ways of conceptualizing self-compassion—responding to oneself in times of suffering characterized by self-kindness versus self-judgment, common humanity versus isolation, and mindfulness versus over-identification or avoidance (Neff, 2003)—suggests it is likely to be particularly relevant in healthcare contexts. Specifically, self-compassion may impact both the general ability to adapt to the pressures of these environments as well as the tendency, ability, or motivation to provide compassionate care. Self-kindness, which refers to treating oneself with warmth, respect, care, and unconditional acceptance (Neff, 2003), may be of particular benefit to healthcare professionals who have a documented tendency toward harsh self-judgment (Bria et al., 2012). Similarly, common humanity—understanding that human suffering, the experience of pain, and imperfections are all part of the shared human experience (Neff, 2003)—may help healthcare professionals reduce the need to present a "perfect" version of themselves, free from mistakes and any struggles of their own (Bynum IV & Sukhera, 2021). Lastly, mindfulness entails a balanced awareness of one's suffering in the present moment (Neff, 2003). Working in systems and professions with unattainable expectations may lead some groups, such as surgeons, to self-blame when errors arise (Shanafelt et al., 2010). Mindfulness may reduce the tendency to over-identify with the negative aspects of one's professional experience, reducing rumination. In sum, while studies linking self-compassion and other-focused care in the healthcare are only beginning to be conducted, the self-compassion construct and how it is thought to "work" may allow it to counteract the negative factors in healthcare (Sinclair et al., 2017).

In this chapter, we address a critical question for studies of self-compassion in applied domains: does (or should) self-compassion benefit other-focused care? We begin by summarizing current evidence for the potential benefits of self-compassion for self- and other-focused outcomes, with the focus resting on studies of healthcare professional samples. We then consider what is known about the mechanisms by which self-compassion is thought to work, reviewing mediational studies as well as theories regarding the mechanisms thought to underpin self-compassion's benefits. We suggest that while the literature linking self-compassion to other-focused care remains empirically underdeveloped, the potential for self-compassion to produce benefits for both the individual and those they work with is clear. Drawing from self-regulation theory (Baumeister & Heatherton, 1996), we delineate a series of possible pathways suited to empirical study. We conclude by suggesting that while ongoing studies of both the outcomes of self-compassion in applied contexts and possible mediating mechanisms are needed, self-compassion represents a way of being in the world and with the self that may be uniquely suited to the challenges of healthcare.

Self-Compassion and Individual Outcomes

Extensive research in both general population and healthcare professional samples suggest that self-compassion predicts better well-being and psychosocial health. Greater trait self-compassion is reliably associated with greater psychological well-being (Zessin et al., 2015) and resilience when faced with major stressors (Sbarra et al., 2012). Meta-analytic findings indicate moderate to strong positive correlations between trait self-compassion and better psychological well-being or mental health, including lower stress, anxiety, and depression (MacBeth & Gumley, 2012; Zessin et al., 2015), and other empirical studies show important links with lower maladaptive perfectionism (Mehr & Adams, 2016), and less rumination (Svendsen et al., 2017). Meta-analyses of self-compassion *interventional* studies show a similar pattern, revealing moderate to large effect-size improvements across outcomes (Ferrari et al., 2019), notably improvements in well-being and reductions in depression, anxiety, and psychological distress (Kirby et al., 2017).

Other data suggest that self-compassion may also predict better physical health and health behaviors (Phillips & Hine, 2019). Of note, greater self-compassion predicts better sleep quality (Brown et al., 2020), fewer physical symptoms (Dunne et al., 2018; Hall et al., 2013; Sirois, 2020; Terry et al., 2013), lower physiological responses to stress (Arch et al., 2014; Breines et al., 2014), and more frequent health-promoting behaviors (Gedik, 2019; Li et al., 2020; Sirois, 2015), such as healthy eating (Adams & Leary, 2007; Schoenefeld

& Webb, 2013), exercise (Magnus et al., 2010), seeking medical care (Terry et al., 2013), and adherence (Sirois & Hirsch, 2019).

While less evidence exists regarding outcomes of specific relevance to samples of healthcare professionals, accumulating evidence in this area shows promising results (Sinclair et al., 2017). Across healthcare samples, greater self-compassion predicts greater resilience (Kemper et al., 2020), better mental health (Olson & Kemper, 2014), such as lower depressive symptoms (McCade et al., 2021), and better quality of life (Dev et al., 2020). Greater trait self-compassion reliably predicts lower burnout, fatigue, and work-related stress in healthcare professional samples (Beaumont et al., 2016a; Crary, 2013; Dev et al., 2020; Finlay-Jones et al., 2015; Kemper et al., 2015). While studies in this area remain cross-sectional and convenience sample-based, the overall pattern and magnitude of the links between self-compassion and mental health outcomes is largely similar to that seen in general population studies.

Beyond indices of mental and physical well-being, self-compassion also has the potential to benefit other important elements of professional functioning in healthcare samples. One study of 200 medical trainees in Canada, for example, found that greater self-compassion predicted the pursuit of more adaptive (versus maladaptive) goals (Babenko & Oswald, 2019). Medical trainees with lower trait self-compassion reported higher mastery avoidance goals, a motivational "style" dominated by the desire to avoid undesirable outcomes, such as being seen as incompetent or failing at certain tasks (Elliot & Dweck, 2013). However, those with greater self-compassion reported lower mastery avoidance goals, potentially indexing a tendency to approach mistakes as opportunities for learning rather than as something to be feared or criticized. Self-compassion has also been associated with greater job satisfaction (Vaillancourt & Wasylkiw, 2020), compassion satisfaction (Buceta et al., 2019), perceived competence (Ying, 2009), and emotional intelligence (Heffernan et al., 2010). At a cross-sectional level then, self-compassion appears to predict important outcomes that are specific to healthcare.

However, interventional work among healthcare samples remains scant. One pilot study tested a 6-week, online self-compassion cultivation program among Australian psychology trainees (Finlay-Jones et al., 2017). This study found pre-post increases in self-compassion and happiness and decreases in depression, stress, and emotion regulatory difficulties; most benefits were maintained at the three-month follow-up (Finlay-Jones et al., 2017). A similar study, again lacking experimental control, found that a six-week, web-based mindful self-compassion program increased self-compassion, reduced self-coldness, alleviated stress, and reduced the symptoms of burnout in practicing psychologists (Eriksson et al., 2018). In nurses, a small study (n = 13) evaluated the 8-week Mindful Self-Compassion (MSC) training, finding increases in self-compassion, mindfulness, resilience, and compassion satisfaction, and reduced burnout and secondary trauma (Delaney, 2018).

Most recently, Neff and colleagues adapted the original MSC program, specifically targeting the challenges in healthcare (Neff et al., 2020). This six-week Self-Compassion for Healthcare Communities (SCHC) program focuses on a "Compassion with Equanimity" component. This particular equanimity focus was aimed at providing a sense of perspective and calm in caregiving interactions. Early findings for this program across two studies in healthcare professionals (including nurses, physicians, social workers, and others) showed improvements in self-compassion and mindfulness and reductions in burnout, stress, exhaustion, and depressive symptoms (with medium to large effect sizes). A subsequent study evaluated a modified version of this program among pediatric nurses (Franco & Christie, 2021). Findings showed that nurses who received the SCHC training reported increases in self-compassion, mindfulness, and compassion satisfaction from pre- to post-training compared to the control group. As in the earlier study, the benefits were maintained at a three-month follow-up (Franco & Christie, 2021).

As noted, studies of self-compassion in healthcare contexts are limited by a reliance on cross-sectional data and/or interventional studies that lack appropriate controls as well as by small sample sizes and high attrition rates. While these limitations remain important (Pavlova & Consedine, 2023), findings nonetheless highlight the potential of self-compassion to enhance well-being, motivation, and professional functioning in healthcare. Many medical professionals enter the field of healthcare because they want to help and often have personal and professional values entailing altruism and compassion for others (Neff et al., 2020). However, despite their dispositional tendency to be compassionate, personal, interpersonal, clinical, and environmental factors can hinder compassion (Fernando & Consedine, 2014a; Fernando & Consedine, 2014b; Sinclair et al., 2016), resulting in reductions in the extent to which caring for others is satisfying (Sprang et al., 2007; Stamm, 2012). What is missing from current research is clarity regarding *why* self-compassion *specifically* (rather than some other intervention) should be of benefit in samples of healthcare professionals and whether it influences other-focused care. We will explore these key questions in the following sections.

Self-Compassion and Other-Focused Care

The evidence for the benefits of self-compassion in healthcare samples is growing. However, the suggestion that the development of self-compassion should lead to increases in other-focused care finds less direct empirical support. Theoretically, several traditions suggest that developing the ability/tendency to be compassionate toward the self ultimately contributes to being compassionate toward others (Gustin & Wagner, 2013). Buddhist writings, for example, suggest that building the capacity to hold suffering in compassionate awareness enables the individual to extend compassion to multiple beings, whether it's for the self, others, or all sentient beings (Hofmann et al., 2011). As noted, however, these assertions have infrequently been subjected to empirical scrutiny and evaluations in healthcare populations are very few indeed.

One early study found that greater trait self-compassion was associated with reports of greater compassion for humanity, empathic concern, and altruism in practicing meditators and community-living adults (Neff & Pommier, 2013). Another study found a positive, small-to-moderate correlation between self-compassion and compassion for others in clinical psychologists and psychology trainees (Yip et al., 2017). In the areas of parent–child and romantic relationships, a recent scoping review suggests that self-compassion is associated with a range of benefits in close interpersonal relationships (Lathren et al., 2021).

Studies evaluating whether self-compassion training can deliver interpersonal benefits are showing promising results. One randomized controlled trial (RCT) evaluated a Compassion Cultivation Training (CCT) Program with 100 adults. This study found that those who received a nine-week CCT (compared to a waitlist control) reported greater increases in compassion for others, receiving compassion from others, as well as in self-compassion (Jazaieri et al., 2013). Another study testing the efficacy of an 8-week pilot Mindful Self-Compassion (MSC) program showed that persons in the intervention group reported greater compassion to others (Neff & Germer, 2013). To this point then, evidence is consistent with the important possibility that self-compassion may enhance other-focused care.

Such an interpretation would, however, be premature. Other cross-sectional studies have found that self-compassion and compassion for others are *un*related (Beaumont et al., 2016b; López et al., 2018) or, in some cases, may be *inversely* related (Mills et al., 2018). A study of 369 palliative care doctors and nurses by Mills et al. (2018), for example, found that while self-compassion predicted greater self-care (r = 0.412), it predicted lower scores on the Santa Clara Brief Compassion Scale (r = −0.122); this result does appear to have been "driven" by associations within the female subsample. Thus, while there is evidence suggesting self-compassion might increase prosocial processes (and the strong theoretical basis for the possibility that the benefits of self-compassion may extend to other-focused care), competing findings are also in evidence. Clearly, there is a need for additional research here. In addition to the need for designs suited to investigating the conditions under which self-compassion does and does not lead to greater care for others, our suggestion here is that we will be better placed to understand core questions regarding self-compassion in healthcare when we have a clearer idea regarding the underlying mechanisms: *why* does self-compassion lead (or not lead) to benefits for the self or for others?

Current Challenges (and Limitations) in Studies Linking Self-Compassion to Other-Focused Care

As intimated, there are several challenges associated with understanding *how* self-compassion interventions work to enhance other-focused care. One initial challenge lies in the fact that many interventions, such as Neff and Germer's (2013) MSC intervention, include components such as the loving-kindness meditation which overtly seek to cultivate compassion for *both* others and the self (Grossman et al., 2004); determining what an intervention is "made" of and thus why/how it might work is often difficult. Interventions including multiple elements and/or a mixed focus on the self and others, making it difficult to determine whether *self-compassion* per se increases other focused care and/or which components of this complex construct might be relevant.

Empirically, a small body of recent work has begun to disentangle the complex interventional components and effects of self-compassion interventions. One recent study, for example, separated self-compassion and compassion for others in three different studies (targeting and comparing specific aspects of self-compassion and compassion for others; Chio et al., 2021). Interestingly, this study found that while cultivating self-compassion in isolation enhanced self-compassion, it did *not* increase compassion for others (Chio et al., 2021). However, when a didactic element including (1) videos that explained self-compassion and other-focused compassion, (2) loving-kindness meditation, and (3) a "universalism" outcome to capture the effects of other-focused concern was added, both self- and other-compassion increased. Such findings might suggest that when self-compassion interventions and/or trainings include direct engagement and promotion of other-oriented values, it may be more effective in enhancing other-focused concern. How ecologically valid such tests are and whether they would work in healthcare populations is unknown at this time.

Compounding this complexity is the fact that most other-focused care outcomes are self-reported. There is a lack of research assessing the hypothesized impact of self-compassion on either behavior or as experienced among the recipients of care (e.g., patients and their families; Sinclair et al., 2017). Paradoxically then, perhaps the most important initial "risk" in this area lies in demonstrating that self-compassion increases feelings of other-focused care, but that such feelings do not readily translate into more compassionate *actions* or the experience of care. One study evaluated whether the development of self-compassion and empathy resulted in greater peer-rated prosociality in an adolescent sample (Marshall et al., 2020). This study found that while self-compassion and empathy were both positively correlated with peer-rated prosocial behavior, only empathy predicted prosocial behavior. Thus, at least in adolescents, greater self-compassion did not predict greater prosocial behavior.

More broadly, while research in other areas (e.g., in romantic relationships) tends to imply that self-compassionate individuals are perceived by their partners as being more caring (Neff & Beretvas, 2013), whether this relationship is evident in healthcare professionals and their patients remain largely unknown at this time (see Baguley et al., 2020 on this issue). Preliminarily, while we might expect that feelings of care will, ultimately, translate into behavior that is experienced as compassionate by patients, there are a very large number of factors that influence the capacity and ability to care (Pavlova et al., 2021). If one purpose of self-compassion interventions in healthcare is to increase other-focused care, we need studies that incorporate objective behavioral measurement (rather than self-report alone) and that treat the experience of feeling cared for among patients as a key outcome variable in our designs.

In summary, while there is clear evidence to suggest that self-compassion training may be beneficial in enhancing other-focused care, exactly *how* this process might work remains largely unknown. Multi-component interventions with mixed measures of self- and other-focus outcomes coupled with the absence of objective measurement make it challenging to determine which components (if any) underpin self-compassion's benefits. An obvious solution to such a challenge is to conduct studies linking self-compassion to distinct individual and other-focused outcomes (including recipients of compassionate care) as well as to evaluate the *specific pathways* that may link self-compassion to particular outcomes. In contributing to this nascent picture, the following section reviews relevant mediation studies, focusing on how self-compassion may offer benefits to healthcare professionals and their patients.

How Might Self-Compassion Work to Enhance Self- and Other-Focused Care? Potential Mediating Mechanisms

As noted, despite evidence for the benefits of self-compassion for the self and others (at least in some samples), the pathways by which self-compassion *works* remain unclear. Both as a trait and in terms of how self-compassion is reflected in interventions, self-compassion is a complicated, multi-componential construct. Perhaps as a part consequence, the active pathways (mediating mechanisms) linking self-compassion to self- and other-outcomes in healthcare provider samples are unclear. Below, we deepen the foundation for considering the dual questions of self- and other-benefit by characterizing two broad classes of mechanism regarding how self-compassion might work: *general resource* vs *compassion-specific* pathways (refer to Fig. 23.1).

General Pathway

As can be seen in the Fig. 23.1, the first class of mechanism relevant to how self-compassion might "work" in healthcare contexts is found in an examination of its general benefits in terms of psychosocial functioning. In theory, the development of self-compassion might lead to greater other-focused care *because* it reduces distress, anxiety, depression, and stress. Hypothetically, the resources the individual was using to manage stress or affective distress might be "freed up" such that caring for others can be accomplished. In common-sense terms, it may be easier to care when the individual practitioner is less stressed and depleted. Consistent with this possibility, most studies testing the potential mediators of self-compassion's effects have been implicitly based in general theories of self-regulation (Baumeister & Heatherton, 1996), notably in ideas regarding the adaptive regulation of emotions (Gratz & Roemer, 2004), stress, and coping (Lazarus, 1966). Below, we briefly review what mediation studies of this possibility in general samples suggest, before

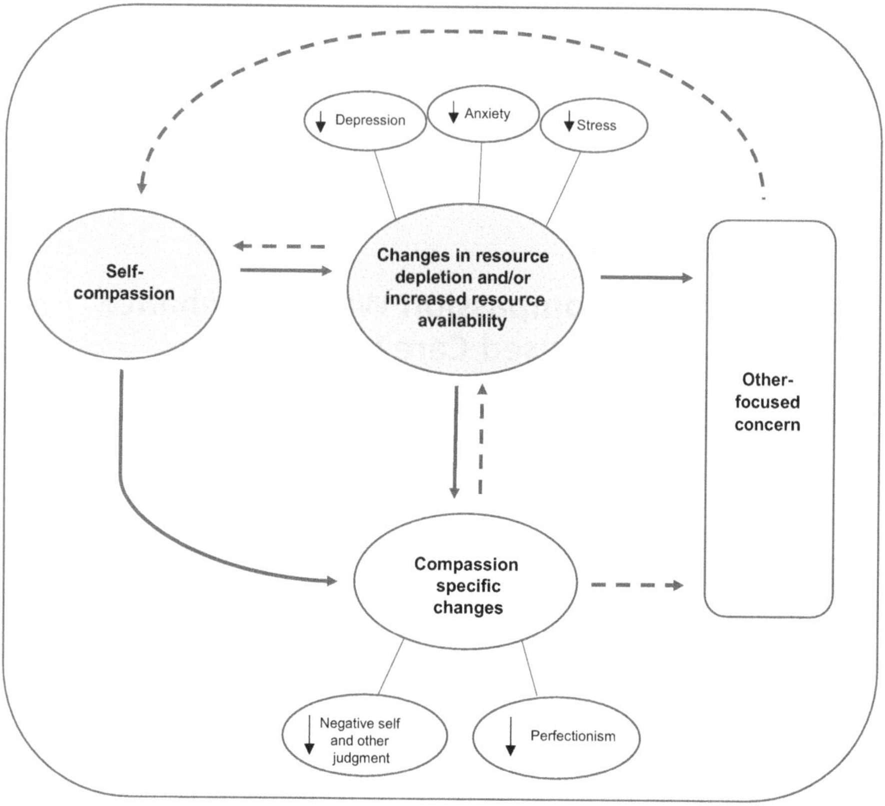

Fig. 23.1 A diagram showing how self-compassion might work to benefit the other-focused care in a healthcare context, including examples of general and specific pathways

considering the few mediational studies of healthcare samples. We then use observations and data from this work to consider how self-compassion might work in terms of increasing *general* regulatory resources[1] (Baumeister & Heatherton, 1996; Baumeister et al., 2007).

There is a growing literature that statistically tests the pathways by which self-compassion may provide benefit. Common mediators investigated in the context of mental health outcomes in general populations include aspects of rumination and worry (Arimitsu & Hofmann, 2015; Fresnics & Borders,

[1] Note. Although self-compassion is generally discussed as potentially increasing "general resource" in this chapter, it is possible that self-compassion may act as a distinct resource. More research is needed to confirm whether self-compassion increases general self-regulation capacity or represents a distinct resource pool.

2017; Hodgetts et al., 2020; Johnson & O'Brien, 2013; Raes, 2010; Tandler et al., 2020), emotion-regulation (Chishima et al., 2018; Meyer & Leppma, 2019), coping (Hamrick & Owens, 2019; Li et al., 2021), perceived stress (Luo et al., 2019), positive and negative affect (Schmidt et al., 2019), subjective happiness (Booker & Dunsmore, 2019), gratitude (Nguyen et al., 2020), and depressive symptoms (Kelliher Rabon et al., 2018). Most works have found statistically significant mediation effects and one recent review concludes by suggesting that emotion regulation strategies might underpin the links between self-compassion and mental health (Inwood & Ferrari, 2018).

At this stage, however, mediation studies linking self-compassion to outcomes in healthcare professionals remain scant. Those that do exist are limited by the issues that characterize mediational analyses in cross-sectional data. One study among nurses found that burnout mediated the relationship between self-compassion and outcomes such as sleep quality and compassion satisfaction (Vaillancourt & Wasylkiw, 2020). Such results imply that self-compassion may protect nurses from burnout, subsequently enabling better sleep and enhanced job satisfaction. Another study evaluated emotion regulation difficulties as a possible mechanism linking self-compassion and stress in psychologists and trainees (Finlay-Jones et al., 2015). Analyses suggested that while self-compassion did not directly influence stress, greater self-compassion was associated with lower stress levels via more adaptive emotion regulation strategies.

As noted, many studies of this kind are conducted within the general framework of self-regulation theory, specifically in the *limited strength model* (Baumeister & Heatherton, 1996; Baumeister et al., 2007). The limited strength model of self-regulation suggests that people have a limited supply of "willpower" that is dedicated to acts of self-control and other operations of the system. In theory, each act of self-control draws from this limited general supply, leaving fewer resources available for subsequent acts that require self-control. According to this influential line of reasoning, when this general resource becomes depleted, people are more likely to experience failures in self-control. While evidence regarding whether individuals can overcome depletion are mixed (Muraven & Slessareva, 2003) and there are ongoing issues with replication (Carter et al., 2015), it is possible that self-compassion may free up self-regulatory resources, prevent depletion, and thus help avoid negative mental health outcomes.

However, it is important to note here that managing distress or stressful situations (both in healthcare and in life more generally) is *assumed* to require the use of finite regulatory resources that are progressively depleted. However, empirical evaluations directly testing this core assumption are entirely absent and empirical evidence in healthcare actually shows that reports of burnout, compassion fatigue, and the barriers to compassion are actually *lower* the longer a practitioner has worked in healthcare (Dev et al., 2019); prima facie, this pattern is inconsistent with a depletion model. Theoretically, it is entirely possible that a healthcare professional is distressed because they are already out of resources rather than, as is more commonly implied, the management of distress consuming general resources. In any case, we clearly need to test the specific pathways that demonstrate the presence (or absence) of the hypothesized mechanisms between self-compassion and different outcomes to truly understand the benefits.

A depletion-based line of reasoning is also clear in the normative interpretations in studies linking self-compassion to physical health outcomes. Several studies have suggested that self-compassion may "free-up" individuals' self-regulation capacity to promote better regulation (e.g., emotion, affect, stress) to promote physical well-being (Finlay-Jones et al., 2015; Hwang et al., 2019; Sirois, 2015). In the modal view, when people are trying to change or adapt more health-promoting behaviors, those with higher self-compassion respond to failures and challenges with acceptance rather than self-criticism or judgment (self-kindness), view setbacks as part of the wider human experience (common humanity), and engage in less rumination or immersion in negative feelings (mindfulness; Adams & Leary, 2007). Such findings are routinely taken to suggest that the benefits gained by "freeing-up" an individual's general self-regulatory capacity is what promotes better outcomes. In theory, the self-regulatory resources that are no longer being consumed in protecting the self from criticism and the associated negative affect can now be devoted to health-promoting self-regulatory behaviors. Again, however, while this perspective is inherently plausible, the possibility is not directly tested.

Nonetheless, a similar line of reasoning might be applied to the question of whether self-compassion can increase other-focused care. While research in this area is scattered (above), it is possible that a "freeing-up" of general self-regulatory capacity may offer interpersonal "resource" benefits and thus increase the ability (or motivation) to engage in other-focused care. Self-regulation is thought to have an important role in forming and maintaining interpersonal relationships, with depleted self-regulatory resources thought to impair interpersonal functioning (Finkel & Campbell, 2001; Finkel et al., 2009). Conversely, either strengthening or freeing up regulatory resources may promote better relationship functioning. For example, one study found that self-control increased the individuals' ability to accommodate in response to a partner's potentially destructive behavior (Finkel & Campbell, 2001). Another study found that individuals whose resources were experimentally depleted (by engaging in an attention-regulation task) were more likely than non-depleted persons to show interpersonal aggression when provoked (Finkel et al., 2009). Although none of these studies directly demonstrate that self-compassion increases resources (or, more technically, reduces the extent to which resources are depleted), they are consistent with the notion that self-compassion might increase either the ability to engage with, understand, and care for others. Given the demands of healthcare environments, one way in which self-compassion training may thus impact other-focused care is by preventing the depletion of resources and thus increasing the individual's capacity to care. As noted, many healthcare professionals are profoundly prosocial and the possibility that reducing depletion might free them to care for others is promising.

Compassion-Specific Pathways

The general self-regulatory or depletion model described above has considerable heuristic value and would seem to map on to the subjective experiences of a highly stressed workforce. However, it is also worth recalling that the development of self-compassion may concurrently change *specific aspects* of psychological and interpersonal functioning that can facilitate other-focused care. Empirically, there may be specific mediating mechanisms (e.g., increased prosocial motivation, reduced judgement of the other, a greater awareness of the "commonalities" between the self and others) that link self-compassion with other-focused care. Below, we briefly survey studies for evidence regarding the changes that comprise and characterize the development of self-compassion that appear to have specific relevance as potential mechanisms linking self-compassion to other-focused care.

To begin, it is worth noting that most of the studies linking self-compassion to various elements of prosociality have been conducted in samples where prosociality has a distinct nature and challenges. While it draws from the same basic psychological systems, other-focused compassion in health settings is distinguished by a number of factors: distinct settings, expectation, or obligation versus being voluntary, by being repeated rather than sporadic, by focusing on strangers rather than family or friends, and by being (indirectly) remunerated. While little is known regarding how or whether such differences matter, suffice to say that compassion for others in healthcare is distinct. These differences noted, a few studies may provide some insight into the *specific* pathways by which self-compassion can lead to greater other-focused care.

Given that seeing patients as having caused or contributed to their own suffering reduces compassion in healthcare (Reynolds et al., 2019), the possibility that self-compassion is accompanied or characterized by lower negative judgments is promising. One study in the context of romantic relationships found that *acceptance of one's own flaws* mediated the effect of self-compassion on acceptance of a partner's flaws, specifically the extent to which the partner procrastinated (Zhang et al., 2020). Another study with adolescents found that *relatedness* (along with trust) mediated the effect of self-compassion on prosocial behavior (Yang et al., 2019). While the populations and study outcomes are distinct, such findings may imply that because self-compassion increases acceptance of one's *own* imperfections (Zhang et al., 2020), there may be "flow on" effect into the ways we accept (versus judge) and relate to others (e.g., via increased common humanity aspect of self-compassion).

As a group that are prone to perfectionism and self-criticism (Bria et al., 2012; Duarte & Pinto-Gouveia, 2017; Enns et al., 2001; Gaufberg et al., 2010), the development of self-compassion among healthcare professionals may thus facilitate the ability or tendency to non-judgmentally accept others and their various sufferings, failings, and challenges. Empirically, we know that seeing patients as responsible for their suffering reduces compassion in healthcare (Fernando & Consedine, 2014a; Reynolds et al., 2019), creating the possibility that the reduction in the tendency to judge one's own failures that characterizes self-compassion may also decrease our judgement of others and thus facilitate the extent to which we care.

In closing, it is worth noting that there is no reason to suspect that either (a) a single mechanism links self-compassion to other-focused care, nor that (b) elements of both general resource and compassion-specific mechanisms do not operate simultaneously or in interaction. Further consideration of how perfectionism might interfere with other focused care provides a useful case study in this regard. Research shows that those with higher self-compassion report lower self-presentational concerns (Long & Neff, 2018; Werner et al., 2012). Controlling self-presentation (Goffman, 1978) is a common way to manage the image that one wishes to project and influence relationships (Jones & Pittman, 1982) and likely evolved as an adaptive mechanism to monitor and regulate social relationships (Trower et al., 1990). A need to "control" self-presentation may be pronounced in healthcare where self-imposed perfectionist standards are compounded by expectations from patients and institutions (Bynum IV & Sukhera, 2021). Thus, while self-compassion might work to reduce self-presentational concerns by increasing self-kindness and/or decreasing self-critical tendencies, changes of this kind may free up resources such that healthcare professionals can direct their attention toward others and their needs, rather than focusing on maintaining the presentation of a particular image.

In summary, while empirical studies of the potential mechanisms are few, theory is clear in suggesting that self-compassion has the potential to enhance other focused care through both general and specific pathways. In terms of general mechanisms, reductions in the need to regulate aversive feelings and/or (self) present in particular ways may free up regulatory capacity for use in prosocial domains. It may also benefit other-focused care by specifically reducing the tendency to judge the suffering of the self (and others) as self-inflicted and thus less deserving of care, a known barrier to compassion in healthcare (Fernando & Consedine, 2014a, 2014b). Although it is unclear whether the development self-compassion is best conceptualized in terms of (a) reducing regulatory resource demands or (b) a different form of resource (or both), self-compassion has the potential to facilitate effective resource management in the service of self- and other-focused care.

Concluding Remarks on Self-Compassion and Other-Focused Care

Patients, families, medical institutions, and professional guidelines as well as professionals themselves expect to medical services with compassion. Too often, however, healthcare providers' own well-being is neglected in training and professional development systems, which may hinder their ability to provide other-focused care. While writers are now advocating for the potential importance of self-compassion in healthcare communities (Neff et al., 2020; Sinclair et al., 2017), there is a lack of empirical data, particularly in relation to how self-compassion interventions might work to benefit other-focused care. Studies remain overwhelmingly cross-sectional, outcomes measurement is self-reported, and the pathways by which self-compassion might lead to other-focused care remains a mystery.

Although self-compassion may be an important potential tool to benefit the self and others, it is important to highlight that self-compassion will not benefit all medical professionals equally. Gilbert (2010) has previously noted that self-compassion can trigger feelings of sadness and grief, resulting from one's attachment styles. For example, those who did not receive care or affection from significant others in the past may find self-compassion overwhelming, shameful, or uncomfortable—also referred to as "backdraft" (Germer,

2009). Hence, it is possible that caring for the self may lead to withdrawal of care from others to protect oneself.

On a similar note, it is possible that self-compassion has the potential to *worsen* personal well-being or *reduce* other-focused concern. Recent studies suggest that one core aspect of self-compassion—mindfulness—has been associated with negative consequences, notably with increased negative affect, psychopathology (Ingram, 1990; Mor & Winquist, 2002), worse mental health (Britton, 2019; Sahdra et al., 2017), emotional blunting, dissociation, and loss of positive emotions (Cebolla et al., 2017; Lindahl et al., 2017; Sierra, 2009; Taylor et al., 2011). As self-compassion interventions often include an aspect of mindfulness, it is possible that increase in self-compassion may also enhance awareness of one's own suffering. Whether such awareness helps or hinders other-focused care is unknown although the balance of probability suggests it is unlikely to help others. Although there is currently no direct evidence implying potential negative consequences of self-compassion interventions (although see Friis et al., 2015), it is important to recognize that increasing self-compassion will not always result in positive outcomes for all individuals or necessarily benefit others.

Secondly, research to date is unclear on the directionality of the links between self-compassion and compassion to others. While being compassionate to oneself in might, in theory, increase compassion to others, studies are mixed. Some imply effects may flow in this direction while others suggest the reverse is more likely. Put simply, being compassionate to others might enable self-compassion. Consistent with this provocative possibility, one study found that by experimentally prompting participants to think of or really give support to others, self-compassion was increased (Breines & Chen, 2013). While the short timeframe of such manipulations must be borne in mind, this possibility is also worth considering in healthcare setting.

Finally, the implementation of self-compassion training in healthcare professionals is not without its challenges. There are both personal and contextual factors that may hinder the development of self-compassion practices. In terms of personal factors, some people may resist training when self-compassion is not correctly understood (e.g., where self-compassion is seen as a form of weakness or self-indulgence) or may be seen as inconsistent with personal values or beliefs systems (Robinson et al., 2016). One study, for example, suggests that resistance to self-compassion arises where people think that *self-kindness* will reduce their likelihood of success or when *self-criticism* is seen as a character strength indexing responsibility (Robinson et al., 2016). This would seem a likely challenge in samples of healthcare professionals.

For contextual factors, research on compassion in healthcare makes it clear that organizational values and institutional structures reinforce particular ways of professional conduct and intra- and inter-personal functioning (Mills et al., 2015). Contexts play a major role in compassionate medical care (Fernando et al., 2016) and different healthcare organizations vary in the extent to which self-compassion and related constructs (e.g., self-care and mindfulness) are normalized, encouraged, and communicated in team dynamics (Egan et al., 2019). Therefore, contextual factors may influence how self-compassion interventions are received and implemented by various healthcare professionals. Although lack of evidence makes it challenging, it seems likely that personal and contextual factors in healthcare will seep into the feasibility and benefits of self-compassion interventions.

To conclude, in this chapter, we discussed the evidence for potential relevance of the widely used self-compassion interventions to the challenges of healthcare. Broadly, the benefits of self-compassion are increasingly accepted, evidence specifically regarding samples of healthcare professionals is only gradually emerging. Both in terms of individual and other-focused outcomes—a key aspect of professional functioning in healthcare—there is some early promise, but there are also inconsistencies and areas of concern. The evidence base is small, outcomes are self-reported, and the search for clarity regarding which components of self-compassion are relevant is ongoing. Our sense here is that future works investigating both the general and the specific pathways linking self-compassion to individual and other-focused outcomes are needed. Such findings will allow us to assess how self-compassion might benefit healthcare professionals to combat the challenges to working in healthcare, ultimately leading to greater compassion toward patients and themselves.

References

Adams, C. E., & Leary, M. R. (2007). Promoting self-compassionate attitudes toward eating among restrictive and guilty eaters. *Journal of Social and Clinical Psychology, 26*(10), 1120–1144. https://doi.org/10.1521/jscp.2007.26.10.1120

Alrawashdeh, H. M., Ala'a, B., Alzawahreh, M. K., Al-Tamimi, A., Elkholy, M., Al Sarireh, F., Abusamak, M., Elehamer, N. M., Malkawi, A., Al-Dolat, W., & Abu-Ismail, L. (2021). Occupational burnout and job satisfaction among physicians in times of COVID-19 crisis: A convergent parallel mixed-method study. *BMC Public Health, 21*(1), 1–18. https://doi.org/10.1186/s12889-021-10897-4

Arch, J. J., Brown, K. W., Dean, D. J., Landy, L. N., Brown, K. D., & Laudenslager, M. L. (2014). Self-compassion training modulates alpha-amylase, heart rate variability, and subjective responses to social evaluative threat in women. *Psychoneuroendocrinology, 42*, 49–58. https://doi.org/10.1016/j.psyneuen.2013.12.018

Arimitsu, K., & Hofmann, S. G. (2015). Cognitions as mediators in the relationship between self-compassion and affect. *Personality & Individual Differences, 74*, 41–48. https://doi.org/10.1016/j.paid.2014.10.008

Babenko, O., & Oswald, A. (2019). The roles of basic psychological needs, self-compassion, and self-efficacy in the development of mastery goals among medical students. *Medical Teacher, 41*(4), 478–481. https://doi.org/10.1080/0142159X.2018.1442564

Baguley, S. I., Dev, V., Fernando, A. T., & Consedine, N. S. (2020). How do health professionals maintain compassion over time? Insights from a study of compassion in health. *Frontiers in Psychology, 11*, 3327. https://doi.org/10.3389/fpsyg.2020.564554

Baumeister, R. F., & Heatherton, T. F. (1996). Self-regulation failure: An overview. *Psychological Inquiry, 7*(1), 1–15. https://doi.org/10.1207/s15327965pli0701_1

Baumeister, R. F., Schmeichel, B. J., & Vohs, K. D. (2007). *Social psychology: Handbook of basic principles* (Vol. 2).

Beaumont, E., Durkin, M., Hollins Martin, C. J., & Carson, J. (2016a). Compassion for others, self-compassion, quality of life and mental well-being measures and their association with compassion fatigue and burnout in student midwives: A quantitative survey. *Midwifery, 34*, 239–244. https://doi.org/10.1016/j.midw.2015.11.002

Beaumont, E., Durkin, M., Hollins Martin, C. J., & Carson, J. (2016b). Measuring relationships between self-compassion, compassion fatigue, burnout and well-being in student counsellors and student cognitive behavioural psychotherapists: A quantitative survey. *Counselling and Psychotherapy Research, 16*(1), 15–23. https://doi.org/10.1002/capr.12054

Booker, J. A., & Dunsmore, J. C. (2019). Testing direct and indirect ties of self-compassion with subjective well-being. *Journal of Happiness Studies: An Interdisciplinary Forum on Subjective Well-Being, 20*(5), 1563–1585. https://doi.org/10.1007/s10902-018-0011-2

Breines, J., Toole, A., Tu, C., & Chen, S. (2014). Self-compassion, body image, and self-reported disordered eating. *Self and Identity, 13*(4), 432–448. https://doi.org/10.1080/15298868.2013.838992

Breines, J. G., & Chen, S. (2013). Activating the inner caregiver: The role of support-giving schemas in increasing state self-compassion. *Journal of Experimental Social Psychology, 49*(1), 58–64. https://doi.org/10.1016/j.jesp.2012.07.015

Bria, M., Baban, A., & Dumitrascu, D. L. (2012). Systematic review of burnout risk factors among European healthcare professionals. *Cognition, Brain, Behavior: An Interdisciplinary Journal, 16*(3), 423–452.

Britton, W. B. (2019). Can mindfulness be too much of a good thing? The value of a middle way. *Current Opinion in Psychology, 28*, 159–165. https://doi.org/10.1016/j.copsyc.2018.12.011

Brown, L., Houston, E. E., Amonoo, H. L., & Bryant, C. (2020). Is self-compassion associated with sleep quality? A meta-analysis. *Mindfulness, 82-91*. https://doi.org/10.1007/s12671-020-01498-0

Brownie, S., Scott, R., & Rossiter, R. (2016). Therapeutic communication and relationships in chronic and complex care. *Nursing Standard, 31*(6), 54. https://doi.org/10.7748/ns.2016.e9847

Buceta, M. I., Bermejo, J. C., & Villacieros, M. (2019). Enhancer elements of compassion satisfaction in healthcare professionals. *An Psicol, 35*(2), 323–331. https://doi.org/10.6018/analesps.35.2.345101

Bynum, W. E., IV, & Sukhera, J. (2021). Perfectionism, power, and process: What we must address to dismantle mental health stigma in medical education. *Academic Medicine, 96*(5), 621–623. https://doi.org/10.1097/ACM.0000000000004008

Carter, E. C., Kofler, L. M., Forster, D. E., & McCullough, M. E. (2015). A series of meta-analytic tests of the depletion effect: Self-control does not seem to rely on a limited resource. *Journal of Experimental Psychology: General, 144*(4), 796. https://doi.org/10.1037/xge0000083

Cebolla, A., Demarzo, M., Martins, P., Soler, J., & Garcia-Campayo, J. (2017). Unwanted effects: Is there a negative side of meditation? A multicentre survey. *PLoS One, 12*(9), e0183137. https://doi.org/10.1371/journal.pone.0183137

Chio, F. H., Mak, W. W., Cheng, R. H., Hsu, A. Y., & Kwan, H. H. (2021). Can compassion to the self be extended to others: The association of self-compassion and other-focused concern. *The Journal of Positive Psychology, 1-11*. https://doi.org/10.1080/17439760.2021.1913638

Chishima, Y., Mizuno, M., Sugawara, D., & Miyagawa, Y. (2018). The influence of self-compassion on cognitive appraisals and coping with stressful events. *Mindfulness, 9*(6), 1907–1915. https://doi.org/10.1007/s12671-018-0933-0

Crary, P. (2013). Beliefs, behaviors, and health of undergraduate nursing students. *Holistic Nursing Practice, 27*(2), 74–88. https://doi.org/10.1097/HNP.0b013e318280f75e

Davison, N., & Williams, K. (2009). Compassion in nursing. 2: Factors that influence compassionate care in clinical practice. *Nursing Times, 105*(37), 18–19.

Delaney, M. C. (2018). Caring for the caregivers: Evaluation of the effect of an eight-week pilot mindful self-compassion (MSC) training program on nurses' compassion fatigue and resilience. *PloS One, 13*(11), e0207261. https://doi.org/10.1371/journal.pone.0207261

Dev, V., Fernando III, A. T., Kirby, J. N., & Consedine, N. S. (2019). Variation in the barriers to compassion across healthcare training and disciplines: A cross-sectional study of doctors, nurses, and medical students. *International Journal of Nursing Studies, 90*, 1–10. https://doi.org/10.1016/j.ijnurstu.2018.09.015

Dev, V., Fernando, A. T., & Consedine, N. S. (2020). Self-compassion as a stress moderator: A cross-sectional study of 1700 doctors, nurses, and medical students. *Mindfulness, 11*(5), 1170–1181. https://doi.org/10.1007/s12671-020-01325-6

Duarte, J., & Pinto-Gouveia, J. (2017). Empathy and feelings of guilt experienced by nurses: A cross-sectional study of their role in burnout and compassion fatigue symptoms. *Applied Nursing Research, 35*, 42–47. https://doi.org/10.1016/j.apnr.2017.02.006

Dunne, S., Sheffield, D., & Chilcot, J. (2018). Brief report: Self-compassion, physical health and the mediating role of health-promoting behaviours. *Journal of Health Psychology, 23*(7), 993–999. https://doi.org/10.1177/1359105316643377

Egan, H., Keyte, R., McGowan, K., Peters, L., Lemon, N., Parsons, S., Meadows, S., Fardy, T., Singh, P., & Mantzios, M. (2019). 'You before me': A qualitative study of health care professionals' and students' understanding and experiences of compassion in the workplace, self-compassion, self-care and health behaviours. *Health Professions Education, 5*(3), 225–236. https://doi.org/10.1016/j.hpe.2018.07.002

Elliot, A. J., & Dweck, C. S. (2013). *Handbook of competence and motivation*. Guilford Publications.

Enns, M. W., Cox, B. J., Sareen, J., & Freeman, P. (2001). Adaptive and maladaptive perfectionism in medical students: A longitudinal investigation. *Medical Education, 35*(11), 1034–1042. https://doi.org/10.1111/j.1365-2923.2001.01044.x

Eriksson, T., Germundsjö, L., Åström, E., & Rönnlund, M. (2018). Mindful self-compassion training reduces stress and burnout symptoms among practicing psychologists: A randomized controlled trial of a brief web-based intervention. *Frontiers in Psychology, 9*, 2340. https://doi.org/10.3389/fpsyg.2018.02340

Fernando, A. T., Arroll, B., & Consedine, N. S. (2016). Enhancing compassion in general practice: It's not all about the doctor. *British Journal of General Practice.* https://doi.org/10.3399/bjgp16X685741

Fernando, A. T., & Consedine, N. S. (2014a). Beyond compassion fatigue: The transactional model of physician compassion. *Journal of Pain Symptom Management, 48*(2), 289–298. https://doi.org/10.1016/j.jpainsymman.2013.09.014

Fernando, A. T., & Consedine, N. S. (2014b). Development and initial psychometric properties of the barriers to physician compassion questionnaire. *Postgraduate Medical Journal, 90*(1065), 388–395. https://doi.org/10.1136/postgradmedj-2013-132127

Fernando, A. T., & Consedine, N. S. (2017). Barriers to medical compassion as a function of experience and specialization: Psychiatry, pediatrics, internal medicine, surgery, and general practice. *Journal of Pain Symptom Management, 53*(6), 979–987. https://doi.org/10.1016/j.jpainsymman.2016.12.324

Ferrari, M., Hunt, C., Harrysunker, A., Abbott, M. J., Beath, A. P., & Einstein, D. A. (2019). Self-compassion interventions and psychosocial outcomes: A meta-analysis of RCTs. *Mindfulness, 10*(8), 1455–1473. https://doi.org/10.1007/s12671-019-01134-6

Finkel, E. J., & Campbell, W. K. (2001). Self-control and accommodation in close relationships: An interdependence analysis. *Journal of Personality Social Psychology, 81*(2), 263. https://doi.org/10.1037/0022-3514.81.2.263

Finkel, E. J., DeWall, C. N., Slotter, E. B., Oaten, M., & Foshee, V. A. (2009). Self-regulatory failure and intimate partner violence perpetration. *Journal of Personality Social Psychology, 97*(3), 483. https://doi.org/10.1037/a0015433

Finlay-Jones, A., Kane, R., & Rees, C. (2017). Self-compassion online: A pilot study of an internet-based self-compassion cultivation program for psychology trainees. *Journal of Clinical Psychology, 73*(7), 797–816. https://doi.org/10.1002/jclp.22375

Finlay-Jones, A. L., Rees, C. S., & Kane, R. T. (2015). Self-compassion, emotion regulation and stress among Australian psychologists: Testing an emotion regulation model of self-compassion using structural equation modeling. *PLoS One, 10*(7), e0133481. https://doi.org/10.1371/journal.pone.0133481

Franco, P. L., & Christie, L. M. (2021). Effectiveness of a one day self-compassion training for pediatric nurses' resilience. *Journal of Pediatric Nursing, 61*, 109–114. https://doi.org/10.1016/j.pedn.2021.03.020

Fresnics, A., & Borders, A. (2017). Angry rumination mediates the unique associations between self-compassion and anger and aggression. *Mindfulness, 8*(3), 554–564. https://doi.org/10.1007/s12671-016-0629-2

Friis, A. M., Consedine, N. S., & Johnson, M. H. (2015). Does kindness matter? Diabetes, depression, and self-compassion: A selective review and research agenda. *Diabetes Spectrum, 28*(4), 252–257. https://doi.org/10.2337/diaspect.28.4.252

Gaufberg, E. H., Batalden, M., Sands, R., & Bell, S. K. (2010). The hidden curriculum: What can we learn from third-year medical student narrative reflections? *Academic Medicine, 85*(11), 1709–1716. https://doi.org/10.1097/ACM.0b013e3181f57899

Gedik, Z. (2019). Self-compassion and health-promoting lifestyle behaviors in college students. *Psychology, Health & Medicine, 24*(1), 108–114. https://doi.org/10.1080/13548506.2018.1503692

Germer, C. (2009). *The mindful path to self-compassion: Freeing yourself from destructive thoughts and emotions*. Guilford Press.

Gilbert, P. (2010). *Compassion focused therapy: Distinctive features*. Routledge.

Gilbert, P. (2014). The origins and nature of compassion focused therapy. *British Journal of Clinical Psychology, 53*(1), 6–41. https://doi.org/10.1111/bjc.12043

Goffman, E. (1978). *The presentation of self in everyday life* (Vol. 21).

Gratz, K. L., & Roemer, L. (2004). Multidimensional assessment of emotion regulation and dysregulation: Development, factor structure, and initial validation of the difficulties in emotion regulation scale. *Journal of Psychopathology and Behavioral Assessment, 26*(1), 41–54. https://doi.org/10.1023/B:JOBA.0000007455.08539.94

Grossman, P., Niemann, L., Schmidt, S., & Walach, H. (2004). Mindfulness-based stress reduction and health benefits: A meta-analysis. *Journal of Psychosomatic Research, 57*(1), 35–43. https://doi.org/10.1016/S0022-3999(03)00573-7

Gustin, L. W., & Wagner, L. (2013). The butterfly effect of caring-clinical nursing teachers' understanding of self-compassion as a source to compassionate care. *Scandinavian Journal of Caring Sciences, 27*(1), 175–183. https://doi.org/10.1111/j.1471-6712.2012.01033.x

Hall, C. W., Row, K. A., Wuensch, K. L., & Godley, K. R. (2013). The role of self-compassion in physical and psychological well-being. *Journal of Psychology: Interdisciplinary and Applied, 147*(4), 311–323. https://doi.org/10.1080/00223980.2012.693138

Hamrick, L. A., & Owens, G. P. (2019). Exploring the mediating role of self-blame and coping in the relationships between self-compassion and distress in females following the sexual assault. *Journal of Clinical Psychology, 75*(4), 766–779. https://doi.org/10.1002/jclp.22730

Heffernan, M., Quinn Griffin, M. T., McNulty, S. R., & Fitzpatrick, J. J. (2010). Self-compassion and emotional intelligence in nurses. *International Journal of Nursing Practice, 16*(4), 366–373. https://doi.org/10.1111/j.1440-172X.2010.01853.x

Hodgetts, J., McLaren, S., Bice, B., & Trezise, A. (2020). The relationships between self-compassion, rumination, and depressive symptoms among older adults: The moderating role of gender. *Aging & Mental Health, 1-10.* https://doi.org/10.1080/13607863.2020.1824207

Hofmann, S. G., Grossman, P., & Hinton, D. E. (2011). Loving-kindness and compassion meditation: Potential for psychological interventions. *Clinical Psychology Review, 31*(7), 1126–1132. https://doi.org/10.1016/j.cpr.2011.07.003

Hwang, Y.-S., Medvedev, O. N., Krägeloh, C., Hand, K., Noh, J.-E., & Singh, N. N. (2019). The role of dispositional mindfulness and self-compassion in educator stress. *Mindfulness, 10*(8), 1692–1702. https://doi.org/10.1007/s12671-019-01183-x

Ingram, R. E. (1990). Self-focused attention in clinical disorders: Review and a conceptual model. *Psychological Bulletin, 107*(2), 156. https://doi.org/10.1037/0033-2909.107

Inwood, E., & Ferrari, M. (2018). Mechanisms of change in the relationship between self-compassion, emotion regulation, and mental health: A systematic review. *Applied psychology: Health and well-being, 10*(2), 215–235. https://doi.org/10.1111/aphw.12127

Jazaieri, H., Jinpa, G. T., McGonigal, K., Rosenberg, E. L., Finkelstein, J., Simon-Thomas, E., Cullen, M., Doty, J. R., Gross, J. J., & Goldin, P. R. (2013). Enhancing compassion: A randomized controlled trial of a compassion cultivation training program. *Journal of Happiness Studies, 14*(4), 1113–1126. https://doi.org/10.1007/s10902-012-9373-z

Johnson, E. A., & O'Brien, K. A. (2013). Self-compassion soothes the savage ego-threat system: Effects on negative affect, shame, rumination, and depressive symptoms. *Journal of Social and Clinical Psychology, 32*(9), 939–963. https://doi.org/10.1521/jscp.2013.32.9.939

Jones, E. E., & Pittman, T. S. (1982). Toward a general theory of strategic self-presentation. In *Psychological perspectives on the self* (Vol. 1, pp. 231–262). Lawrence Erlbaum Associates.

Jones, J., Winch, S., Strube, P., Mitchell, M., & Henderson, A. (2016). Delivering compassionate care in intensive care units: Nurses' perceptions of enablers and barriers. *Journal of Advanced Nursing, 72*(12), 3137–3146. https://doi.org/10.1111/jan.13064

Kelliher Rabon, J., Sirois, F. M., & Hirsch, J. K. (2018). Self-compassion and suicidal behavior in college students: Serial indirect effects via depression and wellness behaviors. *Journal of American College Health, 66*(2), 114–122. https://doi.org/10.1080/07448481.2017.1382498

Kemper, K. J., Mo, X., & Khayat, R. (2015). Are mindfulness and self-compassion associated with sleep and resilience in health professionals? *Journal of Alternative and Complementary Medicine, 21*(8), 496–503. https://doi.org/10.1089/acm.2014.0281

Kemper, K. J., Schwartz, A., Wilson, P. M., Mahan, J. D., Schubert, C. J., Staples, B. B., McClafferty, H., Serwint, J. R., & Batra, M. (2020). Burnout in pediatric residents: Three years of national survey data mindfulness and self-compassion associated with sleep and resilience in health professionals? *Pediatrics, 145*(1), e20191030. https://doi.org/10.1542/peds.2019-1030

Kirby, J. N., Tellegen, C. L., & Steindl, S. R. (2017). A meta-analysis of compassion-based interventions: Current state of knowledge and future directions. *Behavior Therapy, 48*(6), 778–792. https://doi.org/10.1016/j.beth.2017.06.003

Lathren, C. R., Rao, S. S., Park, J., & Bluth, K. (2021). Self-compassion and current close interpersonal relationships: A scoping literature review. *Mindfulness, 1-16.* https://doi.org/10.1007/s12671-020-01566-5

Lazarus, R. S. (1966). *Psychological stress and the coping process*. McGraw-Hill.

Li, A., Wang, S., Cai, M., Sun, R., & Liu, X. (2021). Self-compassion and life-satisfaction among Chinese self-quarantined residents during COVID-19 pandemic: A moderated mediation model of positive coping and gender. *Personality & Individual Differences, 170*, 110457. https://doi.org/10.1016/j.paid.2020.110457

Li, Y., Deng, J., Lou, X., Wang, H., & Wang, Y. (2020). A daily diary study of the relationships among daily self-compassion, perceived stress and health-promoting behaviours. *International Journal of Psychology, 55*(3), 364–372. https://doi.org/10.1002/ijop.12610

Lindahl, J. R., Fisher, N. E., Cooper, D. J., Rosen, R. K., & Britton, W. B. (2017). The varieties of contemplative experience: A mixed-methods study of meditation-related challenges in Western Buddhists. *PLoS One, 12*(5), e0176239. https://doi.org/10.1371/journal.pone.0176239

Long, P., & Neff, K. D. (2018). Self-compassion is associated with reduced self-presentation concerns and increased student communication behavior. *Learning*

Individual Differences, 67, 223–231. https://doi.org/10.1016/j.lindif.2018.09.003

López, A., Sanderman, R., Ranchor, A. V., & Schroevers, M. J. (2018). Compassion for others and self-compassion: Levels, correlates, and relationship with psychological well-being. *Mindfulness, 9*(1), 325–331. https://doi.org/10.1007/s12671-017-0777-z

Luo, Y., Meng, R., Li, J., Liu, B., Cao, X., & Ge, W. (2019). Self-compassion may reduce anxiety and depression in nursing students: A pathway through perceived stress. *Public Health, 174*, 1–10. https://doi.org/10.1016/j.puhe.2019.05.015

MacBeth, A., & Gumley, A. (2012). Exploring compassion: A meta-analysis of the association between self-compassion and psychopathology. *Clinical Psychology Review, 32*(6), 545–552. https://doi.org/10.1016/j.cpr.2012.06.003

Magnus, C. M., Kowalski, K. C., & McHugh, T.-L. F. (2010). The role of self-compassion in women's self-determined motives to exercise and exercise-related outcomes. *Self and Identity, 9*(4), 363–382. https://doi.org/10.1080/15298860903135073

Marshall, S. L., Ciarrochi, J., Parker, P. D., & Sahdra, B. K. (2020). Is self-compassion selfish? The development of self-compassion, empathy, and prosocial behavior in adolescence. *Journal of Research on Adolescence, 30*, 472–484. https://doi.org/10.1111/jora.12492

McCade, D., Frewen, A., & Fassnacht, D. B. (2021). Burnout and depression in Australian psychologists: The moderating role of self-compassion. *Australian Psychologist, 56*(2), 111–122. https://doi.org/10.1080/00050067.2021.1890979

Mehr, K. E., & Adams, A. C. (2016). Self-compassion as a mediator of maladaptive perfectionism and depressive symptoms in college students. *Journal of College Student Psychotherapy, 30*(2), 132–145. https://doi.org/10.1080/87568225.2016.1140991

Meyer, L. P., & Leppma, M. (2019). The role of mindfulness, self-compassion, and emotion regulation in eating disorder symptoms among college students. *Journal of College Counseling, 22*(3), 211–224. https://doi.org/10.1002/jocc.12138

Mills, J., Wand, T., & Fraser, J. (2015). On self-compassion and self-care in nursing: Selfish or essential for compassionate care? (Guest editorial). *International Journal of Nursing Studies, 52*(4), 791–793. https://doi.org/10.1016/j.ijnurstu.2014.10.009

Mills, J., Wand, T., & Fraser, J. A. (2018). Examining self-care, self-compassion and compassion for others: A cross-sectional survey of palliative care nurses and doctors. *International Journal of Palliative Nursing, 24*(1), 4–11. https://doi.org/10.12968/ijpn.2018.24.1.4

Mor, N., & Winquist, J. (2002). Self-focused attention and negative affect: A meta-analysis. *Psychological Bulletin, 128*(4), 638. https://doi.org/10.1037/0033-2909.128.4.638

Muraven, M., & Slessareva, E. (2003). Mechanisms of self-control failure: Motivation and limited resources. *Personality Social Psychology Bulletin, 29*(7), 894–906. https://doi.org/10.1177/0146167203029007008

Neff, K. (2003). The development and validation of a scale to measure self-compassion [empirical study]. *Self and Identity, 2*(3), 223–250. https://doi.org/10.1080/15298860309027

Neff, K. D., & Beretvas, S. N. (2013). The role of self-compassion in romantic relationships. *Self and Identity, 12*(1), 78–98. https://doi.org/10.1080/15298868.2011.639548

Neff, K. D., & Germer, C. K. (2013). A pilot study and randomized controlled trial of the mindful self-compassion program. *Journal of Clinical Psychology, 69*(1), 28–44. https://doi.org/10.1002/jclp.21923

Neff, K. D., Knox, M. C., Long, P., & Gregory, K. (2020). Caring for others without losing yourself: An adaptation of the mindful self-compassion program for healthcare communities. *Journal of Clinical Psychology, 76*(9), 1543–1562. https://doi.org/10.1002/jclp.23007

Neff, K. D., & Pommier, E. (2013). The relationship between self-compassion and other-focused concern among college undergraduates, community adults, and practicing meditators. *Self and Identity, 12*(2), 160–176. https://doi.org/10.1080/15298868.2011.649546

Neff, K. D., Rude, S. S., & Kirkpatrick, K. L. (2007). An examination of self-compassion in relation to positive psychological functioning and personality traits. *Journal of Research in Personality, 41*(4), 908–916. https://doi.org/10.1016/j.jrp.2006.08.002

Nguyen, T. M., Bui, T. T. H., Xiao, X. X., & Le, V. H. (2020). The influence of self-compassion on mindful parenting: A mediation model of gratitude. *Family Journal.* https://doi.org/10.1177/1066480720950421

Olson, K., & Kemper, K. J. (2014). Factors associated with well-being and confidence in providing compassionate care. *Journal of evidence-based complementary alternative medicine, 19*(4), 292–296. https://doi.org/10.1177/2156587214539977

Papadopoulos, I., Taylor, G., Ali, S., Aagard, M., Akman, O., Alpers, L.-M., Apostolara, P., Biglete-Pangilinan, S., Biles, J., García, Á. M., & González-Gil, T. (2017). Exploring nurses' meaning and experiences of compassion: An international online survey involving 15 countries. *Journal of Transcultural Nursing, 28*(3), 286–295. https://doi.org/10.1177/1043659615624740

Pavlova, A., Wang, C. X., Boggiss, A. L., O'Callaghan, A., & Consedine, N. S. (2021). Predictors of physician compassion, empathy, and related constructs: A systematic review. *Journal of General Internal Medicine., 1-12.* https://doi.org/10.1007/s11606-021-07055-2

Pavlova, A., & Consedine, N. S. (2023). Caring for the carer–Self-compassion in the health professions. In *Handbook of Self-Compassion* (pp. 231–250). Springer International Publishing.

Phillips, W. J., & Hine, D. W. (2019). Self-compassion, physical health, and health behaviour: A meta-analysis. *Health Psychology Review, 1-109.* https://doi.org/10.1080/17437199.2019.1705872

Raes, F. (2010). Rumination and worry as mediators of the relationship between self-compassion and depression and anxiety. *Personality and Individual Differences, 48*(6), 757–761. https://doi.org/10.1016/j.paid.2010.01.023

Reynolds, L. M., Powell, P., Lin, Y. S., Ravi, K., Chung, C. Y. K., & Consedine, N. S. (2019). Fighting the flinch: Experimentally induced compassion makes a difference in health care providers. *British Journal of Health Psychology, 24*(4), 982–998. https://doi.org/10.1111/bjhp.12390

Robinson, K. J., Mayer, S., Allen, A. B., Terry, M., Chilton, A., & Leary, M. R. (2016). Resisting self-compassion: Why are some people opposed to being kind to themselves? *Self and Identity, 15*(5), 505–524. https://doi.org/10.1080/15298868.2016.1160952

Sahdra, B. K., Ciarrochi, J., Parker, P. D., Basarkod, G., Bradshaw, E. L., Baer, R., & Realo, A. (2017). Are people mindful in different ways? Disentangling the quantity and quality of mindfulness in latent profiles and exploring their links to mental health and life effectiveness. *European Journal of Personality, 31*(4), 347–365. https://doi.org/10.1002/per.2108

Sbarra, D. A., Smith, H. L., & Mehl, M. R. (2012). When leaving your ex, love yourself: Observational ratings of self-compassion predict the course of emotional recovery following marital separation. *Psychological Science, 23*(3), 261–269. https://doi.org/10.1177/0956797611429466

Schmidt, C. K., Raque-Bogdan, T. L., & Hollern, E. A. (2019). Self-compassion, affect, and body image in college women. *Journal of College Counseling, 22*(2), 152–163. https://doi.org/10.1002/jocc.12127

Schoenefeld, S. J., & Webb, J. B. (2013). Self-compassion and intuitive eating in college women: Examining the contributions of distress tolerance and body image acceptance and action. *Eating Behaviors, 14*(4), 493–496. https://doi.org/10.1016/j.eatbeh.2013.09.001

Seppala, E. M., Hutcherson, C. A., Nguyen, D. T., Doty, J. R., & Gross, J. J. (2014). Loving-kindness meditation: A tool to improve healthcare provider compassion, resilience, and patient care. *Journal of Compassionate Health Care, 1*(1), 1–9. https://doi.org/10.1186/s40639-014-0005-9

Shanafelt, T. D., Balch, C. M., Bechamps, G., Russell, T., Dyrbye, L., Satele, D., Collicott, P., Novotny, P. J., Sloan, J., & Freischlag, J. (2010). Burnout and medical errors among American surgeons. *Annals of Surgery, 251*(6), 995–1000. https://doi.org/10.1097/SLA.0b013e3181bfdab3

Showalter, S. E. (2010). Compassion fatigue: What is it? Why does it matter? Recognizing the symptoms, acknowledging the impact, developing the tools to prevent compassion fatigue, and strengthen the professional already suffering from the effects. *American Journal of Hospice Palliative Medicine, 27*(4), 239–242.

Sierra, M. (2009). *Depersonalization: A new look at a neglected syndrome*. Cambridge University Press.

Sinclair, S., Kondejewski, J., Raffin-Bouchal, S., King-Shier, K. M., & Singh, P. (2017). Can self-compassion promote healthcare provider well-being and compassionate care to others? Results of a systematic review. *Applied psychology: Health and well-being, 9*(2), 168–206. https://doi.org/10.1111/aphw.12086

Sinclair, S., Norris, J. M., McConnell, S. J., Chochinov, H. M., Hack, T. F., Hagen, N. A., McClement, S., & Bouchal, S. R. (2016). Compassion: A scoping review of the healthcare literature. *BMC Palliative Care, 15*(1), 1–16. https://doi.org/10.1186/s12904-016-0080-0

Sirois, F. M. (2015). A self-regulation resource model of self-compassion and health behavior intentions in emerging adults. *Preventive Medicine Reports, 2*, 218–222. https://doi.org/10.1016/j.pmedr.2015.03.006

Sirois, F. M. (2020). The association between self-compassion and self-rated health in 26 samples. *BMC Public Health, 20*(1), 1–12. https://doi.org/10.1186/s12889-020-8183-1

Sirois, F. M., & Hirsch, J. K. (2019). Self-compassion and adherence in five medical samples: The role of stress. *Mindfulness, 10*(1), 46–54. https://doi.org/10.1007/s12671-018-0945-9

Sprang, G., Clark, J. J., & Whitt-Woosley, A. (2007). Compassion fatigue, compassion satisfaction, and burnout: Factors impacting a professional's quality of life. *Journal of Loss Trauma, 12*(3), 259–280. https://doi.org/10.1080/15325020701238093

Stamm, B. H. (2012). Helping the helpers: Compassion satisfaction and compassion fatigue in self- care, management, and policy of suicide prevention hotlines. In A. D. Kirkwood & B. H. Stamm (Eds.), *Resources for community suicide prevention*. Idaho State University.

Svendsen, J. L., Kvernenes, K. V., Wiker, A. S., & Dundas, I. (2017). Mechanisms of mindfulness: Rumination and self-compassion. *Nordic Psychology, 69*(2), 71–82. https://doi.org/10.1080/19012276.2016.1171730

Tandler, N., Kruger, M., & Petersen, L.-E. (2020). Better battles by a self-compassionate partner? The mediating role of personal conflict resolution styles in the association between self-compassion and satisfaction in romantic relationships. *Journal of Individual Differences.* https://doi.org/10.1027/1614-0001/a000333

Taylor, V. A., Grant, J., Daneault, V., Scavone, G., Breton, E., Roffe-Vidal, S., Courtemanche, J., Lavarenne, A. S., & Beauregard, M. (2011). Impact of mindfulness on the neural responses to emotional pictures in experienced and beginner meditators. *NeuroImage, 57*(4), 1524–1533. https://doi.org/10.1016/j.neuroimage.2011.06.001

Terry, M. L., Leary, M. R., Mehta, S., & Henderson, K. (2013). Self-compassionate reactions to health threats. *Personality and Social Psychology Bulletin, 39*(7), 911–926. https://doi.org/10.1177/0146167213488213

Trower, P., Gilbert, P., & Sherling, G. (1990). Social anxiety, evolution, and self-presentation. In *Handbook of social and evaluation anxiety* (pp. 11–45). Springer.

Vaillancourt, E. S., & Wasylkiw, L. (2020). The intermediary role of burnout in the relationship between self-compassion and job satisfaction among nurses. *Canadian*

Journal of Nursing Research, 52(4), 246–254. https://doi.org/10.1177/0844562119846274

Werner, K. H., Jazaieri, H., Goldin, P. R., Ziv, M., Heimberg, R. G., & Gross, J. J. (2012). Self-compassion and social anxiety disorder. *Anxiety, Stress, Coping, 25*(5), 543–558. https://doi.org/10.1080/10615806.2011.608842

West, C. P., Dyrbye, L. N., & Shanafelt, T. D. (2018). Physician burnout: Contributors, consequences and solutions. *Journal of Internal Medicine, 283*(6), 516–529. https://doi.org/10.1111/joim.12752

Yang, Y., Guo, Z., Kou, Y., & Liu, B. (2019). Linking self-compassion and prosocial behavior in adolescents: The mediating roles of relatedness and trust. *Child Indicators Research, 12*(6), 2035–2049. https://doi.org/10.1007/s12187-019-9623-2

Ying, Y.-W. (2009). Contribution of self-compassion to competence and mental health in social work students. *Journal of Social Work Education, 45*(2), 309–323. https://doi.org/10.5175/JSWE.2009.200700072

Yip, S. Y., Mak, W. W., Chio, F. H., & Law, R. W. (2017). The mediating role of self-compassion between mindfulness and compassion fatigue among therapists in Hong Kong. *Mindfulness, 8*(2), 460–470. https://doi.org/10.1007/s12671-016-0618-5

Zessin, U., Dickhäuser, O., & Garbade, S. (2015). The relationship between self-compassion and well-being: A meta-analysis. *Applied Psychology: Health and Well-Being, 7*(3), 340–364. https://doi.org/10.1111/aphw.12051

Zhang, J. W., Chen, S., & Tomova Shakur, T. K. (2020). From me to you: Self-compassion predicts acceptance of own and others' imperfections. *Personality Social Psychology Bulletin, 46*(2), 228–242. https://doi.org/10.1177/0146167219853846

Index[1]

[1] Note: Page numbers followed by 'n' refer to notes.

F. M. Sirois (ed.), *The Palgrave Handbook of Positive Psychology and Health*,
https://doi.org/10.1007/978-3-031-89095-6

The manufacturer's authorised representative in the EU is Springer Nature Customer Service Centre GmbH, Europaplatz 3, 69115 Heidelberg, Germany. If you have any concerns regarding our products, please contact ProductSafety@springernature.com

Printed and bound by CPI Group (UK) Ltd, Croydon, CR0 4YY
01/10/2026
02225953-0020